Handbook of Neuropsychological Assessment

A Biopsychosocial Perspective

CRITICAL ISSUES IN NEUROPSYCHOLOGY

Series Editors

Antonio E. Puente
University of North Carolina, Wilmington

Cecil R. Reynolds
Texas A&M University

Current Volumes in this Series

AGING AND NEUROPSYCHOLOGICAL ASSESSMENT
Asenath La Rue

BRAIN MECHANISMS IN PROBLEM SOLVING AND INTELLIGENCE: A Lesion Survey of the Rat Brain
Robert Thompson, Francis M. Crinella, and Jen Yu

BRAIN ORGANIZATION OF LANGUAGE AND COGNITIVE PROCESSES
Edited by Alfredo Ardila and Feggy Ostrosky-Solis

HANDBOOK OF CLINICAL CHILD NEUROPSYCHOLOGY
Edited by Cecil R. Reynolds and Elaine Fletcher-Janzen

HANDBOOK OF HEAD TRAUMA: Acute Care to Recovery
Edited by Charles J. Long and Leslie K. Ross

HANDBOOK OF NEUROPSYCHOLOGICAL ASSESSMENT: A Biopsychosocial Perspective
Edited by Antonio E. Puente and Robert J. McCaffrey

NEUROPSYCHOLOGICAL EVALUATION OF THE SPANISH SPEAKER
Alfredo Ardila, Monica Rosselli, and Antonio E. Puente

NEUROPSYCHOLOGICAL FUNCTION AND BRAIN IMAGING
Edited by Erin D. Bigler, Ronald A. Yeo, and Eric Turkheimer

NEUROPSYCHOLOGY, NEUROPSYCHIATRY, AND BEHAVIORAL NEUROLOGY
Rhawn Joseph

THE NEUROPSYCHOLOGY OF ATTENTION
Ronald A. Cohen

THE NEUROPSYCHOLOGY OF EPILEPSY
Edited by Thomas L. Bennett

RELIABILITY AND VALIDITY IN NEUROPSYCHOLOGICAL ASSESSMENT
Michael D. Franzen

A Continuation Order Plan is available for this series. A continuation order will bring delivery of each new volume immediately upon publication. Volumes are billed only upon actual shipment. For further information please contact the publisher.

Handbook of Neuropsychological Assessment

A Biopsychosocial Perspective

Edited by

Antonio E. Puente

University of North Carolina at Wilmington
Wilmington, North Carolina

and

Robert J. McCaffrey

University at Albany
State University of New York
Albany, New York

Plenum Press • New York and London

Library of Congress Cataloging-in-Publication Data

Handbook of neuropsychological assessment : a biopsychosocial perspective / edited by Antonio E. Puente and Robert J. McCaffrey.
p. cm. -- (Critical issues in neuropsychology)
Includes bibliographical references and index.
ISBN 0-306-43940-9
1. Neuropsychological tests. 2. Clinical neuropsychology. 3. Neuropsychiatry. I. Puente, Antonio E. II. McCaffrey, Robert J. III. Series.
[DNLM: 1. Neuropsychological Tests. WL 141 H2365]
RC473.N48H36 1992
616.8'0475--dc20
DNLM/DLC
for Library of Congress 92-9129
CIP

ISBN 0-306-43940-9

A Division of Plenum Publishing Corporation
233 Spring Street, New York, N.Y. 10013

Printed in the United States of America

To
Walter Isaac, Ph.D.
(1927–1989)

Contributors

Alfredo Ardila • Instituto Colombiano de Neuropsicologia, Bogotá, Colombia

Joan Ballard • Department of Psychology, Emory University, Altanta, Georgia

Laurence M. Binder • Psychology Service, Veterans Administration Medical Center, Portland, Oregon

Walter B. Branch • Department of Neurology and Pediatrics, Medical College of Georgia, Augusta, Georgia

Morris J. Cohen • Department of Neurology and Pediatrics, Medical College of Georgia, Augusta, Georgia

Eugene R. Delay • Department of Psychology, Regis University, Denver, Colorado

Eugene K. Emory • Department of Psychology, Emory University, Atlanta, Georgia

Marion Eppler • Department of Psychology, Emory University, Atlanta, Georgia

James Gold • Department of Psychology, National Institute of Mental Health, St. Elizabeths Hospital, Washington, D.C.

Gerald Goldstein • Department of Research, Veterans Administration Medical Center, Pittsburgh, Pennsylvania

David E. Hartman • Department of Psychiatry, Cook County Hospital, University of Illinois Medical Center, Chicago, Illinois

Polly Henninger • Division of Biology, California Institute of Technology, Pasadena, California

Arthur MacNeill Horton, Jr. • Division of Clinical Research, National Institute of Drug Abuse, Rockville, Maryland

George W. Hynd • College of Education, Division for the Education of Exceptional Children, University of Georgia, Athens, Georgia

Walter Isaac • Department of Psychology, University of Georgia, Athens, Georgia

Asenath La Rue • Department of Psychiatry and Biobehavioral Sciences, University of California at Los Angeles, Los Angeles, California

Richard Lewine • Departments of Psychiatry and Psychology, Emory University, Atlanta, Georgia

Tyler S. Lorig • Department of Psychology, Washington and Lee University, Lexington, Virginia

Marsha Lucas • Departments of Psychiatry and Psychology, Emory University, Atlanta, Georgia

Sonia Manuel-Dupont • Departments of Communicative Disorders and English, Utah State University, Logan, Utah

Janet R. Matthews • Department of Psychology, Loyola University, New Orleans, Louisiana

Robert J. McCaffrey • Department of Psychology, The University at Albany, State University of New York, Albany, New York

Alice Medalia • Departments of Psychiatry and Neurology, Albert Einstein College of Medicine, Bronx Municipal Hospital Center, Bronx, New York

Peter J. Newman • Illinois State Psychiatric Institute, Chicago, Illinois

Cynthia O'Dell • Department of Psychology, Emory University, Atlanta, Georgia

Susan M. Orsillo • Department of Psychology, The University at Albany, State University of New York, Albany, New York

Feggy Ostrosky-Solis • Facultad de Psicologia, Universidad Nacional Autonoma de Mexico, Mexico City, Mexico

Antonio E. Puente • Department of Psychology, University of North Carolina at Wilmington, Wilmington, North Carolina

Monica Rosselli • Instituto Colombiano de Neuropsicologia, Bogotá, Colombia

Tammy M. Savoie • Department of Psychology, Emory University, Atlanta, Georgia

Jerry J. Sweet • Evanston Hospital and Northwestern University, Evanston, Illinois

B. P. Uzzell • Del Oro Institute, Houston, Texas

Elaine Walker • Departments of Psychiatry and Psychology, Emory University, Atlanta, Georgia

Lisa L. Weyandt • Department of Psychology, University of Rhode Island, Providence, Rhode Island

W. Grant Willis • Department of Psychology, University of Rhode Island, Providence, Rhode Island

Preface

The growth of clinical neuropsychology has been unprecedented. This growth has been oriented more toward the provision of than toward the foundation for services. Thus, while a greater number of psychologists are performing a greater number of neuropsychological procedures, there seems to us an uneven parallel growth between these services and the empirical foundations for them. It should come to no one's surprise that increasingly aggressive attacks on the field have been leveled. Despite these attacks, clinical neuropsychology continues to enjoy exceptional growth within psychology and acceptance by other health practitioners, insurance companies, legislators, judges, juries, and above all, consumers of our services.

Growth without self-reflection is a dangerous enterprise, as is growth without directions. We find it disconcerting that existing and limited "self-analysis" has assumed that neuropsychological dysfunction is immune to the same variables that affect psychological dysfunction. Some attention has been paid to the most obvious ones, such as age, but all others have been ignored and/or misunderstood. This neglect has spawned a body of knowledge replete with questionable data and unfounded conclusions. Hence, it is surprising that clinical neuropsychologists consider themselves to be more scientifically sound than their regular clinical counterparts.

We hope that the present volume helps produce (at a minimum) an increased awareness of how important biopsychosocial variables can be in modulating brain function and dysfunction. At best, we hope that this volume helps produce a more comprehensive paradigm shift in clinical neuropsychology—one that aggressively (yet diplomatically) questions the validity of our knowledge and that places the organism in the context of its life's situation.

Publication lag is a concern for any author. This project is no exception; it was initiated during the early 1980s. The lag, however, was not caused by publishing difficulties but by cognitive ones. The idea of increasing the validity of neuropsychological assessment by increasing clinical sensitivity (and not through syndrome or test knowledge) had to ripen. We trust that the time is right for the message that our contributors present.

A project of this nature hinges on the ideas and work not of a few, but of many. Eliot Werner, Executive Editor at Plenum, has been most patient and supportive as the book's concept changed as frequently as the field for which it is intended. Eliot's expertise in publishing and his knowledge of clinical neuropsychology have been immensely valuable. Our respective departmental chairs, John Williams and Robert A. Rosellini, have been unusually supportive of the use of departmental resources and staff time. We appreciate the opportunity to engage in a project of this nature. Our secretaries—Lydia Woodard, Martha Jo Clemmons, and Mary Anne McDonald—have been patient and efficient throughout the development of this volume. We are especially indebted to our chapter contributors who were prompt and responsive to our deadlines and outside reviews. Additionally, we are grateful to our families—especially to our spouses Linda and Maria—who were supportive throughout the completion of this project.

We dedicate this book to Walter Isaac, our professor while we were graduate students at the University of Georgia, who died before the completion of this volume.

Antonio E. Puente

Wilmington, North Carolina

Robert J. McCaffrey

Albany, New York

Contents

Handbook of Neuropsychological Assessment

A Biopsychosocial Perspective

Historical Perspectives

GERALD GOLDSTEIN

In these introductory remarks, no attempt will be made to summarize the contents of this extensive book, since that would be redundant with the comprehensive overview provided by the editors. Rather, a more historical perspective will be taken here, and I will try to briefly review how the various components of this work fit together into what is now called neuropsychological assessment. The origin of neuropsychological assessment is debatable. Several groups suggest that either they or some historical figure really started it; however, that figure is not always the same person (Goldstein, Hamsher, Goodglass, Reed, & Weinstein, 1985).

THE BEGINNINGS OF NEUROPSYCHOLOGICAL ASSESSMENT

It would probably be fair to say that the field began with an interest in the behavioral changes that take place following brain damage in adults (Goldstein & Scheerer, 1941; Halstead, 1947). Indeed, neuropsychological tests were, and probably still are, popularly known as "tests for brain damage." Thus, one branch of this field developed out of a collaboration with neurologists and neurosurgeons. We tested their patients and wrote our reports or papers, depending on whether we had primarily clinical or research interests at the time. Another branch developed out of a similar kind of collaboration between clinical psychologists and psychiatrists. Psychiatrists wanted to know if clinical psychologists could assess brain-damaged patients with their tests or if they should use those tests in helping to determine whether or not patients were brain damaged. It is my opinion that neuropsychological assessment developed out of a merger between these two areas of practice. The instruments that were

GERALD GOLDSTEIN • Research, Veterans Administration Medical Center, Pittsburgh, Pennsylvania 15206.

HANDBOOK OF NEUROPSYCHOLOGICAL ASSESSMENT: A Biopsychosocial Perspective, edited by Antonio E. Puente and Robert J. McCaffrey. Plenum Press, New York, 1992.

initially used—those available at the time—included portions of the neurological and mental status examination and standard psychological tests. Thus, early neuropsychological practice and research leaned heavily on the Wechsler–Bellevue intelligence scales (Wechsler, 1944), the Rorschach technique (Piotrowski, 1937), the Bender–Gestalt test (Bender, 1938), and other graphics techniques, such as human figure drawings (Machover, 1948). Eventually, these humble beginnings developed into the large collection of instruments described in Lezak's (1983) encyclopedic book, as well as in other collections and handbooks, such as Berg, Franzen, and Wedding's (1987) and Filskov and Boll's (1981; 1986).

NEW APPLICATIONS

Neuropsychological assessment, with its new scientific basis and instruments, has grown to the extent that it is now applied to areas that go well beyond clinical investigation of brain-damaged adults. As will become evident in this volume, there are, first of all, dispositional matters. A person is either very young, young, a mature adult, or elderly. People also have genetic endowments, and events can occur congenitally. The neuropsychological situations at the different life stages, both for the individual with a normal nervous system and the individual who has sustained a disorder affecting the nervous system, are substantially different from one another. Obviously, assessment methods must also be different. One cannot use the same tests on newborn infants that one would use on mature adults.

As can be seen in Chapter 2, the growth of child neuropsychology as a specialty has been remarkable. This area has become more than an extension of adult psychometrics to younger individuals; it has attempted to build foundations in the development of the brain from the prenatal period onward. Areas of study, such as the development of the frontal lobes, hemispheric differences, neural networks, and changes in plasticity of brain function, as well as varying general models of brain function, have contributed in important ways to the neuropsychological assessment of children. An important component of child neuropsychology, covered only briefly in this volume, is the major findings in learning disability, particularly with regard to longitudinal studies, contributed by Rourke (1982); Satz, Taylor, Friel, and Fletcher (1978); Spreen (1987), and their collaborators. There is also a strong scientific foundation for the clinical work derived from life span developmental studies, as can be seen in Chapter 3.

Aside from this longitudinal component, a person is either male or female, relatively rich or poor, right-handed or left-handed, and well-educated or poorly educated. All of these dispositional considerations have been shown to relate to brain function and consequently to neuropsychological function. Thus, we now have subspecialties in clinical neuropsychology for child, adult, and geriatric applications, but we also consider the possible influences of gender, handedness, and socioeducational status on assessment results. In this volume, studies of gender differences, and of relations between handedness, educational status, and sociocultural status and neuropsychological function, are described in Chapters 4, 5, and 6.

DEVELOPMENTS IN PSYCHOMETRICS AND THEIR ASSOCIATED PROBLEMS

One of the important developments in neuropsychological assessment has been the growing effort to construct tests that meet rigorous psychometric standards. As psychological and educational tests, neuropsychological tests should ideally meet standards required for such procedures (Goldstein, 1985). Historically, neuropsychological assessment grew out of extensions of the neurological examination and standardized tests that were not specifically designed for assessment of brain dysfunction. The first battery of tests that was specifically designed for assessment of brain-damaged patients was probably the Goldstein–Scheerer Test Battery (Goldstein & Scheerer, 1941), but it was not standardized and, therefore, not widely used by clinicians until scoring systems for some of the tests were ultimately developed, or the tests themselves were revised so as to permit quantification. Indeed, the widely used Halstead Category test (Halstead, 1947) and Wisconsin Card Sorting test (Grant & Berg, 1948) are derivatives of the Goldstein–Scheerer tests. We now have standardized tests and test batteries specifically designed for assessment of brain-damaged patients.

While this progression has been beneficial for the most part, it has become somewhat problematic since neuropsychological tests began to be used outside of strictly medical settings, particularly in schools and workplaces. They began to border on tests used for classification and placement, sharing many of the problems associated with that area of assessment (Reschly, 1990). Chapter 6, by Ardila, Rosselli, and Ostrosky-Solis, calls our attention to the influence of socioeducational factors on test performance. Those working in school settings are no doubt aware that educational level is correlated with some of our tests, and limited education should not be misinterpreted as brain dysfunction. Furthermore, it now seems clear that simple translation of a test from one language to another does not automatically make the test equally applicable to speakers of either language. We are, therefore, left with two problems. One is that there may be a confounding in medical contexts between socioeducational considerations and health status. The other is that insofar as neuropsychological tests are used for classification and placement, cultural fairness is a pertinent and important issue. As Ardila, Rosselli, and Ostrosky-Solis point out, this problem has not been solved adequately, and we do not yet have satisfactory tests for valid evaluations of people from varying cultures. Thus, one of the clear challenges for neuropsychology is the development of such tests.

NEUROPSYCHOLOGY AND PSYCHOPATHOLOGY

This book has a section on psychopathology, the rationale for which I would like to put in a particular perspective. Having a separate section on psychopathology may be based on the assumption that there is a real distinction between "psychopathological" disorders and the disorders associated with known brain injury or disease traditionally studied by neuropsychologists. With advances in biological psychiatry, that assumption is becoming increasingly less tenable. The untenability is seen most clearly in the case of the schizophrenic disorders, but there is a growing basis for believing that mood and at least some of the anxiety disorders have significant biological components. Historically, it would appear that the neuropsychologists who grew up with neurology were initially skeptical about venturing into psychopathology, whereas those who associated themselves with psychiatrists never saw any difficulties with such a venture in the first place. At present, neuropsychology seems to be solidly embedded in both neurology and psychiatry. This alliance appears to have had implications for clinical practice, research, and interdisciplinary relationships. With regard to clinical practice, neuropsychologists now find themselves in psychiatric facilities in which they are beginning to assess patients with psychiatric disorders that, up until recently, were not of particular interest or apparent relevance to neuropsychologists. While schizophrenia was always a matter of mutual interest, there have recently been important neuropsychological findings for various mood disorders and obsessive–compulsive disorder. I will not document or elaborate on these findings here but will refer the reader to Chapters 8 and 9, in which these exciting new developments are described.

Aside from the impact of the biological revolution in psychiatry, there has also been a paradigmatic shift in neuropsychology. In the past, the implicit or explicit presumption was that the major psychiatric disorders were acquired through experience. In some instances, however, these disorders could give rise to symptoms indistinguishable from symptoms seen in individuals who had sustained structural brain damage. A great deal of research was devoted to the problem of distinguishing between those two conditions. Thus, both schizophrenics and brain-damaged patients had impairments of abstract reasoning or attention, but tests might be devised that would reveal differentiating characteristics within these domains (Goldstein, 1978). This differential diagnosis paradigm has been largely abandoned, most likely because of the identification of abnormalities of brain function and structure in several of the disorders we had thought of as being acquired through experience. Probably the most dramatic transformation of thought appears to have taken place in the case of schizophrenia, culminating in the recent characterization of that disorder as a "brain disease" (Henn & Nasrallah, 1982). Perhaps one of the most interesting transformations took place in the case of autism, which was initially described by Kanner (1943) as having its major etiology in the obsessive and emotionally frigid atmosphere of early family life. Currently, autism is almost universally viewed as a neurobehavioral disorder that is admittedly of unknown cause, but there is increasing evidence for a neurobiological etiology. Sophisticated current thinking about psychopathology views many of the mental disorders as the product of biological and experiential interactions. The implication for neuropsychology is that we now tend to think in terms of the neuropsychological aspects of various disorders rather than in terms of differences between "functional" and "organic" mental disorders. This trend is clearly represented in this book, which has chapters on neuropsychological aspects of anxiety and depressive disorders, as well as schizophrenia.

Another aspect of the psychopathology issue has to do with state–trait considerations. Do transient states of anxiety or depressed mood significantly influence performance on neuropsychological tests? Does motivation influence performance? This book contains two chapters—one on pseudoneurological disorders and the other on deception and malingering—that deal with this important matter. A perhaps more complex state–trait issue has to do with the fact that, unlike the chronic organic mental disorders familiar to neurologists and neuropsychologists, many mental disorders are episodic in nature. The classic case is bipolar mood disorder, but it is now commonly accepted that at least some forms of schizophrenia are episodic in nature, marked by periods of acute symptomatology followed by more quiescent periods. We are only beginning to understand the behavioral and biological characteristics of state–trait phenomena in the mental disorders.

GENERAL MEDICAL APPLICATIONS Of NEUROPSYCHOLOGY

Another new theme can be introduced with a statement to the effect that the brain is a part of the body. Our earlier interest in focal brain lesions produced by stroke, head trauma, or brain tumor perhaps helped us to forget that probably the most common forms of brain disorder are associated with systemic illnesses. Such illnesses often do not produce dramatic symptoms but may progressively impair abilties to the extent that the individual becomes increasingly dysfunctional in performing at least the more complex everyday activities. Aside from that, we are beginning to learn more about the role of general systemic factors in producing focal brain disease. This growth of knowledge is probably seen most clearly in the area of cardiovascular function, where it is quite well-established that hypertension and other cardiovascular disorders are significant risk factors for stroke. Furthermore, processes like hypertension appear to have neuropsychological consequences in and of themselves (King & Miller, 1990).

These considerations appear to have generated an informal alliance between neuropsychologists and those interested in health psychology or behavioral medicine. Thus, some of us have developed an interest in preventive medicine and health maintenance. At a more basic level, we have become interested in how the heart, the liver, the lungs, the endocrine system, the immune system, and other extrabrain structures and systems relate to brain function. At this writing, we are now enmeshed in controversies surrounding our research into acquired immunodeficiency syndrome (AIDS), a generalized disorder of the immune system that appears to negatively affect brain function. We knew for many years that the brain can become infected, but the issues surrounding AIDS appear to be of a different order of magnitude. These matters are considered here in an extensive overview by Lorig (Chapter 14).

Related to the health issue, we have also learned that brain function can become impaired through voluntary or involuntary exposure to harmful environmental agents. The most widely studied of these agents are abused substances, and the most widely studied of those substances is alcohol. There is now an extensive body of literature on neuropsychological aspects of alcoholism, and it is quite common for clinicians to assess patients for the neuropsychological consequences of alcoholism. The literature on other abused substances is less extensive, but there have been studies of heroin, cocaine, and other illicit substances suggesting possible adverse neuropsychological consequences. Alcohol, however, appears to remain the major culprit. At a more basic level, we are beginning to understand just what alcohol does to the brain on a long-term basis (Tarter & van Thiel, 1985). In particular, we have been able to correlate extensiveness of neuropsychological deficit with lesion parameters as ascertained by various imaging techniques.

A second environmental consideration that has now been recognized is neuropsychological toxicology. Some of us more than others are exposed to ambient toxins, largely dependent on where we live or work. Such common substances as paint and pesticides may be toxic to the brain. Extensive research has already been done on various potential toxins, and it is not uncommon to do assessments on individuals because of acute or chronic exposure to these agents.

The third environmental consideration is iatrogenic effects. It is not uncommon in medicine for treatments to have side effects that produce a variety of disorders that were not present before initiation of the treatment. This phenomenon is well-recognized in medicine and is typically considered by physicians when prescribing medication or other treatments. Physicians have become quite aware of this potential trade-off situation and often consider whether or not maintenance of a mild, benign disorder does less harm than aggressive treatment of that disorder. In our own work, we have studied this matter in relation to hypertension, asking several questions concerning whether or not medication for mild hypertension in the elderly impairs quality of life to such an extent that it does patients more harm to provide medication than not to provide it (Goldstein *et al.*, 1990; Materson *et al.*, 1990). In these studies, neuropsychological function was used as one index of quality of life.

In this book, there are two chapters concerning these side effects, one devoted to surgical treatment (Chapter 15) and the other to medication (Chapter 16). With regard to surgery, it may be noted that any general surgery involving the use of anesthesia has potential implications for brain function. Aside from the anesthesia itself, there have been reports of behavioral changes associated with surgery outside of the brain, notably open-heart surgery (Stanton, 1988). When a patient undergoes brain surgery we are obviously interested in the outcome, and we have had the opportunity on several occasions to evaluate patients before and after surgery. Perhaps the first systematic approach was the Greystone studies of psychosurgery (Mettler, 1949), but there have been other opportunities as well. Indeed, one of the factors leading to the development of the Halstead–Reitan neuropsychological test battery was Ward Halstead's studies of patients who had undergone frontal lobe surgery (Halstead, 1947). Surgery for epilepsy has also provided extensive information about brain function.

The neuropsychological consequences of psychoactive drugs are still an unsettled area, particularly with regard to antidepressant medication. Neuroleptics and other antipsychotic drugs have been studied extensively; however, the sophisticated neuropsychologist is now well-aware that these agents may influence test performance, for better or worse, and it is obligatory to consider their potential influence when making clinical interpretations based on the performances of medicated patients.

CONCLUDING REMARKS

All of these considerations indicate that we have come a long way from the days when we were mainly occupied with assessing adults who had sustained focal brain lesions by using clinical tests and examinational methods. Thus, a book of the type we have here reflecting this rather phenomenal growth will surely be worthwhile. Perhaps a final consideration involves reflecting on the growth of neuroscience in general, aside from neuropsychology. Since our field first evolved, scientific knowledge about the brain has grown exponentially. Perhaps most crucially, when the field began, the living brain could not really be visualized. We therefore had to rely on inferential procedures such as the EEG, the physical neurological examination, and behavioral tests to locate areas of pathology. Much of that task has now been taken over by the CT scan and the MRI test, and clinical neuropsychology has turned its interests in other directions. Additionally, the major improvements in what we can see have taught us a great deal about what we cannot see. We cannot see schizophrenia, although we can see interesting structural changes in some patients that may have something to do with it. We often cannot see the subtle effects of closed head injury or of exposure to toxic agents, but behavioral, neurochemical, and psychophysiological consequences of these conditions are becoming increasingly apparent (e.g., Morrow, Steinhauer, Robin, Hodgson, Tortora, & Bober, 1991). Developments in functional imaging are certainly advancing our ability to visualize brain function and structure, but the gap still remains between clinical phenomenology and what can be seen in the brain. As we try to close this gap, conquering the new frontier for neuropsychology appears to require a collaborative effort with neuroscientists involved in structural and functional imaging with the aim of simultaneous assessment of behavioral and imaging data. Such interactions have already provided significant information regarding the relationship between behavior and brain function.

To summarize, this handbook reflects the major developments in the growth of neuropsychological assessment. Beginning with early clinical and laboratory studies of brain-damaged adults and clinical psychological testing for the presence or absence of brain damage, neuropsychological assessment is involved, at a minimum, in the following list of endeavors:

1. in maintaining its traditional role in identification and localization of brain lesions and their behavioral correlates
2. its use as a method of assessing development of brain function over the life span through longitudinal and cross-sectional age-related studies
3. its application in forensic settings to assess competence and to evaluate individuals for disability
4. its use in educational settings to evaluate students for learning disabilities and related academic disorders
5. its use as a relatively common assessment method for psychopathology, particularly with regard to the schizophrenic and mood disorders
6. its use as part of the health status assessment of individuals with numerous general medical disorders, as well as individuals who have suffered exposure to toxic substances
7. its use as part of many ongoing studies of basic brain–behavior relationships in which neuropsychological tests are used as activation procedures while brain function or metabolism is monitored by various scanning methods
8. its use in clinical trials to monitor the effects of drugs or other new treatment procedures
9. its use with other investigative methods in studies of the neurobiology of various disorders such as autism and assorted genetic disorders
10. its use in industrial settings to assess employees' ability levels and possible influences on those levels that may be produced by external agents, such as medication, or internal states, such as fatigue, toxicity, or anoxia
11. its use in educational and vocational rehabilitation settings as a potentially important supplement to the traditional aptitude and achievement tests.

These emerging roles and responsibilities have necessitated engagement in research that addresses itself to problems created by venturing into these new applications. Therefore, we have to be concerned with such matters as the ability range of our tests so that they are appropriate for diverse age groups and for populations with widely varying levels of functioning. We need to understand the impact of socioeducational considerations on these tests and to assure ourselves that our tests are culture-fair. This matter becomes particularly problematic when neuropsychological tests are used for classification, selection, eligibility, or placement. We need to know about the effects of serial testing in order to contribute meaningfully to clinical trials and longitudinal studies in which the same tests are repeated numerous times (Chelune & Goldstein, 1991). We need to know about malingering and other phenomena that might be of importance for our forensic work (see Chapters 11 and 12). This volume was developed to acquaint the reader with many of these new extensions and applications and to provide a review of the areas of investigation needed to support them.

REFERENCES

American Psychological Association, American Educational Research Association, & National Council on Measurement in Education (1985). *Standards for educational and psychological testing.* Washington, D.C.: Author.

Bender, L. (1938). A visual motor gestalt test and its clinical use. *American Orthopsychiatric Association Research Monographs,* No. 3.

Berg, R., Franzen, M., & Wedding, D. (1987). *Screening for brain impairment: A manual for mental health practice.* New York: Springer Publishing.

Chelune, G. J., & Goldstein, G. (1991). Interpreting test–retest changes in neuropsychological practice. Symposium conducted at the annual meeting of the American Psychological Association, San Francisco, California.

Filskov, S. D., & Boll, T. J. (1981). *Handbook of clinical neuropsychology.* New York: Wiley-Interscience.

Filskov, S. D., & Boll, T. J. (1986). *Handbook of clinical neuropsychology, Volume 2.* New York: Wiley-Interscience.

Goldstein, G. (1978). Cognitive and perceptual differences between schizophrenics and organics. *Schizophrenia Bulletin, 4,* 160–185.

Goldstein, G., Hamsher, K. DeS, Goodglass, H., Reed, J., & Weinstein, S. (1985). Some pioneers in the history of clinical neuropsychology in the United States. *International Journal of Neuroscience, 25,* 273–275.

Goldstein, G., Materson, B. J., Cushman, W. C., Reda, D. J., Freis, E. D., Ramirez, E. A., Talmers, F. N., White, T. J., Nunn, S., Chapman, R. H., Khatri, I., Schnaper, H., Thomas, J. R., Henderson, W. G., & Frye, C. (1990). Treatment of hypertension in the elderly. II. Cognitive and behavioral function. *Hypertension, 15,* 361–369.

Goldstein, K., & Scheerer, M. (1941) Abstract and concrete behavior: An experimental study with special tests. *Psychological Monographs, 63,* (Entire No. 239).

Grant, D. A., & Berg, E. A. (1948). A behavioral analysis of degree of reinforcement and ease of shifting to new responses in a Weigl-type card-sorting problem. *Journal of Experimental Psychology, 38,* 404–411.

Halstead, W. C. (1947). *Brain and intelligence: A quantitative study of the frontal lobes.* Chicago: University of Chicago Press.

Henn, F. A., & Nasrallah, H. A. (1982). *Schizophrenia as a brain disease.* New York: Oxford University Press.

Kanner, L. (1943). Autistic disturbances of affective contact. *Nervous Child, 2,* 217–250.

King, H. E., & Miller, R. E. (1990). Hypertension: Cognitive and behavioral considerations. *Neuropsychology Review, 1,* 31–73.

Lezak, M. D. (1983). *Neuropsychological assessment* (2nd ed.). New York: Oxford University Press.

Machover, K. (1948). *Personality projection in the drawing of the human figure.* Springfield, Illinois: C. C. Thomas.

Materson, B. J., Cushman, W. C., Goldstein, G., Reda, D. J., Freis, E. D., Ramirez, E. A., Talmer, F. N., White, T. J., Nunn, S., Chapman, R. H., Khatri, I., Shnaper, H., Thomas, J. R., Henderson,

W. G., & Frye, C. (1990). Treatment of hypertension in the elderly: I. Blood pressure and clinical changes. *Hypertension, 15,* 348–360.

Mettler, F. A. (Ed.) (1949). *Selective partial ablation of the frontal cortex.* New York: Hoeber.

Morrow, L. A., Steinhauer, S. R., Robin, M. J., Hodgson, S., Tortora, S., & Bober, S. (1991). Neurophysiological and neuropsychological impairment following chemical exposure (Abstract). *Journal of Clinical and Experimental Psychology, 13,* 60.

Piotrowski, Z. (1937). The Rorschach inkblot method in organic disturbances of the central nervous system. *Journal of Nervous and Mental Disease, 86,* 525–537.

Reschly, D. J. (1990). Aptitude tests in educational classification and placment. In G. Goldstein & M. Hersen (Eds.), *Handbook of psychological assessment* (2nd ed.). New York: Pergamon Press.

Rourke, B. P. (1982). Central processing deficiencies in children: Toward a developmental neuropsychological model. *Journal of Clinical Neuropsychology, 4,* 1–18.

Satz, P., Taylor, G., Friel, J., & Fletcher, J. M. (1978). Some developmental and predictive precursors of reading disabilities: A six-year follow-up. In A. L. Benton & D. Pearl (Eds.), *Dyslexia: An appraisal of current knowledge.* New York: Oxford University Press.

Spreen, O. (1987). *Learning disabled children growing up: A follow-up into adulthood.* Lisse, Netherlands: Swets & Zeitlinger.

Stanton, B. A. (1988). Neurological, cognitive, and psychiatric sequelae associated with the surgical management of cardiac disease. In R. E. Tarter, D. H. van Thiel, & K. L. Edwards (Eds.), *Medical neuropsychology: The impact of disease on behavior* (pp. 27–73). New York: Plenum Press.

Tarter, R. E., & van Thiel, D. H. (1985). *Alcohol and the brain: Chronic effects.* New York: Plenum Press.

Weschler, D. (1944). The measurement of adult intelligence (3rd ed.). Baltimore: Williams & Wilkins.

I

Constitutional and Demographic Factors

Introduction

In Part I, constitutional and demographic factors affecting clinical neuropsychological assessment are discussed and evaluated in depth. The importance of considering the patient and the context of his or her developmental period is highlighted throughout. This section has three chapters that examine the role of perinatal, childhood, and adult development and aging-related factors in understanding brain function.

Perinatal issues as detailed by Emory *et al.* provide a foundation for the developmental chapters. This is followed by discussion of childhood factors (Cohen *et al.*) and the variables associated with adult development and the aging process (La Rue). The variables of sex and gender (Matthews) and handedness and lateralization (Henninger) are examined next. In both cases, a more comprehensive than usual approach to examining these variables is used. For example, in the former chapter, sex is viewed as a biological variable whereas gender is considered a psychological one.

The role of education and, to a lesser degree, social class and cultural exposure are reviewed by Ardila *et al.* in terms of how they could affect clinical neuropsychological assessment. In addition to socioeducational variables, the role of bilingualism is discussed by Manuel-DuPont *et al.* The study of bilingualism has important implications both in terms of basic brain organization and also as an important factor in the increasingly bilingual population in North America and the world.

1

Perinatal

EUGENE K. EMORY, TAMMY M. SAVOIE, JOAN BALLARD, MARION EPPLER, and CYNTHIA O'DELL

INTRODUCTION

Perinatal factors assume an uncertain role in neuropsychological development. We know that labor is a significant fetal stressor. Drastic shifts in oxygen level during gestation and labor are linked to a continuum of casualty from severe neurological impairments to more subtle disabilities. It is this latter set of disabilities, those of intangible origins, that remain the confounding chapter in developmental neuropsychology. Moreover, it is the infant who experiences perinatal stress, but who will not manifest developmental symptoms of disability until some years later, that causes early identification to be such a difficult task. This endeavor is undertaken by developmental neuropsychological studies of perinatal events. When the clinical neuropsychologist is involved in assessing a child with a benign developmental history who exhibits distinct deficits of an organic nature, pre- or perinatal hypoxia should be suspected. This prescription is grounded in the variable consequences of hypoxic injury and its tendency to produce subclinical, asymptomatic, and latent manifestations during early childhood (Scholz, 1956; Towbin, 1973).

This chapter will review select topics in perinatal medicine that are known, or thought, to cause compromises in the human central nervous system (CNS). It will relate these issues to traumas affecting CNS organization and its functional relationship to early postnatal behavior and development. This relationship is important to the understanding of nonprogressive neurological and

EUGENE K. EMORY, TAMMY M. SAVOIE, JOAN BALLARD, MARION EPPLER, and CYNTHIA O'DELL • Department of Psychology, Emory University, Atlanta, Georgia 30322.

HANDBOOK OF NEUROPSYCHOLOGICAL ASSESSMENT: A Biopsychosocial Perspective, edited by Antonio E. Puente and Robert J. McCaffrey. Plenum Press, New York, 1992.

neuropsychological conditions that have a putative perinatal etiology. The chapter will also discuss neurobehavioral assessment of the young infant and its relation to traditional clinical neuropsychological assessment. Finally, an attempt will be made to link perinatal risk factors to cognitive and intellectual abilities in school-aged children.

HISTORICAL BACKGROUND

The historical foundations of the emerging field that we refer to as "perinatal neuropsychology" have a checkered past without a continuous focused pattern of scientific investigation. Its history, although subsumed under different names, dates back to the bible (Luke 1:44) where the first recorded accounts of the living fetus were acknowledged. But in a more contemporary context, the observation that a connection between prenatal injuries to the CNS, especially oxygen deprivation, and development of intellect and volition was impossible to ignore (Little, 1862) represented the first major breakthrough in the field of perinatal neuropsychology. It would be almost a century before perinatal risk research obtained a solid scientific foothold in Western literature. A number of historical factors contributed to the change in perspective that took place in the 1940s and 1950s. Not the least of these was an understanding of the epidemiology of diseases of childhood and the development of antibiotics and immunizations (Russo & Varni, 1982; Sameroff & Chandler, 1975). Additional changes in sanitation, nutrition, and medical technology virtually eliminated many life-threatening illnesses. Subsequently there began to emerge an identifiable population of chronically ill and developmentally damaged children, many of whom would have died during the first half of the 20th century (Russo & Varni, 1982; Schechler & Halton, 1982).

The politics of poverty and health also played a role in the emergence of risk research as a way to break the cycle of diseases that tended to flourish among low-income and poorly educated families. The substandard living conditions common to many low-income families were seen as a contributor to risk factors known to affect normal growth and development. The "continuum of caretaking casualty" was a concept that attempted to explain why physical and mental health problems tended to perpetuate themselves within certain socioeconomic groups (Sameroff & Chandler, 1975). Research interest followed an emerging political ideology (Riegle, 1972) and perinatal and developmental risk research came into vogue.

Perinatal neuropsychology represents an amalgamation of high-risk infancy research, discoveries in developmental neuroscience (Davidson & Fox, 1982; Fox & Davidson, 1986; Goldman-Rakic, 1985), and the establishment and continuing acceptance of clinical neuropsychology as a professional discipline. It is understandably interdisciplinary with a strong developmental and clinical research emphasis.

BASIC NEUROBIOLOGICAL ISSUES

Chronology of Prenatal Neural Development

The prenatal period extends from the time of fertilization to birth, occurring in humans approximately 270 days after conception. Prenatal life can be divided into three distinct periods: the preovum from 0 to 14 days, embryonic from 14 days to 9 weeks, and fetal from 9 weeks to birth. The ovum is fertilized in about 1 week and attaches itself to the uterine endometrium (mucous membrane) during implantation. Near the third week of gestation the developing embryo enters the neurula stage, when a pear-shaped neural plate emerges from the dorsal ectoderm. In the center of the plate develops a narrow longitudinal neural groove, gradually deepening and eventually folding over onto itself. At the midpoint it begins to close, extending in both the rostral and caudal direction. As the fold closes, its two ends—the anterior and posterior neuropores—remain open until approximately 25 days of gestation (Fig. 1.1). These closures result in a fluid-filled central canal call the neural tube (Fig. 1.2). The process of conversion from an open groove to a sealed tube is called neurulation and is important in both a structural (or anatomical) sense and a functional (or neurobehavioral) sense. It also represents the development of the first organ of the human embryo.

Anomalies in the CNS that occur around 1 month after fertilization are often manifested by particularly serious physiological and neurobehavioral pathology. If the neural tube has difficulty closing, several possible anomalies can occur—i.e., anencephaly, in which the forebrain fails to develop properly because the anterior neuropore does not close, or spina bifida, resulting from caudal difficulty. Although neurulation consumes only 2 weeks of prenatal development, the embryo's susceptibility to teratogenic influences may be highest during this critical period of development (Wilson, 1965).

The fetal period begins around the eighth or ninth week of gestation, with little additional cell differentiation. Vulnerability of the fetus in terms of structural abnormality is decreased due to lack of further cell differentiation. During this time, myelin begins to form, and the weight of the brain rapidly increases.

In the fetal period, the development of the cerebral hemispheres progresses from a smooth surface to form the typical pattern of convolutions and sulci. By the sixth prenatal month, the cortex has developed its six-layer structure and a columnar organization within the cortex eventually develops (Goldman & Nauta, 1977). During this time, changes in the intercerebral commissures (major connection between hemispheres) are closely related to changes in the cerebral cortical layers. However, commissure growth is slow and is related to maturation of the association cortex. At birth the brain weighs approximately 300–350 g. It continues to grow and increases to 1250–1500 g in 4 years, constituting 80% of its adult weight.

Three classes of prenatal neurodevelopmental anomalies can be distin-

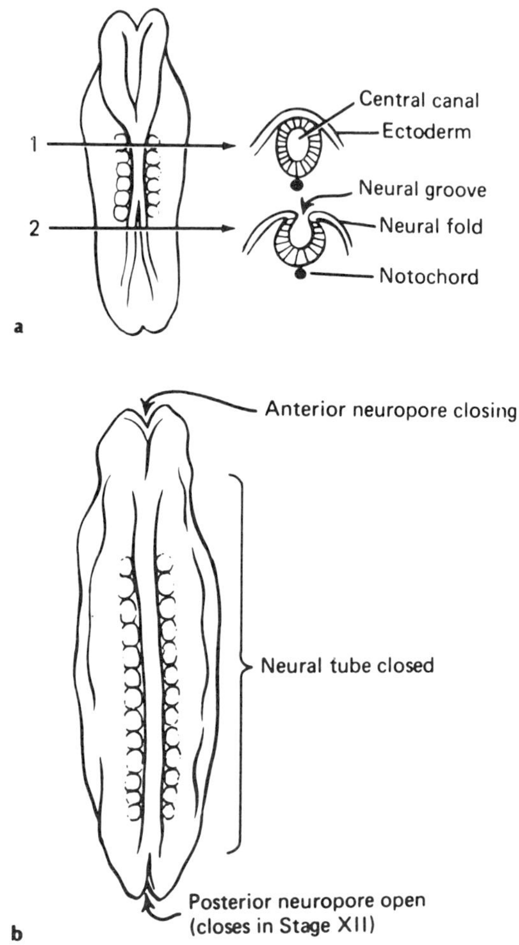

FIGURE 1.1. Beginning of development of the nervous system. (a) start of neurulation, two cross-sectional views. (b) Late stage of neurulation, showing the anterior and posterior neuropores (Lemire, Loeser, Leech, & Alvord, 1975).

guished: those that are incompatible with life, those that are not incompatible with life but severely affect functional behavior, and those that have a widely variable consequence. In some instances a given anomaly may be associated with severe symptoms and in other instances may occur asymptomatically.

Most CNS malformations are defects in the formation of the neural tube during the induction period (3 and 4 weeks of gestation), causing anencephaly or spina bifida. Anencephaly almost always results in death. Spina bifida actually refers to a number of different disorders and their respective degrees of severity. Spina bifida results from an abnormal fusion of the posterior aspect of the developing neural tube. The most severe form is myelomeningocele, in which the saclike bulge contains not only meninges but cerebrospinal fluid as well. These patients often develop hydrocephalus and have other cortical

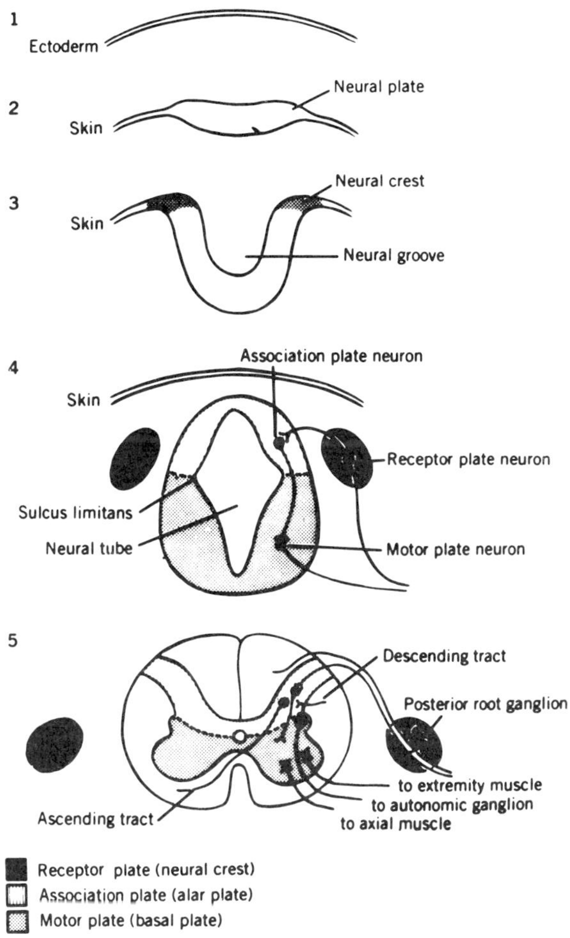

FIGURE 1.2. Stages in the development of a spinal cord segment. Note the development of the alar and basal plates into sensory and motor regions, respectively (Lemire *et al.*, 1975).

abnormalities. Most infants born with myelomeningocele will sustain lifelong physical and mental handicaps (Spreen, Tupper, Risser, Tuokko, & Edgell, 1984).

The major structural abnormality that affects neuropsychological development is hydrocephalus internus and externus (abnormal enlargement of the skull and the brain ventricles or subarachnoid space). Children with hydrocephalus are reported to show an uneven growth of IQ during childhood with nonverbal intelligence developing at a slower rate than verbal intelligence. The development of the vertex and occipital cortex is impaired, blocking the cerebral aqueduct and resulting in visual abnormalities, motor deficits, and seizures. As a result, the child gains little visuospatial experience and develops poor nonverbal intelligence (Spreen *et al.*, 1984).

Development of the newborn with a CNS anomaly depends on the size and location of the defect, particularly in terms of brain development. Microcephaly, porencephaly, and hydrocephalus tend to be associated with developmental retardation. The degree of retardation is highly variable.

There appears to be a strong correlation between malformations of the CNS and the development of brain and intellect. Debate continues over the association between minor physical anomalies—e.g., abnormal head circumference, highly arched palate, single palmar crease, abnormality of the toes and fingers—and the development of intelligence and occurrence of behavior problems (Hynd & Willis, 1988). In school-aged girls, passivity, low activity level, withdrawal, and chronic anxiety are reported to be among the number of anomalies exhibited. In boys, associated hyperactive, disruptive, and impulsive behaviors are evident (Quinn & Rapoport, 1974).

Minor CNS anomalies of only cosmetic significance may adversely affect the child's social interaction, influencing both intelligence and behavior. However, the existence of subtle malformations of the CNS or dysfunction of the brain in such children has not been confirmed.

Normal postnatal neurological development proceeds from the infant acquiring control of his or her eyes, head and neck muscles, upper trunk, hands and arms during the first 4–7 months postnatally. He or she gains increasing command of the torso and fingers and by 8–10 months, sits and crawls alone. A child's first birthday is a key age socially for the parents. The child may stand for brief periods at first, and within a few more weeks stroll gingerly about the house. The next major transition is control of the larynx and the production of words and phrases near 18–20 months. Sphincter control occurs around 24 months and by 3 years, the child is speaking in sentences. Higher-order cognitive development emerges within the next 12 months and includes such concepts as numbers, colors, and form. Broader socialization historically developed after the start of kindergarten when the child learned prosocial skills. However, with the emergence of preschool and dual-career families, many social skills appear at an age earlier than previously supposed (e.g., Knobloch & Pasamanick, 1974). The earliest manifestations of socialization beyond smiling are apparent around the age of 7–9 months when the child may selectively seek physical proximity to a familiar caretaker and later become anxious around unfamiliar adults. Interestingly, almost all children are curious and uninhibited in the presence of unfamiliar infants and young children.

The neurological examination of the older child—while employing traditional assessment of cranial nerve function, sensory systems, skeletal muscles, and gait—will also focus heavily on unique patterns of behavior in the motor, adaptive, language, and social domains (Swaiman, 1989b). Clinically, it is important to recognize what neurological diseases are manifested during the perinatal period. The pattern typified by the onset of neurological conditions can be summarized as follows: (1) traumatic or vascular diseases manifested over a period of minutes or hours, but usually within a day; (2) infectious processes, electrolyte imbalances, and toxic processes having a longer developmental course than trauma and reaching their zenith around the end of the first week of life; (3) and degenerative disorders, neoplastic conditions, and metabolic errors progressing insidiously over a period of several weeks or months during the first year (Swaiman, 1989a).

Prematurity and Low Birth Weight

Prematurity and low birth weight (LBW) are frequently occurring perinatal complications and are commonly associated with high-risk factors. Although the terms *prematurity* and *low birth weight* have been around for some time, their exact meaning is often confused, giving rise to misunderstanding and inaccuracy. Historically, the two terms were used interchangeably (Caputo & Mandell, 1970). They referred to a gestational age of 38 weeks or less and a birth weight of 2500 g or less. More recently, the term *very low birth weight* (VLBW) has been used to designate a birth weight of 1500 g or less. Using the terms *prematurity* and *low birth weight* synonymously leads to some confusion since every premature infant's birth weight is not low, and every LBW infant is not premature. The distinction is an important one as both conditions bear neuropsychological implications. For example, an increased incidence of neurological, intellectual, and behavioral developmental problems occurs in children born prematurely (Fuller, Guthrie, & Alvord, 1983). The incidence of neuropsychological impairments among children born prematurely ranges up to two-thirds (Lubchenco, Horner, Reed, Hix, Metcalf, Cohig, Elliott, & Bourg, 1963). However, earlier studies did not control for age/weight ratios and may have produced uncertain estimates. A more accurate terminology has been introduced, and takes into account the relationship between gestational age and birth weight. The new designations include *small for gestational age* (SGA), *average for gestational age* (AGA), and *large for gestational age* (LGA). These terms distinguish an infant within the statistically normal range for gestational age from an infant whose weight lies outside of the normal range. Although there are additional descriptions related to gestational age/birth weight interactions (Lubchenco, 1976), SGA, AGA, and LGA are most frequently used. The cutoff point for the SGA infant is a birth weight below the 10th percentile for its gestational age. Conversely, the cutoff point for the LGA infant is a birth weight above the 90th percentile for its gestational age. All other infants are regarded as average for gestational age, regardless of their age status (Fig. 1.3). In this way, clinicians and researchers can better determine if an infant's growth is within the expected range for its age. Many SGA babies suffer from what has been called *intrauterine growth retardation* (IUGR). IUGR may be a result of varying prenatal factors, but one factor frequently associated with IUGR is a small or insufficient placenta. These infants, often referred to as "small-for-dates," are suspected of having CNS compromise due to insufficient nutrition and possible oxygen deprivation throughout pregnancy. Such chronic stressors place these babies at exceptionally

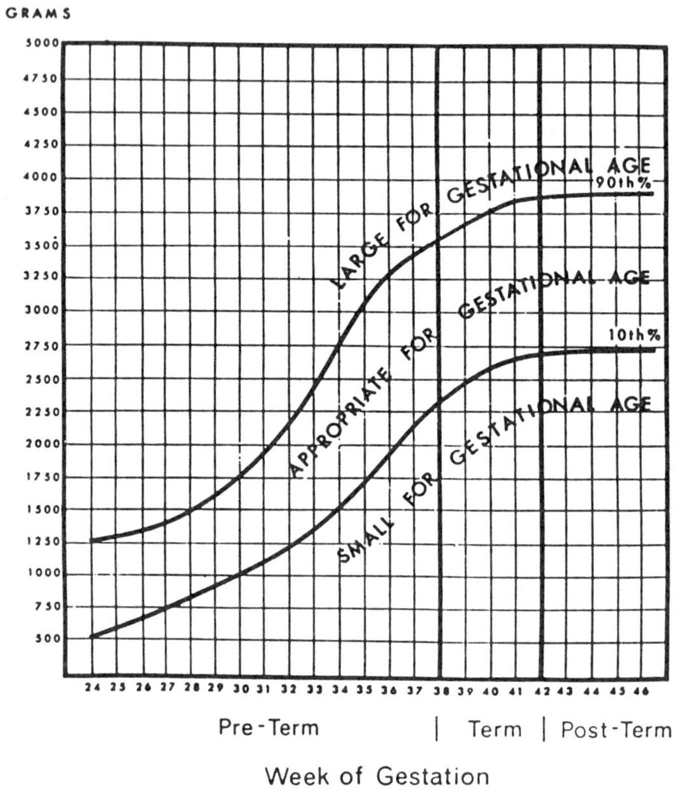

FIGURE 1.3. Classification of newborns by birth weight (BW) and gestational age (GA). GA–BW distribution: GA to be estimated from first day of last menstrual period (LMP) and classified by complete weeks: 37 weeks ÷ 0 days = 37 weeks; 27 weeks ÷ 6 days = 37 weeks. GA: subdivided along abscissa into three categories: Preterm (Pr), All infants less than 38 weeks GA, i.e., 37 weeks ÷ 6 days or less; term (T), All infants between 39th and 42nd weeks GA; post-term (Po), All infants of 42 or more weeks GA. BW: Within each group, three subgroups of infants are defined by BW: LGA, Infants above 90th percentile; AGA, Infants between 90th and 10th percentile; SGA, Infants below 10th perentile. Thus, nine groups of newborn infants are defined and coded as follows:
Pr-LGA, Born before 38th week, BW above 90th percentile.
Pr-AGA, Born before 38th week, BW between 10th and 90th percentile.
Pr-SGA, Born before 38th week, BW below 10th percentile.
T-LGA, Born between 38th and 42nd weeks, BW above 90th percentile.
T-AGA, Born between 38th and 42nd weeks, BW between 10th and 90th percentile.
T-SGA, Born between 38th and 42nd weeks, BW below 10th percentile.
Po-LGA, Born at or after 42nd week, BW above 90th percentile.
Po-AGA, Born at or after 42nd week, BW between 10th and 90th percentile.
Po-SGA, Born at or after 42nd week, BW below 10th percentile.
From "A practical classification of newborn infants by weight and gestational age" by F. C. Battaglia and L. O. Lubchenco, 1967, *Journal of Pediatrics, 71,* p. 159. Reprinted by permission.

high risk for neuropsychological and other developmental difficulties that are otherwise uncorrelated with life-threatening perinatal risk factors (Fig. 1.4). It is important to remember that while many premature infants will also be SGA, full-term infants who weight ≤ 2500 g are also SGA as well as low in birth weight. Premature infants who weigh ≤ 2500 g may not in fact be SGA but simply low in birth weight. The preterm infant may experience adequate growth

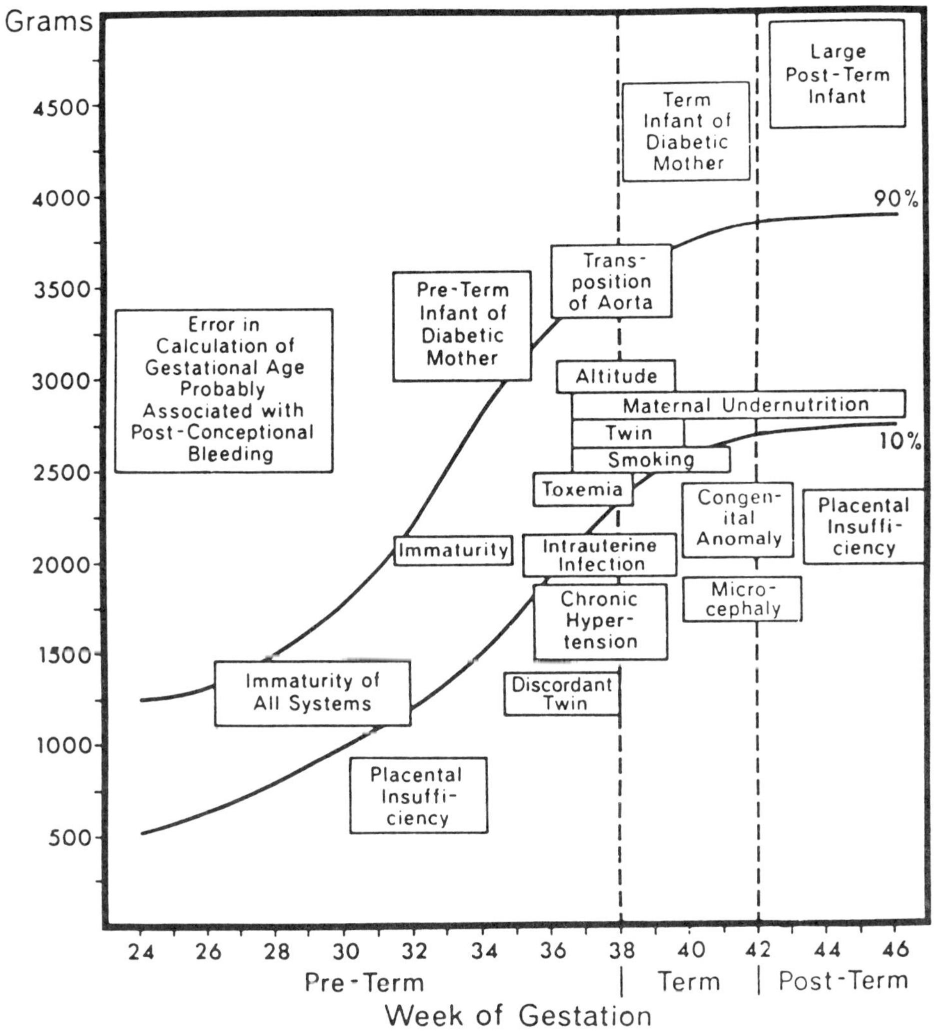

FIGURE 1.4. Deviations of intrauterne growth. Neonatal morbidity by birthweight and gestational age. The boxes indicate the morbidities likely to occur at the various birth weights and gestational ages. From "Factors influencing fetal growth" by L. O. Lubchenco, C. Hansman, & L. Backstrom, in *Aspects of prematurity and dysmaturity* (pp. 149–164) by J. H. P. Jonxis, H. K. A. Visser, & J. A. Troelstra (Eds.), 1968, Leiden, H. W. Stenfert Kroese, N.V., and Springfield, IL: Charles C. Thomas. Adapted by permission.

but has simply been born early. A determination of gestational age cannot therefore be made on the basis of weight alone but rather will include an assessment of posture and flexion of upper and lower extremities (Fig. 1.5).

IUGR has at least two distinct recognizable types. Type I IUGR appears to arise from intrauterine infections, toxins, and possibly very poor maternal diet. These insults are believed to occur in the earlier part of gestation leading to stunted growth of all or most developing organs (Niswander, 1989). This type of IUGR is also referred to as symmetrical growth retardation. An asymmetrical form of growth retardation, referred to as type II IUGR, appears to arise during the third trimester after a relatively normal prior fetal growth. The cause of type II IUGR is related to factors which interfere with placental function. Head and brain size may be normal whereas abdominal viscera and subcutaneous fat are affected. From a neuropsychological perspective, type I IUGR may have more consequences since it also affects brain growth and development.

Historically, LBW infants, many of whom were premature or SGA or both, encountered a number of adversities associated with development. These include poor performance on infant neurobehavior examinations, low intelligence scores during school, and high rates of such developmental deficits as hyperkinesis, autism, language problems, and poor academic achievement (Caputo & Mandell, 1970; Emory, Walker, & Cruz, 1982; Field, 1979; Lubchenco, 1976; Parmelee, 1975; Scarr & Williams, 1973). Recent studies have also found that maturity at birth and birth weight are related to fetal reactivity during labor. Fetuses whose heart rate tends to drop or decelerate with uterine contractions generally have lower birth weight and are less mature than fetuses whose heart rate rises or accelerates with contractions (Emory & Noonan, 1984*a*,*b*). Overall, premature infants, independent of weight percentiles, have a higher incidence of developmental difficulty than healthy term newborns.

An example of the complex interactions that take place among perinatal events is aptly demonstrated by the correlation between fetal heart rate (FHR) decelerations and neonatal neurological morbidity. In a study by Visser, Redman, Huisjes, and Turnbull (1980), terminal antepartum FHR (e.g., late decelerations with low variability) has the poorest neonatal outcome, with fetal acidemia and an umbilical artery pH at elective cesarean of less than 7.15 in 70% of the cases. However, no relationship between pH and morbidity was found in term infants with decelerations; neurologically abnormal infants were preterm with abnormal FHR patterns (Visser, 1989).

The mortality rate for preterm and LBW infants has shown a steady decline. As of the late 1970s, a declining trend of about 25% in infant mortality before 28 days of age was reported for black and while infants born in the United States (Manniello & Farrell, 1977). More infants whose nervous system had been compromised pre- and perinatally were surviving, yet many, especially those at the lower end of the gestational age and birth weight distributions, were exhibiting long-term developmental delays or disabilities. The medical and technical advances that promised better odds for survival of high-risk newborns were, ironically, a major precursor to the proportional rise in long-term infant

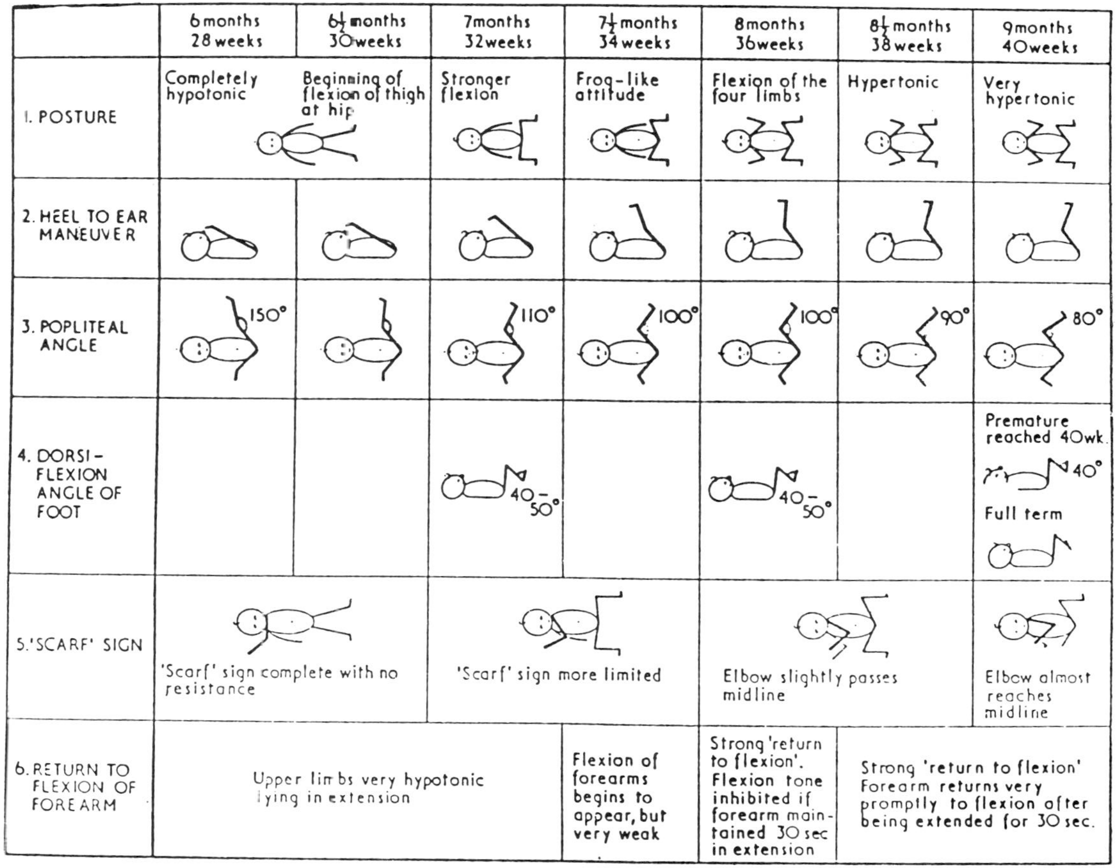

FIGURE 1.5. Passive tone. Increase of tone with maturity illustrated by means of six clinical tests. "Neurological evaluations of the maturity of newborn infants" by A. Amiel-Tison, 1968, *Archives of Disorders of Childhood*, *43*, p. 89. Reprinted by permission.

morbidity. Thus, perinatal factors linked to high mortality are now producing developmental and neuropsychological sequelae among survivors. These medical advances actually anticipated Public Law 94-142 and the rise of developmental neuropsychology. Such events give credence to the notion that a significant percentage of children and adults with neuropsychological impairments of a nonprogressive nature may have sustained CNS compromise during prenatal development (Towbin, 1986). As studies of prematurity and LBW reveal, no single factor is responsible for later neuropsychological impairments except in extreme neonatal pathology. One important factor is that, although the frequency of severe handicaps is greater among LBW and premature infants, most handicapping conditions occur in children born at term gestation and at a normal birth weight (DeSouza & Richards, 1978; Touwen & Huisjes, 1984). Recently, Cohen, Parmelee, Beckwith, and Sigman (1986) suggested that social factors also play a major role in determining the outcome of preterm infants notwithstanding neonatal complications. Mortality and morbidity rates remain higher for African-American babies than for their Caucasian counterparts.

Prematurity and LBW constitute significant developmental deviations in terms of neuropsychological development. Unfortunately, the magnitude of the problem is increasing because of the improved survival rate for many newborns who would have previously expired during the neonatal period.

Anoxia and Hypoxia

Anoxic episodes (termination of oxygen supply) and their immediate consequences are the most common difficulties encountered during the perinatal period and account for the greatest percentage of neurological problems in the neonate. A systematic reduction in oxygen level leads to decreased blood flow to local tissue and, in turn, produces a biochemical switch from aerobic (i.e., occurring in oxygen) generation of energy to less efficient anaerobic (in the absence of oxygen) generation, rapidly depleting the brain's limited reserve of energy (in the form of adenosine triphosphate). An accumulation of biochemical waste products, such as carbon dioxide and lactic acid, generated anaerobically from spent energy supplies, also results. These waste products contribute to the neurological problems created by the anoxic episode.

Gestational causes of anoxia can be described as either maternal or placental. Infectious diseases, diabetes mellitus, and maternal toxemias can all reduce the amount of oxygen available to the fetus as do maternal cardiac arrest, severe anemia or bleeding. If the placenta is underdeveloped for reasons such as maternal malnutrition, then the transport of oxygen to the fetus will be less than optimal. Also, infarction of placental tissue may not permit adequate levels of oxygen to penetrate and reach the fetus (Naeye, 1977).

Parturitional causes of an anoxic episode include abrupt fetal separation from the placenta, placental compression due to uterine hypertonicity, and placenta previa in which the placenta partially or completely blocks the fetus from exiting the uterus. Also, traumatic brain injury may occur during parturition causing an anoxic episode. This typically involves damage to the brain stem, which interferes with CNS control over respiration and other vital systemic functions. Neonates experiencing an anoxic episode during gestation or parturition display clinical signs such as color change and low Apgar scores. They require immediate postnatal intervention.

Consequences of an anoxic episode vary widely according to such factors as cause, duration, age, developmental status, and velocity of the reduction in oxygen level. Thus, it is difficult to generalize clinically about the long-term consequences of anoxia because its consequences can range from immediate death or gross neuropathology through various hypothetical subclinical lesions to the apparent absence of any mental and neurological sequelae.

Anoxia refers to a total lack of oxygen to the fetus or newborn, but hypoxia suggests a partial reduction in the oxygen supply. Hypoxia is therefore the condition most commonly associated with problems of the human fetus in which short- and long-term hypoxic insults are not uncommon. Given that these insults are relatively frequent and result from a host of complications such as respiratory distress syndrome, apnea, or impaired cardiac function, one can appreciate the possible effects of these injuries on subsequent neuropsychological performance (Fig. 1.6).

Hypoxic–ischemic perinatal brain injuries are an immense clinical problem in that they account for a preponderance of severe, nonprogressive neurological deficits occurring secondary to perinatal events (Volpe, 1981). The precise relationship between pathogenic factors and the development of hypoxic–ischemic injuries is largely unknown, although perinatal asphyxia has been implicated in both forms of injury (i.e., hypoxemia and diminished perfusion of the brain; Volpe, 1981). A host of neurological deficits, including mental retardation, seizure disorders, spasticity, choreoathetosis, and ataxia, may follow such injury (Crothers & Paine, 1959; McDonald, 1973; Emory, Tynan, & Dave, 1989). These insults also affect brain structures along the auditory pathway since they are particularly susceptible to damage from asphyxia (Myers, 1975, Murray, 1988). Preterm infants are more likely to sustain injury in the periventricular region, producing hemorrhage and/or infarction (Fig. 1.7).

In full-term infants, cerebral edema, parasagittal cortical infarction, and necrosis of the thalamic and brain stem nuclei are the major foci of injury (Avery, 1985). The importance of gestational age in ascertaining which areas of the brain are most vulnerable to hypoxic/ischemic injury must be appreciated, although neuropsychological assessment of infants who sustain such injuries is primarily concerned with identifying functional impairment that is amenable to treatment (Figs. 1.8 and 1.9).

During labor, uterine contractions create pressure in the cranial cavity, which can disturb blood flow and produce cerebral ischemia. Moreover, uterine contractions may also reduce the level of fetal oxygenation by exacerbating already impaired umbilical cord flow following cord occlusion or placental function related to uteroplacental insufficiency (Martin, Siassi, & Hon, 1974; Chik, Sokol, & Rosen, 1976; Hon, 1975).

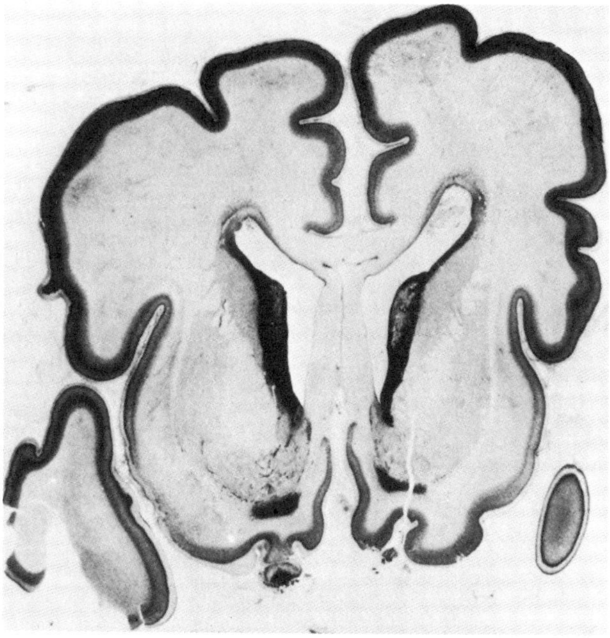

FIGURE 1.6. Cerebrum of premature infants illustrating persistent germinal matrix tissue; the padlike germinal deposits are deeply located, attached to the inner surface of the hemispheric walls, and bulging into the lower lateral portion of the ventricle space on each side. Matrix deposits show minimal hypoxic infarctional lesions, more pronounced on the right, appearing as irregular pale patches of necrosis; thromboses in small veins in the matrix. History of spontaneous delivery at 32 weeks of gestation due to premature detachment of the placenta; infant lived 2 days. Autopsy revealed infarctional damage in other organs in addition to the brain. (Reprinted by permission, A. Towbin.)

Subtle and subclinical damage poses a frequent problem for the clinical neuropsychologist. This problem is aggravated when one is called on to infer cause from a complex set of events such as labor and parturition. Moreover, as many as 50% of brain-damaged infants and children evince no scientifically or clinically significant explanation (Mann, 1986). It appears that selective vulnerability of white matter exists in perinatal brain damage, the principal cause being cord compression. Chronic hypoxia (see Figs. 1.10 and 1.11) may exist without metabolic acidosis, but before pathological evidence of brain damage occurs, clear patterns of cardiovascular instability and electrocorticographic abnormality can be recognized. Interestingly, some abnormality of the umbilical cord is found in 30% of all deliveries. For the clinical neuropsychologist, any perinatal evidence of cord abnormality should raise a suspicion about possible white and gray matter lesions in which brain stem, hypothalamus, and cortical regions represent predilection areas (Mann, 1986).

Information about the FHR pattern in the antepartum (before labor) and intrapartum (during labor) periods could assist clinical neuropsychologists in

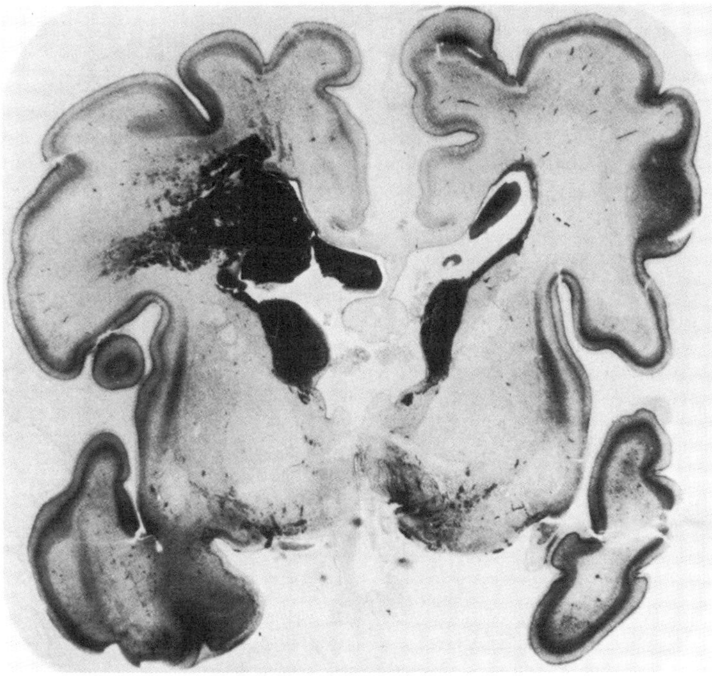

FIGURE 1.7. Deep cerebral hemorrhagic infarction, characteristic pattern of acute hypoxic cerebral damage in the premature fetus and newborn. The area of infarction, deep in the upper portion of the left hemisphere, appears as dark, confluent patches with infiltrating margins, obliterating the deep white matter and extending downward to involve the basal ganglia and germinal matrix tissue. On both sides, the germinal matrix deposit is effaced, replaced by a hemorrhagic mound of infarcted tissue bulging into the lower part of the cerebral ventricles. The case history indicated premature delivery at 35 weeks of gestation; the infant showed increased generalized neurological deterioration with death at 23 h. (Reprinted by permission, A. Towbin.)

determining a likely perinatal etiology for impaired neuropsychological performance in children with a benign history. This is because cardiac rate in the fetus is a direct function of oxygen deprivation. There are several explanations for this phenomenon. First, stroke volume variation in the fetal heart is minimal, and a need for more oxygen is met by an increase in cardiac rate (Battaglia & Meschia, 1986). Therefore, tachycardia in an otherwise healthy fetus may reflect some minor oxygen deprivation. Second, specific patterns of FHR bradycardia are symptomatic of the underlying conditions that produce them. One such condition, uteroplacental insufficiency, perpetuates late decelerations; another, umbilical cord occlusion, causes variable bradycardia (Hon, 1975). Finally, and of great clinical significance is the fact that acute cerebral hypoxic damage in the perinate produces the local process of thrombosis, infarction, and hemorrhage in a manner similar to adult stroke victims (Towbin, 1980). In a parallel sense, the human fetus and newborn with acute or chronic damage suffer strokes that are

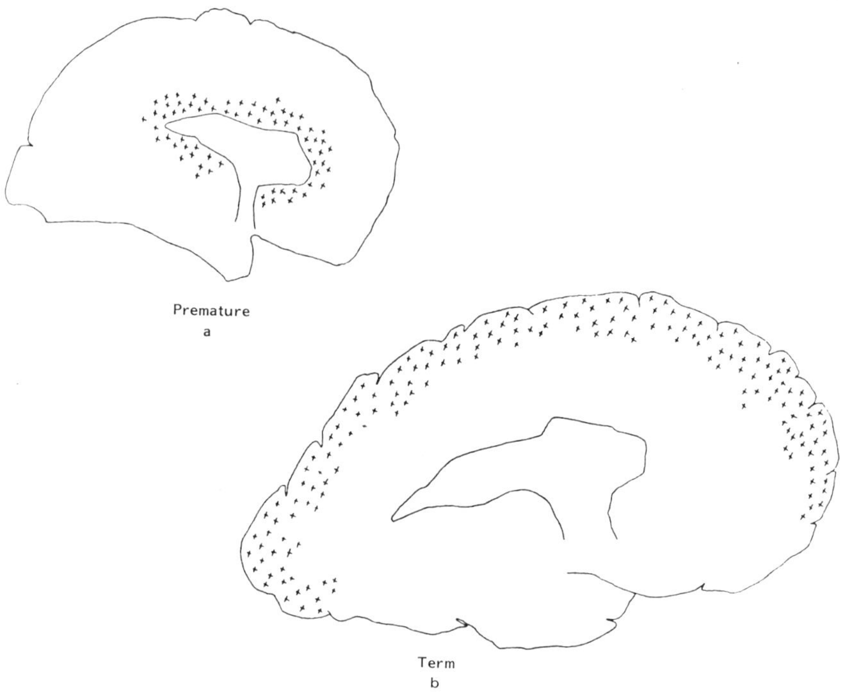

FIGURE 1.8. Two basic patterns of perinatal hypoxic cerebral damage related to gestational age. (a) In the premature, deep, cerebral damage predominates wtih hemorrhagic infarctional destruction of periventricular germinal matrix tissue and adjoining structures. (b) At term, in the mature fetus and newborn, the cerebral cortex with subjacent white matter is the main site of hypoxic infarctional damage.

clinically and pathologically comparable to that of an adult. These circumstances provide the clinical neuropsychologist an insult-based model applicable to developmental neuropsychological assessment of children with histories of hypoxia and respiratory disorders. The missing link from a clinical perspective is the delineation of symptoms, both motor and cognitive, which reflect the maturational level of the child. It is important to recognize that the fetus and term newborn are able to tolerate oxygen deprivation with less severe sequelae than the mature adult (Battaglia & Meschia, 1986; Dawes, 1968). What is required is the calibration of oxygen debt in the fetus and infant that produces damage like that observed in adult patients with acute and chronic hypoxic damage.

In summary, cerebral palsy and severe mental retardation represent extremes at one end of the continuum of developmental disorders. Lesser forms of mental retardation and other neuropsychological disabilities may also trace their origins to the pre- and perinatal periods. Psychometrically based diagnostic assessment of these conditions is a historical tradition in clinical psychology. A suspicion of perinatal trauma is often raised as a causal factor in the patho-

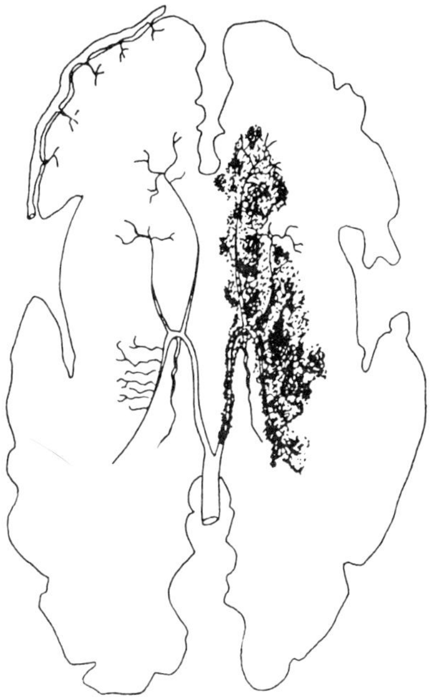

FIGURE 1.9. Mechanism of deep cerebral venous infarction in the premature newborn. The deep cerebral vein on the right is dilated, distended with thrombus, *in vivo* blood clot. The corresponding deep portion of the cerebrum appears with confluent dark patches, areas of hemorrhagic infarction, portions of tissue devitalized and suffused with blood due to interference with local venous damage. Deep venous channels in the premature brain prominently are developed in contrast to the rudimentary superficial cerebral veins. (A. Towbin, *American Journal of Diseases of Children*, 1970.)

genesis of mild and borderline mental retardation, learning disabilities, and other cognitive and neuropsychological deficits claiming a putative organic basis. A common assumption is that the majority of these disorders and disabilities are preventable. Speculation attributes the cause of these disorders to insults incurred during the pre- and perinatal periods (Okazaki, 1983; Towbin, 1977, 1978, 1980).

THEORETICAL ISSUES

A Neuropsychological Perspective

The neuropsychological view of perinatal and obstetrical events acknowledges the diagnostic sensitivity and value of neuropsychological assessment during the formative years. Moreover, perinatal complications are becoming an increasingly investigated topic in neuropsychological research (Gray & Dean, 1988; Emory & Mapp, 1988; Emory, Tynan, & Dave, 1989). The finding of a neuropsychological deficit in the context of a benign developmental history does not, by definition, imply perinatal damage. The critical question is not always whether or not a serious obstetric insult produced neuropsychological sequelae, as in the case of cerebral palsy (CP) or severe mental retardation (MR). Rather, the question is often whether or not subclinical perinatal insults produce

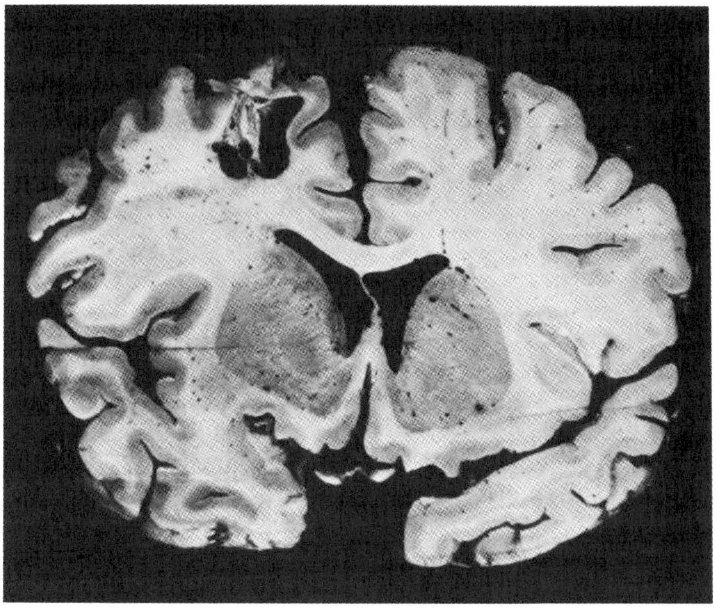

FIGURE 1.10. Focal chronic cystic lesion with scarred margins, pathologically consistent with destruction due to remote hypoxic infarction. History of complicated hypoxic twin birth; other twin died postnatally. Section of cerebrum from surviving twin who lived to the age of 42 years. Moderate neuropsychiatric manifestations throughout life; mild retardation noted in infancy, withdrawn during childhood, depressive during adulthood. Neurologically, this individual showed slight left-sided spasticity and hyperreflexia and had occasional focal epileptic seizures. (Brain section viewed anteriorly; lesion anatomically on the right side of the cerebrum.) (Reprinted by permission, A. Towbin.)

neuropsychological sequelae in the absence of major disorders such as CP or MR. Neuroanatomical lesions and radiographic evidence of neuropathology may not be apparent where subclinical perinatal insult exists, and yet the child exhibits impairment in higher cortical function. Subclinical insults to the perinate that produce clinical sequelae do so because they compromise secondary and tertiary neuropsychological processes. These processes map onto projection areas of primary sensory-motor cortex. Secondary and tertiary neuropsychological processes (Luria, 1973, 1980) involve higher cortical structures at the level of the cerebral hemispheres. Damage to these areas more often includes impairment in high-level coordinated actions, manifested in subtle deficits on psychological and neuropsychological tests. They do not significantly impair gross motor functions and tend to spare basic intellectual functions. Instead they affect cognitive processes involving elaboration, amplification, and integrated perception of incoming sensory information (secondary) and cross-modal integration of information (tertiary) across different sensory modalities and cortical zones (Beaumont, 1983; Luria, 1973). Tertiary functioning also includes inhibition, integrated planning and initiation of cognitive and behav-

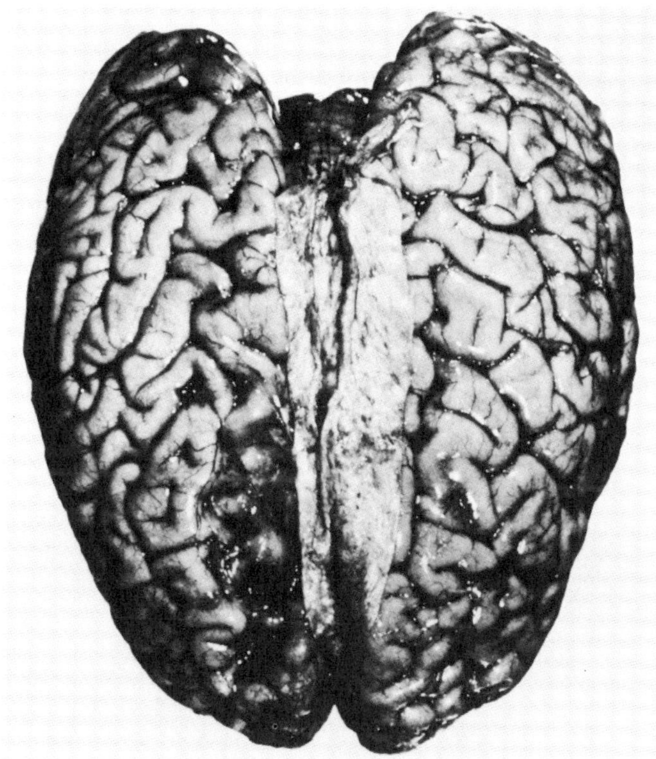

FIGURE 1.11. Chronic cortical cerebral scarring, remote hypoxic lesion related to complicated birth. Right frontal lobe with circumscribed old infarction, depressed area of contracted, distorted convolutions near the midline. The strip of dura on the surface of the cerebrum, lying midline between the hemispheres, contains the superior longitudinal dural sinus, the main channel for venous drainage from the surface of the cerebrum; the lower portion of this channel is patent, appearing as an irregular, open trough gradually narrowing above; the upper part of this venous channel, adjoining the scarred convolutions on the right, is occluded by fibrous tissue, the consequence of a remote thrombosis. Brain specimen from an adult, 42 years old, with history of a hypoxic term delivery. Clinically, slight left-sided spasticity; moderate mental retardation and behavior problem in early life; schizophrenic manifestations in adulthood. (Reprinted by permission, A. Towbin.)

ioral acts. Processing deficits at this level are not likely to be manifested by global impairments of motor or cognitive performance; rather, diffuse brain damage or damage to cerebellar and subcortical structures are more likely to induce such symptoms (Low, Galbraith, Sauerbrei, Muir, Killen, Pater, & Karchmar, 1986).

Perinatal hypoxia in a term fetus primarily affects the cerebral cortex and does not normally extend deeply to affect the basal ganglia (Okazaki, 1983; Towbin, 1977, 1978, 1986). Lesions produced by hypoxia in the term fetus normally involve the cerebral cortex and midbrain structure, the anatomical substrates of secondary and tertiary neuropsychological processing. Neuropsychological deficits arising from damage to these areas are found in children with relatively average intelligence, but with disinhibition syndromes such as hyperactivity and attentional disorders, and more generally, learning disability. Failure to recognize and acknowledge these issues probably accounts for much of the confusion surrounding the perinatal histories of many children who exhibit school-related learning and behavior disorders.

It is implausible to believe that CP developing in a term infant is attributable to massive acute cerebral damage incurred intranatally in an infant who was born in good clinical condition (Towbin, 1986). More plausible is the notion that milder forms of neurological dysfunction, not detectable at birth using traditional assessment, have a unique temporal course and symptom pattern unlike those with massive damage. The problem is complicated by the fact that cases can be found in each group where damage is thought to have occurred before or after the onset of labor. These children, with milder dysfunction, present at school age with slightly below- to above-average intelligence along with behavioral and conduct disturbances. Sociodemographic variables may indirectly act as teratogens for members of the below-average group and are manifested by poor prenatal care or other nonoptimal maternal behavior patterns that compromise the fetal environment. Theoretically, to explain the appearance of neurobehavioral symptoms from prenatal insults during development there should be a three-way interaction among the dimensions of severity, chronicity, and age. In terms of severity and chronicity, mild but chronic fetal hypoxia should be inversely correlated with the severity of neurological and neurobehavioral symptoms at birth. This is largely the result of insidious neuronal damage attributed to physiologic adaptation to hypoxic insult that is compatible with survival. Alone, this condition would probably be insufficient to produce a life-threatening clinical crisis at birth. In high-risk or otherwise complicated labor, the effects are synergistic. Gestational age at birth interacts with chronicity-severity to produce advances and delays in developmental functions similar to those discussed in previous research (Parmelee, 1975).

From the preceding discussion one might inquire as to whether the ideas put forth in this chapter assume a deterministic view of outcome following perinatal insult. Is there no room for recovery or plasticity that might help a traumatized infant compensate for the injuries sustained during pregnancy and delivery? If plasticity implies that an infant who suffers perinatal damage of a neurological nature can overcome such an insult and become a functional adult, then we endorse the notion unequivocally. However, plasticity as a developmental construct rarely addresses the reduction in human potential that occurs after perinatal damage. Therefore, plasticity is only useful in a given frame of reference in that it delineates differences in the recovery of function between developing and mature organisms and the long-term sequelae for each. Our conceptualization of the notion of plasticity refers to relative recovery from trauma or insult depending on the age of the organism at the time of injury as well as the locus and degree of tissue damage. It explicitly assumes some ultimate reduction in individual potential, social and intellectual compensation and competence as an adult notwithstanding.

Perhaps the most relevant point to be made regarding plasticity and recovery of function after perinatal insult is that there is a cost for the organism. It may result in identifiable deficits with clinical manifestations, or with subclinical effects that reduce potential as an adult. But perhaps perinatal insults create a more insidious limitation on compensation after subsequent injuries no matter how mild. Thus, for example, complete recovery from a serious and traumatic perinatal course might be observed without identifiable long-term deficits. However, even a very mild subsequent trauma, a slight bump on the head, may produce drastic enduring deficits appearing out of proportion to the severity of the injury. Such a result would be consistent with clinical studies of patients with closed head injury who recovered but later sustained another slight head injury (Smith, 1984).

APPLICATION TO CLINICAL ASSESSMENT

Multimethod Clinical Neuropsychological Assessment in the Perinatal Period

While logistically difficult, the most telling assessment of potential neurological and later neuropsychological deficits during the perinatal period must include a multilevel hierarchical model. This model consists of four functional domains to assess within-subject consistency across functional domains and over time. The first and most fundamental level of assessment is biochemical. At this level, blood gases related to oxygenation—such as PO_2, PCO_2, pH, HOC_3—determine the level of fetal and neonatal oxygenation. This level of analysis provides the clinician an appraisal of the concentration of oxygen and carbon dioxide at the tissue level and thus helps determine whether a respiratory acidosis exists or, more importantly, whether more basic metabolic acidosis with potential neurological compromise is present. While the clinical neuropsychologist generally will not participate in the assessment of biochemical status, such knowledge contributes to the overall understanding of infant clinical status. The biochemical assessment may also include ACTH and cortisol, which index adrenocortical activity and the stress levels in the infant and fetus. This information provides objective data on tissue oxygenation and organismic stress.

The second level of assessment, in which the clinical neuropsychologist may become involved, is electrophysiological. This assessment is concerned with monitoring biopotentials such as heart rate, EEG activity, and other potentials with known neurological and neuropsychological correlates. Already in use in many hospitals is FHR monitoring, which assists the obstetrician in determining fetal well-being, and brain stem auditory evoked potentials, which assist the electroencephalographer in ascertaining the integrity of the brain stem and hearing acuity in very young infants. These biopotentials have been employed in psychological studies and are shown to be affected by high-risk and complicated birth experiences (Barden & Peltzman, 1980). When correlated with behavior, these techniques are quite useful in diagnosis and treatment planning.

Neurobehavioral Assessment in the Neonatal Period

The third domain of assessment is neurobehavioral. The neurobehavioral level of assessment tends to comprise the clinical neuropsychologist's most important contribution to the evaluation of neuropathology. Self & Horowitz (1979) reported that behavioral assessment of the human newborn had developed along three basic lines. The older and more well known of these procedures was specifically designed to evaluate levels of neurological development in the neonate. The assessment procedures of Andre-Thomas, Chesni, & Saint-Anne Dargassies (1960) and Prechtl & Beintema (1964) distinguish this group. These procedures generally require eliciting a variety of reflexes, among which are Moro, Babinski, tonic-neck-reflex, and other postural reflexes. Central nervous maturity and integrity are inferred from the vigor and latency of these reflexes.

Another dimension of infant assessment is developmental screening. Included in this category are the Apgar (Apgar, 1953) and Denver Developmental Screening Test (DDST) (Frankenburg & Dodds, 1967). The Apgar provides an immediate evaluation of newborn physiologic function after birth. A score of 0–2 is assigned to five signs of newborn responsiveness, e.g., heart rate, respiratory effort, reflex irritability, muscle tone, and color. The research findings on prediction of long-term morbidity are mixed; however, perinatal risk factors tend to be highly correlated with lower Apgar scores as does perinatal mortality (Francis, Self, & Horowitz, 1987).

The Denver scale extends through the preschool years. There is a heavy emphasis on social competence at the higher levels of the scale, and its usefulness in the neonatal period is questionable due to the small number of items. Francis *et al.* (1987) raise serious questions regarding the validity of the DDST because of its underreferral and overreferral rates.

Assessment procedures broadly classed as "behavioral assessments" define a third dimension of infant testing. They can be distinguished from neurological assessments and screening devices by their emphasis on a broader representation of behavioral response systems. Commonly used tests in this category include the Bayley Scales of Infant Development (Bayley, 1969) and the Gesell Developmental Schedule (Knobloch & Pasamanick, 1974). The Bayley Scales have excellent standardization and reliability and modest predictive capacity regarding later IQ (Francis *et al.*, 1987; Siegel, 1979). It is also widely used and provides good data on the child's relative developmental status. For the most part, procedures found in these two latter groups of assessment instruments are standardized on infants at least 4 weeks old.

Neonatal behavioral assessment that relies heavily upon reflexive responses predates other behavioral assessments in current use that increasingly rely on interacting systems and organizational capacities. Uzgiris (1973) argued that a disproportionate amount of infant research focused on specific behaviors. This notion has received some attention in the literature (Bell, Weller, & Waldrop, 1971; Kessen, 1967). Nash (1970) suggests that research be geared toward the interaction of more than one sensory system. Luria (1973, p. 32), citing Vygotsky's earlier work, asserts that it is not only the structure of mental processes that change over time but also their relationship with each other. In other words, interfunctional organization is altered by the process of maturation and experience. In the first stages of development, a complex mental activity rests on a more elementary basis, a "basal function," yet in subsequent stages of development it not only acquires a more complex structure, but also incorporates the close participation of structurally higher forms of activity (Luria, 1973, p. 32). These processes parallel and mirror the development of behavioral response systems. They also have implications for understanding the evolution of infant neurobehavioral assessment. Researchers in the field of infancy seem to recognize the limitations of paradigms that strictly adhere to cause–effect models. Clinicians have known this for decades.

Recent developments in newborn behavioral assessment seem to recognize that many behavioral systems are functional and operating soon after birth. The emphasis on "organized behaviors" and modulation of state reveal an awareness that behavioral competence results from cross-modal and integrative capacities rather than from isolated response capabilities.

One assessment trend that has emerged in newborn research reflects an understanding of the evolution of the CNS and the hierarchical arrangement of cognitive processes (Luria, 1973; Isaacson, 1974). Incorporation of these perspectives into perinatal and newborn research as well as clinical assessment will allow for an integration of genotypic development and phenotypic expression that was not previously known. The early focus on reflexive behavior in infant assessment betrayed an interest in more primitive and basal ganglia functioning. Modern assessment procedures provide for a higher level of phenotypic expression that may be characteristic of the healthy infant. Therefore, just as ontogeny recapitulates phylogeny in fetal development, so does newborn neurobehavioral assessment appear to recapitulate our experience with infant testing. Recent tests incorporate reflexive type responding, which is the basis of some higher level responses.

The fourth area of assessment is social–emotional functioning. Depending on the child's age, this level of analysis may be referred to as either temperament (a term usually reserved for very young children) or personality (more commonly applied to older children and adults). This aspect of clinical neuropsychological assessment is clearly the least developed with regard to children and adults. Some assessment approaches with children have begun to take social–emotional factors into account psychometrically (Rourke, Fisk, & Strang, 1986). However, only within the past decade has there been substantial empirical research on the neuropsychology of emotion (Heilman & Satz, 1983).

Assessment of neurobehavioral status in very young children and infants pays close attention to emotional reactions during early development as reliable markers of the child's overall maturity. Not surprisingly, with the exception of motor development, emotional response represents a major part of the infant's interactive repertoire. The neuropsychological basis for this phenomenon is interpreted as a brain–behavior relationship, mediated by neuroanatomical development. Essentially, the infant and young child manifest relative disinhibition at the cortical level, leaving open the full uninhibited expression of emotional and motoric behaviors. Gradual inhibition of emotional outbursts represents significant neurological maturation and thus should be a key element of infant and child neuropsychological assessment.

Neurobehavioral and Neuropsychological Assessment in Infancy

The neurobehavioral assessment of the neonate and young infant falls into two major categories, (1) spontaneous and (2) respondent behavior. As the term implies, spontaneous behavior involves observable motor activity that is not primarily determined by external stimulus events. This type of behavior involves the assessment of behavioral state regulation and the particular behavioral patterns that occur during the various stages of sleep. Spontaneous behavior may at times seem more vegetative, but it is not simply the result of passive internal processes, but rather active manifestations of self-regulation, inhibitory control, and homeostasis (Kelly, 1981).

The duration and distributional characteristics of individual sleep states in very young infants have been known to correlate with illnesses affecting the CNS. These illnesses commonly disrupt the organizational integrity of infant sleep (Dinges, Davis, & Glass, 1980; Eliasson, Prensky, & Hardin, 1978; Prechtl, Theorell, & Blair, 1973; Watanabe, Miyazaki, Hara, & Hakamada, 1980). From a neuropsychological perspective, the distribution and frequency of sleep states among infants, particularly those who have potential CNS compromise, may represent an important early measure of neurobehavioral integrity; this measure, in turn, reflects the neurological status of the infant as well as predicting later neurological and neuropsychological integrity. Recent evidence reveals that spontaneous sleep startles among healthy infants with high numbers of obstetric complications—as well as preterm and full-term healthy and sick infants—are an especially sensitive neurobehavioral assay of CNS integrity (Emory & Mapp, 1988; Huntington, Zeskind, & Weiseman, 1985). The spontaneous neuronal discharge that presumably generates startles during non-REM sleep in human infants is considered to be a precursor to spontaneous behavior in older subjects. Animal studies (Windle, 1969) indicate that a reduction in spontaneous behavior is the only observable effect among birth-asphyxiated monkeys studied at 4 years of age. Collectively, these findings emphasize that perinatal distress is implicated in the disorganization or reduction of spontaneous behavior during the perinatal period.

Respondent or elicited behavior represents the other main class of behavior used in neurobehavioral and neuropsychological assessment during the neonatal and infancy periods. All of the standardized behavioral assessment techniques, including the Apgar, Brazelton Scale, and Bayley Scales of Infant Development, fall into the category of respondent neurobehavior analysis.

The obvious difficulties and limitations in testing prelinguistic patients are reflected in the special skill and sensitivity required on the part of the clinician. Moreover, higher cortical processes must be inferred to a large extent, since verbal report and instruction are not appropriate. The clinician is therefore confronted with an assessment of state regulation, motor control and maturity, and the influence of stimulation on controlled attention and alertness. Perhaps the most consistent finding, by our group as well as others, is that infants who are immature or are recovering from stressful perinatal experiences will typically exhibit lower scores on attentional and brain-stem reflexive items during the neonatal and infancy period. They may also demonstrate more autonomic lability and physiologic irritability than their nontraumatized counterparts. The behavioral manifestations of attention during such an assessment include alerting behaviors such as widening of eyelids, roving pupils, visual tracking, head rotation, and general lowering of respiratory and motor activity. Much of this behavior is under brain stem control, which may account for why infants who score lower on attentional items also exhibit more abnormal primitive reflexes (e.g. plantar, Babinski, and tonic-neck-reflex) (Emory & Noonan, 1984a). It is evident that lower and higher order reflexive behavior may be adversely affected in clinically compromised and some clinically healthy neonates. As one example of the complementary nature of primitive reflexes and attention, one can simply observe optokinetic nystagmus—an apparently involuntary visual reflex that involves fixation and tracking of objects across the visual field (Gardner & Weitzmann, 1967). Such a reflex is elicited by the stimuli used in neurobehavioral assessment of the neonate, particularly with inanimate and animate visual items. This reflex may form the basis of sustained visual alertness in the developing infants.

Nonoptimal behavioral performance and organization, exhibited by infants who have somewhat protracted physiologic instability arising from distressful labor, is mitigated by the tendency toward recovery, even after relatively severe perinatal insult (Brazelton, 1981; Painter, Depp, & O'Donaghue, 1978). This result implies no significant long-term neurological sequelae for many otherwise stressed infants. However, one should be alerted to subclinical behavioral anomalies during the neonatal period because these "soft signs" may become latent vulnerabilities that lie dormant while primary sensory motor and rudimentary cognitive abilities develop. This explains why some infants and toddlers who have a relatively benign developmental course manifest disorders of attention, behavioral control, and academic performance during the early school years. Such developmental functions depend on the maturation of higher cortical centers which are only minimally tapped by existing assessments during the neonatal and infancy period.

An emerging trend in neurodevelopmental testing of young infants has been referred to as a paradigmatic shift. This shift reflects a focus upon perceptual, cognitive, and memory testing in contrast to traditional assessments of sensorimotor function (Butterbaugh, 1988). These tests of memory and perception may eventually become part of the standardized battery of instruments used in the evaluation of neuropsychological performance among young infants. To think of them in the classical tradition of neuropsychological evaluation, however, appears premature. For example, issues of level of performance and testing-of-limits are never discussed in the context of currently used infant test of memory or novelty preference. Butterbaugh (1988) notes the relative lack of construct validation of recognition memory tests and the unexplained low reliability for recognition memory tests as compared to sensorimotor tests. The possible explanations given, such as inadequate measurement operations, transient situational factors, and/or organismic-related developmental phenomena all appear plausible. A more compelling reason for some of the shortcomings of newer cognitive and perceptual tests of infant neurodevelopmental status is their lack of a clinically relevant conceptual framework.

What is sacrificed in the way of experimental rigor by many "clinical assessment devices" is compensated for by sensitivity and specificity. For example, arousal level and behavioral state are features of neonatal and infant neurobehavioral organization that may be overlooked by recognition memory tests. These regulatory features play a major role in the perception and encoding of information, processes that are fundamental to the performance measures used in recognition memory testing.

If infant test of memory, perception, and cognition are to have a place in clinical neuropsychology, they will need to demonstrate basic discriminant and predictive validity. Their clinical utility can then be recognized and perhaps incorporated into future infant neuropsychological batteries.

SOCIAL–EMOTIONAL FACTORS

Moving beyond the neonatal and early infancy period to early childhood, the repertoire of neuropsychological processes expands, despite the fact that these processes are still not controlled by well-developed linguistic abilities. At later ages, between 12 and 24 months, fine motor skills such as finger manipulation and manipulation of objects, cross-modal and haptic integration, and rudimentary categorization are more precisely assessable. It is important to note the development of social responsiveness and interaction during this period and in early infancy. The domain of social behavior in developmental neuropsychology is accorded minimal consideration during early infancy even though it is highly dependent on an intact and uncompromised nervous system in interaction with the social environment.

Accordingly, social and emotional behavior might be given more attention during the history taking and interview process with young children. For example, stranger anxiety and separation protest in infancy occur with predictable regularity between 1 and 2 years of age. There are probably neural as well as social forces that enhance or attenuate these reactions. Responses and processing of emotional reactions represent another area in which neurological factors play a role. Several studies have suggested impairments in behavioral manifestation of interpersonal responses, chronic emotional difficulties, and affective expression deficits in children and toddlers with right hemisphere damage (Denckla, 1978; Nass & Koch, 1987; Rourke & Strang, 1983; Tranel, Hall, Olson, & Tranel, 1987; Weintraub & Mesulam, 1983). Apparently, justification on clinical grounds, along with limited empirical evidence, support the inclusion of social–emotional factors in neuropsychological assessment with very young children.

Neurobehavioral organization serves as a common pathway for the expression of antecedent and consequential perinatal conditions. These conditions influence behaviors that are symptomatic of nonoptimal circumstances. We are, however, still without a clear and viable risk model that predicts morbidity (Kopp & Parmelee, 1979). Such a model is attainable pending a greater appreciation for the capabilities of the prelinguistic child and an understanding of how fundamental neuromotor and attentional processes influence the development of higher level cognitive skills. It will require an integration of biological and social factors, thus the nature–nurture issue remains an important component of theory development in perinatal neuropsychology.

The nature–nurture issue is closely tied to theories of psychological development, but it has special practical application in perinatal neuropsychology. Sociological and biological phenomena appear to be equally strong predictors of developmental outcome. For example, Parmelee (1986) has argued that in many instances, childhood illnesses can have a beneficial effect on behavioral development. Although this idea appears counterintuitive, in all but the most debilitating illnesses emotional and psychological factors may help to compensate for physical limitations. At the same time, the nonorganic failure-to-thrive syndrome is an excellent example of how biological development can be arrested through limited social stimulation.

Implications for Traditional Clinical Neuropsychological Assessment

There are a few practical considerations for clinical neuropsychologists who choose to incorporate perinatal histories into their assessments. First, for the perinatal history to be of any practical value, it must include more information than the birth weight or gestational age of the child. A prenatal growth chart similar to the one in Fig. 1.3 can help determine if the child was SGA or LGA. Second, a ponderal index (weight-to-length ratio) can be computed for the child if its birth length is known. Knowledge of the anthropometric parameters will help the clinician in formulating an etiological impression of the child's disorder.

Although it may not be possible or practical to obtain prenatal records, information should be obtained from parents with relative ease. The child's medical condition and diagnosis are usually recalled when the condition is a common one such as prematurity, respiratory distress, or jaundice. Knowledge on the part of the clinical neuropsychologist, that multiple nonoptimal perinatal events appear to have a cumulative effect on outcome, is indispensable. Being cognizant of perinatal circumstances also allows the clinician to place the child's social–emotional development into perspective and, therefore, will have far-reaching practical implications. A case in point is where the child's mental abilities exceed their academic performance, partly because a crisis-filled, tenuous, perinatal course has lowered the parents' expectations for intellectual achievement, not because of a learning disability.

In cases where hypoxia is implicated in the perinatal history, a more complete medical record is necessary for detailed information. However, the pattern of cerebral lesions in chronic and acute perinatal hypoxia is such that neuropsychological evaluation should reveal their locus and functional impairment. This is due to the parallel findings of cerebral damage in infants and adults exposed to hypoxic–ischemic injuries (Towbin, 1981).

Abnormal neurological exams in the neonatal and early infancy period point to possible motor and cognitive deficits. A study by Rubin & Balow (1980) confirmed that some continuity exists between abnormal neurological signs in infancy and motor development at 4 years, and between language and intellectual development for up to 12 years. There also appears to be a linear relationship between the severity of intraventricular hemorrhage (IVH) and performance on the Bayley Scales for up to 1 year (Low *et al.*, 1986). Others have also found LBW and IVH to be disproportionately high among children with moderately severe neurological disorders at 3½ years (Williamson, Desmond, Wilson, Murphy, Rozelle, & Garcia-Prats, 1983).

An unresolved problem is whether specific disorders can be predicted from perinatal factors that compromise the CNS. There are the obvious links to mental retardation and cerebral palsy (Naeye & Peters, 1987; Nelson & Ellenberg, 1986). In previous studies of children with congenital heart defects, some of their mental impairments were thought to result from brain insults secondary to chronic hypoxia (Linde, Rasof, & Dunn, 1970; Silbert, Wolff, Mayer, Rosenthal, & Nadas, 1969). Moreover, duration of hypoxia in children with cyanotic heart defects was significantly related to problems in school achievement and intellectual functioning, but was uncorrelated with other risk variables (O'Dougherty, Wright, Gurmezy, Loevenson, & Torres, 1983, 1985). Although overall IQ of these children was within the average range, they often experienced difficulties in school similar to those of children with learning disabilities and attention deficit disorders (O'Dougherty, Neuchterlein, & Drew, 1984; O'Dougherty, Bernston, Boysen, Wright, & Teske, 1988). A similar type of neuropsychological pattern can be caused by mild but chronic hypoxia during gestation. Affected children should be identifiable during the antepartum or intrapartum period because of their previously compromised status and pattern of autonomic responsivity (e.g., FHR during labor, stimulus responsiveness during the antepartum period.) This circumstance portends an eventual clinical role for prenatal neurobehavioral testing.

We have argued that perinatal factors are relevant in clinical neuropsychological assessment. However, a formal bridge from perinatal insult to childhood disorders is often tenuous, especially where minor damage has occurred. Clumsy children, for example, may be those who have suffered mechanical injury to the brain stem or who have minor injury to the umbilical cord and mild impairment in neurological functioning. That the injury has gone unrecognized is aptly demonstrated by their status as "clumsy." While cerebral palsy is considered a disease of the premature infant, those with lesions of a minor degree may present the *formes frustec* of cerebral palsy—tics, awkwardness, and other mild motor dysfunctions (Towbin, 1980).

It would be valuable if more attention were devoted to perinatal histories during school enrollments and when special evaluations are taking place. Ordinarily, there is no special consideration given to prematurity when a child enters school, nor is there any correction for such events when developmental and intellectual quotients are being determined by school psychologists. It appears that the difference between adjusted and unadjusted test scores is generally greater than the standard error of measurement (SEM) of the test. Importantly, Wilson (1987) argues that adjusted scores should be used and illustrates the point in examining the SEM of most IQ tests in relation to chronological age. Matilainen (1987) emphasizes that both corrected and uncorrected ages should be used, especially during the first year of development. When considering that some children have birthdates occurring in the fall, those who are born prematurely will be at a significant psychometric and social disadvantage unless their prematurity is taken into account. Less clear is its association with other disorders.

Recent evidence suggests that psychopathology, especially schizophrenia, may be linked to perinatal complications in offspring at genetic risk. DeLisi, Dauphinais, & Gershon (1988) have discovered a relationship between perinatal complications and reduced size of brain limbic structures in familial schizophrenia. Others have found that ventricular brain ratios may be linked to risk for psychopathology in genetically vulnerable individuals (Silverton, Finello, Mednick, & Schulsinger, 1985). These findings are inconclusive, *but* we know even less about the relationship of perinatal events with disorders of attention and language processing.

What we do know is that clinical neuropsychological assessment is an ever-expanding enterprise, which is beginning to manifest a trend toward including children of younger ages. We currently have standardized batteries that purport to evaluate the child as young as 5 years. As more emphasis is placed on evaluating younger children, one can anticipate a corresponding increase in attention to perinatal complications and their role in early neuropsychological assessment.

ACKNOWLEDGMENTS. Preparation of portions of this chapter was supported by Research Scientist Development Award MH00660 from the National Institute of Mental Health to the first author. The authors express special appreciation to Claire-Anne Maillard for her illustrations.

REFERENCES

Andre-Thomas, M., Chesni, Y., & Saint-Anne Dargassies, S. (1960). The neurological examination of the infant. London: Medical Advisory Committee of the National Spastics Society.

Apgar, V. (1953). A proposal for a new method of evaluation of the newborn infant. *Current Researches in Anesthesia and Analgesia, 32*, 260–267.

Avery, J. (1985). *Neonatology: Pathophysiology and Management of the Newborn* (2nd ed.). Philadelphia: Lippincott.

Barden, T. & Peltzman, P. (1980). Newborn brain stem auditory evoked responses and perinatal events. *American Journal of Obstetrics and Gynecology, 12*, 912–919.

Battaglia, F. C., & Meschia, G. (1986). *An introduction to fetal physiology* (pp. 49–95). New York: Academic Press.

Bayley, N. (1969). *Manual for the Bayley Scales of Infant Development*. New York: Psychological Corporation.

Beaumont, J. G. (1983). *Introduction to neuropsychology*. New York: Guilford Press.

Bell, R., Weller, G., & Waldrop, M. (1971). Newborn and preschooler: Organization of behavior and relations between periods. *Monographs of the Society for Research in Child Development, 36*.

Brazelton, T. B. (1981). Clinical uses of the Brazelton Neonatal Assessment. In M. Coleman (ed.), *Neonatal neurology* (pp. 59–69). Baltimore: University Park Press.

Butterbaugh, G. J. (1988). Selected psychometric and clinical review of neurodevelopmental infant tests. *The Clinical Neuropsychologist, 2*, 350–364.

Caputo, D. & Mandell, W. (1970). Consequences of low birthweight. *Developmental Psychology, 3*, 363–383.

Chik, L., Sokol, R., & Rosen, M. (1976). Prediction of one-minute Apgar score from fetal heart rate. *Obstetrics and Gynecology, 48*, 452–455.

Cohen, S. E., Parmelee, A. H., Beckwith, L., & Sigman, M. (1986). Cognitive development in preterm infants: Birth to 8 years. *Journal of Developmental and Behavioral Pediatrics, 7*, 102–110.

Crothers, B., & Paine, R. S. (1959). *The natural history of cerebral palsy*, Cambridge, Mass.: Harvard University Press.

Davidson, R. J., & Fox, N. A. (1982). Asymmetrical brain activity discriminates between positive versus negative affective stimuli in human infants. *Science, 218*, 1235–1237.

Dawes, G. S. (1968). *Foetal and neonatal physiology*. Chicago: Year Book Medical.

DeLisi, L. E., Dauphinais, I. D., & Gershon, E. S. (1988). Perinatal complications and reduced size of brain limbic structures in familial schizophrenia. *Schizophrenia Bulletin, 14*, 185.

DeSouza, S. W, & Richards, B. (1978). Neurological sequelae in newborn babies after perinatal asphyxia. *Archives of Diseases in Childhood, 53*, 564–569.

Denckla, M. B. (1983). The neuropsychology of social-emotional learning disability. *Archives of Neurology, 40*, 461–462.

Dinges, D., Davis, M., & Glass, P. (1980). Fetal exposure to narcotics: Neonatal sleep as a measure of nervous system disturbance. *Science, 209*, 619.

Eliasson, G., Prensky, A., & Hardin, E. (1978). *Neurological pathophysiology* (2nd ed.). New York: Oxford University Press.

Emory, E. K., & Mapp, J. R. (1988). Effects of respiratory distress and prematurity on spontaneous startle activity in neonates. *Infant Behavior and Development, 11*, 71–81.

Emory, E. K., & Noonan, J. R. (1984a). Fetal cardiac responding: Maturational and behavioral correlates. *Developmental Psychology, 20*, 354–357.

Emory, E. K., & Noonan, J. R. (1984b). Fetal cardiac responding: A correlate of birthweight and neonatal behavior. *Child Development, 55*, 1651–1657.

Emory, E. K., Walker, E., & Cruz, A. (1982). Fetal heart rate. Part I: Factor analysis. *Psychophysiology, 19*, 680–686.

Emory, E. K., Tynan, W. D., & Dave, R. (1989). Neurobehavioral anomalies in neonates with seizures. *Journal of Experimental and Clinical Neuropsychology, 11*, 231–240.

Field, T. (1979). Interaction patterns of preterm and term infants. In T. Field, A. Sostek, S. Goldberg, & H. Shuman (Eds.), *Infants born at risk* (pp. 333–356). New York: Spectrum Publications.

Fox, N. A. & Davidson, R. J. (1986). Taste-elicited changes in facial signs of emotion and the asymmetry of brain electrical activity in human newborns. *Neuropsychologia, 24,* 417–422.

Francis, P. L., Self, P. A.,& Horowitz, F. D. (1987). The behavioral assessment of the neonate: An overview. In J. D. Osofsky (Ed.), *Handbook of child development* (pp. 723–779). New York: Wiley.

Frankenburg, W. K., & Dodds, J. B. (1967). The Denver Developmental Screening Test. *Journal of Pediatrics, 71,* 181–191.

Fuller, P. W., Guthrie, R. D., & Alvord, E. C., Jr. (1983). A proposed neuropathological basis for learning disabilities in children born prematurely. *Developmental Medicine and Child Neurology, 25,* 214–231.

Gardner, R., & Weitzmann, E. (1967). Examination for optokinetic nystagmus in sleep and waking. *Archives of Neurology, 16,* 415–420.

Goldman, P. S., & Nauta, W. J. H. (1977). An intricately patterned prefrontocaudate projection in the rhesus monkey. *Journal of Comparative Neurology, 171,* 369–386.

Goldman-Rakic, P. S. (1985). Toward a neurobiology of cognitive development. In J. Mehler & R. Fox (Eds.), *Neonate cognition: Beyond the blooming buzzing compulsion* (pp. 285–306). Hillside, NJ: Erlbaum.

Gray, J. W., & Dean, R. S. (in press). The effects of perinatal risk factors. *Psychology in the School, 1,* 15–21.

Heilman, K. M., & Satz, P. (Eds.) (1983). *Neuropsychology of human emotion.* New York: Guilford Press.

Hon, E. H. (1975). *An introduction to fetal heart rate monitoring* (2nd ed.). Los Angeles: University of Southern California Medical School Press.

Huntington, L., Zeskind, P. S., & Weiseman, J. (1985). Spontaneous startle activity in newborn infants. *Infant Behavior and Development, 8,* 301–308.

Hynd, G. W., & Willis, W. G. (1988). *Pediatric Neuropsychology* (pp. 21–45, 71–105). New York: Grune & Stratton.

Isaacson, R. L. (1987). *The limbic system.* New York: Plenum Press.

Kelly, D. (1981). Physiology of sleep and dreaming. In E. Kandel & J. Schwartz (Eds.), *Principles of neural science* (pp. 472–485). Amsterdam: Elsevier/North-Holland.

Kessen, W. (1967). Sucking and looking. Two congenital patterns of behavior in the human newborn. In H. Stevenson, E. Hess, & H. Rheingold (Eds.), *Early behavior.* New York: Wiley.

Knobloch, H., & Pasamanick, B. (1974). The Developmental Screening Inventory. In H. Knobloch & B. Pasamanick (Eds.), *Gesell and Amatruda's developmental diagnosis* (3rd ed., pp. 343–355). New York: Harper & Row.

Kopp, K., & Parmelee, A. (1979). Prenatal and perinatal influences on infant behavior. In J. Osofsky (Ed.), *Handbook on infant development* (pp. 29–75). New York: Wiley–Interscience.

Lemire, R. J., Loeser, J. D., Leech, R. W., & Alvord, E. C. (1975) *Normal and abnormal development of the human nervous system.* New York: Harper & Row.

Linde, L. M., Rasof, B., & Dunn, O. J. (1970). Longitudinal studies of intellectual and behavioral development in children with congenital heart disease. *Acta Paediatrica Scandinavica, 59,* 169–176.

Little, W. S. (1862). On the influence of abnormal parturition, difficult labor, premature birth, and asphyxia neonatorum on the mental and physical condition of the child, especially in relation to deformities. *Transaction of the Obstetric Society of London, 3,* 293–344.

Low, J., Galbraith, R., Sauerbrei, E., Muir, D., Killen, H., Pater, E., & Karchmar, E. J. (1986). Motor and cognitive development of infants with intraventricular hemorrhage, ventriculomegaly, or periventricular parenchymal lesions. *American Journal of Obstetrics and Gynecology, 155,* 750–755.

Lubchenco, L. O. (1976). *The high risk infant.* Philadelphia: Saunders.

Lubchenco, L. O., Horner, F. A., Reed, L. H., Hix, I. E., Metcalf, D., Cohig, R., Elliott, H. C., & Bourg, M. (1963). Sequelae of premature birth. Evaluation of premature infants of low birth weights at ten years of age. *American Journal of Diseases of Children, 106,* 101.

Luria, A. (1973). *The working brain: An introduction to neuropsychology.* New York: Basic Books.

Luria, A. R. (1980). *Higher cortical functions in man* (2nd ed.). New York: Basic Books.

Mann, L. I. (1986). Pregnancy events and brain damage. *American Journal of Obstetrics and Gynecology, 155,* 6–8.

Manniello, R. L., & Farrell, P. M. (1977). Analysis of United States neonatal mortality statistics from 1968 to 1974, with specific reference to changing trends in major casualties. *American Journal of Obstetrics and Gynecology, 129,* 667–674.

Martin, C. Siassi, B., & Hon, E. (1974). Fetal heart rate patterns and neonatal death in low birthweight infants. *Obstetrics and Gynecology, 44,* 503–510.
Matilainen, R. (1987). The value of correction for age in the assessment of prematurely born children. *Early Human Development, 15,* 257–264.
McDonald, A. D. (1973). Severely retarded children in Quebec: Prevalence, causes and care. *American Journal of Mental Deficiency, 78,* 205–215.
Murray, A. D. (1988). Newborn auditory brainstem evoked responses (ABRs): Prenatal and contemporary correlates. *Child Development, 59,* 571.
Myers, R. E. (1975). Response of the primate fetus to asphyxia. In E. S. E. Hafez (Ed.), *The mammalian fetus: Comparative biology and methodology* (pp. 320–343). Springfield, Ill.: Thomas.
Naeye, R. L. (1977). Placental infarction leading to fetal neonatal death: A prospective study. *Obstetrics and Gynecology, 50,* 583–588.
Naeye, R. L., & Peters, E. (1987). Antenatal hypoxia and low IQ values. *American Journal of Disabilities of Children, 141,* 50–54.
Nash, J. (1970). *Developmental psychology: A psychobiological approach.* Englewood Cliffs, N.J.: Prentice–Hall.
Nass, R., & Koch, D. (1987). Temperament differences in toddlers with early unilateral right- and left-brain damage. *Developmental Neuropsychology, 3,* 93–99.
Nelson, K. B., & Ellenberg, J. H. (1986). Antecedents of cerebral palsy. Multivariate analysis of risk. *The New England Journal of Medicine, 315,* 81–86.
Niswander, K. R. (1989). Management of growth retardation with a view to preventing neuromotor dysfunction and mental handicaps. In F. Kubli, N. Patel, W. Schmidt, & O. Linderkamp (Eds.), *Perinatal events and brain damage in surviving children* (pp. 108–116). Berlin: Springer-Verlag.
O'Dougherty, M., Wright, F. S., Gurmezy, N., Loevenson, R. B., & Torres, F. (1983). Later competence and adaptation in infants who survive severe heart deficits. *Child Development, 54,* 1129–1142.
O'Dougherty, M., Neuchterlein, K. H., & Drew, B. (1984). Hyperactivity and hypoxic children: Signal detection, sustained attention, and behavior. *Journal of Abnormal Psychology, 93,* 178–191.
O'Doughtery, M., Wright, F. S., Loevenson, R. B., & Torres, F. (1985). Cerebral dysfunction after chronic hypoxia in children. *Neurology, 35,* 42–46.
O'Dougherty, M., Bernston, G. G., Boysen, S. T., Wright, F. S., & Teske, D. (1988). Psychophysiological predictors of attentional dysfunction in children with congenital heart defects. *Psychophysiology, 25,* 305–315.
Okazaki, H. (1983). *Fundamentals of neuropathology.* New York: Igaku-Shoin.
Painter, M. J., Depp, R., & O'Donaghue, P. D. (1978). Fetal heart rate patterns and development in the first year of life. *American Journal of Obstetrics and Gynecology, 132,* 271–276.
Parmelee, A. H. (1975). Neurophysiological and behavioral organization of premature infants in the first months of life. *Biological Psychiatry, 10,* 501–512.
Parmelee, A. H. (1986). Children's illnesses: Their beneficial effects on behavioral development. *Child Development, 57,* 1–10.
Prechtl, H. F. R., & Beintema, D. (1964). *The neurological examination of the full-term newborn infant.* London: Heinemann.
Prechtl, H. F. R., Theorell, K., & Blair, A. W. (1973). Behavioral state cycles in abnormal infants. *Developmental Medicine and Child Neurology, 15,* 606–615.
Prensky, A. L. (1975). Metabolic disorders of genetic origin: Disorders of amino, organic, and nucleic acids and carbohydrate metabolism. In D. B. Tower (Ed.), *The nervous system* (Vol. 2, pp. 205–217). New York: Raven Press.
Quinn, P., & Rapoport, J. (1974). Minor physical anomalies and neurologic status in hyperactive boys. *Pediatrics, 53,* 742–747.
Riegle, K. F. (1972). Influence of economic and political ideologies on the development of developmental psychology. *Psychological Bulletin, 78,* 129–141.
Rourke, B. P., & Strang, J. D. (1983). Subtypes of reading and arithmetic disabilities: A neuropsychological analysis. In M. Rutter (Ed.), *Developmental neuropsychiatry* (pp. 473–488). New York: Guilford Press.
Rourke, B. P., Bakker, D. J., Fisk, J. L., & Strang, J. D. (1985). *Child neuropsychology: An introduction to theory, research and clinical practice* (pp. 9–34). New York: Guilford Press.

Rourke, B. P., Fisk, J. L., & Strang, J. D. (1986). *Neuropsychological assessment of children*. New York: Guilford Press.

Rubin, R. A. & Balow, B. (1980). Infant neurological abnormalities as indicators of cognitive impairment. *Developmental Medicine and Child Neurology, 22*, 336.

Russo, D., & Varni, J. (1982). Behavioral pediatrics. In D. Russo & J. Varni (Eds.), *Behavioral pediatrics: Research and practice*. New York: Plenum Press.

Sameroff, A. J., & Chandler, M. J. (1975). Reproductive risk and the continuum of caretaking casualty. In F. D. Horowitz (Ed.), *Review of child development research* (Vol. 4, pp. 187–244). Chicago: University of Chicago Press.

Scarr, S., & Williams, M. (1973). The effects of early stimulation on low birthweight infants. *Child Development, 44*, 94–101.

Schechler & Halton (1982)

Scholz, W. (1956). Die nicht zu Erweichung fuhrenden unvollstandigen Gewebsnekrosen (Elektive Parenchymnekrose). In F. Henke, O. Lubarsh, & R. Rossle (Eds.), *Handbuch der Speziellen Pathologischen Anatomie und Histologie: Nervensystem* (Vol. 13, Part 1, pp. 1284–1325). Berlin: Springer-Verlag.

Self, P. A., & Horowitz, F. D. (1979). The behavioral assessment of the neonate: An overview. In J. D. Osofsky (Ed.), *Handbook of infant development* (pp. 723–779). New York: Wiley.

Siegel, L. S. (1979). Infant perceptual, cognitive, and motor behaviors as predictors of subsequent cognitive and language development. *Canadian Journal of Psychology, 33*, 382–394.

Silbert, A., Wolff, P. H., Mayer, B., Rosenthal, A., & Nadas, A. S. (1969). Cyanotic heart disease and psychological development. *Pediatrics, 43*, 192–200.

Silverton, L., Finello, K. M., Mednick, S. A., & Schulsinger, F. (1985). Low birth weight and ventricular enlargement in a high-risk sample. *Journal of Abnormal Psychology, 94*, 405–409.

Smith, A. (1984). Early and long-term recovery from brain damage in children and adults: Evolution of concepts of localization, plasticity, and recovery. In C. R. Almli & S. Finger (Eds.), *Early brain damage* (Vol. 1, pp. 299–324). New York: Academic Press.

Spreen, O., Tupper, D., Risser, A., Tuokko, H., & Edgell, D. (1984). *Human developmental neuropsychology*. New York: Oxford University Press.

Stevenson, J. E., Hawcroft, J., Lobascer, M., Smith, I., Wolff, O. H., & Graham, P. J. (1979). Behavioral deviance in children with early treated phenylketonuria. *Archives of Disease in Childhood, 54*, 14–18.

Swaiman, K. F. (1989a). General aspects of the neurologic history. In K. F. Swaiman (Ed.), *Pediatric neurology: Principles and practices* (pp. 3–14). St. Louis: Mosby.

Swaiman, K. F. (1989b). Neurologic examination of the older child. In K. F. Swaiman (Eds), *Pediatric neurology: Principles and practices* (pp. 15–35). St. Louis: Mosby.

Touwen, B. C. L., & Huisjes, H. J. (1984). Obstetrics, neonatal neurology, and later outcome. In C. R. Almli & S. Finger (Eds.), *Early brain damage* (Vol. 1, pp. 169–187).

Towbin, A. (1973). Syndrome of latent cerebral venous thrombosis: Its frequency and relation to age and congestive heart failure. *Stroke, 4*, 410.

Towbin, A. (1977). Trauma in pregnancy-injury to the fetus and newborn. In C. G. Tedeschi, W. G. Eckert & L. G. Tedeschi (Eds.), *Forensic medicine* (Vol. 1, pp. 436–486). Philadelphia: Saunders.

Towbin, A. (1978). Cerebral dysfunctions related to perinatal organic damage: Clinical–neuropathologic correlations. *Journal of Abnormal Psychology, 87*, 617–635.

Towbin, A. (1980). Neuropathologic factors in minimal brain dysfunction. In H. Rie & E. Rie (Eds.), *Handbook of minimal brain dysfunctions: A cortical view* (pp. 169–187). New York: Wiley.

Towbin, A. (1981). Neuropathological aspects: II. Perinatal brain damage and its sequels. In P. Black (Eds.), *Brain dysfunction in children: Etiology, diagnosis, and management* (pp. 47–77). New York: Raven Press.

Towbin, A. (1986). Obstetric malpractice litigation: The pathologist view. *American Journal of Obstetrics and Gynecology, 155*, 927–935.

Tranel, D., Hall, L. E. Olson, S., & Tranel, R. N. (1987). Evidence for a right-hemisphere developmental learning disability. *Developmental Neuropsychology, 3*, 113–127.

Uzgiris, I. (1973). Patterns of cognitive development in infancy. *Merrill-Palmer Quarterly, 19*, 181–204.

Visser, G. H. A. (1989). Antepartum fetal heart rate and movement pattern in relation to oxygenation and neonatal neurological morbidity. In: F. Kubli, N. Patal, W. Schmidt, & S. O. Linderkamp (Eds.), *Perinatal events and brain damage in surviving children* (pp. 131–136). Berlin: Springer-Verlag.

Visser, G. H. A., Redman, C. W. G., Huisjes, H. J., & Turnbull, A. C. (1980). Nonstressed antepartum heart rate monitoring: Implications of decelerations after spontaneous contractions. *American Journal of Obstetrics and Gynecology, 138*, 429–435.

Volpe, J. J. (1981). *Neurology of the newborn*. Philadelphia: Saunders.

Watanabe, K., Miyazaki, S., Hara, K., & Hakamada, S. (1980). Behavioral state cycles, background EEG's and prognosis of newborns with perinatal hypoxia. *Electroencephalography and Clinical Neurophysiology, 49*, 618–625.

Weintraub, S., & Mesulam, M. M. (1983). Developmental learning disabilities and the right hemisphere: Emotional, interpersonal and cognitive components. *Archives of Neurology, 40*, 463–468.

Williamson, W. D., Desmond, M. M., Wilson, G. S., Murphy, M. A., Rozelle, J., & Garcia-Prats, J. A. (1983). Survival of low-birth-weight infants with neonatal intraventricular hemorrhage. *American Journal of Diseases of Childhood, 137*, 1181–1184.

Willis, W. G., & Widerstrom, A. H. (1986). Structure and function in prenatal and postnatal neuropsychological development: A dynamic interaction. In J. E. Obrzut & G. W. Hynd (Eds.), *Child Neuropsychology* (Vol. I). New York: Academic Press.

Wilson, J. G. (1965). Embryological consideration in teratology. In J. G. Wilson & J. Warkany (Eds.), *Teratology: Principles and techniques* (pp. 251–261). Chicago: University of Chicago Press.

Wilson, W. M. (1987). Age adjustment in psychological assessment of children born prematurely. *Journal of Pediatric Psychology, 12*, 445–450.

Windle, W. (1969). Brain damage by asphyxia at birth. *Scientific American, 221*, 76–84.

2

Childhood

MORRIS J. COHEN, WALTER B. BRANCH,
W. GRANT WILLIS, LISA L. WEYANDT,
and GEORGE W. HYND

INTRODUCTION

Childhood neuropsychological assessment can be distinguished from adult neuropsychological assessment by the marked discontinuities that characterize human development (see Fletcher & Taylor, 1984). Many inaccurate assumptions have been made about brain–behavior relationships during childhood that represent generalizations from research that has been conducted with adults. Fortunately, advances in child neuropsychological assessment recently have begun to address a number of these erroneous assumptions (Tramontana & Hooper, 1988). There are a number of theoretical issues germane to this distinction that can facilitate an understanding of the dynamic relationships between brain and behavior that occur throughout the life span. In the first section of this chapter, four of the more cogent issues are discussed including functional brain organization, information processing, cerebral hemispheric lateralization, and plasticity. In the second section, discussion will be directed toward the implication of these issues in the neuropsychological assessment of children and adolescents.

MORRIS J. COHEN and WALTER B. BRANCH • Department of Neurology and Pediatrics, Medical College of Georgia, Augusta, Georgia 30912-3255. W. GRANT WILLIS and LISA L. WEYANDT • Department of Psychology, University of Rhode Island, Providence, Rhode Island 02908. GEORGE W. HYND • College of Education, Division for the Education of Exceptional Children, University of Georgia, Athens, Georgia 30602.

HANDBOOK OF NEUROPSYCHOLOGICAL ASSESSMENT: A Biopsychosocial Perspective, edited by Antonio E. Puente and Robert J. McCaffrey. Plenum Press, New York, 1992.

THEORETICAL ISSUES

Functional Brain Organization

A major premise of child neuropsychological assessment is that classes of behavior (broadly defined to include covert as well as overt activities and functions) involve differential neurological substrata. Specific neurological systems and components have been documented for a variety of motor and sensory capabilities during prenatal as well as postnatal development, but these behavioral classes extend well beyond reflexive and sensory functions, to include higher-order cognitive processes such as attention, information analysis and synthesis, organization and planning, and affective states.

As the brain is highly specialized for function, it is sometimes misconstrued to suggest that particular regions of the brain operate independently. For example, there is a great deal of popular-press literature currently available that dichotomously characterizes the two cerebral hemispheres and classifies individuals as "left-brained" or "right-brained" on the basis of so-called neuropsychological assessment. One reason this oversimplified localizationist literature is problematic is because it frequently forms the basis for ill-founded psychoeducational interventions for children. Such literature also is inconsistent with the view of "functional systems," which is a fundamental concept in neuropsychological assessment that was elaborated by Luria (1980).

Functional Systems of the Brain

There is little doubt that even the neonatal brain comprises a collection of systems that are differentiated by function. The neural substrates for these systems, however, comprise interconnected components rather than discretely localized regions, and they function interdependently toward a unified result. One approach to child neuropsychological assessment is to investigate the integrity of these functional systems through detailed analyses of behavior. This "syndrome analysis" (Luria, 1980) is accomplished by administering a series of tasks to the child in an attempt to identify the common components or interconnections underlying a cluster of symptoms.

Syndrome analysis is consistent with the theory of functional systems because the child's behavior, elicited by some task, is believed to represent the unified result of the integrated activity of the components of the substrate functional system. For example, if a child is unable to perform Behavior X, putatively involving, Components a and b, but able to perform Behavior Y, putatively involving Components b and c, then it is reasonable to speculate that the source of the syndrome involves Component a (Caramazzo, 1984; Shallice, 1979). Of course, in order to use this approach effectively, clinicians must be able to analyze behavior qualitatively according to component neurological substrata. Presently, this task is complicated by a less-than-optimal research base with childhood samples and the possibility that, particularly in the case of higher-order cognitive processes, interrelationships among components of functional systems may covary with ontogenetic development.

Luria (1970) proposed that all functional systems involve components associated with each of three principal "functional units," each of which incorporates distinctive functions that are mutually interdependent. Theoretically, all three units are involved in the performance of any behavior and, given the extensive interconnections within and among these units, each both influences and is influenced by the others. These units comprise subcortical, posterior cortical, and anterior cortical regions of the brain.

Subcortical Unit

The subcortical unit of the brain functionally is specialized for the "maintenance of . . . [an] optimal level of cortical tone . . . essential for the organized course of mental activity" (Luria, 1973, p. 45). This functional concept, or "activating system" (Brodal, 1981), anatomically is associated with the brain stem reticular formation, which is a group of cells within regions of the medulla, pons, and midbrain. The morphological features of this unit implicate its role in all conscious and autonomic activity (Brodal, 1981; Luria, 1973), and support the notion that the subcortical unit is involved in the activation, inhibition, and regulation of the central nervous system. Its system of projection fibers serves to interconnect this unit of the brain with more rostral, as well as caudal neuroanatomical structures, again attesting to the mutual interdependence of the subcortical and the cortical units of the brain.

Cortical Units

Posterior Cortical Unit. The posterior cortical unit of the brain is specialized for the reception, analysis, and storage of information. The neuroanatomical substrate for this unit is the cortex of the parietal, occipital, and temporal lobes. This unit comprises a hierarchy of zones: primary, secondary, and tertiary.

There is one primary zone within each of the three lobes of this unit, and each primary zone essentially is surrounded by a secondary zone. The major tertiary zone within this unit is demarcated by the area where all three lobes overlap, a region that corresponds to the angular gyrus. The functions of the primary and secondary zones within each lobe are limited to a particular modality. For example, zones within the parietal lobes are functionally specialized for the reception, analysis, and storage of kinesthetic and somatosensory information; zones within the occipital lobes for visual information; and zones within the temporal lobes for auditory information. In contrast, the tertiary zones function to synthesize this information across modalities (Luria, 1980).

More specifically, the primary (or projection) zones discriminate among stimuli and influence sensory reception to ensure optimal perception. The secondary (or association, gnostic) zones, in contrast, are relatively more integrative and are adapted to relaying afferent impulses to tertiary zones for further synthesis. Thus, lesions of the primary zones frequently result in specific sensory deficits, whereas lesions of the secondary zones are likely to result in disorganized perceptions within and among complex groups of unimodal stimuli (Luria, 1970). Finally, the tertiary zones are functionally specialized to integrate stimuli across modalities. According to Luria (1973), this integrative function is associated with thinking abstractly and with memorizing information, both of which are cognitive processes that include converting successive stimuli into simultaneously processed groups. Thus, lesions of the tertiary zones of this unit are likely to disrupt simultaneous cognitive processes (Luria, 1980), a holistic kind of thinking.

Anterior Cortical Unit. The anterior cortical unit also comprises three hierarchical zones. In this case, however, it is the tertiary zones that guide the functions of the secondary and primary zones, rather than vice versa as with the posterior cortical unit. The tertiary zones of the anterior cortical unit of the brain are functionally specialized to "play a decisive role in the formation of intentions and programmes, and in the regulation and verification of the most complex forms of human behaviour" (Luria, 1973, p. 84). Such behavior includes speech and higher-order cognitive processes, which partially are characterized by the successive synthesis of information. Secondary zones are functionally specialized to prepare motor programs and to organize movement, whereas the primary zones are functionally specialized to execute the most basic elements of motor activity. The neuroanatomical substrate for this functional unit is the cortex of the frontal lobes.

As already noted, for the developing child, specific functions subserved by Luria's units of the brain, and in particular the anterior cortical tertiary zones (i.e., prefrontal cortex), presently are ill-defined. What little knowledge is available about prefrontal cortical processes derives mainly from research with adults, and primarily adult patients who have sustained frontal-lobe damage (Luria, 1972; Stuss & Benson, 1984). Specific behavior problems that have been associated with frontal-lobe damage in adults include: a defective capacity for self-control, emotional lability, impulsivity, sequencing difficulties, poor planning ability, and perseveration (Beaumont, 1983; Lezak, 1983; Luria, 1972). The capabilities that enable an individual to control these behaviors and to engage in purposeful problem-solving to attain a future goal have been identified as executive functions (Goldberg, 1986 Lezak, 1983; Luria, 1972). Executive functions are thought to facilitate future-oriented behavior by allowing for impulse control, strategic planning, and flexibility of thought and of action.

Despite the obvious psychoeducational implications of executive functions, relatively little information currently is available regarding the nature of these processes in children. Further, the ontogeny of executive functions remains equivocal. Luria (1973), for example, proposed that these processes do not emerge until the prefrontal cortex matures between the ages of 4 and 7 years. In contrast, Golden (1981*a*,*b*) asserted that the frontal lobes, hence executive functions, do not become fully functional until during adolescence. More recently, Welsh and Pennington (1988) argued that executive functions emerge during the first year after birth and continue to develop throughout pubescence and possibly into adulthood. Clearly, more studies that investigate the development of behaviors thought to be subserved by prefrontal regions of the brain are needed to improve our understanding of the nature of executive functions.

Most studies that have attempted systematically to investigate prefrontal functioning in normal children have used cross-sectional designs (i.e., where age and cohort are confounded) and therefore developmental issues have not been addressed directly. Even so, some useful findings have emerged, providing a rich source of developmental hypotheses. For example, Passler, Isaac, and Hynd (1985) examined the performance of boys and girls between ages 6 and 12 years on preseveration, verbal and nonverbal proactive and retroactive inhibition, and verbal and nonverbal conflict tasks. These tasks were chosen because of their association with prefrontal-lobe functioning in adults. Results demonstrated greatest performance gains between ages 6 and 8, with mastery of tasks generally evident by age 12.

Similar results were found by Becker, Isaac, and Hynd (1987) in an investigation of age-related changes in the ability of children to regulate and to inhibit motor action. Tasks involved go–no-go decisions, auditory–sequential and visual-simultaneous conflict, and temporal ordering. A clear age-related increase in these executive-function processes was observed: 8-, 10-, and 12-year-olds performed better than 6-year-olds and 12-year-olds performed better than 8- and 10-year-olds.

Finally, Welsh, Pennington, and Grossier (1991) conducted a normative study of 100 children aged 3 to 12 years, using a battery of neuropsychological measures purported to assess executive function in children (Matching Familiar Figures Test, Motor Sequencing, Tower of Hanoi, Verbal Fluency, Visual Search, and Wisconsin Card Sorting Test). Results were consistent with Passler *et al.* (1985) and with Becker *et al.* (1987), suggesting an early emergence of putative executive functions that may follow a protracted course as a function of age.

Collectively, results from these studies provide a solid basis for the hypothesis that executive functions, typically ascribed to the prefrontal cortical regions (i.e., tertiary region of the anterior cortical unit), are present at an early age, continue to develop throughout childhood, but do not mature until around age 12. Of course, additional research is needed to establish more fully the construct of executive functions in children, and to evaluate psychometric properties of the specific measures employed in these investigations. For example, issues of ceiling effects for scoring procedures, and reliability and validity of tasks should be explored. Even so, results already clearly illustrate a number of potential problems with generalizing adult-based neuropsychological literature to children, as well as with overlooking age-related influences on brain–behavior relationships.

Developmental Issues

Even though its experiential basis primarily was established with adult patients, Luria's (1970) theory of functional brain organization provides a useful framework for conceptualizing child neuropsychological assessments. Given the marked discontinuities in human development, however, a more complete understanding of child and adolescent brain–behavior relationships, especially those that concern higher-order cognitive functions, is not a simple matter of generalization from research with adult samples. Instead, additional research is required that evaluates established theories in consideration of these developmental discontinuities.

For example, the development of primary, secondary, and tertiary cortical zones follows an ontogenetic course. Based on morphological evidence, Luria (1980) suggested that primary cortical zones appear mature by birth, secondary zones by the first few postnatal months, and tertiary zones by the first few postnatal years. Moreover, it is likely that the relationships among these zones covary with chronological age. This possibility was described by Vygotsky as early as 1960, but few studies have directly addressed this hypothesis and there currently is limited empirical evidence to either support or refute this possibility (Merola & Liederman, 1985; Rutter, 1981).

More specifically, in early stages of ontogenetic development, relatively direct and associative sensory processes appear dominant. At later stages, however, more complex integration, related to speech and the higher-order cognitive processes, appears much more pronounced. Thus, one hypothesis is that lesions that are associated with the relatively basic sensory processes and that occur during early childhood may have deleterious effects on the higher-order cognitive processes due to a disturbance in the foundation for those processes. In contrast similar lesions that occur during adulthood (i.e., when the functional systems that subserve the higher-order cognitive processes have been formed) would be expected to have a much more limited effect. This kind of reasoning suggests that during early developmental stages, lesions to primary cortical areas would be expected to also impair the functioning of secondary and tertiary association areas that are subserved by the affected area. Conversely, lesions in the later stages of development would be expected to result in more specific/focal impairment.

Information Processing Modes

The cognitive aspects of Luria's theory of functional brain organization were elaborated by Das, Kirby, and Jarman (1975, 1979), which now has become known as the "Luria–Das" model. The initial research primarily emphasized simultaneous and successive coding processes (e.g., Das, 1972, 1973), although aspects of executive functions (e.g., planning) were not completely neglected (e.g., Ashman & Das, 1980). Thus, this model essentially targeted the two cortical functional units of Luria's theory for its primary foci and attempted to operationalize the cognitive processes putatively subserved by those units. Here, simultaneous synthesis of information has been defined as the process of organizing stimuli into gestalt schemes. The system of relationships among those stimuli is surveyed in a fashion such that the serial order in which individual stimuli are surveyed is unrelated to the perception of the whole. In contrast, successive synthesis of information relies on serial processing. Thus, the system of relationships among stimuli is surveyed consecutively. In this instance, accurate perception depends on synthesizing a series of sequential relationships. This kind of conceptualization focuses on the processes by which stimuli are synthesized rather than the contents (i.e., the nature of the stimuli to be synthesized) or products (i.e., the nature of the synthesized responses) of those processes. Theoretically, the nature of the stimuli to be synthesized minimally influences the mode of information processing. Instead, mode of processing theoretically is more influenced by experiential, sociocultural, and genetic factors as well as the demands of the task (Das & Varnhagen, 1986).

Simultaneous and successive information processing modes originally were discussed by Sechenov as early as 1878, and a long history of research on these constructs (see Kaufman & Kaufman, 1983, for a review) has suggested that they withstand continued tests and analytic techniques (Beller, 1970; Cohen, 1972, 1973; Klatzky & Atkinson, 1971; Patterson & Bradshaw, 1975; Shiffrin & Schneider, 1977). Moreover, these two modes of information processing have emerged for diverse samples of individuals of different cultures; socioeconomic backgrounds; and levels of IQ, development, and achievement (Das *et al.*, 1975, 1979; McCallum & Merritt, 1983).

Neuropsychological Foundation

The robust statistical independence of these two modes of information processing in children (as well as in adults), documented by factor analytic investigations, suggests that they may be subserved by differential neuropsychological foundations. As noted, Luria's (1973, 1980) clinical investigations with adult patients led him to propose relatively greater posterior than anterior cortical involvement for simultaneous synthesis and the reverse (i.e., relatively greater anterior than posterior cortical involvement) for successive synthesis. Specifically, the frontal and temporal lobes process information sequentially, while the parietal and occipital lobes handle information simultaneously. Other investigators have suggested that the neuropsychological foundation for these information processing modes may be related more to the functions of the two cerebral hemispheres (Gazzaniga, 1970; Levy & Trevarthen, 1976; Nebes, 1974). Research has supported relative right cerebral hemispheric specialization for simultaneous synthesis and relative left cerebral hemispheric specialization for successive synthesis. There has ensued some controversy, therefore, about which neural plane (i.e., coronal or sagittal) would provide a better metaphor for understanding the complementary processes of simultaneous and successive synthesis. This issue currently remains equivocal, although there is little dispute that differential cortical substrata are likely to be involved.

One factor that obscures this research is associated with the tendency for clinicians and researchers to administer assessment measures (e.g., K-ABC, WISC-R) that confound operations with modality-specific contents (Willis, 1985). For example, most standardized tasks of simultaneous information processing involve visual contents and motor products, whereas most standardized tasks of successive information processing involve auditory contents and oral products. Given the well-documented differential neuropsychological foundations for visuospatial (i.e., nondominant hemisphere) and language-based (i.e., dominant hemisphere) tasks (Gazzaniga, 1970; Kinsbourne, 1978; Segalowitz, 1983; Springer & Deutsch, 1985), it is not surprising that putative cortical specializations associated with information processing modes are equivocal. Partitioning effects to distinct variables may be particularly important both clinically and experimentally given the possibility that the interactions among those variables (e.g., information processing strategies by stimulus–response modalities) may contribute substantially to differential cerebral organization of functional systems (Willis & Hynd, 1987).

The role of the other major functional unit of Luria's theory, i.e., the subcortical unit which addresses arousal functions, also has been studied from an information processing perspective. For example, Naglieri and Das (1988) reported factor-analytic results and a theoretical elaboration of a model, which they termed "planning–arousal–simultaneous–successive" (PASS). Consistent with Luria's theory, Naglieri and Das cogently argued that the subcortical functional unit of the brain is prerequisite for information processing because of its role in maintaining proper levels of arousal or "cortical tone." The cortical functional units of the brain, of course, also clearly are seen as central to information processing, given the relationship of simultaneous and successive coding processes to the acquisition, storage, and retrieval of information. Finally, the tertiary (or prefrontal) zone, in particular, of the anterior cortical functional unit is implicated in the application of these coding processes for the efficient planning and verification of behavior (i.e., executive functions). As noted, tasks have been identified to operationalize many of these concepts, and their interactive yet distinct nature has been described (see Naglieri & Das, 1988).

The PASS model provides a clear framework for the neuropsychological evaluation of information processing from the perspective introduced by Luria (1973). Given their relationships to assessment, both the PASS model and Luria's theory explicitly acknowledge individual differences in this realm of human performance. In fact, Luria (1980) reported that the component operations that subserve information processing do not mature independently, but instead result from an individual's unique interactions within the environment.

Despite Luria's (1970, 1973, 1980) major theoretical contribution to the PASS model, Luria's own method of neuropsychological assessment differs from the PASS model in one important way. For example, in Luria's method, each case is approached as an individualized experiment, and component operations of tasks are elucidated through a detailed analysis of the syndrome. This syndrome analysis is used to investigate the neuropsychological organization of information processing for a single subject. In contrast, the PASS model was developed through a series of factor analyses that elucidate similar information processing modes within groups.Thus, in the former, individual differences have been used to identify deficits in neuropsychological functioning, and in the latter, individual differences have been used to identify reliable modes of information processing (Das & Varnhagen, 1986). The PASS model, in particular, may prove to be promising for neuropsychological assessment given its psychometric properties, its developmental focus, and its comprehensive perspective.

Cerebral Hemispheric Lateralization

A third theoretical issue germane to childhood neuropsychological assessment concerns processes subserved by the cerebral hemispheres. Functional asymmetries associated with the cortex of the cerebral hemispheres have been a major source of interest to neuropsychologists for many years. These asymmetries, or cerebral hemispheric lateralizations, refer to the relative (as opposed to exclusive) specialization of one cerebral hemisphere for a particular function. It was once thought that only higher-order cognitive functions were subject to lateralization (Luria, 1973; Moscovitch, 1979). Data have emerged, however, to suggest that it seems equally likely that some sensory functions also may be lateralized (Davidoff, 1982).

Theoretical Models

Most models of cerebral lateralization that are relevant to childhood neuropsychological assessment are based on perceptual asymmetries that have been measured through procedures conducted at a behavioral level of analysis. Essentially, these models can be classified as either efferent or afferent (see also Moscovitch, 1986). Efferent models emphasize the role of the cerebral cortex for directing attention and for guiding the perception of environmental stimuli. Thus, it is instructive to consider these models as top-down (or schema-based) models because they suggest a constructive role in the perceptual process. In contrast, afferent models emphasize the largely contralateral sensorineural projection pathways that link a particular receptor organ (e.g., retina of the eye) with the cortical region specialized for the corresponding modality (e.g., visual cortex in the occipital lobes). In this sense, these models often are considered as bottom-up (or data-based) models).

A primary goal of all efferent and afferent models of cerebral hemispheric lateralization is to synthesize principles of cognitive psychology with those of neurology. Efferent models traditionally have been more closely aligned with the cognitive sciences, whereas afferent models traditionally have been more closely aligned with the neurosciences. As Kandel (1985) so aptly articulated, however, the boundary between the disciplines of behavior and biology is arbitrary and changing. Thus, it now appears that our potential to improve our understanding of important issues in clinical neuropsychological assessment during childhood will lie in the interrelationships between these two broad disciplines.

Efferent Models

One of the earliest efferent models of cerebral hemispheric lateralization arose from Kinsbourne's (1970, 1973, 1975) selective activation hypothesis. This hypothesis, which subsequently was incorporated into a revised theory of functional cerebral distance (Kinsbourne & Hicks, 1978), suggested that perceptual asymmetries result from the differential activation of the cerebral hemispheres. This differential activation is due to the involvement of the hemispheres in a secondary task, rather than, for example, to differences in processing capacity. Because the sensorineural projection pathways are organized contralaterally, differential activation of the hemispheres was believes to bias attention in favor of the sensory hemispace that is contralateral to the more activated cerebral hemisphere. Thus, stimuli within that hemispace would be processed more efficiently than stimuli within the ipsilateral hemispace. Currently, the revised model and alternative theories probably better account for the accumulated relevant data, for example, of pervasive interference rather than facilitation effects of secondary tasks (Kinsbourne & Hiscock, 1983), but the selective activation hypothesis is recognized as an important forerunner to other efferent models of cerebral lateralization.

One of these other models was proposed by Friedman and Polson (1981). These investigators conceptualized each cerebral hemisphere as an independent, limited resource system. Resources refer to theoretical mechanisms responsible for the execution of various component operations of a task. In this model, the resources comprised by each cerebral hemisphere are considered to be finite. Thus, the differential executions of operations within a given cerebral hemisphere conceivably could need to compete for a limited supply of resources.

This model assumes that each cerebral hemisphere has the same resource capacity limit, and that increased activation of one hemisphere always is accompanied by an identically increased activation of the opposite hemisphere. Finally, although the hemispheres are conceptualized as separate systems, the products of those systems may become available to the opposite hemisphere as input via commissural transfer. This theory, of course, is in obvious contradistinction to the selective activation hypothesis that holds as its major premise that the hemispheres can be activated differentially.

Evidence to support Friedman and Polson's (1981) model has accrued primarily from studies in which two separate tasks were processed concurrently. Theoretically, when the component operations of one of those tasks, X, primarily are executed in one cerebral hemisphere, there is a relatively limited amount of resources available for the concurrent processing of the second task,

Y, when the component operations associated with Y occur within the homologous hemisphere. Of course, this is not the case when the component operations associated with Y primarily occur within the opposite hemisphere. Thus, perceptual asymmetries associated with Y theoretically reflect hemispheric differences in processing efficiency. Functional lateralization of X, the primary task, therefore, is assumed.

Kinsbourne's (1982) theory of hemispheric lateralization provides an alternative efferent model in marked contrast to the limited capacity conceptualization of Friedman and Polson (1981). From the perspective of Kinsbourne's theory, the assumption of a finite pool of resources is unnecessary. Instead, the brain is conceptualized as a differentiated neural network that comprises interconnected components responsible for particular operations. Given this conceptualization, it follows that task processing necessarily involves a larger portion of the total functional cerebral space than simply its locus of initiation. Consequently, concurrently processed tasks would be predicted to conflict to the extent that their component operations overlap.

This theory of functional cerebral distance (Kinsbourne & Hicks, 1978) received empirical support primarily at a behavioral level of analysis from research specifically designed to test its associated hypotheses and from reinterpretations of data analyzed retrospectively. For example, Kinsbourne and Hicks (1978) reviewed studies of simultaneous imitative effects between contralateral limbs and between speech and manual-motor behaviors. Subsequently, Kinsbourne and Hiscock (1983) reviewed studies of competition between (1) two output processes, (2) an output and a cognitive process, (3) two input processes, and (4) an input and a cognitive process. In these instances, output processes included sequential finger movements, finger oscillation, and expressive speech. Cognitive processes included reading, memory encoding, and visual scanning. Input processes included stimuli contralaterally directed to a particular cerebral hemisphere through dichotic-listening and tachistoscopic tests. Results of this research suggest that relative amounts of motor overflow, transfer, and interference can be explained in terms of degrees of overlap among the component operations involved in task processing.

Thus, Kinsbourne (1982) speculated that highly interconnected cerebral regions, which probably subserve similar processes, may lend themselves to successive (as opposed to simultaneous) use to permit the most efficient processing of a particular task. Conversely, regions of widely disparate functional cerebral distance, which probably subserve dissimilar processes, better may be suited for relatively more simultaneous use with respect to task processing. From this perspective, cerebral lateralization is viewed as a kind of neural separation between complementary component operations that, subsequent to sufficient elaboration, ultimately are aggregated to result in a unitary pattern of behavior. The primary advantage of this initial separation of component operations would be that it protects the distinct, but complementary, contributions of various operations from mutual interference.

These and other efferent theoretical models have some similarities but they also comprise important differences. The available data are insufficient to select one model as most appropriate for organizing the research on cerebral hemispheric lateralization. Issues to be addressed include the so-called independence of the cerebral hemispheres, the extent to which cerebral resources are differentiated, and, perhaps most important, the integrative functions of the cerebral hemispheres associated with higher-order cognitive processes. Some research, for instance, suggests that the particular hemisphere in which the component operations of a task are executed may be less important than the protection that the separate hemispheres provide against interference among those operations (Merola & Liederman, 1985). This is an intriguing hypothesis because it challenges the long-standing view of specific specializations of the cerebral hemispheres. Clearly, further empirical investigation is warranted.

Afferent Models

One assumption of afferent models is that task processing comprises a number of hierarchically arranged components, or operations, each of which receives its input from the previous operation. The execution of particular operations, at least at some stages, further is assumed to occur within the cerebral hemispheres. According to afferent models, there are two possible explanations for the perceptual asymmetries that are elicited from behavioral tests involving dichotic-listening, tachistoscopic, and dichaptic procedures (see Hannay, 1986; Jeeves & Baumgartner, 1986), i.e., efficiency and interhemispheric transfer.

One explanation suggests that each cerebral hemisphere is capable of executing the operations required by the task, but that the hemispheres neither execute those operations identically nor with the same degree of efficiency. For example, if Task X comprises a series of Operations a, b, and c, this explanation suggests that either hemisphere is capable of executing those operations. Any particular operation (e.g., Operation a), however, may be executed differently or more efficiently in one hemisphere (e.g., the dominant hemisphere) than in the other (e.g., the nondominant hemisphere). Thus, if Task X were projected to the dominant hemisphere, which more efficiently executes Operation a, then the behavioral response to Task X would be more favorable than if Task X were projected to the nondominant hemisphere. A perceptual asymmetry would result that favors the dominant cerebral hemisphere, i.e., the contralateral (or right-sided) hemispace. Given the largely (in the case of the visual system, the exclusively) contralateral sensorineural projection pathways, the functional specialization of a cerebral hemisphere for the execution of a particular task would be inferred from the perceptual asymmetry.

An alternative explanation suggests that at least one of the operations required by the task only can be executed in one particular hemisphere. Thus, if a task initially were projected to the cerebral hemisphere that could not execute a component operation, then information would be transferred to the other hemisphere across commissural (i.e., interhemispheric) projection pathways. For example, if Operation a only could be executed in the dominant hemisphere, then if Task X initially were projected to the nondominant hemisphere, information would be transferred to the dominant hemisphere in order to execute Operation a. This explanation assumes that operations that require interhemispheric transfer are executed less rapidly or less accurately than operations that do not require such transfer. In this example, a perceptual asymmetry would result that favors the dominant cerebral hemisphere. Again, given the contralateral sensorineural projection pathways, the functional specialization of a cerebral hemisphere for the execution of a particular task is inferred from the perceptual asymmetry. Thus, for both of these explanations of afferent models, it could be argued that the dominant cerebral hemisphere functionally was specialized for the processing of Task X.

Plasticity

The study of the effects of early brain lesions began with reports by Kennard (1936, 1942). Kennard studied the effects of cortical lesions on motor behavior in primates and came to the conclusion that early damage was associated with better outcome, relative to damage sustained in adulthood. Kennard's findings essentially went unchallenged for decades, and have since become known as the "Kennard principle." Similarly, it was once believed that the cerebral hemispheres were equipotential for the development of language at birth and became progressively more lateralized with development (Lenneberg, 1967). Based largely upon the Kennard principle, the concept of brain "plasticity" was thought to encompass two postulates (Fletcher & Satz, 1983): (1) younger organisms evidence better outcomes following brain injury and (2) there is greater plasticity in the immature CNS which explains the better outcomes. Although some authors find support for the Kennard principle (Smith, 1981; Smith & Sugar, 1975), recent anatomical, physiological, and behavioral research has failed to support Kennard's original findings (Fletcher & Satz, 1983; Hiscock & Kinsbourne, 1987; Passingham, Perry, & Wilkinson, 1983; Rourke, Bakker, Fisk, & Strang, 1983). Plasticity in early childhood is much more complex than such simplistic and global conceptualizations, and such statements must be tempered by the acceptance that several variables are operative that moderate the child's recovery from brain damage. These variables include such factors as premorbid functioning, age at lesion onset, type and size of lesion, location, and subsequent habilitation efforts (Cohen, Hynd, & Hartlage, 1983; Cohen, Prather, & Town, 1990*a*; Cohen, Holmes, Campbell, Smith, & Flanigin, 1990*b*; Pirozzolo & Papanicolaou, 1986).

Although the exact physiological mechanisms underlying recovery of function and brain plasticity remain unclear, numerous physiological and behavioral/functional processes have been postulated to account for recovery processes (Chelune & Edwards, 1981; Cohen *et al.*, 1990*a,b*; Rourke *et al.*, 1983). Physiological mechanisms include axonal regenerative and collateral sprouting, and denervation supersensitivity, while behavioral mechanisms include functional diaschisis, inhibitory release theories, and functional reorganization.

As an example of the modern view of brain plasticity, investigations by Woods and Teuber (1973) and Rasmussen and Milner (1977) indicate that early damage to the language centers of the left hemisphere lead to a functional shift in language abilities to the right hemisphere. However, this transfer of skills is not without a price. The phenomenon of crowding (Lansdell, 1962, 1969) occurs in which the nonverbal skills normally subserved by the right hemisphere show impairments. In addition, studies by Dennis and Whitaker (1976, 1977) reveal that although transfer of language function can occur in children who have undergone hemidecortication in the first year of life, these children nonetheless exhibit subtle deficiencies in language.

Further, it has become increasingly apparent that the brain simultaneously chooses and molds the environment, through behavior, and is shaped by the environment, through environmental stimulation. From animal studies it is well known that early and/or specific environmental manipulation significantly influence such morphological factors as characteristics of neurons in the visual system (Greenough, 1976; Hirsch & Spinelli, 1971; Kratz, Sherman, & Kalil, 1979), dendritic branching (Greenough, 1976), cerebellar parameters (Pysh & Weiss, 1979), and total brain weight (Rosenzweig, Bennett, & Diamond, 1972). What is unclear are the effects of early environmental manipulation on higher cortical functions and cognition. Given the vast number of variables that appear to play a role in recovery of function, it is clear that more brain plasticity and habilitation research is needed before child neuropsychologists can comfortably make predictive statements about long-term outcome following early brain insult.

APPLICATION TO CLINICAL ASSESSMENT

Neuropsychological assessment of children and adolescents necessitates that the psychologist possess a strong knowledge of developmental issues and inferences, as well as of tests that are appropriate for this age group. However, approximately two-thirds of self-declared neuropsychologists routinely perform assessments of children and adolescents without acquiring such a knowledge base (Adams, 1988).

While it is beyond the scope of this chapter to discuss the various battery (Golden, 1988*a*,*b*; Reitan, 1974; Selz, 1981) and eclectic approaches (Benton, Hamsher, Varney, & Spreen, 1983; Gaddes, 1980; Hynd & Cohen, 1983; Knights & Norwood, 1979; Obrzut, 1981; Spreen & Gaddes, 1979) that are currently being used in the assessment of children and adolescents, the reader is referred to the sources listed above and others (Hynd & Obrzut, 1981; Obrzut & Hynd, 1986*a*; Rourke *et al.*, 1983; Rutter, 1983; Teeter, 1986; Tramontana & Hooper, 1987) for such discussion. Instead, it is the intent of the present authors to use the remainder of this chapter to discuss the clinical implication of the theoretical issues previously discussed.

Developmental Issues

Differential diagnosis is a process through which classes of presenting symptoms are reviewed and systematically excluded to reach a parsimonious diagnostic decision about a person's presenting complaints. For the adult neuropsychologist, differential diagnosis involves differentiating: (1) acute versus chronic, (2) static versus progressive, and (3) functional/psychiatric versus organic/biological processes in conjunction with providing data characterizing the focal versus diffuse nature of the patient's presenting symptom cluster. While these issues are equally germane to child neuropsychological assessment, additional confounds present in the form of ontogenetic differences in behavior, and relatively greater variability within a given age group. Finally, the child neuropsychologist is oftentimes called upon to help differentiate between acquired versus neurodevelopmental disorders. As a result, paramount importance must be given to the use of test instruments that are sensitive to developmental changes in behavior. Unfortunately, many child neuropsychological assessment instruments in use today have not been designed with developmental considerations in mind (Welsh & Pennington, 1988). Thus, the two major neuropsychological test batteries most commonly employed with children, the Luria–Nebraska Children's Revision and the Halstead–Reitan Test Batteries (including the younger child's version, the Reitan–Indiana Neuropsychological Test Battery for Children), are downward extensions of their corresponding adult versions, with modifications for children (Teeter, 1986). While clearly these tests represent advances in the neuropsychological examination of the child, they do not fully reflect the enormous functional differences between the fully developed adult brain and the rapidly developing child's brain.

These differences are best highlighted with reference to the assessment of frontal lobe functioning. Of the different neuroanatomical divisions of the brain, perhaps none has captured the attention of neuroscience researchers as have the frontal lobes. In spite of the recent proliferation of research addressing frontal lobe functioning in children, however, the frontal lobes remain perhaps the least understood division of the cortex (Welsh & Pennington, 1988). This lack of understanding is due in large part because most of what is known about frontal lobe functioning is derived from studies of adults with focal lesions.

As previously discussed, Luria (1973) believed that the prefrontal region of the frontal lobes does not mature until ages 4–7, while Golden (1981*a*,*b*) postulated that this same region does not begin development until adolescence, and further asserted that children with frontal lobe damage remain symptomless until ages 12–15 or older. Golden (1981*a*,*b*) stated that this is the reason the children's version of the Luria–Nebraska Neuropsychological Test Battery does not attempt to assess frontal lobe functioning. In contrast, Welsh and Pennington (1988), drawing upon the Piagetian and nonhuman primate literature, maintained that the frontal region of the brain appears to be a silent area in children simply because we assess this region using traditional adult criteria. Thus, the notion of the frontal lobes being so-called "silent" areas stems from two implicit assumptions regarding frontal lobe assessment: (1) the behaviors that are traditionally thought of as being frontally mediated behaviors are defined in terms of adult levels of performance, and (2) the assessment instruments we employ with children are by-and-large, downward extensions of adult neuropsychological tests. This contention is further supported by the work of Boucugnami and Jones (1989), the neurophysiological/rCBF studies of Lou and colleagues (Lou, Henriksen, Bruhn, Borner, & Nielsen, 1989), and the preliminary animal work of Cohen, Holmes, and Diamond (1989), which indicate that early insult to frontal lobe structures does not remain "silent" but in fact underlies much of the behavioral dysfunction seen in "attention deficit hyperactivity disorder" including perseveration, self-directed attention, inhibitory capacity, and hyperactivity.

Assessment of Premorbid Level of Functioning

Poor performance on tests that purport to measure the neuropsychological status of developing brains may be reflective of two non-mutually exclusive factors: the loss of previously acquired abilities through brain injury or the lack of development of abilities. The implications of this developmental variability are enormous, especially in relation to the child's premorbid level of functioning in comparison with the child's present neuropsychological profile (Goldstein & Levin, 1987). For example, the child who exhibited problematic behavior and academic learning difficulties before a head injury may be functioning at baseline levels postinjury, if these behaviors and learning problems continue at their preinjury levels. In such a case it may be improper to conclude that the child's injury "caused" the abnormal behavior and aberrant learning problems. Similarly, consider the case of the academically bright child who demonstrates only average intellectual performance upon neuropsychological evaluation postinjury. It would likewise be improper to conclude that this child suffered no lasting intellectual impairment as a result of his or her injury. Careful consideration of the child's preinjury level of functioning would lessen the probability of the neuropsychologist making these types of errors in judgment.

At present there is no adequate psychometric test, inventory, or rating scale that would provide the examiner a reasonably valid indicator of the child's premorbid level of intellectual/cognitive functioning. To greater and lesser degrees, clinical judgment plays a role in assessing preinjury functioning. Wechsler tried to devise a system for estimating an individual's premorbid level of intellectual functioning that was based upon "hold" versus "no hold" subtests from the WAIS (Wechsler, 1944). Wechsler believed that the Digit Symbol, Block Design, Digit Span, Arithmetic, and Picture Arrangement subtests of the WAIS (the "don't hold" subtests) were more likely to be depressed relative to the Information and Vocabulary subtests (the "hold" subtests) in cases of brain injury (Groth-Marnat, 1984). Wechsler's "hold" versus "no hold" classification scheme, however, is not widely used in clinical practice (Reynolds & Gutkin, 1979).

In an attempt to predict the premorbid intellectual status of children, Reynolds and Gutkin (1979) used stepwise multiple regression to analyze the standardization sample data from the WISC-R. The authors used the demographic variables of father's occupational status, sex, race, urban versus rural residence, and geographic region of residence to predict verbal, performance, and full-scale IQ scores. The following multiple correlations were obtained: Verbal IQ $R = 0.44$, Performance IQ $R = 0.37$, and Full Scale IQ $R = 0.44$. Although the demographic variables contributed significantly to the variance accounted for, the total variance accounted for ranges only from 14% to 19%. As a result, large standard errors of estimates for each IQ score were obtained. Klesges and Sanchez (1981) and Klesges (1982) note that Reynolds and Gutkin (1979) fail to provide empirical evidence as to the utility of the formulas, and in an attempt to cross-validate the formulas (Klesges & Sanchez, 1981) no evidence was found to support the clinical usefulness of the formulas.

The effects of preinjury neuropsychological and behavioral functioning on postinjury neuropsychological and behavioral performance can be illustrated by examples from divergent sources in the literature. For example, Craft, Shaw, and Cartlidge (1972) examined premorbid personality characteristics in head-injured children. Using the children's classmates as controls, they found a higher incidence of teacher-reported premorbid behavioral problems in the head-injured children, as compared with the children's classmate controls. Similarly, Brown, Chadwick, Shaffer, Rutter, and Traub (1981) and Rutter (1981) found that mildly injured children, as defined as posttraumatic amnesia (PTA) of at least 1 hr but less than 7 days, demonstrated a higher rate of premorbid behavioral and academic disturbances than more severely head-injured children. However, even more interesting was the discovery that the mildly head injured group's problematic behavior did not change postinjury. Based on these data, Rutter (1981) suggests that the development of postinjury sequelae may in part reflect preinjury personality characteristics of the child.

Similarly, out of 18 children suffering from "head trauma" who were evaluated by Fuld and Fisher (1977), "only three children . . . could be described as academically and socially normal before their accidents" (p. 497). The other 15 children had preinjury problems such as learning difficulties, mental retardation, and severe delinquency. Taken together, these studies suggest that premorbid behavioral and neuropsychological functioning may have a significant effect upon interpretation of neuropsychological data at the time of postinjury neuropsychological assessment.

Much useful information regarding premorbid behavioral and intellectual functioning may be obtained from the setting where most children and adolescents spend the majority of their waking lives, their schools. School records including end-of-year standardized achievement testing, report cards, previous psychological testing, special education records, and interviews with teachers can provide a wealth of information about the academic and behavioral functioning of the child undergoing a neuropsychological evaluation. Often, reports by teachers can provide an objectivity that many parents lack, and a basis for comparison, albeit oftentimes subjective, with other students of similar age/grade level, and across settings (i.e., home/school).

Finally, interview with the parents and review of the child's developmental and medical history is absolutely essential if the examiner is to be successful in addressing the common referral questions of chronicity, progression, organicity, focality, and long-term outcome. This involves obtaining an accurate understanding of the chief complaints including onset and progression over time, results from previous evaluations and treatment of the problem, thorough review of the family history (emphasizing neurological, psychiatric, social, and learning problems), pregnancy, labor and delivery, developmental milestones, and medical history (emphasizing sensory/motor impairments, childhood diseases/syndromes, reoccurring illnesses, hospitalizations, and medication history). Despite the significance of such data to any form of psychological assessment, it is the experience of the present authors as well as that of our colleagues that a thorough history taking is oftentimes found to be lacking in the school and clinical psychology evaluations previously done on new patient referrals.

Qualitative Observations during Assessment

In most instances, the information gathered through careful observation of the child or adolescent during the evaluation can oftentimes be as informative as the quantitative analysis of the test data in formulating answers to the referral questions. For example, how easily the child separates from parents, quality of eye contact with the examiner, and the willingness to try and stick with difficult items can provide valuable information about the self-concept and emotionality of the child.

The assessment of language is supplemented greatly by qualitative observation and analysis of articulation, fluency, prosody, the presence of echolalia, and the ability to comprehend and use language in a social context (i.e., the evaluation). Specifically, such observations serve to supplement the quantitative performance on formal language testing and thereby help the examiner determine if in fact language is developing at an abnormal rate and if so, what aspects of language development are being affected. For example, a qualitative analysis of articulation (i.e., difficulty with sound creation versus sound blending) can provide important clues to localization of dysfunction in addition to determining if the difficulty is merely a normal developmental variant. Finally, observations during testing of distractibility, difficulty sustaining attention, impulsivity, verbal or motor perseveration, error awareness and the ability to self-correct one's own behavior, and social disinhibition may be indicators, and oftentimes are the only indicators, of frontal lobe dysfunction in children.

The Neuropsychological Examination

Whether the child neuropsychologist ascribes to one of the traditional battery approaches to assessment or takes an eclectic approach, it is absolutely essential that the test instruments employed do a thorough job of sampling all of the cognitive components that taken together make up what is traditionally referred to as higher cortical functioning. Specifically, the child neuropsychologist must pick up where the neurological exam traditionally ends and provide the documentation that verifies the developmental integrity of each of Luria's cortical units/analyzers.

Perhaps the best place to begin the neuropsychological assessment of children and adolescents is with intelligence testing. First, administration of the WISC-III, or other individually administered intelligence test such as the KABC or Stanford–Binet Fourth Edition, provides the trained child neuropsychologist with an estimate of a child's intellectual potential or psychometric "g," which can be used as a reference point in making interpretations about performance on other instruments that are designed to assess specific abilities. Second, administration of the IQ test provides the child neuropsychologist with a vehicle from which to sample the waterfront of higher cortical functioning, and with the aid of analytical approaches such as that described by Kaufman (1979), to begin formulating hypotheses about the child's cortical strengths and weaknesses which will require further verification. Third, administration of intelligence testing is almost always required by state Departments of Education in making a diagnosis of learning disability, mental handicap, and "slow learner" (which is sometimes less obvious). In this regard, the child neuropsychologist must provide the parents with a finished product that will be usable by the child's school system so that one of the major goals of assessment can be accomplished, that being appropriate classroom placement and remediation of the identified disability.

The assessment of language involves the evaluation of both the auditory as well as the sensory-motor cortical analyzers. According to Luria (1980), it is the auditory analyzer in the temporal lobe of the dominant hemisphere (Heschl's gyrus and Wernicke's area) that is involved with the receptive aspects of language including auditory perception and speech sound discrimination, as well as the giving of meaning to spoken words and sentences. In contrast, the sensory-motor analyzer in the frontal lobe of the dominant hemisphere (motor strip involving tongue/mouth and Broca's area) mediates speech sound creation as well as the blending of sounds to create words and sentences. Therefore, language assessment of children should involve the use of standardized norm-referenced tests designed to adequately assess auditory acuity, auditory discrimination, articulation, fluency/word finding, comprehension of single words, and sentence repetition, as well as the child's ability to formulate and comprehend spoken commands and sentences. In order to be complete, the language assessment should also attempt to assess the right hemisphere's contribution to language which involves the comprehension of emotional gesture, as well as the comprehension and expression of the prosodic aspects of language.

The assessment of visuospatial perception/construction involves evaluation of both the sensory-motor and visual cortical analyzers in the occipital and parietal lobes. Together, these areas are involved in visual and tactile–kinesthetic perception, visual discrimination, orientation in space, and constructional praxis. Assessment of these higher cortical functions in children should once again involve the use of standardized norm-referenced tests to adequately assess visual acuity and visual fields, visual spatial/tactile perception and discrimination, fine motor functioning, spatial orientation, and constructional praxis.

Like their adult counterparts, children and adolescents are vulnerable to hypoxic–ischemic events, viral encephalopathies, closed head injuries, and other insults to the brain that frequently affect the anterior and mesial aspects of the temporal lobes. As a result, it is not uncommon to find disorders of memory following closed head injury (Levin, Eisenberg, Kobayashai, & Wiig, 1982) and infection (Maertens, Cohen, & Krawiecki, 1987) in children. Therefore, a comprehensive examination of memory functions in children and adolescents is absolutely essential.

While there is a lack of standardized norm-referenced memory batteries available for children, subtests from various tests of intelligence and learning aptitude can be used to provide the child neuropsychologist with a means of assessing immediate recall of auditory/verbal and visual spatial/nonverbal material. In addition, traditional adult memory assessment instruments such as the Rey Auditory Verbal Learning Test, the Rey Complex Figure, and the Selective Reminding Test (Lezak, 1983; Kolb & Wishaw, 1990) can be used qualitatively to make judgments about the child's efficiency in storing and accessing material from long-term memory.

In order to adequately assess memory, the child neuropsychologist must also direct his/her assessment to the highly related construct of attention, which perhaps is the foundation for memory/learning. According to Luria (1980), the subcortical unit of the brain is responsible for maintaining the optimal "cortical tone" necessary for organized mental activity. Anatomically, we are referring to the brain stem reticular formation as well as the activation and inhibitory pathways leading to and from the frontal lobes. In order to thoroughly assess attention, tasks should be selected that sample three major components. Immediate attention refers to the ability to orient to a given task and involves complex scanning and tracking ability. Sustained attention, or vigilance, is the ability to maintain optimum arousal and orientation over time, and selective attention involves the ability to selectively attend or focus on certain key aspects of one's environment while at the same time filtering out what is left. Given the high frequency of referrals of children to mental health centers for "attention deficit hyperactivity disorder" (Safer & Allen, 1976; Lambert, Sandoval, & Sassone, 1978) and the high reported incidence of attentional disorders following head injury in children (Chadwick, Rutter, Shaffer, & Shrout, 1981), tests of attention must become an important component of the neuropsychological assessment of children and adolescents.

Finally, the child/adolescent neuropsychological evaluation would not be complete without a detailed assessment of academic achievement and screening of emotional/behavioral disturbance. Assuming normal classroom exposure, achievement testing is absolutely essential if the neuropsychologist is going to diagnose the presence of specific learning disabilities. In addition, achievement testing shortly after brain insult can also serve to provide the neuropsychologist with an additional mechanism for evaluating the child's ability to learn and store material into long-term memory prior to the insult, provided that the child's history is not consistent with the presence of a developmental learning disability or mental retardation. Screening for social/emotional disturbance is also necessary in making a diagnosis of a specific learning disability in that the neuropsychologist must demonstrate that the learning problem is not secondary to such a disturbance. In addition, behavior rating scales, such as the Achenbach Child Behavior Checklist (Achenbach & Edelbrock, 1983) or the Conners Parent and Teacher Rating Scales (Conners, 1982), completed by the child's parents and teachers as well as clinical interview/projective assessment, are useful in verifying the presence of disordered behavior and social–emotional impairment that is characteristic of many brain impairments. For example, as previously stated, perhaps the first evidence of frontal lobe dysfunction in children will take the form of behavioral deficits including motoric and verbal perseveration, attention, disinhibition, hyperactivity, poor organization and planning ability, as well as an inability to monitor and self-correct one's behavior.

A Functional System Approach to Interpretation

According to Luria's (1980) functional system approach, a given behavior (functional system) is produced not by a single localized area of the brain, but by many interrelated areas/components working in concert. Thus, insult to a specific component or part of a functional system results in a characteristically abnormal performance of that behavior which will be qualitatively different depending upon which component of the functional system is affected. The insult will also affect other functional systems that require the affected component for normal performance. Finally, functional systems that do not require the specific component for normal performance will remain essentially unaffected. Thus, the child neuropsychologist not only must be proficient in test administration and interpretation from a quantitative (norm-referenced) standpoint, but also skilled at qualitative analysis (observation) of how a child or adolescent passes or fails test items, as well as how the various functional systems necessary for successful classroom and adaptive functioning are performed.

Several examples will be given to illustrate this method of interpretation. Suppose a child demonstrated significantly impaired performance on a paper-and-pencil constructional task such as the Bender-Gestalt. Concluding that the child exhibited poor visual–motor integration leaves the task of interpretation half done. The child neuropsychologist should then attempt to determine what component(s) is responsible for the poor performance; in other words, what part of the functional system is dysfunctional. Is the poor performance primarily due to a visual-spatial perceptual problem, or a motor output problem, or both? If the answer is not readily apparent from a qualitative analysis of the child's performance, then additional testing of visual-spatial perception and fine motor functioning will be necessary.

A further example involves the use of the digit span subtest from the WISC-R. While many authors regard this test as measuring auditory short-term memory (Sattler, 1988; Kaufman, 1979), some authors have suggested that the extra component of requiring the subject to repeat digits backwards involves an additional cognitive process (Gardner, 1981; Jensen & Figueroa, 1975). Thus, assuming adequate attention, poor performance on this subtest can be attributed to a temporal lobe memory disorder, or to a frontal lobe disinhibition syndrome (Luria, 1980; Stuss & Benson, 1984; Stuss, Benson, Kaplan, Weir, Naser, Lieberman, & Ferril, 1983). Once again, this will necessitate that the examiner present the child with additional executive function and memory tasks in order to adequately characterize the dysfunction.

A Functional System Approach to the Assessment of Learning Disabilities

The comprehensive description of neuropsychological functioning is of paramount importance in the evaluation of learning disabilities. Historically, these disorders have been presumed to be due to underlying CNS dysfunction even though the overwhelming majority of learning-disabled individuals do not have diagnosable brain lesions resulting from traumatic injury or obvious congenital abnormalities such as porencephaly, agenesis of the corpus callosum, and hydrocephalus to name a few. However, neuropathological studies of patients with developmental dyslexia and developmental dysphasia (Galaburda & Kemper, 1979; Galaburda, Sherman, Rosen, Aboitiz, & Geschwind, 1985; Cohen, Campbell, & Yaghmai, 1989) consistently demonstrate the presence of developmental anomalies in the cerebral cortex consisting of neuronal ectopias, and architectonic dysplasias located mainly in the parasylvian regions and affecting predominantly the left cerebral hemisphere. In addition, all of the brains showed a deviation from the standard pattern of cerebral asymmetry characterized by symmetry of the planum temporale. The significance of the finding of cerebral symmetry has been supported by computer tomography (Haslam, Dalby, Johns, & Rademaker, 1981; Hier, LeMay, Rosenberger, & Perlo, 1978; Rosenberger & Hier, 1980) and magnetic resonance imaging studies (Rumsey, Dorwart, Vermess, Denckla, Kruesi, & Rapoport, 1986; Hynd, Semrud-Clikeman, Lorys, Novey, & Eliopulos, 1990), which have shown high incidence of abnormal cerebral symmetry in dyslexics. Taken together, these studies appear to indicate that a neurodevelopmental abnormality during midgestation, the period of neuronal migration from the germinal matrix to the cerebral cortex, underlies the typical case of learning disability. Thus, a functional system approach to interpretation readily lends itself to the neuropsychological assessment of learning-disabled children and adolescents. In this instance, the ultimate goal of the neuropsychological assessment is not to localize a specific lesion site, but rather to accurately describe the child's pattern of neuropsychological strengths and weaknesses and relate them to the specific learning disability or learning disabilities with which the child presents.

For example, in the case of developmental dyslexia the child neuropsychologist should begin assessment by dissecting the functional system of reading into its higher cortical components. In so doing, we find that several cortical areas within both hemispheres become actively involved in the reading process. Specifically, the visual analyzer in the occipital/parietal cortex is necessary for carrying out letter discrimination, letter-string discrimination, as well as word-string discrimination. The auditory analyzer in the temporal lobe is involved in letter-sound discrimination as well as word and sentence comprehension, and the sensory-motor analyzer in the frontal lobe and motor strip mediates letter-sound production, sound blending, as well as subvocalization and/or vocalization of words and sentences. Thus, when all of these components are working in concert and at optimal efficiency, the examiner will observe a normal reading pattern. However, as previously stated, if one or more of these components is dysfunctional, qualitatively different patterns of disordered reading will emerge. In fact, this sort of functional system analysis to higher cortical functioning is greatly supported by recent research in the area of developmental dyslexia, which indicates that the disorder is heterogeneous in nature and comprised of at least three major subtypes (Boder, 1971; Fisk & Rourke, 1979; Hynd and Cohen, 1983; Mattis, French, & Rapin, 1975; Petrauskas & Rourke, 1979; Pirozzolo, 1979; Satz & Morris, 1981). As expected, based upon a functional system analysis, these three subgroups demonstrate strikingly different patterns of neuropsychological test performance. Children in subtype I (language disorder/dysphonetic) typically exhibit significantly lower verbal as compared with performance IQ scores on intelligence testing, in conjunction with receptive and expressive language delay, word finding/fluency problems, auditory discrimination problems, and poor short-term auditory/verbal memory. This is contrasted by relative strengths in the areas of constructional praxis, visual discrimination, and visual memory. Qualitative analysis of their reading and spelling errors reveals marked difficulty in phonetic word attack and sound blending when asked to read and spell words that are not in sight word vocabulary.

Children in subtype II (visual-spatial/dyseidetic) typically exhibit significantly lower performance as compared with verbal IQ scores in conjunction with deficits in constructional praxis, visual spatial perception, and visual memory. In contrast, relative strengths are noted in the areas of expressive and receptive language development, and auditory/verbal memory. Qualitative analysis of their reading and spelling patterns reveals that this subtype is able to generate close phonetic approximations to words not in sight word vocabulary.

However, they frequently confuse visually similar letters and words, and letter reversals are commonly noted in their written work.

Finally, the third subtype of dyslexic children (mixed) typically exhibit fairly good consolidation between their IQ score with neuropsychological deficits noted in the linguistic as well as the visual spatial areas. Qualitative analysis of their reading and spelling patterns reveals poor phonetic word attack and sound blending skills in conjunction with frequent visual spatial errors. Thus, evidence from this subtyping research strongly supports Luria's theoretical model of higher cortical functioning via functional systems.

Recommendations: Making the Data Work for the Patient

In this chapter we have examined some of the theoretical and clinical issues that are relevant to the neuropsychological investigation of children and adolescents. Through the delineation of intact and impaired functional systems, the child neuropsychological evaluation encompasses more than simply detecting the presence or absence of brain damage. Perhaps the most crucial aspect of the evaluation, and arguably the component with the smallest research base, centers around making appropriate recommendations for the remediation and/or compensation of deficits associated with neuropsychological impairment. This encompasses the blending of theoretical issues, clinical experience, and good commonsense judgment.

In the realm of child and adolescent neuropsychological assessment, this typically involves recommendations for special education and other remedial programs such as occupational therapy, physical therapy, and speech/language therapy. With this in mind, the child neuropsychologist must be knowledgeable of the state and local guidelines that govern special education placement as well as the availability of other public and private resources.

In addition, the child neuropsychologist would be remiss if he/she did not offer recommendations as to the most appropriate mode of instruction for children with neuropsychological impairments. For example, if a child exhibits the language disorder/dysphonetic type of learning disability, a whole word or language experience approach, deemphasizing phonics, may be most appropriate for that child. Similarly, a child who exhibits the visual-spatial/dyseidetic learning disability may be taught best by emphasizing phonetic methods and deemphasizing visual-spatial or pictorial strategies (Hynd & Cohen, 1983; Hooper & Willis, 1989; Hooper, Willis, & Stone, in press; Hynd, 1986).

At times, the child neuropsychologist may make referrals to medial or other allied health professionals for further evaluation. The child neuropsychologist must be knowledgeable of the range of services provided by these professionals. Similarly, child neuropsychologists often play an important role in linking parents of brain-injured and learning-disabled children with local, state, and national advocacy groups.

Finally, the brain-injured child or adolescent may place significant social and emotional burdens on family members (Lezak, 1988). Some parents will readily acknowledge the present and future limitations of their brain-injured child, while others cling to ill-founded beliefs that their son or daughter will someday be a normal, fully integrated member of society. While not all child neuropsychologists conduct counseling and therapy sessions within their own practice, an assessment of the family dynamics involved may necessitate appropriate referral to a family or marriage therapist, preferably one who is sensitive to the issues involved in the care of a brain-injured child.

SUMMARY

This chapter has presented an overview of the key theoretical and clinical issues germane to childhood neuropsychological assessment. It was emphasized that the neuropsychological assessment of children differs vastly from adult neuropsychological assessment, due in large part to the enormous and rapid neurophysiological, intellectual, social, and behavioral changes that characterize child development. As a result, adult-based theories and procedures oftentimes have limited applicability to the neuropsychological assessment of children (e.g., frontal lobe assessment). Fortunately, recent advances in child neuropsychology have begun to address this problem. As a result, we have attempted to familiarize the reader with current thinking on the issues of brain organization, information processing, cerebral hemispheric lateralization, and plasticity.

In addition, the clinical implications of these theoretical issues were discussed. These included a qualitative analysis of behavioral observations, consideration of premorbid level of functioning, a functional system approach to assessment, and appropriate, neuropsychologically based treatment recommendations. The field of child neuropsychology must continue to develop its own theories and clinical assessment procedures, rather than rely on those that are simply downward extensions of adult theories and procedures. Only in this way can the field of child neuropsychological assessment continue to advance and achieve meaningful contributions toward a more complete understanding of neuropsychological development.

REFERENCES

Achenbach, T. M., & Edelbrock, C. S. (1983). *Manual for the Child Behavior Checklist and Revised Child Behavior Profile*. Burlington: Department of Psychiatry, University of Vermont.

Adams, K. M. (1988). Neuropsychology is not just in the eye of the provider. *Professional Psychology: Research and Practice, 19*, 488–489.

Ashman, A. F., & Das, J. P. (1980). Relation between planning and simultaneous–successive processing. *Perceptual and Motor Skills, 51*, 371–382.

Beaumont, J. G. (1983). *Introduction to neuropsychology*. New York: Guilford Press.

Becker, M. G., Isaac, W., & Hynd, G. W. (1987). Neuropsychological development of nonverbal behaviors attributed to "frontal lobe" functioning. *Developmental Neuropsychology, 3*, 275–298.

Beller, H. K. (1970). Parallel and serial stages in matching. *Journal of Experimental Psychology, 84,* 213–219.
Benton, A. L., Hamsher K., Varney, N. R., & Spreen, O. (1983). *Contributions to neuropsychological assessment.* New York: Oxford University Press.
Boder, E. (1971). Developmental dyslexia: Prevailing diagnostic concepts and a new diagnostic approach. In H. R. Myklebust (Ed.), *Progress in learning disabilities* (Vol. II, pp. 293–321). New York: Grune & Stratton.
Boucugnami, L. L., & Jones R. W. (1989). Behaviors analogous to frontal lobe dysfunction in children with attention deficit disorder. *Archives of Clinical Neuropsychology, 4,* 161–173.
Brodal, A. (1981). *Neurological anatomy in relation to clinical medicine* (3rd ed.). New York: Oxford University Press.
Brown, G., Chadwick, O., Shaffer, D., Rutter, M., & Traub, M. (1981). A prospective study of children with head injuries: III. Psychiatric sequelae. *Psychological Medicine, 11* 63–78.
Caramazzo, A. (1984). The logic of neuropsychological research and the problem of patient classification in aphasia. *Brain and Language, 21,* 9–20.
Chadwick, O., Rutter, M., Shaffer, D., & Shrout, P. E. (1981). A prospective study of children with head injuries II. Specific cognitive deficits. *Journal of Clinical Neuropsychology, 3,* 101–120.
Chelune, G. J., & Edwards, P. (1981). Early brain lesions: Ontogenetic–environmental considerations. *Journal of Consulting and Clinical Psychology, 49,* 777–786.
Cohen, G. (1972). Hemispheric differences in a letter classification task. *Perception and Psychophysics, 11,* 139–142.
Cohen, G. (1973). Hemispheric differences in serial versus parallel processing. *Journal of Experimental Psychology, 97,* 349–356.
Cohen, M. J., Hynd, G., & Hartlage, L. C. (1983). A shift in language lateralization: One case for and one case against. *Clinical Neuropsychologist, 5,* 129–135.
Cohen, M. J., Holmes, G. L., & Diamond, B. (1989, October). Behavioral effects of hypoxia in the developing rat brain. Paper presented at the 18th annual meeting of the Child Neurological Society, San Antonio.
Cohen, M. J., Campbell, L. R., & Yaghami, F. (1989). Neuropathological abnormalities in developmental dysphasia. *Annals of Neurology, 25,* 567–570.
Cohen, M. J., Prather, A., & Town, P. (1990*a*). Neurodevelopmental differences in emotional prosody in normal children with left and right temporal lobe epilepsy. *Brain and Language, 38,* 122–134.
Cohen, M. J., Holmes, G. L., Campbell, L. R., Smith, J. R., & Flanigin, H. F. (1990*b*). Memory performance following unilateral electrical stimulation of the hippocampus in a child with right temporal lobe epilepsy. *Journal of Epilepsy, 3,* 115–122.
Conners, C. K. (1982). Parent and teacher rating forms for the assessment of hyperkinesis in children. In P. A. Keller & L. G. Ritter (Eds.), *Innovations in clinical practice: A source book* (Vol. I, pp. 257–264). Sarasota, Fla.: Professional Research Exchange.
Craft, A. W., Shaw, D. A., & Cartlidge, N. E. (1972). Head injuries in children. *British Medical Journal, 4,* 200–203.
Das, J. P. (1972). Patterns of cognitive ability in nonretarded and retarded children. *American Journal of Mental Deficiency, 77,* 6–12.
Das, J. P. (1973). Structure of cognitive abilities: Evidence for simultaneous and successive processes. *Journal of Educational Psychology, 65,* 103–108.
Das, J. P., & Varnhagen, C. K. (1986). Neuropsychological functioning and cognitive processing. In J. E. Obrzut & G. W. Hynd (Eds.), *Child neuropsychology* (Vol. I, pp. 117–140). New York: Academic Press.
Das, J. P., Kirby, J. R., & Jarman, R. F. (1975). Simultaneous and successive synthesis: An alternative model for cognitive abilities. *Psychological Bulletin, 82,* 87–103.
Das, J. P., Kirby, J. R., & Jarman, R. F. (1979). *Simultaneous and successive cognitive processes.* New York: Academic Press.
Davidoff, J. B. (1982). Studies with non-verbal stimuli. In J. G. Beaumont (Ed.), *Divided visual field studies of cerebral organization* (pp. 30–55). New York: Academic Press.
Dennis, M., & Whitaker, H. A. (1976). Language acquisition following hemidecortication: Linguistic superiority of the left over the right hemisphere. *Brain and Language, 3,* 404–433.

Dennis, M., & Whitaker, H. A. (1977). Hemispheric equipotentiality and language acquisition. In S. J. Segalowitz & F. A. Gruber (Eds.), *Language development and neurological theory* (pp. 93–107). New York: Academic Press.

Fisk, J. L., & Rourke, B. F. (1979). Identification of subtypes of learning disabled children at three age levels: A neuropsychological, multivariate approach. *Journal of Clinical Neuropsychology, 1,* 289–310.

Fletcher, J. M., & Satz, P. (1983). Age, plasticity, and equipotentiality: A reply to Smith. *Journal of Consulting and Clinical Psychology, 51,* 763–767.

Fletcher, J. M., & Taylor, H. G. (1984). Neuropsychological approaches to children: Towards a developmental neuropsychology. *Journal of Clinical Neuropsychology, 6,* 39–56.

Friedman, A., & Polson, M. C. (1981). Hemispheres as independent resource systems: Limited capacity processing and cerebral specialization. *Journal of Experimental Psychology: Human Perception and Performance, 7,* 1031–1058.

Fuld, P. A., & Fisher, P. (1977). Recovery of intellectual ability after closed head injury. *Developmental Medicine and Child Neurology, 1,* 495–502.

Gaddes, W. H. (1980). *Learning disabilities and brain function.* Berlin: Springer-Verlag.

Galaburda, A. M., & Kemper, T. C. (1979). Cytoarchitectonic abnormalities in developmental dyslexia: A case study. *Annals of Neurology, 6,* 94–100.

Galaburda, A. M., Sherman, G. F., Rosen, G. D., Aboitiz, F., & Geschwind, N. (1985). Developmental dyslexia: Four consecutive patients with cortical anomalies. *Annals of Neurology, 18,* 222–233.

Gardner, R. A. (1981). Digits forward and digits backward as two separate tests: Normative data on 1567 school children. *Journal of Clinical Child Psychology,* summer, 131–135.

Gazzaniga, M. S. (1970). *The bisected brain.* Englewood Cliffs, NJ: Prentice–Hall.

Goldberg, E. (1986). Varieties of perseveration: A comparison of two taxonomies. *Journal of Clinical and Experimental Neuropsychology, 8,* 710–726.

Golden, C. J. (1981*a*). A standardized version of Luria's neuropsychological tests. In S. B. Filskov & T. J. Boll (Eds.), *Handbook of clinical neuropsychology.* New York: Wiley.

Golden, C. J. (1981*b*). The Luria–Nebraska Children's Battery: Theory and formulation. In G. W. Hynd & J. E. Obrzut (Eds.), *Neuropsychological assessment and the school-age child: Issues and procedures* (pp. 277–302). New York: Grune & Stratton.

Goldstein, F. C., & Levin, H. S. (1987). Epidemiology of pediatric closed head injury: Incidence, clinical characteristics, and risk factors. *Journal of Learning Disabilities, 20,* 518–525.

Greenough, W. T. (1976). Enduring brain effects of differential experience and training. In M. R. Rosenzweig & E. L. Bennett (Eds.), *Neural mechanisms of learning and memory.* Cambridge, Mass.: MIT Press.

Groth-Marnat, G. (1984). *Handbook of psychological assessment.* New York: Van Nostrand–Reinhold.

Hannay, H. J. (Ed.). (1986). *Experimental techniques in human neuropsychology.* New York: Oxford University Press.

Haslam, R. H., Dalby, J. T., Johns, R. D., & Rademaker, A. W. (1981). Cerebral asymmetry in developmental dyslexia. *Archives of Neurology, 38,* 679–682.

Hier, D. B., LeMay, M., Rosenberger, P. B., & Perlo, V. P. (1978). Developmental dyslexia: Evidence for a subgroup with a reversal of cerebral asymmetry. *Archives of Neurology, 35,* 90–92.

Hirsch, H. V. B., & Spinelli, D. N. (1971). Modification of the distribution of receptive field orientation in cats by selective visual exposure during development. *Experimental Brain Research, 13,* 509–527.

Hiscock, M., & Kinsbourne, M. (1987). Specialization of the cerebral hemispheres: Implications for learning. *Journal of Learning Disabilities, 20,* 130–143.

Hooper, S. R., & Willis, W. G. (1989). *Learning disability subtyping: Neuropsychological foundations, conceptual models, and issues in clinical differentiation.* Berlin: Springer-Verlag.

Hooper, S. R., Willis, W. G., & Stone, B. H. (in press). Neuropsychological issues and approaches to treatment of children with learning disorders. In R. S. Dean & E. S. Batchelor (Eds.), *Pediatric neuropsychology: Interfacing assessment and treatment in the rehabilitation of neurological disorders.* Elmsford, NY.: Pergamon Press.

Hynd, C. R. (1986). Educational intervention in children with developmental learning disorders. In J. E. Obrzut & G. W. Hynd (Eds.), *Child neuropsychology* (Vol. II, pp. 265–297). New York: Academic Press.

Hynd, G. W., & Cohen, M. J. (1983). *Dyslexia: Neuropsychological theory, research, and clinical differentiation*. New York: Grune & Stratton.

Hynd, G. W., & Obrzut, J. E. (Eds.). (1981). *Neuropsychological assessment and the school-age child: Issues and procedures*. New York: Grune & Stratton.

Hynd, G. W., Semrud-Clikeman, M., Lorys, A. R., Novey, E. S., & Eliopulos, D. (1990). Brain morphology in developmental dyslexia and attention deficit disorder/hyperactivity. *Archives of Neurology, 47*, 919–926.

Jeeves, M., & Baumgartner, G. (Eds.). (1986). Methods in neuropsychology [Special issue]. *Neuropsychologia, 21* (1).

Jensen, A. R., & Figueroa, R. A. (1975). Forward and backward digit span interaction with race and IQ: Predictions from Jensen's theory. *Journal of Educational Psychology, 67*, 882–893.

Kandel, E. R. (1985). Cellular mechanisms of learning and the biological basis of individuality. In E. R. Kandel & J. H. Schwartz (Eds.), *Principles of neural science* (2nd ed., pp. 816–833). Amsterdam: Elsevier.

Kaufman, A. S. (1979). *Intelligent testing with the WISC-R*. New York: Wiley.

Kaufman, A. S., & Kaufman, N. L. (1983). *Kaufman Assessment Battery for Children: Interpretive manual*. Circle Pines, Minn.: American Guidance Service.

Kennard, M. (1936). Age and other factors in motor recovery from precentral lesions in monkeys. *Journal of Neurophysiology, 1*, 447–496.

Kennard, M. (1942). Cortical reorganization of motor function: Studies on series of monkeys of various ages from infancy to maturity. *Archives of Neurology and Psychiatry, 47*, 227–240.

Kinsbourne, M. (1970). The cerebral basis of lateral asymmetries in attention. *Acta Psychologica, 33*, 193–201.

Kinsbourne, M. (1973). The control of attention by interaction between the cerebral hemispheres. In S. Kornblum (Ed.), *Attention and performance IV* (pp. 239–256). New York: Academic Press.

Kinsbourne, M. (1975). The mechanism of hemispheric control of the lateral gradient of attention. In P. M. A. Rabbit & S. Dornic (Eds.), *Attention and performance V* (pp. 81–97). New York: Academic Press.

Kinsbourne, M. (Ed.). (1978). *Asymmetrical function of the brain*. London: Cambridge University Press.

Kinsbourne, M. (1982). Hemispheric specialization and the growth of human understanding. *American Psychologist, 37*, 411–420.

Kinsbourne, M., & Hicks, R. E. (1978). Functional cerebral space: A model for overflow, transfer and interference effects in human performance: A tutorial review. In J. Requin (Ed.), *Attention and performance VII* (pp. 345–362). Hillsdale, NJ: Erlbaum.

Kinsbourne, M., & Hiscock, M. (1983). Asymmetries of dual-task performance. In J. B. Hellige (Ed.), *Cerebral and hemisphere asymmetry* (pp. 255–334). New York: Praeger.

Klatzky, R., & Atkinson, R. (1971). Specialization of the cerebral hemispheres in scanning for information in short-term memory. *Perception and Psychophysics, 10*, 335–338.

Klesges, R. C. (1982). Confusing clinical and statistical significance? A reply to Reynolds and Gutkin. *Journal of Consulting and Clinical Psychology, 50* 772–774.

Klesges, R. C., & Sanchez, V. C. (1981). Cross-validation of an index of premorbid intellectual functioning in children. *Journal of Consulting and Clinical Psychology, 49*, 141.

Knights, R. M., & Norwood, J. W. (1979). *A neuropsychological test battery for children: Examiner's manual*. Ottawa: Knights Psychological Consultants.

Kolb, B., & Wishaw, I. Q. (1990). *Fundamentals of human neuropsychology* (3rd ed.). San Francisco: Freeman.

Kratz, K. E., Sherman, S. M., & Kalil, R. (1979). Lateral geniculate nucleus in darkreared cats: Loss of y cells without changes in cell size. *Science, 203*, 1353–1355.

Lambert, N. M., Sandoval, J., & Sassone, D. (1978). Prevalence of hyperactivity in elementary school children as a function of social system definers. *American Journal of Orthopsychiatry, 48*, 446–463.

Lansdell, H. (1962). Laterality of verbal intelligence in the brain. *Science, 135*, 922–923.

Lansdell, H. (1969). Verbal and nonverbal functions in right-hemisphere speech. *Journal of Comparative and Physiological Psychology, 69*, 734–738.
Lenneberg, E. H. (1967). *Biological foundations of language*. New York: Wiley.
Levin, H., Eisenberg, H. M., Kobayashi, K., & Wiig, E. R. (1982). Memory and intellectual ability after head injury in children and adolescents. *Neurosurgery, 11*, 668–673.
Levy, J., & Trevarthen, C. (1976). Metacontrol of hemispheric function in human split-brain patients. *Journal of Experimental Psychology: Human Perception and Performance, 2*, 299–312.
Lezak, M. D. (1983). *Neuropsychological assessment* (2nd ed.). New York: Oxford University Press.
Lezak, M. (1988). Brain damage is a family affair. *Journal of Clinical and Experimental Neuropsychology, 10*, 111–123.
Lou, H. C., Henriksen, L., & Bruhn, P. (1984). Focal cerebral hypoperfusion in children with dysphasia and/or attention deficit disorder. *Archives of Neurology, 41*, 825–829.
Lou, H. C., Henriksen, L., Bruhn, P., Borner, H., & Nielsen, J. B. (1989). Striatal dysfunction in attention deficit and hyperkinetic disorder. *Archives of Neurology, 46*, 48–52.
Luria, A. R. (1970). Functional organization of the brain. *Scientific American, 222*, 66–78.
Luria, A. R. (1972). *The man with a shattered world*. New York: Basic Books.
Luria, A. R. (1973). *The working brain: An introduction to neuropsychology*. New York: Basic Books.
Luria, A. R. (1980). *Higher cortical functions in man*. New York: Basic Books.
Maertens, P., Cohen, M. J., & Krawiecki, N. (1987). The use of neuropsychological evaluation in the medical management of subdural empyema. *Archives of Clinical Neuropsychology, 2*, 145–154.
Mattis, S., French, J. H., & Rapin, I. (1975). Dyslexia in children and young adults: Three independent neuropsychological syndromes. *Developmental Medicine and Child Neurology, 17*, 150–163.
McCallum, R. S., & Merritt, F. M. (1983). Simultaneous–successive processing among college students. *Journal of Psychoeducational Assessment, 1*, 85–93.
Merola, J. M., & Liederman, J. (1985). Developmental changes in hemispheric independence. *Child Development, 56*, 1184–1194.
Moscovitch, M. (1979). Information processing and the cerebral hemispheres. In M. S. Gazzaniga (Ed.), *Handbook of behavioral neurobiology* (Vol. II, pp. 379–446). New York: Plenum Press.
Moscovitch, M. (1986). Afferent and efferent models of visual perceptual asymmetries: Theoretical and empirical implications. *Neuropsychologia, 24*, 91–114.
Naglieri, J. A., & Das, J. P. (1988). Planning–arousal–simultaneous–successive (PASS): A model for assessment. *Journal of School Psychology, 26*, 35–48.
Nebes, R. D. (1974). Hemispheric specialization in commissurotomized man. *Psychological Bulletin, 81*, 1–14.
Obrzut, J. E. (1981). Neuropsychological procedures with school-age children. In G. W. Hynd & J. E. Obrzut (Eds.), *Neuropsychological assessment and the school-age child: Issues and procedures* (pp. 237–275). New York: Grune & Stratton.
Obrzut, J. E., & Hynd, G. W. (Eds.). (1986*a*). *Child neuropsychology: An introduction to theory and research*. New York: Academic Press.
Obrzut, J. E., & Hynd, G. W. (1986*b*). Child neuropsychology: An introduction to theory and research. In G. W. Hynd & J. E. Obrzut (Eds.), *Child neuropsychology* (Vol. I, pp. 1–12). New York: Academic Press.
Passingham, R. E., Perry, V. H., & Wilkinson, F. (1983). The long-term effects of removal of sensorimotor cortex in infant and adult rhesus monkeys. *Brain, 106*, 675–705.
Passler, M. A., Isaac, W., & Hynd, G. W. (1985). Neuropsychological development of behaviors attributed to frontal lobe functioning in children. *Developmental Neuropsychology, 1*, 349–370.
Patterson, K., & Bradshaw, J. L. (1975). Differential hemispheric mediation of nonverbal visual stimuli. *Journal of Experimental Psychology: Human Perception and Performance, 1*, 246–252.
Petrauskas, R., & Rourke, B. P. (1979). Identification of subgroups of retarded readers: A neuropsychological multivariate approach. *Journal of Clinical Neuropsychology, 1*, 17–37.
Pirozzolo, F. J. (1979). *The neuropsychology of developmental reading disorders*. New York: Oxford University Press.
Pirozzolo, F. J., & Papanicolaou, A. C. (1986). Plasticity and recovery of function in the central

nervous system. In J. E. Obrzut & G. W. Hynd (Eds.), *Child neuropsychology* (Vol. I, pp. 141–154). New York: Academic Press.

Pysh, J. J., & Weiss, G. H. (1979). Exercise during development induces an increase in Purkinje cell dendritic tree size, *Science, 206,* 230–232.

Rasmussen, T., & Milner, B. (1977). The role of early left-brain injury in determining lateralization of cerebral speech functions. *Annals of the New York Academy of Sciences, 299,* 255–369.

Reitan, R. M. (1974). *Clinical neuropsychology: Current status and applications.* New York: Winston.

Reynolds, C. R., & Gutkin, T. B. (1979). Predicting the premorbid intellectual status of children using demographic data. *Clinical Neuropsychology, Second Quarter,* 36–38.

Rosenberger, P. B., & Hier, D. B. (1980). Cerebral asymmetry and verbal intellectual deficits. *Annals of Neurology, 8,* 300–304.

Rosenzweig, M. R., Bennett, E. L., & Diamond, M. C. (1972). Brain changes in response to experience. *Scientific American, 226,* 22–29.

Rourke, B. P., Bakker, D. J., Fisk, J. L., & Strang, J. D. (1983). *Child neuropsychology: An introduction to theory, research, and practice.* New York: Guilford Press.

Rumsey, J. M., Dorwart, R., Vermess, M., Denckla, M. B., Kruesi, M. J. P., & Rapoport, J. L. (1986). Magnetic resonance imaging of brain anatomy in severe developmental dyslexia. *Archives of Neurology, 43,* 1045–1046.

Rutter, M. (1981). Psychological sequelae of brain damage in children. *American Journal of Psychiatry, 139,* 21–33.

Rutter, M. (1983). *Developmental neuropsychiatry.* New York: Guilford Press.

Safer, D., & Allen, R. (1976). *Hyperactive children: Diagnosis and management.* Baltimore: University Park Press.

Sattler, J. M. (1988). *Assessment of children.* San Diego: Jerome Sattler.

Satz, P., & Morris, R. (1981). Learning disability subtypes: A review. In F. J. Pirozzolo & M. C. Wittrock (Eds.), *Neuropsychological and cognitive processes in reading* (pp. 109–141). New York: Academic Press.

Sechenov, I. (1878). *Selected physiological and psychological work.* Moscow: Foreign Languages Publishing House.

Segalowitz, S. J. (1983). *Two sides of the brain.* Englewood Cliffs, NJ: Prentice–Hall.

Selz, M. (1981). Halstead–Reitan neuropsychological test batteries for children. In G. W. Hynd & J. E. Obrzut (Eds.), *Neuropsychological assessment and the school-age child: Issues and Procedures* (pp. 195–235). New York: Grune & Stratton.

Shallice, T. (1979). Case study approach in neuropsychological research. *Journal of Clinical Neuropsychology, 1,* 183–212.

Shiffrin, R. M., & Schneider, W. (1977). Controlled and automatic human information processing: II. Perceptual learning, automatic attending, and a general theory. *Psychological Review, 84,* 127–190.

Smith, A. (1981). On the organization, disorganization, and reorganization of language and other brain functions. In Y. Levrun & O. Zangwill (Eds.), *Lateralization of language in the child.* Lisse: Swets & Zeitlinger.

Smith, A., & Sugar, O. (1975). Development of above normal language and intelligence 21 years after left hemispherectomy. *Neurology, 25,* 813–818.

Spreen, O., & Gaddes, W. H. (1979). Developmental norms for 15 neuropsychological tests age 6–15. *Cortex, 5,* 170–190.

Springer, S. P., & Deutsch, G. (1985). *Left brain, right brain.* San Francisco: Freeman.

Stuss, D. T., & Benson, F. (1984). Neuropsychological studies of the frontal lobes. *Psychological Bulletin, 95,* 3–28.

Stuss, D. T., Benson, F., Kaplan, E., Weir, W. S., Naser, M. A., Lieberman, I., & Ferril, D. (1983). The involvement of the orbital-frontal cerebrum in cognitive tasks. *Neuropsychologia, 21* 235–248.

Teeter, P. A. (1986). Standard neuropsychological batteries for children. In G. W. Hynd, & J. E. Obrzut (Eds.), *Child neuropsychology* (Vol. II, pp. 187–227). New York: Academic Press.

Tramontana, M., & Hooper, S. (1987). *Neuropsychological assessment with children.* New York: Plenum Press.

Tramontana, M. G., & Hooper, S. R. (Eds.). (1988). *Assessment issues in child neuropsychology*. New York: Plenum Press.
Vygotsky, L. S. (1960). *Development of the higher mental functions*. Moscow: Izd. Akad. Ped. Nauk ASFSR.
Wechsler, D. (1944). *Measurement of adult intelligence*. Baltimore: Williams & Wilkins.
Welsh, M. C., & Pennington, B. F. (1988). Assessing frontal lobe functioning in children: Views from developmental psychology. *Developmental Neuropsychology, 4*, 199–230.
Welsh, M. C., Pennington, B. F., & Grossier, B. F. (1991). A normative-developmental study of executive function: A window on prefrontal function in children. *Developmental Neuropsychology, 7*, 131–149.
Willis, W. G. (1985). Successive and simultaneous processing: A note on interpretation. *Journal of Psychoeducational Assessment, 4*, 343–346.
Willis, W. G., & Hynd, G. W. (1987). Lateralized interference effects: Evidence for a processing style by modality interaction. *Brain and Cognition, 6*, 112–126.
Woods, B. T., & Teuber, H.-L. (1973). Early onset of complementary specialization of cerebral hemispheres in man. *Transactions of the American Neurological Association, 98*, 113–117.

3

Adult Development and Aging

ASENATH LA RUE

INTRODUCTION

This chapter continues the discussion of developmental aspects of neuropsychological assessment, examining age-related changes in the last half of the life span. Old age, like early development, is a time of rapid change within all levels of the organism. Many late-life changes are poorly understood, but there are enough descriptive data to indicate that advanced age is a critical individual difference parameter.

In clinical neuropsychological assessment, it is important to make allowances for normative aging changes in differential diagnosis and to become familiar with prominent old-age mental disorders. It is also important to recognize that aging can exaggerate the neuropsychological impact of other psychiatric, neurologic, and medical conditions.

Perhaps the most beneficial contribution that a neuropsychologist can make to the welfare of older patients is to determine whether current cognitive or emotional problems are consistent with normal aging. Psychologists are most likely of all health care professionals to have had training in normal development and to have worked in research or clinical settings with healthy individuals. This basic training provides a conceptual framework for understanding aging changes and for developing criteria to judge when performance is age-consistent. Many clinical neuropsychological measures are poorly normed in the upper age ranges (Albert, 1981) or have dubious relevance to everyday activities of older people (Schaie & Schaie, 1977). Therefore, to work effectively with elderly patients, familiarity with the broader literature on normal aging is required.

ASENATH LA RUE • Department of Psychiatry and Biobehavioral Sciences, University of California at Los Angeles, Los Angeles, California 90024-1759.

HANDBOOK OF NEUROPSYCHOLOGICAL ASSESSMENT: A Biopsychosocial Perspective, edited by Antonio E. Puente and Robert J. McCaffrey. Plenum Press, New York, 1992.

This chapter comments briefly on the scope of aging and age-related problems and notes some fundamental issues in the study of adult development and aging. Summaries of neurobiological and cognitive changes in normal aging are then presented, followed by brief overviews of dementia and geriatric depression. The final section summarizes implications of current knowledge for clinical assessment of older patients.

OLDER ADULTS: DEMOGRAPHY, HEALTH, AND SOCIAL IMPACT

For the first time in history, most people in societies such as our own can plan on growing old. The average life expectancy for a woman born in the United States today is 78.2 years and for a man, 71.2 years (National Center for Health Statistics, 1986). Even those who are currently "old" can expect to live many more years; i.e., average life expectancy at age 65 is 18.6 years for women and 14.6 years for men (National Center for Health Statistics, 1986). About 21% of the current U.S. population is at least 55 years old and 12% are 65 or older (U.S. Bureau of the Census, 1987). Older adults are the only segment of the population predicted to grow substantially in the next 50 years, so that by the year 2030, one in three Americans will be 55 or older, and one in five at least 65 (U.S. Senate Special Committee on Aging, 1987–1988).

As growing old has become more predictable, interest in aging has increased and attitudes toward older people are changing in a positive way (Gatz & Pearson, 1988). Middle-aged people are now more curious about what it is like to be old and many have begun to make changes in their life-styles in an attempt to ensure a healthy and independent old age.

However, health problems of the elderly have also assumed a new importance. Neurodegenerative disorders of later life such as Alzheimer's disease have gained increasing attention, as both professionals and the general public have come to appreciate the emotional and monetary costs of these long-term and currently irreversible conditions. Chronic medical disorders are also prevalent in upper age groups. More than four out of five people 65 and older have at least one chronic medical illness and many have multiple conditions. Older people are hospitalized twice as often as younger adults, make more outpatient visits to physicians, and use twice as many prescription drugs (National Center for Health Statistics, 1987). Medical care of the elderly is very costly, with people 65 and over accounting for one-third of this country's health care expenditures; costs would be greater if unpaid assistance of relatives and friends were to be included (U.S. Senate Special Committee on Aging, 1987–1988).

The aged are at much greater risk for significant cognitive impairment than younger adults. In the community, about 4.9% of people 65 or older have cognitive deficits, compared to only 0.6% of people between the ages of 18 and 64 (Regier, Boyd, Burke, Rae, Myers, Kramer, Robins, George, Karno, & Locke, 1988). In medical hospital settings, between one-third and one-half of elderly patients have either transient or persistent cognitive problems (Rapp, Parisi,

Walsh, & Wallace, 1988; Small & Fawzy, 1988). Rates of psychiatric hospitalization for organic mental disorder also increase dramatically with advancing age (La Rue, Dessonville, & Jarvik, 1985). In addition, many older people suffer from depression, paranoid disorder, pain syndromes, and sleep disturbance (La Rue & McCreary, 1991). Overall, older people continue to be poorly served by the mental health system (Roybal, 1988). According to an American Psychological Association survey, less than 5% of psychological services are delivered to clients over the age of 65 and fewer than 1% of psychologists report a primary focus in aging (VandenBos & Stapp, 1983).

ISSUES IN THE STUDY OF AGING

Who Is Old?

Americans often change their opinion about who is old depending on their own current age. The chronological delimiters of "young," "middle-aged," and "elderly" also vary across research investigations. By societal tradition, age 65 has taken on a common significance in denoting who is old. This tradition dates from the 1880s in Germany, when Otto von Bismarck identified 65 as the qualifying age for certain social welfare benefits (Butler & Lewis, 1973). This is still the primary starting age for Social Security and Medicare benefits in the United States. As legislators are increasingly aware, however, a much greater percentage of people are now living past 65 than was the case in the 1880s.

Most neurobiological and cognitive age changes appear to develop in a continuous fashion. The rate of change often accelerates at some point in the late-life span, but the point of inflection differs for different cellular, organ, and behavioral/functional systems. Chronological age provides a rough marker for these developmental events, even though specific chronological boundaries for old age are arbitrary. For example, studies that focus on young-old groups (e.g., people in their 60s) frequently come to different conclusions about the pattern and extent of aging changes than those with much older subjects (e.g., people in their 80s or 90s).

Early normative investigations of neuropsychological measures excluded elderly adults or used very small unrepresentative samples of older people. Recent studies have done a better job of including the elderly in standardization and validation samples. In general, however, very old people (age 80 and above) are not included, or are represented in insufficient numbers to provide acceptable norms. For example, in the revised versions of the Wechsler Adult Intelligence Scale (WAIS-R; Wechsler, 1981) and the Wechsler Memory Scale (WMS-R; Wechsler, 1981), 70 to 74 years is the oldest age bracket in the normative tables.

Variability in Older Adult Groups

Life-span development has been compared to an opening fan, implying that the uniqueness of the individual increases with the passage of time. There are many studies of aging that seem to support this idea, reporting larger standard deviations for older adult samples than for younger groups. This common outcome raises doubts about the feasibility of identifying normative age functions and of inferring age trajectories for individuals from group results.

Recently, greater attention has been paid to the possibility that variance may be inflated due to inclusion of medically ill subjects in aged samples. In studies of regional cerebral blood flow, for example, higher values are observed for completely healthy older adults compared to those who have risk factors for cerebrovascular illness (e.g., hypertension), who, in turn, have higher values than those with a history of transient ischemic attacks (Meyer & Shaw, 1984). Similar differences between optimally healthy and risk-factored subjects have been noted on electrophysiological and reaction time measures (e.g., Birren, Butler, Greenhouse, Sokoloff, & Yarrow, 1963) and have been mentioned as a cause of conflicting results in recent positron emission tomography studies (see Metter, 1988). In many aging studies, health screening has been superficial, and as a result, the extent of medical illness cannot be determined.

Some geriatric specialists argue that only optimally healthy subjects (i.e., with no identified illnesses, no suggestion of subclinical pathology, and no medications) should be included in studies of normal aging (e.g., Albert, Heller, & Milberg, 1988). Others point out that results of these studies may not generalize to average old people; if used as normative reference points, such studies could result in a majority of older people being classified as ill or impaired.

This issue is hard to resolve. Rates of chronic medical illness are strongly correlated with increasing age in the adult population. In addition, neurobiological changes associated with normal aging often overlap with signs of illness. For example, neuropathological diagnoses of Alzheimer's disease are based on counts of cerebral neuritic plaques and neurofibrillary tangles; however, both of these findings are also observed in normal aged brains. Diagnoses are made according to quantitative criteria that may not be valid for subjects of very advanced aged (see Crystal, Dickson, Fuld, Masur, Scott, Mehler, Masdeu, Kawas, Aronson, & Wolfson, 1988).

A realistic view is that a spectrum of aging functions may be needed for both biological and psychological variables, with separate trajectories established for groups that differ in physical health or other important individual difference parameters. Until sufficient data exist to establish these functions, care must be taken to examine sample characteristics in aging studies and to select appropriate normative groups for interpreting clinical findings.

Cross-sectional and Longitudinal Studies

Most aging studies use cross-sectional research designs, comparing separate groups of younger and older adults at a particular point in time. The limitations of this approach have been discussed in detail by Baltes, Reese, and

Nesselroade (1977), Schaie and Hertzog (1985), Nesselroade and Labouvie (1985), and others. The primary problem is that groups differing in age often differ in many other factors as well. Of particular concern is the confounding of age and generation (birth cohort) effects. Each generation is exposed to unique combinations of experience as they age, ranging from major events (e.g., wars) to changing technology (e.g., television, computers) to shifting dietary and exercise patterns. The cumulative effects of these experiences cannot be adequately controlled by matching age groups on a few characteristics such as education or occupation.

Longitudinal studies, providing serial assessments of the same individuals over months or years, are another source of data on normal aging. The major limitations of this design concern selective attrition. Especially at very advanced ages, subjects who remain in a study through many successive testings are likely to be exceptional individuals, having fewer physical health problems and scoring higher initially on many cognitive measures. An additional problem is that age trajectories from a single longitudinal study may not generalize to other samples.

In the area of cognition and aging, cross-sectional studies generally lead to larger estimates of aging change than longitudinal studies. The usual interpretation is that cross-sectional studies overestimate the amount of change that individuals experience as they age, whereas longitudinal studies tend to underestimate these changes. Cognition and aging is one of the few topics where there are sufficient data from both designs to permit integration and development of a consensus view. Neurobiological aging studies are predominantly cross-sectional, either out of necessity or convenience; as a result, there is little basis for knowing how biological aging functions are biased by this method.

NORMAL AGING

Neurobiological Changes

Age differences have been reported on many neurobiological indices. Detailed reviews of these differences can be found in Finch and Schneider (1985, Albert (1984), Albert and Moss (1988), and other sources.The present overview is restricted to some of the most prominent changes observed in aging humans. Normal findings are briefly contrasted with those of patients with autopsy-confirmed Alzheimer's disease or with the clinical syndrome of dementia associated with this disease (dementia of the Alzheimer type, DAT).

Neuroanatomical Changes

Table 3.1 summarizes age-related neuroanatomical findings (see Kemper, 1984, for a review). One of the best-documented changes is an overall decrease in brain weight or volume with age. In a study correcting for cohort trends,

TABLE 3.1. Selected Neurobiological Age Differences[a]

Measure	Direction of change	Comments
Neuroanatomy		
Brain weight/volume	Decrease	Cohort differences
Ratio of gray to white matter	Increase	Reflects myelin loss
Width of gyri	Increase	Noted on autopsy and CT
Size of ventricles	Increase	Noted on autopsy and CT
Neuron number	Decrease	Varies by region; small neurons may increase
Dendritic arborization	Inconsistent	Decreased in motor cortex
Amlyoid deposition	Increase	
Neuritic plaques	Increase	
Neurofibrillary tangles	Increase	Few in cortex
Granulovacuolar degeneration	Increase	Rare in cortex
Neurotransmitters		
Cholinergic metabolism	Inconsistent	
Cholinergic receptor binding	Decrease	
Dopamine metabolism	Decrease	Especially in striatum
Norepinephrine metabolism	Decrease	
Monoamine oxidase	Increase	
Brain metabolism		
Glucose metabolic rate	Inconsistent	May vary by region
Cerebral blood flow	Inconsistent	May vary by region
Discourse production	Variable	Speech more verbose, repetitive, imprecise
Electrophysiology		
Dominant EEG frequency	Decrease	Little change in optimally healthy aged
Alpha reactivity	Decrease	
Cortical coupling	Increase	May suggest less regional specialization
Latency of brain-stem and sensory evoked responses	Increase	Partly due to decreased nerve conduction speed
Amplitude of sensory evoked responses	Increase	May suggest decreased cortical inhibition
Latency of event-related potentials (P-300)	Increase	Slowing of central decision processes

[a]From *Concise Guide to Geriatric Psychiatry* (pp. 14–15) by J. E. Spar and A. La Rue, 1990, Washington D.C.: American Psychiatric Press. Copyright 1990 by American Psychiatric Press, Inc. Adapted by permission.

Miller, Alston, and Corsellis (1980) reported no change in the volume of cerebral hemispheres between the ages of 20 and 50 years, followed by a 2% decrease per decade through age 98 for both men and women. Increases in the ratio of gray to white matter in the cerebral hemispheres suggest an age-related loss of myelin (Miller *et al.*, 1980), which is greatest in regions where myelinization is completed relatively late in the developmental cycle (e.g., association and limbic cortices, as opposed to motor, visual, and auditory regions). Other gross changes in brain morphology that have been observed on autopsy are gyral atrophy and ventricular dilation. Gyral atrophy is most extensive in the convexities of the frontal lobes, parasagittal region, and temporal and parietal lobes, and is not highly correlated with ventricular dilation (Kemper, 1984). Atrophic changes in aging brains have also been documented using computerized tomographic (CT) procedures. Nearly all CT studies report increased ventricular size with advancing age, but there are discrepancies across studies in the age at which significant enlargement is observed (see Albert & Stafford, 1988, for a review). Some of these discrepancies may be due to variations in subject selection criteria and in the methods used to measure ventricle size. Studies of optimally healthy older adults, and those using automated or highly standardized measurement procedures, generally show that ventricular size does not substantially increase until about the seventh decade.

Age-related neuronal loss has been reported for all areas of the human neocortex, although some regions show more loss with age than others. In an early and widely cited study, Brody (1955) reported cell losses ranging from 32% to 49% in the precentral gyrus, superior temporal gyrus, and visual cortex when 70- to 95-year-olds were compared to adolescents, with no appreciable loss in the postcentral gyrus. Based on a review of more recent cytoarchitectural studies, Kemper (1984) indicates that in the cortex, the most pronounced losses are in the frontal polar cortex (area 10), premotor cortex (area 6), and an association region in the temporal lobe (area 21). The temporal limbic region (area 38) and association areas of the somesthetic and visual cortex (areas 40 and 18, respectively) also show losses in cell count with age, but to a lesser degree. Neuronal loss has been observed in all areas of the hippocampal formation, but in the amygdala, as well as subcortical forebrain, brain stem, and cerebellar formations, age-related change is more selective (Kemper, 1984). Terry and Hansen (1988) suggest that neuronal shrinkage, rather than loss, may be the predominant finding in normal human aging. In a study of brains of 51 subjects between ages of 20 and 100 years, declines in the number of large neurons were largely offset by increases in small, presumably shrunken, neurons.

Scheibel and colleagues (e.g., Scheibel, Lindsay, Tomiyasu, & Scheibel, 1975, 1976) described a characteristic pattern of degenerative changes in dendritic processes with age, with swelling of the cell body and apical shaft preceding loss of horizontal dendritic processes, followed, in turn, by loss of basal and apical dendritic branches. These changes were most clearly noted in the large Betz cells of the motor cortex, but were also observed in the hippocampal region and in neocortical pyramidal cells. However, Buell and Coleman (1979) found that in normal aging, growing dendritic trees predominate over regressing trees in the parahippocampal region.

Other widely studied microscopic changes include accumulation of intra- and intercellular structures presumed to reflect pathological processes. These include deposition of amyloid in cerebral blood vessels and brain tissue, development of neuritic plaques and neurofibrillary tangles, and granulovacuolar degeneration. Brain amyloid deposition has been linked to immunological change, although its precise immunological significance is not known. Glenner (1979) hypothesized that amyloid may leak through the blood–brain barrier, allowing plasma proteins to enter the intercellular space, initiating changes that lead to formation of neuritic plaques and neurofibrillary tangles. Many other possible roles of amyloid are being actively researched (Marx, 1989).

Although plaques and tangles are commonly observed in the brains of older people with normal cognitive function, both are noted in greater concentrations in the brains of patients with Alzheimer's disease and some other neurodegenerative disorders. Also, in normal aging, tangles and granulovacuolar degeneration are rarely observed in the neocortex (Matsuyama & Nakamura, 1978).

In his summary of age-related neuroanatomical changes, Kemper (1984) divided findings into three groups. Included in the first group are decreased brain weight, loss of neurons, loss of myelin, gyral atrophy, ventricular dilation, and amyloid accumulation. All show relatively strong correlations with age and each is further accentuated in Alzheimer's disease; however, there is considerable overlap in distributions for normal aging and this form of dementia. Changes in the second group, including granulovacuolar degeneration and neurofibrillary tangles, also increase with age, but they are noted only in small numbers and restricted distribution in the brains of healthy older adults. In Alzheimer's disease, these findings are more widespread throughout the brain and much more numerous. Senile plaques are included in a third group where frequency and distribution in aging and Alzheimer's are intermediate to changes in the first and second groups.

Neurotransmitter Changes

Of the many different neurotransmitters that have been identified, only a few have been studied extensively with respect to human aging. This discussion focuses on the cholinergic and catecholaminergic neurotransmitter systems, since changes in these systems may be important for understanding age-related changes in cognition (for reviews, see Bartus, Dean, Beer, & Lippa, 1982; Kubanis & Zornetzer, 1981; Rogers & Bloom, 1985).

Indirect evidence of the role of the cholinergic neurotransmitter system for cognitive function in aging is provided by studies of normal young adults in which temporary problems with learning and memory and performance IQ have been induced by administering drugs that block uptake of the neurotransmitter acetylcholine (ACh) at the receptor. These deficits are similar in some respects to those observed in normal aging, suggesting, perhaps, a common cholinergic basis (see Drachman & Leavitt, 1974, for a discussion).

Because ACh is difficult to measure, most investigations of age differences have monitored levels of the synthetic enzyme choline acetyltransferase (CAT) as a marker for cholinergic metabolism. Some studies have reported significant decreases in CAT in normal elderly adults compared to young control subjects in the cortex, striatum, and hippocampus; however, others studying the same brain regions have found no age difference in CAT (Rogers & Bloom, 1985). Bartus and colleagues (1982) suggest that age-related changes in CAT may be small and, therefore, hard to measure, and that investigators examining large brain sites (e.g., the cortex or the hippocampus) may inadvertently sample different cell populations. In contrast to the literature on normal aging, virtually all studies examining CAT in Alzheimer's patients have reported reliable declines compared to control samples (Bartus *et al.*, 1982; Rogers & Bloom, 1985). More consistent evidence for age-related changes has been obtained for cholinergic receptor binding. In advanced old age, there are either fewer operative receptors (especially muscarinic receptors) remaining on cholinergic cells or fewer cholinergic cells overall (Rogers & Bloom, 1985). The presence of Alzheimer's disease does not appear to add to age-related receptor loss (Bartus *et al.*, 1982).

As noted in Table 3.1, levels of catecholamine neurotransmitters, dopamine (DA) and norepinephrine (NE), reliably decline with age. Pronounced decreases in DA and tyrosine hydroxylase (TH), the enzyme that stimulates synthesis of catecholamines, have been observed in the human brain, particularly in the striatum (McGeer & McGeer, 1975, 1976; Rogers & Bloom, 1985). Old-age declines in NE have been reported for brain stem assays which include the locus coeruleus (Kubanis & Zornetzer, 1981; Rogers & Bloom, 1985) and in human septum and substantia nigra. Monoamine oxidase (MAO), an enzyme that breaks down catecholamines, may increase with age by as much as 50% (Robinson, Nies, Davies, Bunney, Davis, Colburn, Bourne, Shaw, & Coppen, 1972). The number of catecholaminergic receptors, and the responsiveness of these receptors to environmental stressors (e.g., shock or other painful stimuli), appear to decrease with age in several brain regions (Kubanis & Zornetzer, 1981). However, even in old age, catecholaminergic neurons appear to possess some reserve capacity, and may increase their firing rates to compensate for declining cell numbers (Carlsson, 1986).

Behavioral effects of altered catecholamine function have been studied much more extensively in animals than in humans. In rodent species, changes in NE have been implicated in decreased neural plasticity, inability to curb arousal, altered feedback control of the hypothalamic–pituitary–adrenal system, and problems with selective attention (see Kubanis & Zornetzer, 1981, for a review). Alterations in these functions could, in turn, result in changes in learning and memory or other complex cognitive processes (Kubanis & Zornetzer, 1981).

Brain Metabolism

A number of procedures have been developed in recent decades that permit *in vivo* examination of metabolic processes in the human brain, most notably regional cerebral blood flow (rCBF) and positron emission tomography (PET). These offer the opportunity of observing brain regions that are activated by performance of specific cognitive acts and of studying the functional interplay between different areas of the brain. Metter (1988) provides an excellent description of these methods as applied to the study of aging, and Phelps and Mazziotta (1985) give an informative overview of emission tomographic methods and their application to a wide range of brain–behavior questions.

Many recent investigations of rCBF use a procedure in which radioactive xenon gas is either injected or inhaled. The xenon is carried throughout the brain by blood flow and its distribution in various areas is monitored with multiple detectors placed over the skull. Cerebral blood flow can also be measured by positron emission techniques (Phelps & Mazziotta, 1985). One of the assumptions made in studying rCBF is that changes in neuronal metabolism are directly reflected in cerebral blood flow, with lessened blood flow indicating lower metabolic rates.

PET also involves the injection or inhalation of small quantities of radioactive tracers. Many different tracers have been developed (see Phelps & Mazziotta, 1985), but the most common in aging studies has been 2-deoxy-2-[^{18}F]fluoro-D-glucose (FDG), a glucose compound labeled with a radioactive form of fluorine. Glucose provides the primary energy source for most brain metabolic processes, and brain tissues use FDG as if it were ordinary glucose. As a result, FDG accumulates most rapidly in tissues where there is a high metabolic rate. As the radioactive substance decays in these tissues, it emits positrons that are recorded by detectors and computer-analyzed, providing quantitative estimates of metabolic rates for various brain regions.

In studies of normal older adults, declines in global and regional blood flow measurements have been reported in some investigations (e.g., Kuhl, Metter, Riege, & Phelps, 1982; Kuhl, Metter, Riege, & Hawkins, 1984), but many others have found no changes with age (e.g., Duara, Grady, Haxby, Ingvar, Sokoloff, Margolin, Manning, Cutler, & Rapoport, 1984). Metter (1988) attributes some of the inconsistency to subject selection procedures. For example, Kuhl and colleagues excluded subjects with neurologic disorders, moderate hypertension, and severe heart disease, but may have included individuals with milder levels of illness. Therefore, age-related declines may have reflected hypertensive and atherosclerotic changes. By contrast, Duara and colleagues only accepted subjects who had no evidence of any disease, i.e., optimally aging individuals.

Age differences in glucose metabolism also vary from study to study. Kuhl *et al.* (1982) reported about a 20% decrease in global metabolic rates for glucose from age 24 to 74 years and a reduction in the normal trend toward high metabolic rates in the frontal region. Other PET studies have found no significant age differences (Duara *et al.*, 1984; de Leon, George, Ferris, Christman, Fowler, Gentes, Brodie, Reisberg, & Wolf, 1984). Metter (1988) concludes that the overall pattern of brain glucose metabolism is the same for young and old adults, and quantitative age differences are small, if present at all.

Cerebral Electrophysiology

Electroencephalographic (EEG) recordings measure the ongoing electrical activity of the brain. Typically, EEG is measured with multiple scalp electrodes to permit simultaneous evaluation of activity in several brain regions. Several aspects of EEG output can be monitored, including frequency, amplitude, consistency across time, and symmetry across brain regions. These parameters can be rated clinically (by visual inspection of the EEG tracings) or by computer-assisted methods (e.g., brain electrical activity mapping, BEAM).

The most consistently reported EEG change late in life is a diffuse slowing of the dominant alpha rhythm from a mean frequency of 10 cps to 8 or 9 cps (Obrist, 1963, 1975; Wang & Busse, 1969). The extent of slowing is related to general health, being greatest among persons with cardiac or cerebrovascular disease. Other age-associated findings include increased occurrence of slower rhythms (delta and theta activity, representing $\leq$ 4 cps and 5 to 7 cps, respectively), a high incidence of focal findings (affecting approximately one-third of normal elderly persons), and decreased alpha reactivity or blocking (Duffy & McAnulty, 1988).

Although EEG slowing is a correlate of normal aging, age differences are small compared to those observed with dementia. A majority of patients with primary degenerative dementia (generally, DAT) show slowing into the theta range, compared to only about 7% of normal aged persons (Wang & Busse, 1969). Delta activity is also much more common in dementia than in normal aging (Wang & Busse, 1969).

Recent studies with optimally healthy older adults suggest that only minimal age-related EEG change occurs in the absence of chronic or acute medical illness (Duffy & McAnulty, 1988). Mean alpha frequencies in the range of 9.5 to 9.8 Hz (similar to values reported for young and middle-aged adults) have been reported for very healthy older people, with delta and theta activity either decreasing in old age (Katz & Horowitz, 1982) or showing no age-related change (Giaquinto & Nolfe, 1986).

Other commonly used electrophysiological measures include evoked potentials (EPs) and event-related potentials (ERPs). Unlike the clinical EEG, these measures are correlated in time with the processing of specific stimuli and are believed to reflect certain cognitive operations, particularly sensory discrimination and decision making (see John, Karmel, Corning, Easton, Brown, Ahn, John, Harmoney, Prichep, Toro, Gerson, Bartlett, Thatcher, Kaye, Valdes, & Schwartz, 1977). Very early components of the EP (occurring at 20 msec or less after stimulation) represent the activity of brain stem or thalamic structures. Age differences have been reported for both auditory brain stem evoked responses and somatosensory evoked responses, with longer latencies observed at older ages (see Duffy & McAnulty, 1988, for a review). Much of this change has been attributed to decreased speed of nerve conduction. EPs observed between 30 and 100 msec after stimulation are thought to reflect cortical activation from sensory pathways. Latencies for these components are also prolonged in old age. Analysis of amplitudes suggests that elderly adults may be stimulus "augmenters"; that is, they tend to show increased amplitudes of brain response to more intense stimulation. This augmentation may imply reduced cortical inhibition in old age (Dustman, Snyder, & Schlehuber, 1981).

Late components of the cortical response to stimulation reflect not only automatic effects of stimulus registration but internal reactions (e.g., recognition or surprise) as well. The term event-related potential (ERP) has been adopted to refer to these components. The most widely studied ERP is the P300. This is a positive peak in the waveform that occurs in young adults at about 300 to 500 msec after stimulation, particularly when the subject detects a rare stimulus within a series of more familiar stimuli (the so-called "oddball paradigm").

A number of studies using auditory oddball paradigms have observed an increase in mean latency and a decrease in mean amplitude of the P300 across the adult life span (e.g., Beck, Swanson, & Dustman, 1980; Brown, Marsh, & La Rue, 1983; Goodin, Squires, Henderson, & Starr, 1978). Most investigations suggest that there is an accelerated rate of increase in P300 latency at advanced ages (e.g., Brown *et al.*, 1983; Mullis, Holcomb, Diner, & Dykman, 1985). However, a study of optimally healthy elderly subjects reported only a slight age-related increase in P300 latency (Duffy, Albert, McAnulty, & Garvey, 1984). In young adults, larger P300 amplitudes are observed from parietal recording sites than from frontal sites; in the elderly, amplitudes are about equal for these two regions (e.g., Mullis *et al.*, 1985). This has been interpreted as suggesting selective frontal lobe aging (Duffy & McAnulty, 1988).

Summary of Neurobiological Changes

Neuroanatomically, old and young brains appear to differ in many ways. Older brains are smaller, have decreased quantities of white matter, contain fewer large neurons in several regions, and contain more numerous neuropathological markers, including amyloid deposition, neuritic plaques, neurofibrillary tangles, and granulovacuolar degeneration. Differences in neurotransmitter levels and associated enzymes have also been observed. Most of the evidence for these changes comes from autopsy studies, and there are many conflicting results. Important methodological factors that may affect outcomes include the time between death and the freezing of tissue specimens, the duration and severity of preterminal illness, subjects' drug and nutritional histories, and specific assay and staining techniques (Rogers & Bloom, 1985; Selkoe & Kosik, 1984).

To date, the evidence for normal aging changes in rCBF and brain glucose metabolism is not impressive, particularly when physically healthy subjects are studied. This presents a somewhat different, and less negative, picture of human brain aging. However, the data base with these techniques is still small and methods are constantly being improved; as further studies are completed, a better estimate of the extent and pattern of age changes is likely to emerge.

Electrophysiological data suggest that slowing occurs with advancing age in the rate at which the brain registers sensory information and makes decisions about differences between stimuli. There may also be age differences in modes of cognitive processing (e.g., diminished cortical inhibitory ability). However, some age-related slowing may be due to effects of illness (see Duffy & McAnulty, 1988).

At present, it is difficult to know which neurobiological aging changes are primary and which are secondary. Also, as discussed below, research assessing the functional significance of these changes is very preliminary.

Cognitive Performance

There is an extensive literature on cognitive performance in normal aging which is discussed in detail in Birren and Schaie (1990), Botwinick (1984), and Poon (1980, 1986). Major age differences are listed in Table 3.2 and briefly discussed below.

TABLE 3.2. Age Differences in Cognitive Performance

Measure	Direction of change	Comment
Intelligence		
Crystallized	Stable/ increase	May decline slightly at advanced ages
Fluid	Decline	Begins between 55 and 70; onset varies for cohorts and individuals
Attention		
Simple attention span	Stable	
Selective attention	Decrease	
Concentration	Decrease	
Flexibility	Decrease	Related to fluid intelligence
Divided attention	Inconsistent	
Language		
Everyday communication	Stable	Except with sensory deficit
Phonologic, syntactic knowledge	Stable	Less use of complex syntax
Lexical knowledge	Stable	
Naming	Decrease	Trouble accessing lexicon
Word fluency	Decrease	
Discourse comprehension	Stable	Some decline if complex
Learning and memory		
Sensory memory	Decrease	Registration time increased
Primary memory	Stable	
Secondary memory	Decrease	Less optimal encoding; retrieval problems
Tertiary memory	Inconsistent	
Visuospatial ability		
Judgment of line orientation	Decrease	Stable in healthy aged
Recognition of embedded or incomplete figures	Decrease	
Copying complex figures	Decrease	
Three-dimensional construction	Decrease	
Reasoning and problem-solving		
Self-rated ability	Increase	
Concept identification	Decrease	Less decline for practical concepts
Inquiry	Decrease	Redundant questions
Solving logical problems	Decrease	
Practical reasoning	Variable	May differ for novel versus familiar tasks

Intelligence

An influential model of the effects of normal aging on basic intellectual abilities is the fluid/crystallized conceptualization proposed by Cattell (1963) and subsequently expanded and revised by Horn (e.g., Horn, 1970, 1982). Briefly stated, Cattell (1963) hypothesized that human intellectual abilities could be divided into two broad categories: (1)those dependent on accumulation of formal and informal educational experiences over the course of a lifetime ("crystallized" abilities, Gc), and (2) those reflecting maturational growth and decline of neural structures ("fluid" abilities, Gf). In normal aging, crystallized abilities were expected to improve or remain stable with the passage of time, but fluid abilities were predicted to decline due to decremental changes in the central and peripheral nervous system. Subsequent revisions of the model have treated crystallized and fluid intelligence as overarching (second-order) constructs, and have identified a number of more specific (first-order) intellectual components that vary in relation to age. These include short-term acquisition and retrieval functions, tertiary storage and retrieval functions, and clusters of abilities related to sensory function and cognitive speed.

The primary data base for the fluid/crystallized model is provided by cross-sectional studies of standardized intelligence measures. Different subtests from these batteries are assumed to measure different components in the fluid/crystallized model (Horn, 1985). On the Wechsler intelligence scales (Wechsler, 1955, 1981), for example, Information, Comprehension, Similarities, and Vocabulary are considered measures of crystallized intelligence, performance subtests as fluid intellectual measures, and Digit Span and Arithmetic as measures of short-term acquisition and retrieval.

The possibility that cross-sectional studies may exaggerate intellectual declines due to the confounding of cohort and age effects has received much attention in the literature (see Baltes & Schaie, 1974). Using data from the Seattle Longitudinal Aging Study, in which several birth cohorts have been followed over a period of years, Schaie and colleagues have been able to demonstrate that different cohorts vary in their rates of intellectual change across specific age intervals (see Schaie, 1983, for a review). However, the most recent analyses of data from this study (Hertzog & Schaie, 1986, 1988) suggest that the basic trend toward declining fluid intelligence holds across generations. Decline generally begins at some point between age 55 and 70, with individual differences in the age of transition. This is considerably later in life than was initially postulated in the Cattell/Horn model, lending support to the notion of intellectual stability through the middle years and into early old age.

It has also been questioned whether the declines on fluid intelligence might not be artifactual; i.e., resulting from factors such as reduced sensory acuity, differential familiarity with testing, or simple differences in motor speed. However, correlations between measures of intelligence and visual or auditory acuity have been found to be relatively low in normal aging (Sands & Meredith, 1989), and removing time constraints does not raise total scores of old subjects to the levels of young people (e.g., Storandt, 1977). Older adults' performance on fluid intellectual tests improves considerably with training or unstructured practice (e.g., Willis & Schaie, 1986), indicating that declines are not immutable. However, younger people also benefit from practice on these tasks (e.g., Erber, Botwinick, & Storandt, 1981). Considered together, these studies suggest that fluid intelligence tests are genuinely difficult for older adults. Reduced speed of solution, and problems in grappling with the novelty of procedures, are an integral part of the age-related decrement (see Botwinick, 1984; Salthouse, 1985).

Occasional questions have also been raised about the stability of scores on crystallized intelligence measures. For example, Botwinick and Storandt (1974) expanded the scoring categories for the Vocabulary subtest from the Wechsler Adult Intelligence Scale (WAIS; Wechsler, 1955) and found that elderly subjects were less likely than young adults to give perfect synonyms as responses and more likely to describe examples or uses of the words. Thus, if a more stringent approach were taken to scoring, even Vocabulary scores might be interpreted as showing some decremental age effects. These findings are consistent with other mild age differences in language ability.

Finally, it is important to note that in longitudinal studies of very old subjects (e.g., people in their 80s or older), it is not unusual to observe slight declines on a number of crystallized intelligence measures (see Jarvik & Bank, 1983). This may be due to the fact that a greater proportion of older subjects are experiencing "terminal decline" (i.e., an accelerated loss of performance statistically linked with nearness to death) or may simply suggest that the slope of aging change accelerates in advanced old age.

Attention

On very simple attention tasks such as forward digit span or the mental control subscales of the Wechsler Memory scales (1945, 1987), age differences are absent or small, at least through the early 70s. However, more demanding or complex attention tasks often show marked age effects. For example, on the Trail Making Test, Part B, where a person must shift between series of numbers and letters in completing a visuomotor tracking task, older people are much slower than younger adults (e.g., Davies, 1968), and many score in the range associated with brain damage in younger groups (Heaton, Grant, & Matthews, 1986).

The possible importance of attention in explaining intellectual decline was recently illustrated in a study by Stankov (1988) in which adults in the age range of 20 to 70 years completed a lengthy battery of intelligence and attention tests. Factor analyses suggested three distinct dimensions of attention (concentration, flexibility, search), all of which correlated negatively with age (*r*s ranged from -0.43 to -0.48). Controlling for attentional factors through part-correlation procedures significantly altered the relationship between age and fluid and crystallized intelligence factors. That is, partialling out attentional variance virtually eliminated the age-related decline in Gf and led to an increased estimate of Gc improvement with age. In effect, these data suggest that if older individuals could attend as well as the young, many of the aging declines we have come to anticipate on intelligence testing would be eliminated (see also Hoyer & Plude, 1980).

Learning and Memory

When older people complain about their cognitive abilities, they usually mention problems with memory (Williams, Denney, & Schadler, 1983). Research substantiates many of these complaints but indicates that some aspects of memory are more affected by age than others (see Botwinick, 1984; Craik, 1977; Kausler, 1982; Poon, 1986, for detailed reviews).

Sensory and Primary Memory. Experimental investigations, using very brief presentations of complex stimuli, provide evidence for age-related slowing in sensory memory (e.g., Cerella, Poon, & Fozard, 1982; Walsh, Till, & Williams, 1978). This suggests that older adults require more time than younger people to establish an accurate internal representation of external events. However, since the magnitude of age differences is quite small, sensory memory changes probably have little impact on practical function. Age changes in primary (short-term) memory appear to be negligible. That is, older adults perform about as well as young people on tasks requiring conscious maintenance of a small amount of information over short periods of time (e.g., digit span, word span).

Secondary (Long-Term) Memory. Secondary memory is the area in which the greatest differences between young and old have been reported. This type of memory refers to the acquisition, retention, and retrieval of information over intervals ranging from a few minutes to days or weeks.

Craik (1977) has championed a depth-of-processing interpretation of age effects in secondary memory, in which normal older people are assumed to engage in less extensive and less efficient initial processing of material that they are attempting to learn. Less successful processing results in a degraded memory trace that is subsequently more difficult to retrieve. There is an extensive experimental literature consistent with this notion (see Perlmutter & Mitchell, 1982). For example, older people are less likely than the young to spontaneously use association strategies when learning a list of words (Hulicka & Grossman, 1967). In addition, training studies (e.g., Canestrari, 1968; Hulicka & Grossman, 1967; Treat, Poon, & Fozard, 1981) show marked short-term benefits of instructing older subjects in the use of such mnemonic strategies as visual imagery and verbal associations or the method of loci (Robertson-Tchabo, Hausman, & Arenberg, 1976).

Retrieval deficits may also contribute to secondary memory problems. Recognition memory exceeds free recall at all ages, but the magnitude of difference is often greater for the old than the young (e.g., Craik & McDowd, 1987; Kaszniak, Poon, & Riege, 1986). This suggests that older people may be less efficient than the young at retrieving information that they know.

Recent studies have begun to ask *why* older subjects have less effective encoding and retrieval processes. One hypothesis is that older people have more limited resources in terms of energy and attention; therefore, they will encounter the greatest problems on tasks that require a substantial outlay of effort (e.g., Hasher & Zacks, 1979; Craik & McDowd, 1987). Free recall of specific details is an effortful process, requiring the subject to engage in self-initiated activity during both the learning and retrieval phases; by contrast, in a recognition test, appropriate mental operations are cued by the re-presentation of external stimuli (Craik & McDowd, 1987).

The differential effort hypothesis receives some support from studies in which subjects are asked to perform a secondary task (generally, choice reaction time) at the same time while attempting to recognize or recall a list of words (Macht & Buschke, 1983; Craik & McDowd, 1987). Disproportionate slowing during recall is noted for older subjects, suggesting greater "energy costs" of recall processes in old age.

Investigators concerned about the validity of laboratory tests have hypothesized that memory for activities might be a more natural task for elderly subjects than recalling arbitrary lists of words or geometric designs. The first studies to examine this possibility reported an absence of age differences on free recall of simple subject-performed activities like drawing a circle or clapping hands (e.g., Backman, 1985). This finding generated great interest in the field, because it was one of the few demonstrations of equality of memory for young and old adults. However, on longer list of actions, age-related deficits have subsequently been observed (Cohen, Sandler, & Schroeder, 1987; Guttentag & Hunt, 1988). This type of research is only one aspect of a broader line of investigation focusing on "everyday memory" and aging (see West, 1986, for a review). The variability in tasks and procedures limits the generalizations that can be drawn from these studies (West, 1986). It is safe to state, however, that on many "everyday" tasks as well as many "artificial" ones, older subjects often perform more poorly than younger comparison groups. Even in areas of expertise such as bridge-playing, age-related deficits in recall have been observed (e.g., Charness, 1981).

Although the finding of age differences on secondary memory tasks is one of the most robust outcomes in the study of normal aging, substantial subgroup and individual differences have been observed. For example, Craik, Byrd, and Swanson (1987) found that volunteers in their 70s from affluent retirement communities performed as well as young college undergraduates on tests of verbal fluency, paired associate learning, and verbal free recall. And, within a large group of elderly community residents, Arbuckle, Gold, and Andres (1986) found that education and intellectual activity were better predictors of performance on memory tests than chronological age.

Tertiary (Remote) Memory. Anecdotally, older adults' recall of people and events from early in their lives is often very impressive. When asked to describe how their memories operate, many older people will comment on the clarity of remote memories in contrast to the events of the last few days or weeks.

Literature on tertiary (remote) memory is mixed with respect to the existence of age-related change. In part, this is because this aspect of memory is very difficult to measure. On tests of recall of faces or names of famous people, or important historical events, it is impossible to control for degree of initial exposure to the material, or for subsequent rehearsal (Craik, 1977).

Using one of the best public events questionnaires devised to date, Howes and Katz (1988) recently reported significant age differences in remote recall between young, middle-aged, and elderly groups. The elderly subjects had a fairly constant level of recall across all of the time periods (spanning an interval of 50 years), but they performed worse than middle-aged subjects for time periods that both age groups had lived through.

Bahrick, Bahrick, and Wittlinger (1975) took a more personal approach to the study of tertiary memory, examining recall and recognition for high-school graduating classmates over intervals of 3 to nearly 50 years. On recognition and matching tasks, for either names or pictures of faces, approximately 90% accuracy was observed for at least 15 years after graduation, and performance on picture recognition remained high through 35 years after graduation. A significant drop in performance was noted after 48 years, but even the oldest subjects were able to recognize the names and photos of about 70% of their former classmates.

Overall, the research on tertiary memory suggests the presence of age effects, but the reliability of this finding varies, most likely because of differences in the method used to measure remote remembering.

Language

In the absence of significant auditory or visual impairment, everyday communication is well maintained in old age (Bayles & Kaszniak, 1987). Age does not appear to erode a person's knowledge of the sounds of language and rules for their combination (phonologic knowledge). Syntactic knowledge, i.e., knowing how to meaningfully combine words, is also well-maintained, although some studies report age differences in the correct use of grammar and syntax (Bayles & Kaszniak, 1987), and in spontaneous speech, older people may avoid the use of grammatical forms and syntactic structures that place a heavy demand on memory (Kynette & Kemper, 1986).

Word knowledge is another area of comparative strength for older adults, as suggested by vocabulary testing and lexical decision tasks (e.g., Bowles & Poon, 1985). If young and old subjects are presented with strings of letters and asked to decide which are actual words, no age differences are observed in either accuracy or speed. However, if given definitions of target words and asked to supply the names, old adults are slower and less accurate than younger subjects (Bowles & Poon, 1985). This suggests a breakdown with age in access to lexical knowledge.

Problems with lexical access are also suggested by studies of confrontation naming, where young adults generally outperform elderly subjects (e.g., Albert *et al.*, 1988; Borod, Goodglass, & Kaplan, 1980). Semantic association errors, circumlocutions, and perceptual errors all increase with age, but phonologic errors do not (Albert *et al.*, 1988). Each common error type suggests that older people possess correct word information, but they seem to have difficulty retrieving precise words within a semantic field. In effect, these data confirm what older patients will often report during testing, i.e., that they know the item, but just cannot think of its name.

On verbal fluency testing, older people generally produce fewer words in a limited time than younger subjects (e.g., Albert *et al.*, 1988; Benton & Hamsher, 1976; Borod *et al.*, 1980). Age effects are generally small in absolute magnitude, but the downward trend with increasing age is quite consistent, particularly if subjects are over the age of 70.

In discourse, older adults often produce more verbose and elaborate responses than middle-aged individuals. For example, when asked to write a description of a picture, Obler (1980) found 70- and 80-year-olds produced more complex, embedded sentences; in oral description, there was greater personalization, repetition of items, redundancy, and use of indefinite terms such as "something" in the speech of older adults compared to middle-aged people. Age differences in comprehension of discourse have also been documented, particularly if the listener must recall story content or draw an inference based on the material presented (Cohen, 1979; Ulatowska, Hayaski, Cannito, & Fleming, 1986).

Visuospatial Abilities

Performance on simple tests of visual perception such as judging line orientation may not be greatly affected by age. In one study of healthy and well-educated subjects, most people in their 80s (92%) scored within two standard deviations of the norm for people in their 50s (Benton, Eslinger, & Damasio, 1981).

Complex visual perception tasks produce larger age effects. Older adults perform worse than middle-aged or young adults on visual-closure tests that require the identification of figures from incomplete drawings (Danziger & Salthouse, 1978; Read, 1988), and on embedded figure tasks, where a simple geometric pattern must be identified within a complex random design (Axelrod & Cohen, 1961; Capitani, Sala, Lucchelli, Soave, & Spinnler, 1988). Older people also find it harder to match pictures of unfamiliar faces (Benton *et al.*, 1981; Benton, Van Allen, Hamsher, & Levi, 1978) and to critique their copies of three-dimensional designs (Plude, Milberg, & Cerella, 1986).

Age-related declines in visuospatial abilities are also suggested by studies of fluid intelligence, where many of the pertinent tasks (e.g., WAIS performance subtests) involve visuoperceptual or visuomotor activities.

Reasoning and Problem Solving

Most older adults believe that their problem-solving abilities improve with age (Denney & Palmer, 1981). However, research does not concur with self-appraisal. This discrepancy appears to stem from the fact that older people and researchers have different things in mind when they refer to problem solving. When queried about what they meant by problem solving, older people indicated "everyday problems," such as financial difficulties (Denney & Palmer, 1981). By contrast, most laboratory studies have focused on tasks requiring specific forms of logical reasoning, often presented in abstract terms.

Older adults have more difficulty than younger people in forming and inferring concepts. When instructed to ask questions that will help them identify which of several pictures an examiner has in mind (the "Twenty Questions" game), older people ask more questions that eliminate only one alternative at a time, as opposed to those that eliminate categories of alternatives (Denney & Denney, 1982). In more explicit categorization or classification tasks, elderly subjects are more likely than young adults to arrange stimuli to form designs, rather than grouping according to superordinate concepts; they also are more likely to group objects on the basis of functional relationships (e.g., a knife slicing an orange) as opposed to abstract semantic relationships (e.g., orange and banana grouped as fruits). Similarly, when presented with a series of stimuli that differ in multiple dimensions (e.g., shape, color, size) and asked to infer a particular dimension as "correct" based on feedback from the examiner, older people have been reported to perform very poorly; many appear to respond randomly on such tasks and to receive no benefit from feedback provided across the trials (Offenbach, 1974).

Problems with concept formation may be reduced on tasks that involve more familiar stimuli (Arenberg, 1968). However, even on more familiar tasks, declines begin to become apparent for people in their 70s. In longitudinal analyses, Arenberg (1982) found that older participants made many repetitious selections, particularly on tasks that they were unable to solve correctly. This suggested a form of information overload, with older subjects finding it hard to review their past selections and plan the next step in situations where they had already made many previous choices. Redundant inquiry and disorganization have also been noted on problem-solving tasks. For example, Welford (1958) presented young and middle-aged people with a task simulating the servicing of radios. While attempting to discover the correspondence between terminals on a box (the "radio") and those drawn on a circuit diagram, older adults took many more redundant meter readings, suggesting to Welford that they had difficulty making sense of the results of their inquiry.

Some age-related deficits in reasoning may be due to educational differences or other confounded factors. In a study comparing middle-aged and elderly people on Piagetian problem-solving tasks (e.g., discovering factors that affect oscillation of a pendulum or swing), younger and older samples were matched for educational level as well as for physical health (La Rue & Waldbaum, 1980). The two age groups did not differ in their use of concrete versus formal operational reasoning. However, education and health effects were significant; people with a high school education or less, and those with health problems, produced more concrete solutions than college-educated, optimally healthy subjects.

Although logical problem solving is not an area of strength for most old people, performance improves with practice and training (e.g., Sanders, Sterns, Smith, & Sanders, 1975). In fact, in this area of cognitive performance, opportunities for unstructured practice may provide longer-lasting benefits than specific logical training (Blackburn, Papalia-Finlay, Foye, & Serlin, 1988).

Summary of Cognitive Changes with Normal Aging

In later life, some aspects of cognitive performance remain stable while others reliably decline. Tasks that require demonstration of verbal-cultural knowledge in an unpaced format show minimal normal aging change, whereas novel tasks, often requiring visuospatial processing, speeded perceptual-motor integration, or logical reasoning, generally result in age declines. In the Cattell–Horn model, the former types of tasks are assumed to tap crystallized intelligence, and the latter, fluid intelligence.

Primary and tertiary memory are relatively stable with age, but substantial deficits are noted in secondary memory. Some of these deficits may be due to a passive learning style; i.e., older people use mnemonic and organizational strategies less often than younger adults, which, in turn, may reflect diminished effort and attentional resources.

Some normal older people have more cognitive problems than others. Important moderating factors include age itself (with greater problems observed in the 70s and 80s than in the 60s), educational/SES level (some advantaged older people outscore young adults), and physical health (even moderate, stable health problems are predictive of lower cognitive scores).

A distinguishing feature of cognitive performance in normal older adults is plasticity. Even in areas of comparative weakness (e.g., secondary memory and concept formation), impressive gains in performance are observed with training and practice.

RELATING NEUROBIOLOGICAL AND BEHAVIORAL CHANGE

Biological and behavioral aging research has proceeded on parallel tracts, with biological changes studied by different researchers, using different methods and models, than behavioral changes. For neuropsychologists, however, the few studies that have interrelated biological and behavioral variables are of particular interest.

Historically, the principal data base in human neuropsychology has been obtained by studying individuals with acquired brain injury, and in particular, those with discrete brain lesions. The value of this literature for understanding normal brain function has long been a matter of debate. In aging where changes develop slowly across a broad range of neurobiological measures, it may be particularly difficult to extrapolate from lesion investigations.

Nonetheless, the literature contains some attempts to interpret normal aging changes in light of performance of brain-damaged patients. A right-hemisphere hypothesis has been advanced (e.g., Klisz, 1978) based on similarities in cognitive performance between normal older people and patients with right-hemisphere lesions. There are several problems with this interpretation. The data base for this comparison was limited to studies using the WAIS and the Halstead–Reitan Neuropsychological Battery (Reitan & Davison, 1974), neither of which adequately evaluates learning and memory; it is unlikely that patients with focal right-hemisphere deficits would have similar learning and memory deficits as normal older adults. Also, in neurobiological studies, there is little evidence that age changes are lateralized to the right hemisphere. A frontal-deficit hypothesis of normal aging changes has also been advanced (e.g., Albert & Kaplan, 1980; Hochanadel & Kaplan, 1984; Mittenberg, Seidenberg, O'Leary, & DiGiulio, 1988). Older people make some of the same types of errors on neuropsychological tests as patients with frontal lesions (Albert & Kaplan, 1980; Hochanadel & Kaplan, 1984). Also, in an investigation comparing performance of younger and older subjects on tests designed to evaluate frontal, temporal, and parietal functions, the strongest correlations were observed between age and frontal measures (Mittenberg *et al.*, 1988). In addition, there are occasional findings in the neurobiological literature suggestive of prominent frontal lobe aging (e.g., neuronal loss in the superior frontal cortex, scattered reports of frontal glucose hypometabolism, and augmented EP amplitude in older subjects). However, findings such as neuronal loss, plaques and tangles, and neurotransmitter changes occur in many other brain regions as well. Also, relationships between the frontal lobes and behavioral functions are exceedingly complex and difficult to evaluate with a few psychometric measures. In this author's opinion, it is premature to try to attribute normal aging changes in cognition to selective frontal impairment.

Researchers specializing in aging have emphasized the importance of studying multiple brain regions and multiple neurobiological measures in relation to cognitive change. This is difficult work because it entails the combined methodological problems of both neurobiological and behavioral research, in addition to the problems resulting from multiple correlational comparisons.

There have been several cross-validation studies relating measures of cognitive performance to neuropathological findings (see Fuld, 1986, for a review). Usually, both pathological and normal control groups have been included in this research. An example of this type of study was recently reported by Katzman, Terry, DeTeresa, Brown, Davies, Fuld, Renbing, and Peck (1988). Subjects were 137 very old (mean age 85.5 years) residents of a nursing home who were given brief cognitive testing on a yearly basis; after death, autopsies were performed examining cell counts, numbers of neuritic plaques and neurofibrillary tangles, and levels of CAT and somatostatin. The cognitive tests consisted of a shortened version of the Information–Memory–Concentration test (Blessed, Tomlinson, & Roth, 1968; Katzman, Brown, Fuld, Peck, Schechter, & Schimmel, 1983) and a multitrial object recall test (Fuld, 1981). Neuroanatomical and neurochemical data were obtained from eight brain regions: midfrontal, superior temporal, and inferior parietal cortex, cingulate gyrus, visual cortex, hippocampus, amygdala, substantia innominata, substantia nigra, locus coeruleus, and cerebellar vermis.

Subjects were separated into four groups on the basis of their cognitive and neuropathological findings. There were two cognitively normal groups, one without evidence of Alzheimer brain pathology (n = 19) and another with moderate findings consistent with Alzheimer's disease such as elevated numbers of neuritic plaques and reduced CAT (n = 10). There were also two cognitively impaired groups, with and without evidence of Alzheimer brain changes (n = 76 and 32, respectively). The most intriguing aspect of the results concerned the cognitively normal subjects whose brains contained evidence of Alzheimer's changes. Brains in this group were heavier on the average than any other group, and they also contained more large neurons in several brain regions. The investigators speculated that these subjects may have had "incipient Alzheimer's disease" but did not show it behaviorally because of greater brain reserve. A second important finding was that, in general, brains of demented and nondemented patients in this very-old sample did not differ by as great a margin as has been noted in younger samples. A final, humbling, result was that for 11% of the clinically demented subjects, there was no evidence on autopsy of Alzheimer-type pathology or other cerebral pathology that might have been the cause of poor performance.

This study illustrates that most older people with severe cognitive impairments have brain changes consistent with Alzheimer's disease. However what it says about normal aging is less clear. A broad range of neuropathological findings was observed in patients with normal cognitive performance. How some functioned well despite indications of Alzheimer changes is a question that warrants further study.

Recent biobehavioral investigations using PET techniques have emphasized the importance of considering functioning, interactive brain systems when attempting to explain behavioral outcomes (Riege, Harker, & Metter, 1986). This idea is certainly not new (Luria, 1974); however, technical advances have made it possible to study these dynamic brain–behavior relations in a more direct and quantitative way. This is till very difficult to do, however, and there are relatively few investigations focusing on normal aging. One example that illustrates the complexity of this endeavor is a study by Riege, Metter, Kuhl, and Phelps (1985) who examined glucose metabolism in multiple brain regions for 23 subjects (aged 27 to 78 years) who also completed an extensive battery of memory measures. Eighteen different brain regions were examined and compared to performance on 18 different cognitive tests. Older subjects generally performed poorly on memory tests compared to younger adults. By contrast, age was unrelated to regional glucose metabolic rates, except in an area of the left inferior frontal lobe (at or near Broca's area), where hypometabolism was observed in older subjects. Metabolic rates in this region correlated significantly with performance on tasks requiring retrieval of words, sentences, and designs from secondary memory. Intercorrelations between metabolic rates for frontal and subcortical regions decreased in strength with age, suggesting that for older adults, there may be reduced interaction between these regions during memory activities.

This study was carefully conducted and findings were assessed in a thorough and statistically cautious manner. However, the number of subjects was very small (e.g., there were only eight people in the old-age group) compared to the number of variables measured. Other aspects of methods may also have affected results. For example, PET and cognitive testing were conducted on different days, separated by an interval of up to 1 week. In addition, subjects were evaluated in an eyes-open resting state during PET that may have affected levels of activity observed in different regions (see Metter, 1988). Finally, limits in the PET procedure per se must be appreciated; e.g., regions of interest for computing metabolic rates were identified by subjective visual analysis of PET records, and the scanner provided relatively poor resolution of hippocampal structures that may be crucial for learning and memory.

As these two investigations illustrate, research interrelating neurobiological and behavioral changes in human aging is still very preliminary. Neuroanatomical cross-validation studies document a rough correlation between behavioral performance and neuroanatomical findings across a normal to severely impaired range, but many exceptions are observed (e.g., cognitively normal old people with brain changes consistent with Alzheimer's disease). In addition, the mechanisms by which specific neuroanatomic findings may relate to behavioral impairments are poorly understood. Techniques such as PET provide greater potential for measuring the brain in action, but there have been few studies focusing on normal aging and many technical limitations that remain to be overcome.

DEMENTIA OF THE ALZHEIMER TYPE

Autopsy studies indicate that at least 50% of elderly, cognitively impaired patients have brain changes consistent with Alzheimer's disease, either alone or in combination with cerebrovascular pathology (e.g., Katzman *et al.*, 1988; Tomlinson, Blessed, & Roth, 1970). Currently, there are no medical tests that can confirm the presence of Alzheimer's disease prior to death. Instead, patients are diagnosed as having dementia of the Alzheimer type (DAT), provided that their behavior and clinical laboratory findings meet specified criteria (American Psychiatric Association, 1987; McKhann, Drachman, Folstein, Katzman, Price, & Stadlan, 1984). Neuropsychological assessment is routinely included in diagnostic work-ups for possible dementing illness.

Detailed discussions of neurobiological and neuropsychological findings in DAT can be found in Albert and Moss (1988), Bayles and Kaszniak (1987), Poon (1986), Scheibel and Wechsler (1986), and Wurtman (1985). Relative to normal aging, the number of large neurons in cortical and subcortical regions may be reduced in DAT by 40% or more, CAT levels decline by 50 to 90%, and neurofibrillary tangles are observed in the cortex in addition to the hippocampus (see Katzman *et al.*, 1988; Wurtman, 1985). Brain amyloid is observed in nearly all DAT cases, and neuritic plaques and granulovacuolar degeneration are typically more numerous and widely dispersed throughout the brain (see Kemper, 1984; and preceding section on Neurobiology of Aging).

The cognitive deficits of DAT vary with duration or severity of illness (see Burke, Miller, Rubin, Morris, Coben, Duchek, Wittels, & Berg, 1988; Hughes, Berg, Danziger, Coben, & Martin, 1982; Reisberg, Ferris, de Leon, & Crook, 1982; Reisberg, Ferris, de Leon, Sinaiko, Franssen, Kluger, Mir, Borenstein, George, Shulman, Steinberg, & Cohen, 1988, for examples of severity rating scales). Marked impairment of recent (secondary) memory is the first symptom that most relatives or clinical observers report (e.g., Sim & Sussman, 1962), and in formal testing of a mildly impaired patient, this is the area in which the most pronounced impairment is likely to be observed. The memory deficit is quantitatively more severe than that associated with normal aging (e.g., Hart, Kwentus, Hamer, & Taylor, 1987*a*; La Rue, D'Elia, Clark, Spar, & Jarvik, 1986*a*; Miller, 1971; Wilson, Bacon, Fox, & Kaszniak, 1983), affects acquisition or storage as well as retrieval (Hart *et al.*, 1987*a*; La Rue *et al.*, 1986*a*), occurs on automatic as well as effortful processing tasks (Shimamura, Salmon, Squire, & Butters, 1987), and is generally not responsive to cueing or organization (Granholm & Butters, 1988; Weingartner, Kaye, Smallberg, Ebert, Gillin, & Sitaram, 1981*a*). Other common early signs of DAT include word-finding problems and deficits on perceptual-motor integrative tasks that clearly exceed norms established for healthy aging. In moderately impaired patients, a broader pattern of deficits emerges, with many other language, visuospatial, and reasoning impairments observed. At least mild impairments of immediate (primary) memory can be seen on careful testing (e.g., Wilson *et al.*, 1983) and retrieval from remote (tertiary) memory becomes less reliable. There may also be personality changes, with specific symptoms varying between individuals and stages of illness (Petry, Cummings, Hill, & Shapira, 1988; Rubin, Morris, Storandt, & Berg, 1986).

Research indicates that there may be variability in the pattern of cognitive impairments in early stages of illness (e.g., Martin, Browers, Cox, Teleska, Fedio, Foster, & Chase, 1986). By far the most common pattern is pronounced secondary memory impairment accompanied by both anomic language changes and visuospatial or perceptual-motor impairments. However, for some patients, language changes may occur in isolation of visuospatial impairments, or vice versa. Whether these performance patterns reflect different forms of the disease, perhaps with different biological or genetic substrates, is an unresolved question (see critical review by Jorm, 1985). There has also been considerable discussion concerning early versus late-onset illness. Until a few years ago, dementia with presenile onset (before age 60 to 65) was considered a separate disease from "senile dementia." As autopsy data accumulated confirming the presence of common pathological markers in both groups, the one-disease model became the accepted view. However, there are indications that early onset disease may have a higher genetic loading (e.g., Heston, Mastri, Anderson, & White, 1981) and that clinical symptoms may be more severe than those of late-onset DAT (e.g., Filley, Kelly, & Heaton, 1986). The role of other individual difference factors (e.g., premorbid ability level, education, gender) has not been clearly documented.

Several studies comparing mildly impaired DAT patients with age-matched normal controls show that acceptable group discrimination can be achieved with brief neuropsychological screening batteries. For example, Storandt, Botwinick, Danziger, Berg, and Hughes (1984) reported highly accurate classification based on a combination of three well-known measures, Logical Memory from the Wechsler Memory Scale (Wechsler, 1945), verbal fluency (Benton & Hamsher, 1976), and Trails A (Reitan, 1958), Eslinger, Damasio, Benton, and Van Allen (1985) achieved comparable discrimination with the Iowa Screening Battery for Mental decline, composed of a brief measure of temporal orientation, the revised Visual Retention Test (Benton, 1974), and verbal fluency (Benton & Hamsher, 1976). It is important to recognize, however, that these batteries simply screen for the presence of dementia and do not specifically identify DAT. In a replication study using the same battery as Storandt and colleagues, much lower rates of classification were noted when patients with other organic disorders (e.g., multi-infarct dementia, alcoholic dementia, Parkinson's disease) were contrasted with DAT patients (Tierney, Snow, Reid, Zorzitto, & Fisher, 1987).

There have been occasional attempts to identify test outcomes that may be specific to DAT. For example, Fuld (1984) proposed that a particular pattern of WAIS subtests might be useful in distinguishing DAT patients from those with multi-infarct dementia. However, the pattern had low specificity even in Fuld's original data, and replication studies have generally failed to support the diagnostic utility of the pattern (Filley, Kobayashi, & Heaton, 1987). The presence of intrusion errors has also been described as a possible behavioral marker for DAT (Fuld, Katzman, Davies, & Terry, 1982), but these too are commonly observed in other brain disorders.

At present, cognitive test findings must be combined with history and laboratory findings to make an accurate clinical diagnosis of DAT. When the full set of recommended procedures is used in clinical diagnosis (McKhann *et al.*, 1984), fairly high rates of confirmation of Alzheimer-type brain changes are likely to be observed on autopsy (Fox, Penn, Clasen, Martin, Wilson, & Savoy, 1986; Tierney, Fisher, Anthony, Zorzitto, Snow, Reid, & Nieuwstraten, 1988).

Although Alzheimer's disease is the most likely etiology for persistent cognitive impairment in old age, there are many other possible causes (see National Institute on Aging Task Force, 1980). Impairments can result from improper medication, severe affective or other psychiatric disorder, cerebro- and cardiovascular events, and a host of chronic medical illnesses. Situational changes (e.g., hospitalization), pain, and sensory deficits can also cause either acute or gradual declines in cognitive performance, especially when superimposed on other normal aging changes.

DEPRESSION IN OLDER ADULTS

Depression is another common disorder in older people, affecting as many as 15% of community-resident people over the age of 65 (Blazer & Williams, 1980) and 25% or more of older people hospitalized because of medical illness (Small & Fawzy, 1988; Rapp *et al.*, 1988). Depression appears to affect older people in much the same way as younger adults and many of the same treatments can be used with younger and older patients to alleviate depressive symptoms (see Jarvik, Mintz, Steuer, & Gerner, 1982; La Rue *et al.*, 1985; Thompson, Gallagher, & Breckenridge, 1987). However, certain features of depression may be more prevalent or pronounced in older patients, and as a result, there may be an increased rate of diagnostic errors.

Older patients' scores on depression rating scales may be inflated by endorsement of somatic symptoms. In part, this reflects the higher level of actual medical illness among older people. In addition, however, older patients may be prone to "masked depression," in which somatic complaints are exaggerated and psychological symptoms underreported. Despite these problems, recent studies indicate that standard depression rating scales can be effectively used to screen for geriatric depression (e.g., Norris, Gallagher, Wilson & Winograd, 1987), and that use of such scales may help to curb oversight of depression in older medical patients (Rapp *et al.*, 1988).

Older depressed patients may also experience striking cognitive deficits. This is by no means the predominant pattern, since many studies show minimal cognitive impairment in older depressed patients relative to age-matched controls (see Niederehe, 1986, for a review). However, for 10% to 20% of depressed older adults, cognitive problems are severe enough to rival the deficits produced by organic dementia (McAllister, 1983; Rabins, 1983). This combination of cognitive and affective symptoms has been referred to as depressive pseudodementia (Caine, 1981; Wells, 1979), or more accurately, as dementia syndrome of depression (Folstein & McHugh, 1978). Correct diagnosis of dementia syndrome of depression is complicated by the fact that many patients with Alzheimer-type or multi-infarct dementia develop depressive symptoms (e.g., Liston, 1977; Reifler, Larson, & Hanley, 1982). Thus, combinations of cognitive and depressive symptoms can have different underlying causes.

Dementia syndrome of depression can only be clearly identified on a post hoc basis; that is, when cognitive performance returns to normal as depression lifts. However, monitoring of certain clinical features may facilitate identification of patients with this condition. According to Wells (1979), depressive pseudodementia is likely to be characterized by some or all of the following features: a history of prior depressive episodes; mood disturbance antedating cognitive problems in the current episode; abrupt onset and rapid progression of cognitive deficits; circumscribed as opposed to global impairment on mental status examination; frequent "don't know" answers on cognitive testing; and incongruity between performance on testing and everyday cognitive function.

These guidelines have not been validated in any large-scale longitudinal investigations. However, one recent study (Reynolds, Hoch, Kupfer, Buysse, Houck, Stack, & Campbell, 1988) compared pretreatment clinical characteristics for patients diagnosed with depressive pseudodementia or primary degenerative dementia (most likely, DAT). Pseudodemented subjects were selected on the basis of several criteria, including a positive response to treatment with antidepressant medication with parallel cognitive benefits. Compared to the patients with dementia, those with pseudodementia had initially presented with milder global cognitive impairment, more severe depressive symptomatology, and fewer problems with everyday activities such as finding one's way around familiar streets. On a quantitative mental status exam, pseudodemented patients had as many problems as the "true" demented patients on delayed recall, repetition of a phrase, and following the three-stage command, but they outperformed the demented group on orientation, registration, calculations, and language and visuographic items.

This study and many others show that certain patients with mixed symptoms of depression and dementia improve substantially with treatment and maintain these gains for at least a year or two (e.g., La Rue, Spar, & Hill, 1986*b*; Post, 1966; Rabins, Merchant, & Nestadt, 1984). However, it is unlikely that brief screening instruments will prove sufficient to reliably distinguish these patients from those who have depressive symptoms in addition to mild dementia of the Alzheimer or multi-infarct type. More extensive neuropsychological evaluation can sometimes be helpful in this differentiation.

There is a rapidly expanding literature on cognition in depression (see Johnson & Magaro, 1987, and Weingartner & Silberman, 1982, for reviews). Most recent work has focused on learning and memory, examining performance on effortful as opposed to automatic tasks (Hasher & Zacks, 1979). Depressed patients generally perform poorly compared to age-matched controls on tasks that require significant spontaneous effort, e.g., learning and recall of unorganized lists of words (e.g., Hart *et al.*, 1987*a*; Roy-Byrne, Weingartner, Bierer, Thompson, & Post, 1986; Weingartner, Cohen, Murphy, Martello, & Gerdt, 1981*b*); by contrast, they often show no impairment on less direct or demanding memory procedures, e.g., judging how often they have recently encountered a particular stimulus (Roy-Byrne *et al.*, 1986), recognizing short lists of words (Cummings & Benson, 1984), learning highly organized word lists (Weingartner *et al.*, 1981*b*), or incidental recall (Hart, Kwentus, Wade, & Hamer, 1987*b*). These findings have been interpreted as suggesting that, in depression, memory impairment is directly related to the capacity for sustained effort (e.g., Weingartner *et al.*, 1981*b*), which, in turn, may be mediated by catecholaminergic deficiency (e.g., Reus, Silberman, Post, & Weingartner, 1979) or other dysfunctions of subcortical brain structures (Caine, 1981; Cummings & Benson, 1984). This pattern of memory deficit stands in contrast to that observed in DAT and other cortical dementias, where impairment has been noted on certain automatic as well as effortful memory tasks (Shimamura *et al.*, 1987). However, it is not unlike the pattern observed in normal aging, as discussed above.

Whether the effortful/automatic distinction will prove useful for clinical identification of dementia syndrome of depression is not known. Depressed inpatients have problems with multiple aspects of learning and memory (La Rue, 1989) and many other cognitive tasks as well. It is still advisable to observe treatment response to clarify diagnosis. In our own work on this topic, we found that cognitively impaired depressed patients benefited as much from treatment as those who were cognitively intact, but that a longer and more aggressive course of treatment was required to achieve equivalent benefit (La Rue *et al.*, 1986*b*).

SUMMARY AND IMPLICATIONS FOR CLINICAL ASSESSMENT

Normal aging involves many neurobiological changes. The significance of any single change for explaining behavioral developments is largely a matter of speculation. The next decade of research is likely to provide exciting new advances in knowledge of brain–behavior relations in humans of all ages, but at present, it is important to recognize that procedures such as CT or PET scans cannot substitute for neuropsychological assessment of functional abilities.

Decline is clearly present in normal cognitive aging. However, some aspects of cognition decline more than others. Areas showing relatively pronounced changes include fluid intellectual abilities, sustained and complex attentional processes, secondary memory, accessing of word knowledge, visuospatial abilities, and reasoning and problem-solving. Areas of relative preservation include crystallized verbal intelligence, simple attention, primary and tertiary memory, and everyday communication through language. A distinctive feature of normal older-adult cognition is plasticity, with improvements commonly noted as a result of cueing, training, or even unstructured practice. In clinical neuropsychological assessment, it is important to learn to recognize the distinctive features of normal aging, so that illness will not be overdiagnosed. Referring to normative tables is not a substitute for understanding age-related patterns, in part because age norms are still absent or unrepresentative for many measures, and more importantly, because static norms do not encompass expected benefits of practice, training, or testing of limits.

There are marked individual differences in rates of cognitive aging. These are related in part to other well-known individual difference parameters such as level of education or socioeconomic status. Physical health is another crucial mediator; even those with subclinical change may show deficits relative to optimally healthy people. These observations underscore the need to select normative reference points with caution and careful attention to the individual. Unless the person being evaluated is truly exceptional in terms of educational background and physical health, it is probably inappropriate to compare his or her performance to norms reported in studies of optimally aging people. Also, in a person with cognitive deficits and chronic medical illness (e.g., cardiovascular disease or chronic obstructive pulmonary disease), it is best to compare performance to medical neuropsychological norms before concluding that impairments reflect an independent, neurodegenerative condition such as Alzheimer-type dementia.

Normal aging changes overlap with those observed in dementia, neurobiologically and behaviorally. Cognitive changes in DAT are typically more pronounced quantitatively, and in some cases, qualitative analysis will also provide clear demarcation (e.g., as when multiple intrusion errors are observed). However, in very early stages of DAT, neuropsychological differentiation from advanced normal aging may be difficult. In such cases, careful consideration must be given to the risk/benefit ratio for different types of diagnostic errors. On the whole, it is probably most important to minimize false-positive errors, since mistakes of this type can have serious detrimental consequences for older adults in terms of restricting independence and access to medical treatment. In some situations, however, false-negative errors may cause unnecessary stress on family members who are attempting to cope with behaviors of the patient that they cannot understand or manage in usual ways.

Aging may compound the cognitive deficits that accompany depression. Whether this represents a true interaction of aging and depressive illness, or simply additive effects of separate processes, is unclear. However, in assessing any older depressed adult with cognitive problems, the hypothesis of depressive pseudodementia must be given the benefit of the doubt. This possibility is strengthened with a subject's performance is clearly compromised by diminished effort or attention. However, 10 to 20% of older depressed inpatients will have impairments even on simple tasks that require little effort. Particularly in these cases, it is important to track response to treatment before forming firm diagnostic impressions.

Finally, even for older adults where diagnostic impressions are quite clear, neuropsychological testing may play an important role in treatment and management decisions, Neuropsychological tests provide one of the best means of monitoring the effectiveness of specific pharmacologic and behavioral treatments and can help to identify individuals who may benefit from rehabilitation or more basic supportive activities such as adult day-care.

REFERENCES

Albert, M. L. (Ed.). (1984). *Clinical neurology of aging*. New York: Oxford University Press.

Albert, M. S. (1981). Geriatric neuropsychology. *Journal of Consulting and Clinical Psychology*, *49*, 835–850.

Albert, M. S., & Kaplan, E. (1980). Organic implications of neuropsychological deficits in the elderly. In L. W. Poon & J. L. Fozard (Eds.), *New directions in memory and aging* (pp. 403–432). Hillsdale, N.J.: Erlbaum.

Albert, M. S., & Moss, M. B. (Eds.). (1988). *Geriatric neuropsychology*. New York: Guilford Press.

Albert, M. S., & Stafford, J. L. (1988). Computed tomography studies. In M. S. Albert & M. B. Moss (Eds.), *Geriatric Neuropsychology* (pp. 211–227). New York: Guilford Press.

Albert, M. S., Heller, H. S., & Milberg, W. (1988). Changes in naming ability with age. *Psychology and Aging*, *3*, 173–178.

American Psychiatric Association. (1987). *Diagnostic and statistical manual of mental disorders (DSM-III-R)* (3rd ed., revised). Washington D.C.: Author.

Arbuckle, T. Y., Gold, D., & Andres, D. (1986). Cognitive functioning of older people in relation to social and personality variables. *Psychology and Aging, 1*, 55–62.

Arenberg, D. (1968). Concept problem solving in young and old adults. *Journal of Gerontology, 23*, 279–282.

Arenberg, D. (1982). Changes with age in problem solving, In F. I. M. Craik & S. Trehub (Eds.), *Aging and cognitive processes* (pp. 221–236). New York: Plenum Press.

Axelrod, S., & Cohen, L. D. (1961). Senescence and embedded-figure performance in vision and touch. *Perceptual and Motor Skills, 12*, 283–288.

Backman, L. (1985). Further evidence for the lack of adult age differences on free recall of subject-performed tasks: The importance of motor action. *Human Learning, 4*, 79–87.

Bahrick, H. P., Bahrick, P. O., & Wittlinger, R. P. (1975). Fifty years of memory for names and faces: A cross-sectional approach. *Journal of Experimental Psychology: General, 104*, 54–75.

Baltes, P. B., & Schaie, K. W. (1974). Aging and IQ: The myth of the twilight years. *Psychology Today, 7*, 35–40.

Baltes, P. B., Reese, H. W., & Nesselroade, J. R. (Eds.). (1977). *Life-span developmental psychology: Introduction to research methods*. Monterey, Calif.: Brooks/Cole.

Bartus, R. T., Dean, R. L., III, Beer, B., & Lippa, A. S. (1982). The cholinergic hypothesis of geriatric memory dysfunction. *Science, 217*, 408–417.

Bayles, K. A., & Kaszniak, A. W. (1987). *Communication and cognition in normal aging and dementia*. Boston: College-Hill.

Beck, E. C., Swanson, C., & Dustman, R. E. (1980). Long latency components of the visually evoked potential in man: Effects of aging. *Experimental Aging Research, 6*, 523–542.

Benton, A. L. (1974). *Revised Visual Retention Test* (4th ed.). New York: Psychological Corporation.

Benton, A. L., & Hamsher, K. (1976). *Multilingual Aphasia Examination*. Iowa City: University of Iowa Press.

Benton, A. L., Van Allen, M. W., Hamsher, K., & Levin, H. S. (1978). *Test of facial recognition*. Iowa City: University of Iowa Hospitals.

Benton, A. L., Eslinger, P. J., & Damasio, A. R. (1981). Normative observations on neuropsychological test performances in old age. *Journal of Clinical Neuropsychology, 3*, 33–42.

Birren, J. E., & Schaie, K. W. (Eds.). (1990). *Handbook of the psychology of aging* (3rd ed.). New York: Academic Press.

Birren, J. E., Butler, R. N., Greenhouse, S. W., Sokoloff, L., & Yarrow, M. R. (1963). Interdisciplinary relationships: Interrelations of physiological, psychological and psychiatric findings in healthy elderly men. In J. E. Birren, R. N. Butler, S. W. Greenhouse, L. Sokoloff, & M. R. Yarrow (Eds.), *Human aging: A biological and behavioral study* (pp. 283–305). Washington, D.C.: U.S. Government Printing Office.

Blackburn, J. A., Papalia-Finlay, Foye, B. F., & Serlin, R. C. (1988). Modifiability of figural relations performance among elderly adults. *Journal of Gerontology: Psychological Sciences, 43*, P87–P89.

Blazer, D. G., & Williams, C. D. (1980). Epidemiology of dysphoria and depression in an elderly population. *American Journal of Psychiatry, 137*, 439–444.

Blessed, G., Tomlinson, B. E., & Roth, M. (1968). The association between quantitative measures of dementia and of senile change in the cerebral grey matter of elderly subjects. *British Journal of Psychiatry, 114*, 797–811.

Borod, J. C., Goodglass, H., & Kaplan, E. (1980). Normative data on the Boston Diagnostic Aphasia Examination, Parietal Lobe Battery, and the Boston Naming Test. *Journal of Clinical Neuropsychology, 2*, 209–215.

Botwinick, J. (1984). *Aging and behavior* (3rd ed.). Berlin: Springer.

Botwinick, J., & Storandt, M. (1974). Vocabulary ability in later life. *Journal of Genetic Psychology, 125*, 303–308.

Bowles, N. L., & Poon, L. W. (1985). Aging and retrieval of words in semantic memory. *Journal of Gerontology, 40*, 71–77.

Brody, H. (1955). Organization of the cerebral cortex—III. A study of aging in the human cerebral cortex. *Journal of Comparative Neurology, 102*, 511–556.

Brown, W. S., Marsh, J. T., & La Rue, A. (1983). Exponential electrophysiological aging: P3 latency. *Electroencephalography and Clinical Neurophysiology, 55,* 277–285.
Buell, S. J., & Coleman, P. D. (1979). Dendritic growth in the aged human brain and failure of growth in senile dementia. *Science, 206,* 854–856.
Burke, W. J., Miller, J. P., Rubin, E. H., Morris, J. C., Coben, L. A., Duchek, J., Wittels, I. G., & Berg, L. (1988). Reliability of the Washington University Clinical Dementia Rating. *Archives of Neurology, 45,* 31–32.
Butler, R. N., & Lewis, M. I. (Eds.). (1973). *Aging and mental health: Positive psychosocial approaches.* St. Louis: Mosby.
Caine, E. (1981). Pseudodementia: Current concepts and future directions. *Archives of General Psychiatry, 38,* 1359–1364.
Canestrari, R. E., Jr. (1968). Age changes in acquisition. In G. A. Talland (Ed.), *Human aging and behavior* (pp. 169–188). New York: Academic Press.
Capitani, E., Sala, S. D., Lucchelli, F., Soave, P., & Spinnler, H. (1988). Perceptual attention in aging and dementia measured by Gottschaldt's Hidden Figure Test. *Journal of Gerontology: Psychological Sciences, 43,* P157–P163.
Carlsson, A. (1986). Brain neurotransmitters in normal and pathological aging. In A. B. Scheibel & A. F. Wechsler (Eds.), *The biological substrates of Alzheimer's disease* (pp. 193–203). New York: Academic Press.
Cattell, R. B. (1963). Theory of fluid and crystallized intelligence: A critical experiment. *Journal of Educational Psychology, 54,* 1–22.
Cerella, J., Poon, L. W., & Fozard, J. L. (1982). Age and iconic read-out. *Journal of Gerontology, 37,* 197–202.
Charness, N. (1981). Visual short-term memory and aging in chess players. *Journal of Gerontology, 36,* 615–619.
Cohen, G. (1979). Language comprehension in old age. *Cognitive Psychology, 11,* 412–429.
Cohen, R. L., Sandler, S. P., & Schroeder, K. (1987). Aging and memory for words and action events: Effects of item repetition and list length. *Psychology and Aging, 2,* 280–285.
Craik, F. I. M. (1977). Age differences in human memory. In J. E. Birren & K. W. Schaie (Eds.), *Handbook of the psychology of aging* (pp. 384–420). Princeton, N.J.: Van Nostrand–Reinhold.
Craik, F. I. M., & McDowd, J. M. (1987). Age differences in recall and recognition. *Journal of Experimental Psychology: Learning, Memory, and Cognition, 13,* 474–479.
Craik, F. I. M., Byrd, M., & Swanson, J. M. (1987). Patterns of memory loss in three elderly samples. *Psychology and Aging, 2,* 79–86.
Crystal, H., Dickson, D., Fuld, P., Masur, D., Scott, R., Mehler, M., Masdeu, J., Kawas, C., Aronson, M., & Wolfson, L. (1988). Clinico-pathologic studies in dementia: Nondemented subjects with pathologically confirmed Alzheimer's disease. *Neurology, 38,* 1682–1687.
Cummings, J. L., & Benson, D. F. (1984). Subcortical dementia: Review of an emerging concept. *Archives of Neurology, 41,* 874–879.
Danziger, W. L., & Salthouse, T. A. (1978). Age and the perception of incomplete figures. *Experimental Aging Research, 4,* 67–80.
Davies, A. (1968). The influence of age on Trail Making Test performance. *Journal of Clinical Psychology, 24,* 96–98.
de Leon, M. J., George, A. E., Ferris, S. H., Christman, D. R., Fowler, J. S., Gentes, C. I., Brodie, J., Reisberg, B., & Wolf, A. P. (1984). Positron emission tomography and computed tomography assessments of the aging human brain. *Journal of Computer Assisted Tomography, 8,* 88–94.
Denney, N. W., & Denney, D. R. (1982). The relationship between classification and questioning strategies among adults. *Journal of Gerontology, 37,* 190–196.
Denney, N. W., & Palmer, A. M. (1981). Adult age differences on traditional and practical problem-solving measures. *Journal of Gerontology, 36,* 323–328.
Drachman, D. A., & Leavitt, J. (1974). Human memory and the cholinergic system. *Archives of Neurology, 30,* 113–121.
Duara, R., Grady, C., Haxby, J., Ingvar, D., Sokoloff, L., Margolin, R. A., Manning, R. G., Cutler, N. R., & Rapoport, S. I. (1984). Human brain glucose utilization and cognitive function in relation to age. *Annals of Neurology, 16,* 702–713.

Duffy, F. H., & McAnulty, G. (1988). Electrophysiological studies. In M. S. Albert & M. B. Moss (Eds.), *Geriatric neuropsychology* (pp. 262–289). New York: Guilford Press.

Duffy, F. H., Albert, M. S., McAnulty, G., & Garvey, A. J. (1984). Age-related differences in brain electrical activity of healthy subjects. *Annals of Neurology, 16,* 430–438.

Dustman, R. E., Snyder, E. W., & Schlehuber, C. J. (1981). Life-span alterations in visual evoked potentials and inhibitory function. *Neurobiology of Aging, 2,* 187–192.

Erber, J. T., Botwinick, J., & Storandt, M. (1981). The impact of memory on age differences in Digit Symbol performance. *Journal of Gerontology, 36,* 586–590.

Eslinger, P. J., Damasio, A. R., Benton, A. L., & Van Allen, M. (1985). Neuropsychologic detection of abnormal mental decline in older persons. *Journal of the American Medical Association, 253,* 670–674.

Filley, C. M., Kelly, J., & Heaton, R. K. (1986). Neuropsychologic features of early- and late-onset Alzheimer's disease. *Archives of Neurology, 43,* 574–576.

Filley, C. M., Kobayashi, J., & Heaton, R. K. (1987). Wechsler Intelligence Scale profiles, the cholinergic system, and Alzheimer's disease. *Journal of Clinical and Experimental Neuropsychology, 9,* 180–186.

Finch, C. E., & Schneider, E. L. (Eds.). (1985). *Handbook of the biology of aging* (2nd ed.). Princeton, N.J.: Van Nostrand–Reinhold.

Folstein, M. F., & McHugh, P. R. (1978). Dementia syndrome of depression. In R. D. Katzman, R. D. Terry, & K. L. Bick (Eds.), *Alzheimer's disease: Senile dementia and related disorders* (pp. 87–96). New York: Raven Press.

Fox, J. H., Penn, R., Clasen, R., Martin, E., Wilson, R., & Savoy, S. (1986). Pathological diagnosis in clinically typical Alzheimer's disease. *New England Journal of Medicine, 313,* 1419–1420.

Fuld, P. A. (1981). *The Fuld Object-Memory Evaluation.* Chicago: Stoelting Instrument Company.

Fuld, P. A. (1984). Test profile of cholinergic dysfunction and of Alzheimer-type dementia. *Journal of Clinical Neuropsychology, 6,* 380–392.

Fuld, P. A. (1986). Pathological and chemical validation of behavioral features of Alzheimer's disease. In L. W. Poon (Ed.), *Handbook for clinical memory assessment of older adults* (pp. 302–306). Washington, D.C.: American Psychological Association.

Fuld, P. A., Katzman, R., Davies, P., & Terry, R. O. (1982). Intrusions as a sign of Alzheimer dementia: Chemical and pathological verification. *Annals of Neurology, 11,* 155–159.

Gatz, M., & Pearson, C. G. (1988). Ageism revised and the provision of psychological services. *American Psychologist, 43,* 184–188.

Giaquinto, S., & Nolfe, G. (1986). The EEG in the normal elderly: A contribution to the interpretation of aging and dementia. *Electroencephalography and Clinical Neurophysiology, 63,* 540–546.

Glenner, G. G. (1979). Congophilic microangiopathy in the pathogenesis of Alzheimer's syndrome (presenile dementia). *Medical Hypotheses, 5,* 1231–1236.

Goodin, D. S., Squires, K. C., Henderson, B. H., & Starr, A. (1978). Age-related variations in evoked potentials to auditory stimuli in normal human subjects. *Electroencephalography and Clinical Neurophysiology, 44,* 447–458.

Granholm, E., & Butters, N. (1988). Associative encoding and retrieval in Alzheimer's and Huntington's disease. *Brain and Cognition, 7,* 335–347.

Guttentag, R. E., & Hunt, R. R. (1988). Adult age differences in memory for imagined and performed actions. *Journal of Gerontology: Psychological Science, 43,* P107–P108.

Hart, R. P., Kwentus, J. A., Hamer, R. M., & Taylor, J. R. (1987*a*). Selective reminding procedure in depression and dementia. *Psychology and Aging, 2,* 111–115.

Hart, R. P., Kwentus, J. A., Wade, J. B., & Hamer, R. M. (1987*b*). Digit Symbol performance in mild dementia and depression. *Journal of Consulting and Clinical Psychology, 55,* 236–238.

Hasher, L., & Zacks, R. T. (1979). Automatic and effortful processes in memory. *Journal of Experimental Psychology: General, 108,* 356–388.

Heaton, R. K., Grant, I., & Matthews, C. G. (1986). Differences in neuropsychological test performance associated with age, education, and sex. In I. Grant & K. M. Adams (Eds.), *Neuropsychological assessment of neuropsychiatric disorders* (pp. 100–120). New York: Oxford University Press.

Hertzog, C., & Schaie, K. W. (1986). Stability and change in adult intelligence: 1. Analysis of longitudinal covariance structures. *Psychology and Aging, 1,* 159–171.

Hertzog, C., & Schaie, K. W. (1988). Stability and change in adult intelligence: 2. Simultaneous analysis of longitudinal means and covariance structures. *Psychology and Aging, 3,* 122–130.

Heston, L. L., Mastri, A. R., Anderson, V. E., & White, J. (1981). Dementia of the Alzheimer type. *Archives of General Psychiatry, 38,* 1085–1090.

Hochanadel, G., & Kaplan, E. (1984). Neuropsychology of normal aging. In M. L. Albert (Ed.), *Clinical neurology of aging* (pp. 231–244). New York: Oxford University Press.

Horn, J. L. (1970). Organization of data on life-span development of human abilities. In L. R. Goulet & P. B. Baltes (Eds.), *Life-span developmental psychology: Research and theory* (pp. 423–466). New York: Academic Press.

Horn, J. L. (1982). The aging of human abilities. In B. B. Wolman (Ed.), *Handbook of developmental psychology* (pp. 847–870). Englewood Cliffs, N.J.: Prentice–Hall.

Horn, J. L. (1985). Remodeling old models of intelligence. In B. B. Wolman (Ed.), *Handbook of intelligence* (pp. 267–300). New York: Wiley.

Howes, J. L., & Katz, A. N. (1988). Assessing remote memory with an improved public events questionnaire. *Psychology and Aging, 3,* 142–150.

Hoyer, W. J., & Plude, D. J. (1980). Attentional and perceptual processes in the study of cognitive aging. In L. Poon (Ed.), *Aging in the 1980s: Psychological issues* (pp. 227–239). Washington, D.C.: American Psychological Association.

Hughes, C. P., Berg, L., Danziger, W. L., Coben, L. A., & Martin, R. L. (1982). A new clinical scale for the staging of dementia. *British Journal of Psychiatry, 140,* 566–572.

Hulicka, I. M., & Grossman, J. L. (1967). Age group comparisons for the use of mediators in paired-associate learning. *Journal of Gerontology, 22,* 46–51.

Jarvik, L. F., & Bank, L. (1983). Aging twins: Longitudinal psychometric data. In K. W. Schaie (Ed.), *Longitudinal studies of adult psychological development* (pp. 40–63). New York: Guilford Press.

Jarvik, L. F., Mintz, J., Steuer, J., & Gerner, R. (1982). Treating geriatric depression: A 26-week interim analysis. *Journal of the American Geriatrics Society, 30,* 713–717.

John, E. R., Karmel, B. Z., Corning, W. C., Easton, P., Brown, D., Ahn, H., John, M., Harmoney, T., Prichep, L., Toro, A., Gerson, I., Bartlett, F., Thatcher, R., Kaye, H., Valdes, P., & Schwartz, E. (1977). Neurometrics. *Science, 196,* 1393–1409.

Johnson, M. H., & Magaro, P. A. (1987). Effects of mood and severity of memory processes in depression and mania. *Psychological Bulletin, 101,* 28–40.

Jorm, A. F. (1985). Subtypes of Alzheimer's dementia. A conceptual analysis and critical review. *Psychological Medicine, 15,* 543–553.

Kaszniak, A. W., Poon, L. W., & Riege, W. (1986). Assessing memory deficits: An information-processing approach. In L. W. Poon (Ed.), *Handbook for clinical memory assessment of older adults* (pp. 168–188). Washington, D.C.: American Psychological Association.

Katz, R., & Horowitz, G. R. (1982). Electroencephalogram in the septuagenarian: Studies in a normal geriatric population. *Journal of the American Geriatrics Society, 3,* 273–275.

Katzman, R., Brown, T., Fuld, P., Peck, A., Schechter, R., & Schimmel, H. (1983). Validation of a short orientation–memory–concentration test of cognitive impairment. *American Journal of Psychiatry, 140,* 734–739.

Katzman, R., Terry, R., DeTeresa, R., Brown, T., Davies, P., Fuld, P., Renbing, X., & Peck, A. (1988). Clinical, pathological, and neurochemical changes in dementia: A subgroup with preserved mental status and numerous neocortical plaques. *Annals of Neurology, 23,* 138–144.

Kausler, D. H. (1982). *Experimental psychology and human aging.* New York: Wiley.

Kemper, T. (1984). Neuroanatomical and neuropathological changes in normal aging and in dementia. In M. L. Albert (Ed.), *Clinical neurology of aging* (pp. 9–52). New York: Oxford University Press.

Klisz, D. (1978). Neuropsychology and medical disorders. In M. Storandt, I. C. Seigler, & M. F. Elias (Eds.), *The clinical psychology of aging* (pp. 71–95). New York: Plenum Press.

Kubanis, P., & Zornetzer, S. F. (1981). Age-related behavioral and neurobiological changes: A review with an emphasis on memory. *Behavioral and Neural Biology, 31,* 115–172.

Kuhl, D. E., Metter, E. J., Riege, W. H., & Phelps, M. E. (1982). Effects of human aging on patterns of local cerebral glucose utilization determined by the F-18 fluoro-deoxyglucose method. *Journal of Cerebral Blood Flow and Metabolism*, *2*, 163–171.

Kuhl, D. E., Metter, E. J., Riege, W. H., & Hawkins, R. A. (1984). The effect of normal aging on patterns of local cerebral glucose utilization. *Annals of Neurology*, *15*, S133–S137.

Kynette, D., & Kemper, S. (1986). Aging and the loss of grammatical forms: A cross-sectional study of language performance. *Language and Communication*, *6*, 65–72.

La Rue, A. (1989). Patterns of performance on the Fuld Object Memory Evaluation in elderly inpatients with depression or dementia. *Journal of Clinical and Experimental Neuropsychology*, *11*, 409–422.

La Rue, A., & McCreary, C. (1991). Emerging issues in the health care of the elderly. In J. Sweet, R. Rozensky, & S. Tovian (Eds.), *Handbook of clinical psychology in medical settings* (pp. 223–248). New York: Plenum Press.

La Rue, A., & Waldbaum, A. (1980, February). Aging vs. illness as predictors of Piagetian problem solving in older adults. Paper presented at a meeting of the 10th Annual Interdisciplinary International Conference on Piagetian Theory and the Helping Professions, Los Angeles.

La Rue, A., Dessonville, C., & Jarvik, L. F. (1985). Aging and mental disorders. In J. E. Birren & K. W. Schaie (Eds.), *Handbook of the psychology of aging* (2nd ed., pp. 664–702). Princeton, N.J.: Van Nostrand–Reinhold.

La Rue, A., D'Elia, L. F., Clark, E. O., Spar, J. E., & Jarvik, L. F. (1986*a*). Clinical tests of memory in dementia, depression, and healthy aging. *Psychology and Aging*, *1*, 69–77.

La Rue, A., Spar, J., & Hill, C. (1986*b*). Cognitive impairment in late-life depression: Clinical correlates and treatment implications. *Journal of Affective Disorders*, *11*, 179–184.

Liston, E. H. (1977). Occult presenile dementia. *Journal of Nervous and Mental Disease*, *164*, 263–267.

Luria, A. (1974). *The working brain*. London: Penguin.

Macht, M. L., & Buschke, H. (1983). Age differences in cognitive effort in recall. *Journal of Gerontology*, *38*, 695–700.

Martin, A., Browers, P., Cox, C., Teleska, P., Fedio, P., Foster, N. L., & Chase, T. H. (1986). Towards a behavioral typology of Alzheimer's patients. *Journal of Clinical and Experimental Neuropsychology*, *8*, 594–610.

Marx, J. L. (1989). Brain protein yields clues to Alzheimer's disease. *Science*, *243*, 1664–1666.

Matsuyama, H., & Nakamura, S. (1978). Senile changes in the brain in the Japanese: Incidence of Alzheimer's neurofibrillary change and senile plaque. In R. Katzman, R. D. Terry, & K. L. Bick (Eds.), *Alzheimer's disease: Senile dementia and related disorders* (pp. 287–297). New York: Raven Press.

McAllister, T. W. (1983). Overview: Pseudodementia. *American Journal of Psychiatry*, *140*, 528–533.

McGeer, E. G., & McGerr, P. L. (1975). Age changes in the human for some enzymes associated with metabolism of catecholamines, GABA, and acetylcholine. In J. M. Ordy & K. R. Brizzee (Eds.), *Neurobiology of aging* (pp. 287–305). New York: Plenum Press.

McGeer, E. G., & McGeer, P. L. (1976). Neurotransmitter metabolism and the aging brain. In R. D. Terry & S. Gershon (Eds.), *Neurobiology of aging* (pp. 389–404). New York: Raven Press.

McKhann, G., Drachman, D., Folstein, M., Katzman, R., Price, D., & Stadlan, E. M. (1984). Clinical diagnosis of Alzheimer's disease: Report of the NINCDS–ADRDA Work Group. *Neurology*, *34*, 939–944.

Metter, E. J. (1988). Positron tomography and cerebral blood flow studies. In M. S. Albert & M. B. Moss (Eds.), *Geriatric neuropsychology* (pp. 228–261). New York: Guilford Press.

Meyer, J. S., & Shaw, T. G. (1984). Cerebral blood flow in aging. In M. L. Albert (Ed.), *Clinical neurology of aging* (pp. 178–196). New York: Oxford University Press.

Miller, A. K. H., Alston, R. L., & Corsellis, J. A. N. (1980). Variations with age in the volumes of grey and white matter in the cerebral hemispheres of man: Measurements with an image analyser. *Neuropathology of Applied Neurobiology*, *6*, 119–132.

Miller, E. (1971). On the nature of the memory disorder in presenile dementia. *Neuropsychologia*, *9*, 75–81.

Mittenberg, W., Seidenberg, M., O'Leary, D. S., & DiGiulio, D. V. (1988, January). Changes in cerebral functioning associated with normal aging. Paper presented at a meeting of the International Neuropsychological Society, New Orleans.

Mullis, R., Holcomb, P., Diner, B., & Dykman, R. A. (1985). The effects of aging on the P3 component of the visual event-related potential. *Electroencephalography and Clinical Neurophysiology, 62,* 141–149.

National Center for Health Statistics. (1986). *Health, United States, 1986* (DHHS Publication PHS 87-1232). Washington, D.C.: Department of Health and Human Services.

National Center for Health Statistics. (1987). Family use of health care, United States, 1980. *National Medical Care Utilization and Expenditure Survey* (DHHS Publication 87-20210). Washington, D.C.: Department of Health and Human Services.

National Institute on Aging Task Force. (1980). Senility reconsidered. *Journal of the American Medical Association, 244,* 259–263.

Nesselroade, J. R., & Labouvie, E. W. (1985). Experimental design in research on aging. In J. E. Birren & K. W. Schaie (Eds.), *Handbook of the psychology of aging* (2nd ed., pp. 35–60). Princeton, N.J.: Van Nostrand–Reinhold.

Niederehe, G. (1986). Depression and memory impairment in the aged. In L. W. Poon (Ed.), *Handbook for clinical memory assessment of older adults* (pp. 226–237). Washington, D.C.: American Psychological Association.

Norris, J. T., Gallagher, D., Wilson, A., & Winograd, C. H. (1987). Assessment of depression in geriatric medical outpatients: The validity of two screening measures. *Journal of the American Geriatric Society, 35,* 989–995.

Obler, L. K. (1980). Narrative discourse style in the elderly. In L. K. Obler & M. L. Albert (Eds.), *Language and communication in the elderly* (pp. 75–90). Lexington, Mass.: Heath.

Obrist, W. D. (1963). The electroencephalogram of healthy aged males. In J. E. Birren, R. N. Butler, S. W. Greenhouse, L. Sokoloff, & M. Yarrow (Eds.), *Human aging: A biological and behavioral study* (pp. 79–93). Washington, D.C.: U. S. Government Printing Office.

Obrist, W. D. (1975). Cerebral physiology of the aged: Relation to psychological function. In N. R. Burch & H. L. Altschuler (Eds.), *Behavior and brain electrical activity* (pp. 421–430). New York: Plenum Press.

Offenbach, S. I. A. (1974). A developmental study of hypothesis testing and cue selection strategies. *Developmental Psychology, 10,* 484–490.

Perlmutter M., & Mitchell, D. B. (1982). The appearance and disappearance of age differences in adult memory. In F. I. M. Craik & S. Trehub (Eds.), *Aging and cognitive processes* (pp. 127–143). New York: Plenum Press.

Petry, S., Cummings, J. L., Hill, M. A., & Shapira, J. (1988). Personality alternations in dementia of the Alzheimer type. *Archives of Neurology, 45,* 1187–1190.

Phelps, M. E., & Mazziotta, J. C. (1985). Positron emission tomography: Human brain function and biochemistry. *Science, 228,* 799–809.

Plude, D. J., Milberg, W. P., & Cerella, J. (1986). Age differences in depicting and perceiving tridimensionality in simple line drawings. *Experimental Aging Research, 12,* 221–225.

Poon, L. W. (Ed.). (1980). *Aging in the 1980s.* Washington, D.C.: American Psychological Association.

Poon, L. W. (Ed.). (1986). *Handbook for clinical memory assessment of older adults.* Washington, D.C.: American Psychological Association.

Post, F. (1966). Somatic and psychic factors in the treatment of elderly psychiatric patients. *Journal of Psychosomatic Research, 10,* 13–19.

Rabins, P. V. (1983). Reversible dementia and the misdiagnosis of dementia: A review. *Hospital and Community Psychiatry, 34,* 830–835.

Rabins, P. V., Merchant, A., & Nestadt, G. (1984). Criteria for diagnosing reversible dementia caused by depression: Validation by 2-year follow-up. *British Journal of Psychiatry, 144,* 488–492.

Rapp, S. R., Parisi, S. A., Walsh, D. A., & Wallace, C. E. (1988). Detecting depression in elderly medical inpatients. *Journal of Consulting and Clinical Psychology, 56,* 509–513.

Read, D. E. (1988). Age-related changes in performance on a visual-closure task. *Journal of Clinical and Experimental Neuropsychology, 10,* 451–466.

Regier, D. A., Boyd, J. H., Burke, J. D., Jr., Rae, D. S., Myers, J. K., Kramer, M., Robins, L. N., George, L. K., Karno, M., & Locke, B. Z. (1988). One-month prevalence of mental disorders in the United States. *Archives of General Psychiatry, 45*, 977–986.

Reifler, B. V., Larson, E., & Hanley, R. (1982). Coexistence of cognitive impairment and depression in geriatric outpatients. *American Journal of Psychiatry, 139*, 623–629.

Reisberg, B., Ferris, S. H., de Leon, M. J., & Crook, T. (1982). The global deterioration scale for assessment of primary degenerative dementia. *American Journal of Psychiatry, 139*, 1136–1139.

Reisberg B., Ferris, S. H., de Leon, M. J., Sinaiko, E., Franssen, E., Kluger, A., Mir, P., Borenstein, J., George, A. E., Shulman, E., Steinberg, G., & Cohen, J. (1988). Stage-specific behavioral, cognitive, and in vivo changes in community residing subjects with age-associated memory impairment and primary degenerative dementia of the Alzheimer type. *Drug Development Research, 15*, 101–114.

Reitan, R. M. (1958). Validity of the Trail Making Test as an indicator of organic brain damage. *Perceptual and Motor Skills, 19*, 199–206.

Reitan, R. M., & Davison, L. A. (Eds.). (1974). *Clinical neuropsychology: Current status and applications.* New York: Winston/Wiley.

Reus, V. I., Silberman, E., Post, R. M., & Weingartner, H. (1979). D-Amphetamine: Effects on memory in a depressed population. *Biological Psychiatry, 14*, 345–356.

Reynolds, C. F., Hoch, C. C., Kupfer, D. J., Buysse, D. J., Houck, P. R., Stack, J. A., & Campbell, D. W. (1988). Bedside differentiation of depressive pseudodementia from dementia. *American Journal of Psychiatry, 145*, 1099–1103.

Riege, W. H., Metter, E. J., Kuhl, D. E., & Phelps, M. E. (1985). Brain glucose metabolism and memory functions: Age decrease in factor scores. *Journal of Gerontology, 40*, 459– 467.

Riege, W. H., Harker, J. O., & Metter, E. J. (1986). Clinical validators: Brain lesions and brain imaging. In L. W. Poon (Ed.), *Handbook for clinical memory assessment of older adults* (pp. 314–336). Washington, D. C.: American Psychological Association.

Robertson-Tchabo, E. A., Hausman, C. P., & Arenberg, D. (1976). A classical mnemonic for old learners: A trip that works. *Educational Gerontology, 1*, 215–226.

Robinson, D. S., Nies, A., Davies, H. M., Bunney, W. E., Davis, J. M., Colburn, R. W., Bourne, H. R., Shaw, D. M., & Coppen, A. J. (1972). Ageing, monoamines and monoamine-oxidase levels. *Lancet, 1*, 290–291.

Rogers, J., & Bloom, F. E. (1985). Neurotransmitter metabolism and function in the aging central nervous system. In C. E. Finch & E. L. Schneider (Eds.), *Handbook of the biology of aging* (2nd ed., pp. 645–691). Princeton, N.J.: Nostrand–Reinhold.

Roybal, E. R. (1988). Mental health and aging: The need for an expanded federal response. *American Psychologist, 43*, 189–194.

Roy-Byrne, P. P., Weingartner, H., Bierer, L. M., Thompson, K., & Post, R. M. (1986). Effortful and automatic cognitive processes in depression. *Archives of General Psychiatry, 43*, 265–267.

Rubin, E. H., Morris, J. C., Storandt, M., & Berg, L. (1986). Behavioral changes in patients with mild senile dementia of the Alzheimer's type. *Psychiatry Research, 21*, 55–62.

Salthouse, T. A. (1985). Speed of behavior and its implications for cognition. In J. E. Birren & K. W. Schaie (Eds.), *Handbook of the psychology of aging* (2nd ed., pp. 400–426). Princeton, N.J.: Van Nostrand–Reinhold.

Sanders, J. A. C., Sterns, H. L., Smith, M., & Sanders, T. E. (1975). Enhancement of conjunctive concept attainment in older adults. *Developmental Psychology, 11*, 824–829.

Sands, L. P., & Meredith, W. (1989). Effects of sensory and motor functioning on adult intellectual performance. *Journal of Gerontology, 44*, P56–P58.

Schaie, K. W. (1983). The Seattle Longitudinal Study: A 21-year exploration of psychometric intelligence in adulthood. In K. W. Schaie (Ed.), *Longitudinal studies of adult psychological development* (pp. 64–135). New York: Guilford Press.

Schaie, K. W., & Hertzog, C. (1985). Measurement in the psychology of adulthood and aging. In J. E. Birren & K. W. Schaie (Eds.), *Handbook of the psychology of aging* (2nd ed., pp. 61–92). Princeton, N.J.: Van Nostrand–Reinhold.

Schaie, K. W., & Schaie, J. P. (1977). Clinical assessment and aging. In J. E. Birren & K. W. Schaie (Eds.), *Handbook of the psychology of aging* (pp. 692–723). Princeton, N.J.: Van Nostrand–Reinhold.

Scheibel, A. B., & Wechsler, A. F. (Eds.). (1986). *The biological substrates of Alzheimer's disease*. New York: Academic Press.

Scheibel, M. E., Lindsay, R. D., Tomiyasu, U., & Scheibel, A. B. (1975). Progressive dendritic changes in aging human cortex. *Experimental Neurology, 47*, 392–403.

Scheibel, M. E., Lindsay, R. D., Tomiyasu, U., & Scheibel, A. B. (1976). Progressive dendritic changes in the aging human limbic system. *Experimental Neurology, 53*, 420–430.

Selkoe, D., & Kosik, K. (1984). Neurochemical changes with aging. In M. L. Albert (Ed.), *Clinical neurology of aging* (pp. 53–75). New York: Oxford University Press.

Shimamura, A. P., Salmon, D. P., Squire, L. R., & Butters, H. (1987). Memory dysfunction and word priming in dementia and amnesia. *Behavioral Neuroscience, 101*, 347–351.

Sim, M., & Sussman, I. (1962). Alzheimer disease: Its natural history and differential diagnosis. *Journal of Nervous Mental Disorders, 135*, 489–499.

Small, G. W., & Fawzy, F. I. (1988). Psychiatric consultation for the medically ill elderly in the general hospital: Need for a collaborative model of care. *Psychosomatics, 29*, 94–103.

Stankov, L. (1988). Aging, attention, and intelligence. *Psychology and Aging, 3*, 59–74.

Storandt, M. (1977). Age, ability level, and method of administering and scoring the WAIS. *Journal of Gerontology, 32*, 175–178.

Storandt, M., Botwinick, J., Danziger, W. L., Berg, L., & Hughes, C. P. (1984). Psychometric differentiation of mild senile dementia of the Alzheimer type. *Archives of Neurology, 41*, 497–499.

Terry, R. D., & Hansen, L. A. (1988). Some morphometric aspects of Alzheimer disease and of normal aging. In R. D. Terry (Ed.), *Aging and the brain* (pp. 109–114). New York: Raven Press.

Thompson, L. W., Gallagher, D., & Breckenridge, J. S. (1987). Comparative effectiveness of psychotherapies for depressed elders. *Journal of Consulting and Clinical Psychology, 55*, 385–390.

Tierney, M. C., Snow, W. G., Reid, D. W., Zorzitto, M. L., & Fisher, R. H. (1987). Replication and extension of the findings of Storandt and coworkers. *Archives of Neurology, 44*, 720–722.

Tierney, M. C., Fisher, R. H., Anthony, J. L., Zorzitto, M. L., Snow, W. G., Reid, D. W., & Nieuwstraten, P. (1988). The NINCDS–ADRDA work group criteria for the clinical diagnosis of probable Alzheimer's disease: A clinicopathologic study of 57 cases. *Neurology, 38*, 359–364.

Tomlinson, B. E., Blessed, G., & Roth, M. (1970). Observations on the brains of nondemented old people. *Journal of Neurological Science, 11*, 205–242.

Treat, N. J., Poon, L. W., & Fozard, J. L. (1981). Age, imagery, and practice in paired-associate learning. *Experimental Aging Research, 7*, 337–342.

Ulatowska, H. K., Hayaski, M. M., Cannito, M. P., & Fleming, S. G. (1986). Disruption of reference. *Brain and Language, 28*, 24–41.

U.S. Bureau of the Census. (1987). Estimates of the population of the United States, by age, sex and race: 1980–1986. *Current Population Reports* (Series P-25, No. 1000). Washington, D.C.: Author.

U.S. Senate Special Committee on Aging. (1987–1988). *Aging America: Trends and projections*. Washington, D.C.: Department of Health and Human Services.

VandenBos, G. R., & Stapp, J. (1983). Service providers in psychology: Results of the 1982 APA Human Resources Survey. *American Psychologist, 38*, 1330–1352.

Walsh, D. A., Till, R. E., & Williams, M. V. (1978). Age differences in peripheral perception processing: A monoptic backward masking investigation. *Journal of Experimental Psychology: Human Perception and Performance, 4*, 232–243.

Wang, H. S., & Busse, E. W. (1969). EEG of healthy old persons—A longitudinal study: I. Dominant background activity and occipital rhythm. *Journal of Gerontology, 24*, 419–426.

Wechsler, D. (1945). A standardized memory scale for clinical use. *Journal of Psychology, 19*, 87–95.

Wechsler, D. (1955). *Wechsler Adult Intelligence Scale*. New York: Psychological Corporation.

Wechsler, D. (1981). *Wechsler Adult Intelligence Scale—Revised*. New York: Psychological Corporation.

Wechsler, D. (1987). *Wechsler Memory Scale—Revised*. New York: Psychological Corporation.

Weingartner, H., & Silberman, E. (1982). Models of cognitive impairment: Cognitive changes in depression. *Psychopharmacology Bulletin, 18*, 27–42.

Weingartner, H., Kaye, W., Smallberg, S. A., Ebert, M. H., Gillin, J. C., & Sitaram, N. (1981*a*). Memory failures in progressive idiopathic dementia. *Journal of Abnormal Psychology, 90,* 187–196.
Weingartner, H., Cohen, R. M., Murphy, D. L., Martello, J., & Gerdt, C. (1981*b*). Cognitive processes in depression. *Archives of General Psychiatry, 38,* 42–47.
Welford, A. T. (1958). *Aging and human skill.* London: Oxford University Press.
Wells, C. E. (1979). Pseudodementia. *American Journal of Psychiatry, 136,* 895–900.
West, R. L. (1986). Everyday memory and aging. *Developmental Neuropsychology, 2,* 323–344.
Williams, A., Denney, N. W., & Schadler, M. (1983). Elderly adults' perception of their own cognitive development during the adult years. *International Journal of Aging and Human Development, 16,* 147–158.
Willis, S. L., & Schaie, K. W. (1986). Training the elderly on the ability factors of spatial orientation and inductive reasoning. *Psychology and Aging, 1,* 239–247.
Wilson, R. S., Bacon, L. D., Fox, J. H., & Kaszniak, A. W. (1983). Primary memory and secondary memory in dementia of the Alzheimer type. *Journal of Clinical Neuropsychology, 5,* 337–344.
Wurtman, R. J. (1985). Alzheimer's disease. *Scientific American, 252,* 62–74.

4

Sex and Gender

JANET R. MATTHEWS

SEX AND GENDER

The terms *sex* and *gender* are difficult to separate in much of the literature. Unger (1979) suggested that the term *sex* had been used to cover too wide a range of conditions. She recommended use of the term *gender* for "those nonphysiological components of sex that are culturally regarded as appropriate to males or to females" (Unger, 1979, p. 1086). She also noted that it is important for researchers to be careful when stating that observed "sex" differences lead to "gender" differences without examining differences in the environment and socialization processes of the subjects. As environmental and socialization differences are seldom cited in the research articles used in this chapter, only the term *sex* will tend to be used.

Some general texts in the field of neuropsychology do address both sex and gender issues (Kolb & Whishaw, 1990; Wedding, Horton, & Webster, 1986) but these topics do not tend to be emphasized. The phrase *sex differences* appears in the index of many texts on neuropsychological assessment (e.g., Franzen, 1989; Incagnoli, Goldstein, & Golden, 1986; Lezak, 1983). These texts address sex differences in performance on specific tests that tend to be included in neuropsychological assessment batteries.

The question that must be asked is whether this topic is missing from many texts because it is irrelevant to neuropsychological assessment or whether it has been omitted because it has yet to be investigated adequately by the discipline. This chapter will attempt to answer that question by considering historical references to sex and gender issues in the fields of neurology and neuropsychology, the basic neurobiological issues that underlie this area, and the applications that have been made to neuropsychological assessment up to this time.

JANET R. MATTHEWS • Department of Psychology, Loyola University, New Orleans, Louisiana 70118.

HANDBOOK OF NEUROPSYCHOLOGICAL ASSESSMENT: A Biopsychosocial Perspective, edited by Antonio E. Puente and Robert J. McCaffrey. Plenum Press, New York, 1992.

HISTORICAL FOUNDATIONS

Baumeister (1988) stated that there has been an active investigation of sex differences in the field of psychology and that this approach was necessary to overcome a previously male-dominated literature. He suggested that small sex differences found in the past have led to exaggeration of the effect and potential gender discrimination. When considering the scientific importance of reported gender differences, he questioned the benefit due to the fact that subjects are not assigned at random to sex and there are often too many potential explanations of these gender differences to make the data useful. By contrast, Rothblum (1988) proposed that greater attention be given to gender issues with both similarities and differences receiving attention in the presentation of research data. Consideration of the literature in health and neuropsychology leads to the suggestion that gender issues in these specialties have not received the attention that Baumeister (1988) and Rothblum (1988) report for the psychological general literature.

Blechman and Brownell (1988) noted that there is minimal information available in the literature on women's health and behavior. Since neurobiological problems are a subset of health and behavior issues, it might be assumed that this literature contains little of importance to the study of sex issues. According to Woods and Hebben (1988), sex differences have not received much attention from neurology when considering incidence, prevalence, etiology, or prognosis of neurological problems. In their review of methodological considerations that are important when conducting research in clinical neuropsychology, Parsons and Prigatano (1978) noted that although sex differences are considered important in many facets of human life, this variable had been ignored by most researchers up to that point in time. They suggested that future research either needed to match groups for the number of male and female subjects or to have a sufficient number of one sex to reach a large *N* and to be able to analyze these data separately. They also suggested that data from small samples of one sex be compared to the large sample of the other sex to see if any obtained effects were similar for the small sample. There are indications that some attention has been given to these suggestions (e.g., Golden & Vincente, 1983; Goldstein & Tarter, 1986). Bloom and Lazerson (1988) state that psychologists agree that females, on average, are more verbally fluent than males and that males, on average, possess more acute visual-spatial abilities. They tie these differences to difference in brain function by sex.

Early Studies

Much of the early research on the impact of brain insult on behavior was conducted in military and VA settings. Since the vast majority of these patients were male, it is not surprising that sex issues did not arise. Another reason some of the early studies may not have considered sex as an issue is that even in non-VA settings, many of the patients studied were those who had been injured in military combat situations. This activity has been limited, to a great extent, to males.

Early studies conducted in non-military-related hospital settings often used temporal lobe surgery patients as subjects. This type of surgery is most often conducted to alleviate epilepsy (Springer & Deutsch, 1985). Epilepsy, although a symptom of multiple problems, has been reported more frequently in males than in females. Another major category of neurological disease contributing early data is stroke, which also has a considerably higher male than female rate of occurrence (Weinfeld, 1981). With the more recent development of such specialty facilities as head trauma units, long-term rehabilitation centers for brain-injured persons, and neuropsychology centers, it is time to replicate some of the early studies and use sex as a variable since female patients are now more readily available. Spreen, Tupper, Risser, Tuokko, and Edgell (1984) noted that care needs to be taken in the interpretation of sex differences that may be found in neuropsychological investigations because studies that report variation between sexes may have more individual variation within a sex group than between the sexes. It is also important to remember that reported sex differences may be the result of the socialization process rather than any physiological variability and thus fall under Unger's (1979) definition of gender rather than sex.

THEORETICAL AND BASIC NEUROBIOLOGICAL ISSUES

In this section, theories about the relationship between sex and neurobiological development are presented. These theories are illustrated by the presentation of research findings on sex differences in verbal and general cognitive skills as well as brain structure.

Although some theorists have addressed gender issues (e.g., Harris, 1978; McGee, 1979), their writings comprise a small segment of the neuropsychological and neurobiological literature to date. There is an insufficient data base at this stage to comment on gender issues.

Cognitive Development

Some researchers have suggested that females show better verbal skills than do males (Hoyenga & Hoyenga, 1979; Klooz & Rosenbaum, 1988; Maccoby & Jacklin, 1974). It is important, when examining this literature, to consider the range of performance within each sex group because there is often considerable overlap of the two samples even though their mean group differences are significant. A gender-related factor that has been hypothesized to be of importance to this suggested difference in verbal abilities is estrogen level. Hoyenga and Hoyenga (1979) reported that males who have high estrogen levels and feminized bodies tend to score high on verbal fluency tests. They also noted that the sex chromosome may play a role in the development of verbal skills since individuals who have extra sex chromosomes, such as those with Klinefelter's syndrome (XXY), tend to have lowered scores on standard IQ tests that require cognitive processing of material. Sex hormones have also been tied to visual-spatial abilities. Hier and Crowley (1982) found that males who suffer from a rare genetic deficiency that leads to a lack of testosterone production at puberty score below the reported male average on visual-spatial tasks.

Another source of data suggesting differential sex influences on cognitive development comes from an examination of the performance of children and adolescents who are clinically deviant in their rate of growth. Rovet (1983) compared subjects with idiopathic precocious puberty to a clinically delayed group and a matched control sample. Each subject was given the age-appropriate Wechsler test of intelligence. Verbal ability was assessed using the Vocabulary and Similarities subtests of the Wechsler and a sentence verification task presented using 35-mm slides. This latter task required the subject to judge whether a sentence about a picture was true or false. Spatial ability was judged based on the Block Design and Object Assembly subtests of the Wechsler and a slide-presented mental rotation task. The mental rotation task required the subject to judge whether stimulus pairs that were differently oriented had the same or different three-dimensional shape. Dichotic listening was assessed by simultaneously presenting to each ear recorded pairs of digit sequences. The sequences were of either three digits or four digits. Sex by condition differences were found. On spatial abilities, precocious females did better than matched controls while matched controls did better than precocious males. Among the delayed development subjects, females did less well than controls while males did not differ from controls. On IQ test performance, precocious puberty females and delayed development males did better than the opposite two categories. These data lend support for the hypothesis that the physical characteristics associated with atypical puberty have a differential impact by sex on cognitive abilities. Further research is needed to provide information on the specific physical processes involved in this difference.

Neuroanatomical Differences

Possible differences in male and female brain function may be traced to structural differences. In one of the early human studies of this issue, deLacoste-Utamsing and Holloway (1982) reported that the splenium of the corpus callosum was larger and more bulbous in females than males in 14 autopsied brains. A later replication study (Holloway & deLacoste, 1986) reported a significantly larger corpus callosum in the female than male brain but their sample has been criticized as not being representative of the population (Witelson & Kigar, 1988). Most other studies of the splenial area in adults have reported no sex differences (Dementer, Ringo, & Doty, 1985; Witelson, 1985). In a fetal brain study (deLacoste, Holloway, & Woodward, 1986), the females were reported to show a larger callosal area than the males but this difference was not statistically significant.

Peters (1988) stated that the literature supports the concept that male brains are generally larger than female brains. This size difference has been tied to average difference in overall body size with larger bodies having larger brains. Based on this information, it would then be expected that the female callosal area should be smaller than that of the male rather than what has been found in the limited available data (Kolb & Whishaw, 1990).

The female cerebral cortex has been found to be typically thicker on the left side and the male cortex thicker on the right side (Wada, Clarke, & Hamm, 1975; Witelson & Palie, 1973). Sex hormone level is one suggested explanation for this observed difference. Data in the animal literature support the concept that estradiol, a derivative of testosterone, increases the rate of neuronal loss in the cortex. Females have been found to have a larger number of estradiol receptors in the right hemisphere while males have a larger number of these receptors in the left hemisphere. The animal literature supports the hypothesis that there is a critical period of neuronal growth during which these hormones also act to organize the central nervous system in differential ways by sex. While many of these studies have investigated rats, there are also data from hamsters, rhesus monkeys, and gerbils that support the hypothesis of sex-related structural differences in the brain (DeLisi, Dauphinais, & Hauser, 1989). It is possible that these structural differences may apply to the human brain as well and form an early foundation for structural differences of the brain by sex.

Research with learning-disabled children has also provided support for sex differences in brain development (Younes, Rosner, & Webb, 1983). When a group of 119 learning-disabled children ages 5 to 18 years and 152 controls ages 5 to 15 years were evaluated on a 46-component neurological examination, males were found to be more immature than females within each category. A neuroimmaturity index (NI) was constructed based on test findings. When age was controlled, males were found to have a higher NI than females. Consideration of individual test performance revealed that males had their greatest difference from females on writing and spelling tasks.

Data from studies of gender differences in the cognitive effects of alcoholism have also been used to support the hypothesis of structural differences between the male and female brain. In a sample of 15 female and 15 male alcoholics matched for age and drinking history, both groups showed expected neuropsychological deficits compared to controls (Sparadeo, Zwick, & Butters, 1983). When these subjects were retested following a 30-day period of sobriety, the male alcoholics continued to score in the impaired range while the female alcoholics' scores were no longer different from those of the controls. One potential explanation of these data is that the female brain is less susceptible than the male brain to structural damage from alcohol. Similar results have also been reported for a sample of subjects recovering from alcohol-attributed deficits as determined by CT scans (Jacobson, 1986). Although these data may support structural differences in the male and female brain, other researchers reporting similar findings (Hesselbrock, Weidenman, & Reed, 1985) have raised the issue of personality variables, which may also influence performance by such subjects. They found that evidence of an antisocial personality pattern interacted with sex in their sample of 172 males and 72 females in an inpatient treatment program sample. These data suggest the need to include personality measures before making hypotheses about sex differences.

Fleet and Heilman (1985) suggested that sex differences in language lateralization lead to differential probabilities by sex of stuttering following unilateral lesion with men more likely than women to stutter following left-hemisphere lesion and women more likely than men to stutter following right-hemisphere lesion. To support their hypothesis, they reported case history data on a 42-year-old, right-handed female who had a right-hemisphere infarct. She had no history of stuttering. Following the infarct, stuttering without aphasia was present. Family history revealed that both her father and brother had developmental stuttering. Related to these data is the fact that females have been found to have significantly faster rates of neural transmission than males (Newman, Bunderson, & Brey, 1985).

Data that can be viewed as supportive of sex differences in the functional organization of the brain have been reported for healthy subjects. When subjects were matched for age, Warkentin, Rodriguez, and Rosadini (1988) found that females showed a significantly higher global cerebral blood flow than males did. They also found sex-specific differences in regional cerebral blood flow. Males in this sample showed the traditionally expected difference of right frontal flow being greater than left frontal flow. The females in this sample, however, had higher flows in the left central and right temporal areas. This difference in regional cerebral blood flow is suggestive of sex differences in functional organization but the specifics of these differences have yet to be determined. Larue (1986) also found sex differences in cerebral blood flow. Her subjects had unilateral lesions due to ischemic brain disease. The females were found to have both a higher mean blood flow and a higher flow to gray matter than the males. This finding obtained despite the fact that the females tended to have greater cortical loss due to atrophy than the males.

Piazza (1980) investigated possible sex differences in the processing of nonverbal auditory stimuli. Ear asymmetry for melodies and familiar sounds was assessed. The female subjects showed a significant left ear advantage. Although the males also demonstrated a slight left ear advantage, the difference was not significant. These data support the hypothesis that lateralization for at least some nonverbal auditory stimuli may be greater for females than for males.

According to Levy (1984), the right hemisphere is dominant for language in about 30 to 40% of left-handers. At least some theories have related handedness to testosterone (Geschwind & Galaburda, 1985) suggesting that this is one of the reasons more males than females are left-handed. Their hypothesis proposes that a high level of testosterone will slow the maturation of the left hemisphere relative to the right hemisphere. This differential hemispheric development results in a higher rate of left-handed males. Research on handedness and brain development has also found that inverted writers, regardless of hand dominance, perform differently from noninverted writers on a variety of neurological tests. Such performance differences suggest differential brain function between these two groups but the specifics of this difference remain speculative (Levy & Reid, 1978; Levy & Wagner, 1984). Although handedness and sex have been related in the neurological literature, the concept of inversion by gender has not been actively explored. The relationship of handedness and inversion to specific brain functions needs considerable investigation. The topic of handedness is covered in detail in Chapter 5.

There are many other individual studies in the literature from neurology, physical anthropology, and neurobiology that have a bearing on this topic. The material cited here is merely a selection from that growing literature. What is important is that researchers are considering sex and gender issues. For the future of this research area, it is important for researchers in various disciplines to remain aware of the theories and data generated by each specialty.

APPLICATION TO CLINICAL ASSESSMENT

This section will address research data on the differential performance of males and females on standard tests used in neuropsychological evaluations. Because current data provide conflicting results, representative literature both supporting and not supporting gender differences on measures such as the Wechsler intelligence scales and the Halstead–Reitan (HRNB) battery are presented.

Laterality and Wechsler Performance

There is research evidence suggesting that the effect of unilateral damage to the brain has a different impact depending upon the sex of the individual. Using previously reported Wechsler–Bellevue scores for 15 female and 16 male patients with unilateral lesions, Inglis and Lawson (1981) found a laterality effect for the males but not for the females.

Research by Lansdell (1961, 1968) found that following left temporal lobectomies, males and females had differential patterns of impairment when compared to controls of their own sex. Impaired males did less well on proverb interpretation (Lansdell, 1961) and on the verbal subtests of the Wechsler–Bellevue (Lansdell, 1968) but this "traditional" reaction was not found in the females. Following right temporal lobectomies, the nonverbal abilities of the males as measured on the Wechsler–Bellevue subtests were more impaired than the verbal abilities but again the results did not obtain for the females (Lansdell, 1968). McGlone (1977, 1978) reported similar findings. In her research with stroke and tumor patients, she found that females showed loss of verbal abilities only after bilateral insult. All of her patients were right-handed adults. Not only were problems with verbal skills found more often in left-hemisphere-damaged males but the level of deficit was greater for the males than the females. Using data from the WAIS, she found no differences in scores on the nonverbal subtests by either sex or side of damage. Significant differences were found, however, when the score on the nonverbal items was compared to that on the verbal items. For the males, left side damage impaired the verbal IQ more than the nonverbal IQ and the opposite was found for right side damage. This difference was not found in the females. Such data could be used to support the hypothesis that there is greater specialization of brain function in males than in females (Woods & Hebben, 1988).

Inglis and his colleagues (Inglis, Ruckman, Lawson, MacLean, & Monga, 1982) attempted to replicate McGlone's findings by assessing 100 adults, 80 of whom had suffered unilateral cerebrovascular accident. All patients in this study were tested with the WAIS. As would be expected from McGlone's findings, left-hemisphere-damaged males had lower verbal IQs (VIQ) than performance IQs (PIQ) and right-hemisphere-damaged females showed small but not significant VIQ–PIQ differences in the same direction as the males. When they compared these brain-damaged subjects to controls (Inglis, Ruckman, Lawson, MacLean, & Monga, 1983), they found further support for their hypothesis that females, more than males, utilize left-hemisphere processing for tasks that are viewed as nonverbal in nature. Using a sample of 83 males and 32 females with unilateral brain damage, Sundet (1986) also found significant VIQ–PIQ discrepancies for males but not for females when tested with the WAIS.

Bornstein and Matarazzo (1984) critically reviewed studies of the influence of sex differences on Wechsler scores following unilateral lesions by reanalyzing previously reported data. They omitted studies that used the same patient data as well as the data from patients for whom the EEG abnormalities were bilateral but more prominent in one hemisphere. Despite their attempts to attain sample comparability, they noted that lesion etiology was heterogeneous. They suggested that the rate of lesion progression may be an important factor in brain compensation as reflected in Wechsler performance and yet this factor could not be assessed adequately from available data. Despite the fact that some studies found sex differences, they concluded that the data did not support the use of such differences with individual patients, that the number of patients who did not meet the suggested sex differences was clinically important, and that future studies needed to consider more closely group comparability.

In a study that followed the suggestions of Bornstein and Matarazzo (1984), Yeo, Turkheimer, and Bigler (1984) used information from CT scans to match their groups on lesion size and location prior to data analysis. The CT data were analyzed by a computerized procedure to quantify specific brain parameters. The lesion size was expressed as a ratio of the volume of the lesion to the volume of the subject's brain. The location of the lesion was the centerpoint as determined by a three-dimensional coordinate system. When these subjects were given a neuropsychological battery, they found significant sex by location differences with left-lesioned males showing greater impairment than left-lesioned females and right-lesioned males showing less impairment than right-lesioned females. From these data, Yeo and his colleagues concluded that since the subjects were matched for locus and extent of lesion as well as etiology, differences supported a hypothesis of sex differences in brain organization.

Challenges to Gender Differences

The data from McGlone (1977, 1978) and others have not gone unchallenged. Herring and Reitan (1986) suggested that these studies are confounded. They noted that when multiple univariate analyses of variance are conducted, there is the potential for an inflated alpha level if adjustment procedures are not used. They also called into question the equivalency of McGlone's groups since only a subset of the whole sample was used when the sex by lesioned hemisphere effects were examined.

When Herring (1984) investigated the performance of unilaterally lesioned subjects on the HRNB, his results did not support a conclusion of sex differences in cerebral organization or in higher cognitive abilities. While reporting sex differences in Digit Symbol (females were superior), Tactile Finger Recognition (females were superior), and Finger Oscillation (males were superior), he concluded that these differences were too small to justify a hypothesis of differential lateralization.

Snow and Sheese (1985) tested McGlone's gender difference concept using the WAIS with 28 males and 17 females with unilateral damage due to infarcts. Their data did not support a sex difference. Bornstein (1984) investigated the question of differential cognitive impairment by sex using the WAIS-R with a sample of 63 patients with unilateral lesions. Both males and females showed the same VIQ–PIQ discrepancies and in the same directions as previous research had found for males only. Bornstein suggested the WAIS-R, although overlapping the formerly used WAIS to a great extent, may be slightly more difficult than its predecessor. With this increase in difficulty level, the WAIS-R may be more sensitive to VIQ–PIQ differences than was the WAIS. Since Bornstein's sample was also somewhat younger than McGlone's (1977, 1978) sample, it may be that sex differences in reaction to impairment change across the adult period. Bornstein concluded, however, that data up to that time did not support a concept of sex differences in the functional organization of the brain.

In an attempt to further investigate the sex question in functional organization of the brain, Herring and Reitan (1986) administered the Wechsler–Bellevue to three groups of subjects. One group consisted of 48 people with evidence of right cerebral hemisphere damage with an equal number of subjects with left cerebral hemisphere damage. The control group consisted of 28 subjects described as neurologically normal. There were an equal number of males and females within each group. Their data did not support a sex effect as they found no consistent evidence of sex by lesioned hemisphere. This study differed from those reporting sex differences (Inglis *et al.*, 1982; McGlone, 1977, 1978) in the version of the Wechsler test used and in the use of a statistical procedure to adjust the alpha level because of the multiple comparisons being made. When Snow, Freedman, and Ford (1986) surveyed the existing literature on the impact of lateralized brain injury on individual task performance, they concluded that the literature supported a sex effect with the Wechsler–Bellevue but not with the WAIS. Without data comparing all three versions of the Wechsler scale on VIQ–PIQ differences, it cannot be determined to what extent this factor influenced the Herring and Reitan data or the general concept of sex issues and intellectual impairment.

When sex issues and specific aspects of intellectual development are considered in nonimpaired children, additional data of importance are found. Data from impaired adults could be viewed as supportive of differential reaction to trauma by sex or to differences in gender development that are accentuated by trauma. When a sample of neurologically normal third, fifth, and seventh grade children were given the Vocabulary and Block Design subtests of the WISC-R, sex differences were not found (Regard, Strauss, & Knapp, 1982). Further exploration with a similar population using the entire test would be helpful.

A sample of 137 male and 113 female adult epileptics were found to have sex differences on 12 of 33 comparisons of test scores (Kupke, Lewis, & Rennick, 1979). Males tended to perform better than females on measures of gross motor skill, visual-spatial abilities, and quantitative skills. Females performed better than males on measures of verbal and psychomotor ability. Since these data are similar to those found with neurologically unimpaired subjects, they might be viewed as supporting the hypothesis of sex differences in localization of function. Further research in this area, while also supporting sex differences in localization of function, has raised questions about the range of visuospatial abilities for which this difference occurs (Lewis & Kamptner, 1987).

Literature Summaries

When analyzing the growing literature on sex influences on brain organization, McGlone (1986) stated that her prior theory (McGlone, 1980) regarding greater asymmetrical organization of the male than female brain should be rejected as too simplistic. To replace her earlier theory, she suggested some working hypotheses to guide future investigations. These hypotheses centered on the use of new methods for specifying the site and size of the dysfunction as well as the importance of replication studies in a wide range of laboratories.

Yeo (1989) concluded that both literature reviews and meta analyses provide support for the position that the reported sex differences following lesions occur more often than would be expected by chance. The data suggest that it is unlikely these differences are due to strategy and therefore gender rather than sex variables.

In another analysis of the existing literature, Anderson (1987) concluded that in the majority of studies of adults, males are more lateralized than females for verbal processing and visuospatial processes while females are more lateralized for nonverbal auditory processes. Bryden (1981) also concluded that the literature supports the hypothesis of more lateralized male brains at least for verbal dichotic and verbal tachistoscopic studies with additional but less strong support from measures of visual and tactile senses.

Not all investigators agree with Anderson's analysis of the current literature. Some researchers suggest that Anderson's conclusions are the result of a Type 1 error (Springer & Deutsch, 1985). Since most journals are not willing to publish "no difference" results, the literature supporting sex differences in lateralization may only represent a small percentage of the actual research that has been conducted on this topic. When considering the "Type 1" error issue for these studies, it may be noted that very few studies report a significant sex difference in lateralization with the females being more lateralized than the males. Perhaps this fact is one of the reasons that, given the current literature base, the hypothesis of sex differences in laterality is considered by many to remain viable.

Spatial, Sensory, and Visual Factors

Witelson (1976) studied 200 children between the ages of 6 and 13 using a dichotic stimulation test. All of these children were described as being strongly right-handed. Findings supported an interaction of hand and sex for these subjects. For the males, the performance with the left hand was significantly better than with the right hand. For the females, this differential performance did not occur. When these subjects were administered a dichotic digits task, they did not show differential hearing advantage. Witelson's data support the hypothesis that there may be sex differences in spatial abilities and that such differences occur in childhood.

If there are differences in spatial abilities, neuropsychologists will need to consider these factors when norming assessment tools. Further investigation is also needed to better determine whether there is a physiological basis for these reported gender differences. These reported differences have been hypothesized to result from either a recessive gene on the X chromosome or hormonal effects on the organization and function of the brain (Dean, 1985; Kolb & Whishaw, 1990; Wedding, Horton, & Webster, 1986).

Responsiveness to sound is often included as part of a neuropsychological evaluation. Therefore, it is important for the assessor to note that numerous studies have reported sex differences in pure tone thresholds, sound localization, and tolerance of noise (Baker, 1987). Several studies have also provided support for the concept that among females there is variability of response to a number of sensory tasks, including auditory tasks, as a result of menstrual variation (Diamond, Diamond, & Mast, 1972; Parlee, 1983). Parlee's (1983) review of the literature produced data suggesting menstrual rhythm is also related to performance on tasks of vision, olfaction, taste, and touch. Research has yet to determine the mechanism leading to these menstrual differences in performance. Not all authors concur with the position that sex differences in auditory processing have been supported in the literature. Spreen *et al.* (1984) stated that sex differences in development have not been found for auditory receptivity.

Much of the research on visual acuity has reported better performance by males than females (Baker, 1987). This sex difference has been found to occur as early as age 6 (Young, Beattie, Newby, & Swindal, 1954). When visual organization is measured, however, sex differences may not occur. Hilgert and Treloar (1985) found no relationship between scores on the Hooper Visual Organization Test and sex in a sample of 54 elementary school students who had been referred for psychometric evaluation. A range of visual tasks are used as part of a neuropsychological evaluation. Some of these tasks are measures of visual ability while others are intended to evaluate specific abilities but are highly visual in form. A tool often included in evaluations is the Stroop Color and Word Test (SCW). The SCW is described as a measure of cognitive efficiency or verbal fluency (Golden, 1978) but requires certain visual skills for completion. To investigate whether there would be a gender difference in performance on this type of task, Stroop stimuli were presented laterally to 40 subjects (Simon, Paullin, Overmyer, & Berbaum, 1985). No gender differences in performance were found. When Connor and her colleagues (Connor, Franzen, & Sharp, 1988) administered the SCW to 40 college undergraduates in the standard test presentation style, they also found no sex effect. Their data support the prior findings on visual organization. Since these data are based on small samples of normals, there is a need for further investigation with larger and more diverse groups.

Test Batteries

Erlandson (1987) investigated the effect of sex on performance on the Luria–Nebraska Neuropsychological Battery (LNNB). Data on 144 subjects were found to support a hypothesis of sex differences in both visuospatial and verbal abilities. Special cutoff scores by sex were developed for these subjects. When these new cutoff scores were applied to the original data, there was a significant increase in the hit rate.

The LNNB has also been used to assess the neuropsychological function of psychiatric patients as theories have been developed to tie unilateral hemispheric dysfunction to specific psychiatric disorders (Boklage, 1977; Gur, 1977). Using a sample of schizophrenic and manic–depressive patients, Frazier, Silverstein, and Fogg (1989) reported that sex differences are either associated with, or influence, complex cognitive–perceptual skills. These gender differences alone, however, do not account for lateralization differences. There was also some evidence of bilateral involvement. Specifically, female major depressive patients showed significantly greater deficits than male major depressive patients on the right-hemisphere empirical scale. Gender-related differences were not found among their schizophrenic sample.

Subject variables, including sex, were investigated for their relationship to scores on the HRNB in a group of 288 seizure disorder patients between the ages of 15 and 52 (Seidenberg, Gamache, Beck, Smith, Giordani, Berent, Sackellares, & Boll, 1984) using a stepwise regression analysis. On the HRNB, sex was found to be a significant factor only for grip strength and tapping. As the authors note, generalizability of their data is limited by the fact that adult seizure patients are unique among brain-damaged patients due to the fact that the problem is often both chronic and episodic. Comparable studies using various patient populations are needed. Gordon and O'Dell (1983) used a subset of the HRNB, yielding 14 scores, with a college student sample and reported similar data for grip strength and tapping. This study used data from prior research (Gordon, O'Dell, & Bozeman, 1981) on 50 college students and then added to the subject pool for the second study. Although they also found females to perform significantly better than males on left-hand fingertip number writing, left-hand finger agnosia, and Tactual Performance Test memory and location scores, they stated that these differences were not clinically relevant.

Extending the data base by age and educational level, Yeudall and his colleagues (Yeudall, Fromm, Reddon, & Stefanyk, 1986; Yeudall, Reddon, Gill, & Stefanyk, 1987) provided normative data from a neurologically intact sample on a range of neuropsychological tests. One of the variables examined in these studies was sex. In their 1986 study, 225 subjects ranging in age from 15 to 40 years were given 12 neuropsychological tests that Yeudall stated he used in addition to the Halstead–Reitan test battery to improve accuracy of diagnosis. Sex differences were not found for Language Modalities Test for Aphasia, Memory-for-Designs, Coloured Progressive Matrices, Controlled Word Association, L. J. Tactile Recognition, and Wisconsin Card Sorting. Sex differences were reported for Symbol-Gestalt, Minute Estimation, Written Word Fluency, Purdue Pegboard, Williams Clinical Memory, and Symbol Digit Modalities. In a sample of 50 male and 50 female 12- to 13-year-old black subjects, Knuckle and Asbury (1986) found females to be superior to males on the Purdue Pegboard. They also found these female subjects to outperform the male subjects on the Benton Visual Retention Test and the Symbol Digit Modalities Test. Such differences suggest the need to consider sex norms not only for these tests but for other tests that measure similar abilities. In an attempt to add to the normative base on neuropsychological tests, these researchers also evaluated their subjects on the HRNB (Yeudall *et al.*, 1987). Sex differences were not found for Name Writing, Speech-Sounds Perception, Trail Making, Halstead Category, Tactual Performance Test, Seashore Rhythm, Tactile Form Recognition, Finger-Tip Number Writing Perception, and Face-Hand. Sex differences were found for Finger Tapping, Dynamometer, and Finger Localization for the preferred hand on double stimulation.

Although gender effects were not found on the Tactual Performance Test in the Yeudall *et al.* (1987) study, they have been reported with neurologically sound college students (Chavez, Schwartz, & Brandon, 1982; Kupke, 1983). In a sample of 26 male and 26 female students (Chavez *et al.*, 1982), females had significantly higher Localization scores than males. Opposite-sex pairs of examiners and subjects yielded superior performance on both memory and location scores when compared to same-sex pairs with 40 male and 40 female college students. Without comparable data from a neurologically impaired sample and a larger sample size, the strength of this sex-of-examiner effect remains in question.

A number of studies have reported sex differences in finger tapping performance (Brandon, Chavez, & Bennett, 1986; Buckelew & Hannay, 1986; Chavez, Trautt, Brandon, & Steyaert, 1983; Gordon & O'Dell, 1983; Harris, 1982; Morrison, Gregory, & Paul, 1979; Yeudall *et al.*, 1987). Not only do females produce significantly fewer taps than males, but the particular finger tapping instrument used may also influence performance level. In an investigation of the performance of normal undergraduates (Chavez *et al.*, 1983), use of the Western Psychological Services' finger tapping apparatus resulted in significantly more taps than when the Halstead apparatus was used, suggesting that norms developed on one apparatus may not be applicable to another. Significant sex differences were found regardless of the apparatus used with females producing fewer taps than males who used the same apparatus.

A characteristic that has been considered relative to finger tapping which complicates the data base on this topic is ethnic background. When comparing the performance of Anglo and non- Anglo juvenile offenders, Andrew (1977) found significant differences in finger tapping performance between Anglo females and non-Anglo females with the former being slower on the task. The performance of the non-Anglo females was not significantly different from the males. These data raise issues regarding the relationship between ethnicity and sex as they relate to neuropsychological test performance. The current literature provides little information on this subject.

SUMMARY

One question that has been raised in the literature is whether or not sex and gender variables should continue to be considered in psychological research studies. The data available at this time suggest that sex is slowly becoming a factor in neuropsychological research but that gender issues have generally not been addressed. Further investigation of these factors is justified in the field of clinical neuropsychological assessment. There is no way to determine the number of investigations that have failed to find sex and gender differences due to the policy of not publishing "no difference" data.

The current data base suggests that some neuroanatomical structures and assessment tools have been investigated more carefully than others. Future research on sex and gender issues needs to consider a wider range of subjects with larger samples. Since factors such as psychiatric diagnosis and ethnic background have been raised as potentially relevant to considerations of differential performance by gender on at least some tests, it would be useful if future researchers would provide information about these factors when reporting their data. In the field of neuropsychological assessment, there seems to be a tendency to focus on the more "objective" data from specialty measures rather than the more traditional personality measures or use of the diagnostic classification nomenclature. As a research field, there has been progress since the suggestion was made by Parsons and Prigatano (1978) that we had been ignoring gender differences in our research. A considerable improvement is needed before we will have sufficient data to have it become clinically useful to us. Not only will these investigations need to address a wider range of tests, larger samples of neurologically impaired and nonimpaired subjects of all ages, and various personality diagnoses, but these investigators would benefit from an awareness of the range of related literature that is available from other disciplines. Among those other disciplines are neurology, physical anthropology, and neurobiology. Due to the nature of this subject, it is imperative that researchers have a broad base and that practicing clinicians become sensitive to the implications of the current data as well as its limitations.

REFERENCES

Anderson, N. S. (1987). Cognition, learning, and memory. In M. A. Baker (Ed.), *Sex differences in human performance* (pp. 37–54). New York: Wiley.

Andrew, J. (1977). Delinquents and the Tapping Test. *Journal of Clinical Psychology, 33,* 786–791.

Baker, M. A. (1987). Sensory functioning, In M. A. Baker (Ed.), *Sex differences in human performance* (pp. 5–36). New York: Wiley.

Baumeister, R. F. (1988). Should we stop studying sex differences altogether? *American Psychologist, 43,* 1092–1095.

Blechman, E. A., & Brownell, K. D. (1988). *Handbook of behavioral medicine for women*. Elmsford, N.Y.: Pergamon Press.

Bloom, F. E., & Lazerson, A. (1988). *Brain, mind, and behavior* (2nd ed.). San Francisco: Freeman.

Boklage, C. E. (1977). Schizophrenia, brain asymmetry development, and twinning: Cellular relationship with etiological and possible prognostic implications. *Biological Psychiatry, 12,* 19–35.

Bornstein, R. A. (1984). Unilateral lesion and the Wechsler Adult Intelligence Scale—Revised: No sex differences. *Journal of Consulting and Clinical Psychology, 52,* 604–608.

Bornstein, R. A., & Matarazzo, J. D. (1984). Relationship of sex and the effects of unilateral lesions of the Wechsler intelligence scales. *The Journal of Nervous and Mental Disease, 172,* 707–710.

Brandon, A. D., Chavez, E. L., & Bennett, T. L. (1986). A comparative evaluation of two neuropsychological finger tapping instruments: Halstead–Reitan and Western Psychological Services. *International Journal of Clinical Neuropsychology, 8,* 64–65.

Bryden, M. P. (1981). *Laterality: Functional asymmetry in the intact brain*. New York: Academic Press.

Buckelew, S. P., & Hannay, H. J. (1986). Relationships among anxiety, defensiveness, sex, task difficulty, and performance on various neuropsychological tasks. *Perceptual and Motor Skills, 63,* 711–718.

Chavez, E. L., Schwartz, M. M., & Brandon, A. (1982). Effects of sex of subject and method of block presentation on the Tactual Performance Test. *Journal of Consulting and Clinical Psychology, 50,* 600–601.

Chavez, E. L., Trautt, G. M., Brandon, A., & Steyaert, J. (1983). Effects of test anxiety and sex of subject on neuropsychological test performance: Finger Tapping, Trail Making, Digit Span and Digit Symbol tests. *Perceptual and Motor Skills, 56,* 923–929.

Connor, A., Franzen, M. D., & Sharp, B. (1988). Effects of practice and differential instructions on Stroop performance. *International Journal of Clinical Neuropsychology, 10,* 1–4.

Dean, R. S. (1985). Foundation and rationale for neuropsychological bases of individual differences. In L. C. Hartlage & C. F. Telzrow (Eds.), *The neuropsychology of individual differences: A developmental perspective*. New York: Plenum Press.

deLacoste, M. C., Holloway, R. L., & Woodward, D. J. (1986). Sex differences in the fetal human corpus callosum. *Human Neurobiology, 5,* 93–96.

deLacoste-Utamsing, C., & Holloway, R. L. (1982). Sexual dimorphism in the human corpus callosum. *Science, 216,* 1431–1432.

DeLisi, L. E., Dauphinais, D., & Hauser, P. (1989). Gender differences in the brain: Are they relevant to the pathogenesis of schizophrenia? *Comprehensive Psychiatry, 30,* 197–208.

Dementer, S., Ringo, J., & Doty, R. W. (1985). Sexual dimorphism in the human corpus callosum? *Society for Neuroscience Abstracts, 11,* No. 254.12.

Diamond, M., Diamond, A. L., & Mast, M. (1972). Visual sensitivity and sexual arousal levels during the menstrual cycle. *Journal of Nervous and Mental Disease, 155,* 170–176.

Erlandson, G. L. (1987). Gender differences, diagnostic validity and the Luria–Nebraska Neuropsychological Battery (Doctoral dissertation, The University of Wisconsin–Milwaukee, 1987). *Dissertation Abstracts International, 48,* 83A.

Fleet, W. S., & Heilman, K. M. (1985). Acquired stuttering from a right hemisphere lesion in a right-hander. *Neurology, 35,* 1343–1346.

Franzen, M. D. (1989). *Reliability and validity in neuropsychological assessment.* New York: Plenum Press.

Frazier, M. F., Silverstein, M. L., & Fogg, L. (1989). Lateralized cerebral dysfunction in schizophrenia and depression: Gender and medication effects. *Archives of Clinical Neuropsychology, 4,* 33–44.

Geschwind, N., & Galaburda, A. M. (1985). Cerebral lateralization: Biological mechanisms, associations, and pathology: I. A hypothesis and a program for research. *Archives of Neurology, 42,* 428–459.

Golden, C. J. (1978). *Stroop Color and Word Test: A manual for clinical use.* Chicago: Stoelting.

Golden, C. J., & Vincente, P. J. (1983). *Foundations of clinical neuropsychology.* New York: Plenum Press.

Goldstein, G., & Tarter, R. E. (1986). *Advances in clinical neuropsychology* (Vol. 3). New York: Plenum Press.

Gordon, N. G., & O'Dell, J. W. (1983). Sex differences in neuropsychological performance. *Perceptual and Motor Skills, 56,* 126.

Gordon, N. G., O'Dell, J. W., & Bozeman, N. (1981). Variation in neuropsychological performance as a function of sex. *Journal of Psychology, 109,* 127–131.

Gur, R. E. (1977). Motoric laterality imbalance in schizophrenia. *Archives of General Psychiatry, 34,* 33–37.

Harris, L. J. (1978). Sex differences in spatial ability: Possible environmental, genetic, and neurological factors. In M. Kinsbourne (Ed.), *Asymmetrical function of the brain.* London: Cambridge University Press.

Harris, M. D. (1982). The effects of depression, test artifacts, and sex on neuropsychological tests (Doctoral dissertation, Washington State University, 1981). *Dissertation Abstracts International, 42,* 2986B.

Herring, S. L. (1984). Neuropsychological performances of male and female subjects with unilateral cerebral lesions (Doctoral dissertation, The University of Arizona, 1983). *Dissertation Abstracts, 44,* 3236B.

Herring, S., & Reitan, R. R. (1986). Sex similarities in verbal and performance IQ deficits following unilateral cerebral lesions. *Journal of Consulting and Clinical Psychology, 54,* 537–541.

Hesselbrock, M. E., Weidenman, M. A., & Reed, H. B. (1985). Effects of age, sex, drinking history, and antisocial personality on neuropsychology of alcoholics. *Journal of Studies on Alcohol, 46,* 313–320.

Hier, D., & Crowley, W. (1982). Spatial ability in androgen-deficient men. *New England Journal of Medicine,* May 20.

Hilgert, L. D., & Treloar, J. H. (1985). The relationship of the Hooper Visual Organization Test to sex, age, and intelligence of elementary school children. *Measurement and Evaluation in Counseling and Development, 17,* 203–206.

Holloway, R. L., & deLacoste, M. C. (1986). Sexual dimorphism in the human corpus callosum: An extension and replication study. *Human Neurobiology, 5,* 87–91.

Hoyenga, K. B., & Hoyenga, K. T. (1979). *The question of sex differences: Psychosocial, cultural and biological issues*. Boston: Little, Brown.

Incagnoli, T., Goldstein, G., & Golden, C. J. (1986). *Clinical applications of neuropsychological test batteries*. New York: Plenum Press.

Inglis, J., & Lawson, J. S. (1981). Sex differences in the effects of unilateral brain damage on intelligence. *Science, 212*, 693–695.

Inglis, J., Ruckman, M., Lawson, J. S., MacLean, A. W., & Monga, T. N. (1982). Sex differences in the cognitive effects of unilateral brain damage. *Cortex, 18*, 257–275.

Inglis, J., Ruckman, M., Lawson, J. S., MacLean, A. W., & Monga, T. N. (1983). Sex differences in the cognitive effects of unilateral brain damage: Comparison of stroke and normal control subjects. *Cortex, 19*, 551–555.

Jacobson, R. (1986). The contributions of sex and drinking history to the CT brain scan changes in alcoholics. *Psychological Medicine, 16*, 547–559.

Klooz, N. A., & Rosenbaum, G. (1988, August). Lateralization of function in aging men and women. Paper presented at the meeting of the American Psychological Association, Atlanta.

Knuckle, E. P., & Asbury, C. A. (1986). WISC-R discrepancy score directions and gender as reflected in neuropsychological test performance of black adolescents. *Journal of Research and Development in Education, 20*, 44–51.

Kolb, B., & Whishaw, I. Q. (1990). *Fundamentals of human neuropsychology* (3rd ed.). San Francisco: Freeman.

Kupke, T. (1983). Effects of subject sex, examiner sex, and test apparatus on Halstead Category and Tactual Performance Tests. *Journal of Consulting and Clinical Psychology, 51*, 624–626.

Kupke, T., Lewis, R., & Rennick, P. M. (1979). Sex differences in the neuropsychological functioning of epileptics. *Journal of Consulting and Clinical Psychology, 47*, 1128–1130.

Lansdell, H. (1961). The effects of neurosurgery on a test of proverbs. *American Psychologist, 16*, 448.

Lansdell, H. (1968). The use of factor scores from the Wechsler Bellevue Scale of Intelligence in assessing patients with temporal lobe removals. *Cortex, 4*, 257–268.

Larue, L. J. (1986). Lateralized sex differences in human cognitive functioning (Doctoral dissertation, Rutgers University, 1986). *Dissertation Abstracts International, 47*, 965A.

Levy, J. (1984). A review, analysis, and some new data on hand-posture distributions in left-handers. *Brain and Cognition, 3*, 105–127.

Levy, J., & Reid, M. (1978). Variations in cerebral organization as a function of handedness, hand posture in writing, and sex. *Journal of Experimental Psychology: General, 107*, 119–144.

Levy, J., & Wagner, N. (1984). Handwriting, posture, visuomotor integration, and lateralized reaction time parameters. *Human Neurobiology, 3*, 157–161.

Lewis, R. S., & Kamptner, N. L. (1987). Sex differences in spatial task performance of patients with and without unilateral lesions. *Brain Cognition, 6*, 142–152.

Lezak, M. D. (1983). *Neuropsychological assessment* (2nd ed.). New York: Oxford University Press.

Maccoby, E. E., & Jacklin, C. N. (1974). *The psychology of sex differences*. Stanford: Stanford University Press.

McGee, M. G. (1979). Human spatial abilities: Psychometric studies and environmental, genetic, hormonal, and neurological influences. *Psychological Bulletin, 86*, 889–918.

McGlone, J. (1977). Sex differences in the cerebral organization of verbal functions in patients with unilateral brian lesions. *Brain, 100*, 775–793.

McGlone, J. (1978). Sex differences in functional brain symmetry. *Cortex, 14*, 122–128.

McGlone, J. (1980). Sex differences in human brain symmetry: A critical survey. *The Behavioral and Brain Sciences, 3*, 215–263.

McGlone, J. (1986). The neuropsychology of sex differences in human brain organization. In G. Goldstein & R. E. Tarter (Eds.), *Advances in clinical neuropsychology* (Vol. 3, pp. 1–30). New York: Plenum Press.

Morrison, M. W., Gregory, R. J., & Paul, J. J. (1979). Reliability of the Finger Tapping Test and a note on sex differences. *Perceptual and Motor Skills, 48*, 139–142.

Newman, P. W., Bunderson, K., & Brey, R. H. (1985). Brain stem electrical responses of stutterers and normals by sex, ears, and recovery. *Journal of Fluency Disorders, 10*, 59–67.

Parlee, M. B. (1983). Menstrual rhythms in sensory processes: A review of fluctuations in vision, olfaction, audition, taste, and touch. *Psychological Bulletin, 93*, 539–548.

Parsons, O. A., & Prigatano, G. P. (1978). Methodological considerations in clinical neuropsychological research. *Journal of Consulting and Clinical Psychology, 46*, 608–619.

Peters M. (1988). Corpus callosum. *Canadian Journal of Psychology, 42*, 313–324.

Piazza, D. M. (1980). The influence of sex and handedness in the hemispheric specialization of verbal and nonverbal tasks. *Neuropsychologia, 18*, 163–176.

Regard, M., Strauss, E., & Knapp, P. (1982). Children's performance on verbal and non-verbal fluency tasks. *Perceptual and Motor Skills, 55*, 839–844.

Rothblum, E. D. (1988). More on reporting sex differences. *American Psychologist, 43*, 1095.

Rovet, J. (1983). Cognitive and neuropsychological test performance of persons with abnormalities of adolescent development: A test of Waber's hypothesis. *Child Development, 54*, 941–950.

Seidenberg, M., Gamache, M. P., Beck, N. C., Smith, M., Giordani, B., Berent, S., Sackellares, J. C., & Boll, T. J. (1984). Subject variables and performance on the Halstead Neuropsychological Test Battery: A multivariate analysis. *Journal of Consulting and Clinical Psychology, 52*, 658–662.

Simon, J. R., Paullin, C., Overmyer, S. P., & Berbaum, K. (1985). Reaction time to word meaning and ink color of laterally-presented Stroop stimuli: Effects of handedness and sex. *International Journal of Neuroscience, 28*, 21–33.

Snow, W. G., & Sheese, S. (1985). Lateralized brain damage, intelligence, and memory: A failure to find sex differences. *Journal of Consulting and Clinical Psychology, 53*, 940–941.

Snow, W. G. Freedman, L., & Ford, L. (1986). Lateralized brain damage, sex differences, and the Wechsler Intelligence Scales: A reexamination. *Journal of Clinical and Experimental Neuropsychology, 8*, 179–189.

Sparadeo, F. R., Zwick, W. R., & Butters, N. (1983). Cognitive functioning of alcoholic females: An exploratory study. *Drug and Alcohol Dependence, 12*, 143–150.

Spreen, O., Tupper, D., Risser, A., Tuokko, H., & Edgell, D. (1984). *Human developmental neuropsychology*. New York: Oxford University Press.

Springer, S. P., & Duetsch, G. (1985). *Left brain, right brain* (rev. ed.). San Francisco: Freeman.

Sundet, K. (1986). Sex differences in cognitive impairment following unilateral brain damage. *Journal of Clinical and Experimental Neuropsychology, 8*, 51–61.

Unger, R. K. (1979). Toward a redefinition of sex and gender. *American Psychologist, 34*, 1085–1094.

Wada, J., Clarke, R., & Hamm, A. (1975). Asymmetry of frontal speech zones in 100 adult and 100 infant brains. *Archives of Neurology, 32*, 239–246.

Warkentin, S., Rodriguez, G., & Rosadini, G. (1988). Gender differences in regional cerebral blood flow. *Journal of Clinical and Experimental Neuropsychology, 10*, 332 (Abstract).

Wedding, D., Horton, A. M., & Webster, J. (Eds.). (1986). *The neuropsychology handbook: Behavioral and clinical perspectives*. Berlin: Springer.

Weinfeld, F. (1981). The Nation survey of stroke. *Stroke, 12*, 52–53.

Witelson, S. F. (1976). Sex and the single hemisphere: Specialization of the right hemisphere in spatial processing. *Science, 193*, 425–427.

Witelson, S. F. (1985). On hemisphere specialization and cerebral plasticity from birth: Mark II. In C. Best (Ed.), *Hemispheric function and collaboration in the child* (pp. 33–85). New York: Academic Press.

Witelson, S. F., & Kigar, D. L. (1988). Anatomical development of the corpus callosum in humans: A review with reference to sex and cognition. In D. L. Molfese & S. J. Segalowitz (Eds.), *Brain lateralization in children: Developmental implications* (pp. 35–57). New York: Guilford Press.

Witelson, S. F., & Palie, W. (1973). Left hemisphere specialization for language in the newborn: Neuroanatomical evidence of asymmetry. *Brain, 96*, 641–646.

Woods, B. T., & Hebben, N. (1988). Neurological function and dysfunction. In E. A. Blechman & K. D. Brownell (Eds.), *Handbook of behavioral medicine for women* (pp. 145–159). Elmsford, N.Y.: Pergamon Press.

Yeo, R. A. (1989). Individual differences. In E. D. Bigler, R. A. Yeo, & E. Turkheimer (Eds.), *Neuropsychological function and brain imaging* (pp. 295–316). New York: Plenum Press.

Yeo, R. A., Turkheimer, E., & Bigler, E. (1984). The influence of sex and age on unilateral cerebral lesion sequelae. *International Journal of Neuroscience, 24,* 299–301.

Yeudall, L. T., Fromm, D., Reddon, J. R., & Stefanyk, W. O. (1986). Normative data stratified by age and sex for 12 neuropsychological tests. *Journal of Clinical Psychology, 42,* 918–946.

Yeudall, L. T., Reddon, J. R., Gill, D. M., & Stefanyk, W. O. (1987). Normative data for the Halstead–Reitan neuropsychological tests stratified by age and sex. *Journal of Clinical Psychology, 43,* 346–367.

Younes, R. P., Rosner, B., & Webb, G. (1983). Neuroimmaturity of learning disabled children: A controlled study. *Developmental Medicine and Child Neurology, 25,* 574–579.

Young, F A., Beattie, R. J., Newby, F. J., & Swindal, M. T. (1954). The Pullman study—A visual survey of Pullman school children. *American Journal of Optometry and Archives of American Academy of Optometry, 31,* 192–203.

5

Handedness and Lateralization

POLLY HENNINGER

INTRODUCTION

To accurately assess the nature and extent of brain injury, is it important to know the patient's handedness? Evidence from both clinical and normal populations indicates that the organization of brain functions differs for right- and left-handers. In general, left-handers are less lateralized for linguistic, visuospatial, and other cognitive and affective processes, and are likely to show bilateral representation of cognitive functions. Lack of standardization in the measurement of handedness and the influence of other variables such as familial sinistrality, sex, and reasoning ability on brain organization make it difficult to specify for any particular individual. However, awareness of the identified modifiers of brain organization and knowledge of findings on handedness relating to lateralized functions can assist the neuropsychologist in making more accurate diagnoses and inferences. This chapter will present current research findings on laterality and handedness and apply them to issues of clinical concern.

Lateralization

Lateralization refers to the specialization of a function or activity in one side of the organism. It is observed in asymmetries of motor, perceptual, and cognitive functions. These asymmetries reflect differential specialization of the two cerebral hemispheres. Specifically, language, analytic processes, and motor activities on the right side of the body are lateralized to the left cerebral hemisphere, and nonverbal, visuospatial processes, and motor activities on the left side of the body are lateralized to the right hemisphere. Several terms are

POLLY HENNINGER • Division of Biology 156-29, California Institute of Technology, Pasadena, California 91125.

HANDBOOK OF NEUROPSYCHOLOGICAL ASSESSMENT: A Biopsychosocial Perspective, edited by Antonio E. Puente and Robert J. McCaffrey. Plenum Press, New York, 1992.

used to describe lateralized cognitive processing. *Hemispheric specialization* refers to the fact that each hemisphere is specialized for certain types of processing. Asymmetric performance on a perceptual task indicates hemispheric specialization for the type of processing elicited by that task with preferential ability in the domain of the contralateral hemisphere. *Cerebral dominance*, an older term that originally implied left hemisphere dominance refers both to the differential ability of the two hemispheres to do their respective types of processing and also to the notion that one hemisphere dominates and directs behavior. Thus, the left hemisphere dominates and directs behavior during verbal activities; the right hemisphere is more likely to dominate during nonverbal, visuospatial activities. *Hemisphericity* is the notion that a given individual relies more on one mode of processing, and therefore more on one hemisphere than the other, for most activities, regardless of their analytic or synthetic nature. This differential utilization is presumed to be reflected in the individual's "cognitive style." A tendency to approach problems verbally or analytically is presumed to differentially activate the left hemisphere and indicate left-sided hemisphericity whereas a tendency to deal with information holistically or spatially is believed to differentially activate the right hemisphere and indicate right-sided hemisphericity. When people use the term *laterality*, they usually are referring to *hemispheric specialization*.

Most higher-order cognitive functions are lateralized, that is, they are represented differentially in the two hemispheres with one hemisphere being more involved in any particular operation. The extent to which one hemisphere dominates depends upon a complex interaction of stimulus, task, response, and individual difference variables. Except in very simple tasks, both hemispheres are involved in processing. Nonetheless, each hemisphere is specialized for particular functions, and when a hemisphere is damaged, the person cannot perform, or performs poorly, tasks subserved by those functions. This is most evident in aphasia, the loss of the ability to express or understand language, and in apraxia, the loss of the ability to carry out familiar, articulated movements following damage, in most people, to the left hemisphere. It is also evident in the common loss of visuospatial nonverbal functions following damage to the right hemisphere.

Laterality of function is relative and not absolute. For example, although the left hemisphere is specialized for the production of language, the right hemisphere also has linguistic abilities. While the left hemisphere is responsible for phonology, syntax, and semantics, the right hemisphere produces the intonation and emotion in the speaker's voice and comprehends the same in the speech of others (Springer & Deutsch, 1989). Studies of commissurotomy subjects have shown that the right hemisphere has considerable linguistic capability (e.g., Zaidel, 1976), more than is typically recognized. To complicate the matter further, the extent of linguistic representation in the right hemisphere differs among individuals (Myers, 1984), and the extent of right hemisphere involvement in a task varies depending upon its perceptual, motor, and cognitive demands (Henninger, 1989*a*). Lastly, interhemispheric collaboration is an integral part of cognitive processing. Although one area may initiate processing, information is passed to other parts of the brain, most notably from one hemisphere across the callosum to the other, for continued processing or output. Part of the challenge in diagnosing a patient's brain damage is differentiating between problems that reflect damage to a specific location and problems that reflect the fact that the brain functions as a whole, like a machine with numerous interconnecting gears, in which an insult anywhere can disrupt processing. What appears to be a right hemisphere deficit actually may be a problem in interhemispheric transfer to the left hemisphere for output. For example, a patient's inability to name a picture representing a shape palpated by his left hand could reflect a right hemisphere deficit in shape recognition or it could indicate a problem in callosal transfer to the left hemisphere for output.

It is difficult to infer hemispheric damage from differential performance on any one task in the brain-injured person. Multiple influences on brain organization, the varying cognitive requirement of a task, and individual differences in problem solving make it difficult to isolate the lateralized contribution of each hemisphere to complex cognitive tasks in the normal brain. However, converging evidence from perceptual, motor, and cognitive tasks involving functions specific to either hemisphere can be used to infer damage.

Handedness

Handedness, the preferential usage of one hand over the other for skilled and unskilled manual activities, is the clearest example of lateralization. Human beings are overwhelmingly right-handed with approximately 90% of the population using the right hand for writing and other unimanual skilled activities. Right-handedness is slightly greater in women, with the margin of difference in various surveys ranging from 1% to 4% (Harris & Carlson, 1988). Right-handedness reflects left-hemispheric specialization for manual functions, which in turn reflects left hemisphere specialization in humans.

The hemispheres are differentiated in their functional potential from birth for the abilities and specializations that become increasingly apparent with age (e.g., Levy, 1976). Although the neural substrate for handedness is present from birth (Witelson, 1987), bimanual activity is characteristic of infancy with a gradual increase in unimanual activity during early childhood (Miller, 1982). Hand use takes time to consolidate; handedness is established by about 3 years of age (Ingram, 1975). Continued differentiation between the hands increases with age, particularly for tasks requiring a relatively high degree of coordination and muscle control (Durost, 1934). Similarly, lateralization of cognitive functions becomes more differentiated with age as the cognitive operations required become more symbolic and complex (Bates, O'Connell, Vaid, Sledge, & Oakes, 1986).

The relationships between handedness and representation of function are neither clear nor direct. Although right-handedness is the best predictor of left hemispheric representation of language, left-handedness does not indicate reversed representation, simply different representation of language. The brains of most right-handed people appear to be organized similarly, with the left hemisphere being specialized for linguistic functions and the right for spatial functions. This complementary specialization appears to be true for most right-handed men, but many people, particularly non-right-handers, do not show it. They show either bilateral or noncomplementary representation (Bryden, Hecaen, & DeAgostini, 1983). The fact that different handedness groups show different patterns of hemispheric asymmetries suggests that handedness is a behavioral marker for patterns of brain organization. Lastly, hemisphericity differences between handedness groups, with left-handers overrepresented among artists, musicians, and mathematicians, suggest differences in preferred cognitive style.

One of the reasons that it is difficult to predict the cerebral organization of left-handers is that there are different types of left-handers. There are those who are naturally (genotypically) left-handed and those who are disguised right-handers. The latter are individuals who, because of early insult to the brain, have switched handedness and now write with their left hand. If an injury or disease occurs in the former, the reaction will be different than if it occurs in the latter (Satz, Soper, & Orsini, 1988). These left-handers differ in their brain organization and perhaps in their aptitudes from natural left-handers. Furthermore, in addition to strong and weak natural left-handers, there are people who are ambidextrous (equal manual skill in both hands) or show ambiguous handedness (change handedness on a task) (Satz *et al.*, 1988), or conditional handedness (change handedness predictably under specified conditions) (Henninger, submitted for publication). Little research exists on these individuals but it appears they may have quite distinctive brain organization.

Left-handedness has ramifications. Although most studies that have compared the cognitive abilities of right- and left-handers in the general population have not found differences (see Hardyck, Petrinovich, & Goldman, 1976, for a review), left-handers are overrepresented in fields that depend on abilities presumably subserved by the right hemisphere: architecture (e.g., Peterson & Lansky, 1974), engineering (D'Amico & Kimura, 1987), music (Peterson, 1979), visual arts (Mebert & Michel, 1980). Also, left- and mixed handers are disproportionately represented among many clinical populations: the learning-disabled (Gordon, 1986), the delinquent (Gabrielli & Mednick, 1980; Feehan, Stanton, McGee, Silva, & Moffitt, 1990), those with autoimmune diseases (Geschwind & Behan, 1982), alcoholism (Bakan, 1973), autism (Dawson, 1988), schizophrenia (McCreadie, Crorie, Barron, & Winslow, 1982), early dementia (Alzheimer type) (Seltzer, Burres, & Sherwin, 1984), tardive dyskinesia (McCreadie *et al.*, 1982), and mental retardation (Kinsbourne, 1988), in most cases, presumably because of pathology in the left hemisphere. Left-handedness is associated also with early breast cancer in women (Kramer, Albrecht, & Miller, 1985). Differences in aptitudes, interest, cognitive profiles, and clinical problems in right- and left-handers may reflect differences in brain organization. Knowledge of handedness may suggest different courses of treatment.

Much of our knowledge about handedness derives from work in the past decade, and many of the issues are not yet sufficiently resolved to make credible inferences to clinical practice. Within the next decade, quite different classifications may emerge. The major neuropsychological batteries are not separately normed for right- and left-handers (Golden, Hammeke, & Purisch, 1980; Reitan and Wolfson, 1985). The sparse amount of evidence led Filskov and Catanese (1986) to conclude that special evaluation of test results of left-handers need not be considered, except to assume that higher scores will be obtained by the preferred hand on psychomotor tasks, and to explore the possibility of bilateral or right-hemisphere representation of language when inconsistent neuropsychological test findings are found. However, knowledge of individual differences in brain structure and organization is increasing, and the evidence of differences between right- and left-handers suggests that in the future, testing of laterality will become important for adequate assessment. Awareness of the issues involved will direct the practitioner toward the potential areas in which assessment of handedness may prove to be important.

HISTORICAL FOUNDATIONS

Laterality

The idea of localization without regard to hemisphere is first mentioned in the Hippocratic writings, ca. 400 B.C. (Benton, 1965). In contrast, the concept of hemispheric dominance is relatively recent. It arose out of Broca's observation in 1861 of an association between aphasia and lesions of the left frontal lobe, culminating in his famous dictum in 1865: "nous parlons avec l'hemisphere gauche" (we speak with the left hemisphere). For a number of decades the concept of cerebral dominance was only concerned with language functions (speaking, understanding, writing, and reading). In 1868, Jackson proposed his idea of the "leading" hemisphere, referring to the hemisphere dominant for speech, and the right hemisphere became known as the minor or subordinate hemisphere (Springer & Deutsch, 1989). Cerebral dominance was extended to other behaviors such as skilled motor activity and abilities related to body image as additional clinical evidence indicated that lesions of the left hemisphere were associated with losses in these abilities also.

In the 1940s, neurologists and psychologists called attention to the fact that deficits such as impairment in visual space perception, constructional apraxia, or inattention to one visual half-field seemed to occur with much higher frequency in patients with lesions of the right hemisphere than in those with lesions of the left (Benton, 1965). The broadening of the concept of cerebral dominance to include abilities of the right hemisphere allowed the question of a relationship between handedness and cerebral dominance for language to reemerge.

In the 1960s, the introduction of the complete commissurotomy operation in which the corpus callosum and the minor commissures separating the two cerebral hemispheres are surgically severed for the treatment of intractable epilepsy allowed more direct measurements of lateralized functions. Extensive testing of the disconnected hemispheres of the commissurotomized patients revealed that each hemisphere was fully conscious, could learn independently, performed cognitive operations differently, and retained only the information to which it was exposed (Sperry, 1974). Experiments with these patients indicated that the left hemisphere was specialized for verbal, analytic, auditory processes and the right hemisphere was specialized for visuospatial processes. Later studies revealed that although one hemisphere might be specialized for a task, the other hemisphere might take control of processing (Levy & Trevarthen, 1976).

In addition to clinical studies of brain-lesioned and brain-altered subjects, studies of normal subjects using perceptual techniques have brought knowledge of lateralized processing in the intact brain. The two most commonly used techniques have been the dichotic testing technique for testing lateralized auditory processes and tachistoscopic presentation for testing visual processes. In a dichotic presentation, two competing stimuli are presented simultaneously to each ear. The subject reports, orally or manually, what he or she hears. Typically the subject reports the information from one ear faster or more accurately. The resulting ear advantage is interpreted as an advantage for the contralateral hemisphere for the processing involved. Kimura (1961*a*,*b*) showed that there was a close relation between performance of dichotic listening tasks and speech lateralization: individuals with left hemispheric speech tended to be more accurate in reporting verbal information presented to the right ear; individuals with right hemispheric speech tended to be more accurate in reporting verbal information presented to the left ear. The dichotic technique is the best technique for testing language lateralization in the normal subject (Bryden, 1988) and can be used in neuropsychological assessment. However, variables other than language lateralization, such as attentional strategies or hemisphericity, affect performance and results should be interpreted cautiously. Tachistoscopic presentation depends on the observation that sensory inputs from the left visual half-field (LVH) of each eye are projected directly to the right hemisphere and sensory inputs from the right visual half-field (RVH) of each eye are projected directly to the left hemisphere. With rapid presentation of the stimuli in which the subject does not have time to move his or her eyes, stimulation can be directed to one hemisphere. Tachistoscopic presentation provides a means of testing lateralization of printed language. Perceptual techniques have confirmed lateralized processing in normal subjects of verbal, visuospatial, musical, emotional, mathematical, and other stimuli and of many verbal and nonverbal processes.

Handedness

Interest in handedness long predates knowledge of brain functions. Since ancient times, right and left have been associated with opposite attributes of moral, religious, and political significance. These have included male and female, good and evil, day and night, straight and crooked (Corballis, 1980). Connotations related to left consistently have been negative and connotations related to right consistently positive. Left-handers are frequently referred to as "sinistrals," a word etymologically related to "sinister." In other languages also the terms for left or left-handed have contained at least one derogatory meaning (Springer & Deutsch, 1989). The Bible repeatedly refers to the right hand as the hand of moral preference. Jesus sits at the right hand of God. As Hardyck and Petrinovich (1977) point out, honors, virtues, and powers are ascribed to the right hand and there is not one honorable reference in the Bible to the left hand. Folk wisdom linked left-handedness to a variety of undesirable personal characteristics including those of criminals, degenerates, prostitutes, and people with aggressive tendencies (Harris & Carlson, 1988). Whatever the reasons, left-handedness was considered inferior and this bias may have played a role in the left-handed patient's life.

With the idea of cerebral dominance and left hemispheric specialization being uniquely human came the notion that right-handedness reflects left hemispheric specialization. A left-hander was less specialized and perhaps less evolved. Handedness was first associated with brain organization by Broca (1865, as cited by Dimond, 1972) who suggested that both speech and manual dexterity are attributable to the inborn superiority of the left hemisphere in right-handers. He also speculated that there might be individuals in which this was reversed (left-handers). Although he also maintained that it was not necessary that speech and handedness be linked, the notion that the hemisphere controlling speech is one the side opposite to the preferred hand became known as Broca's rule and was influential for many years. Evidence contradicting this principle came from a study of epileptic patients by Penfield and Roberts (1959) who found that dysphasia following surgery on the right hemisphere was not significantly more frequent in the left-handed than in the right-handed. They concluded that the left hemisphere is dominant for speech in the vast majority of left- and right-handers. Studies that have followed have shown a more complex picture, i.e., that the pattern of cerebral speech dominance in left-handers is more variable. For example, Gloning, Gloning, Haub, and Quatember (1969), in comparing right-handed and non-right-handed patients with verifiable unilateral lesions, found that non-right-handed patients show less marked dominance for language and that among the non-right-handers, significant differences are found in the language functions disturbed depending upon which hand is used for writing.

THEORETICAL AND BASIC NEUROBIOLOGICAL ISSUES

Handedness and Laterality of Function

Language Laterality

Regardless of how language representation is measured, it differs between right- and left-handers and varies more among the latter. Most right-handers have language unilaterally represented in the left hemisphere. Three positions have been advanced with respect to hemispheric speech lateralization in left-handers (Satz, 1980). The first is a variable unilateral position that assumes that speech representation is lateralized either in the left or the right hemisphere in left-handers, with the majority being left-sided (approximately two-thirds). The second is a variable unilateral and bilateral representation with three types of speech representation: left, right, and bilateral. These two positions postulate that the majority of left-handers have left-sided representation of speech. The third is a bilateral and variable unilateral position that postulates a much greater representation of bilateral speech. Generally, only left-handedness has been associated with bilateral speech representation.

What is meant by bilateral representation? Does it mean double representation, i.e., that the same function is represented twice, once in each hemisphere? Or does it mean divided representation with some aspects, i.e., language expression, lateralized to one hemisphere and other aspects, i.e., language comprehension, represented in the other hemisphere? The findings of opposite hemispheric representation in some left-handers for speech output and comprehension (Naeser & Borod, 1986) strongly suggest that bilaterality means divided representation. Similarly, amytal studies (studies using the Wada technique in which sodium amytal is injected unilaterally into the carotid artery and the verbal difficulties or muteness that follow indicate language representation in the contralateral hemisphere) have found that bilateral speech representation is reflected by speech interruption with injection to either hemisphere rather than a lack of speech interruption with injection to either side (Milner, 1974). This interpretation is supported by anatomical findings of a larger callosum in non-right-handers (Witelson, 1989) and would be compatible with more fibers in the callosum.

In contrast, research using sodium amytal has also found that some ambidextrous subjects do not become mute or lose consciousness with injection to either hemisphere (Serafetinides, Hoare, & Driver, 1965). Perhaps ambidexterity reflects duplicate representation of function. It is likely that in most cases of left- or mixed handedness, bilateral representation of function reflects an integrated system drawing upon both hemispheres. However, it is possible that in some cases, i.e., stutterers, it reflects the development of a secondary language center in the right hemisphere resulting in duplicate representation of function.

Aphasia Studies. Studies of left-handers show that the lesions that determine language difficulties are more frequently in the left hemisphere, but they can be in either hemisphere (Hecaen & Sauguet, 1971). The frequency of aphasia is greater in the left-handed (Satz, 1979) but it is more likely to be transient than in the right-handed (Gloning & Quatember, 1966). Regardless of the hemisphere injured, severity is milder and recovery is more rapid and more complete in the left-handed (Luria, 1966), although not all studies have found recovery to be more rapid (e.g., Newcombe & Ratcliff, 1973). This higher incidence of aphasia with better prognosis of recovery suggests incomplete lateralization of speech in the majority of the left-handers (Gloning & Quatember, 1966) which results in greater sensitivity to lesions, with either more tissue that can compensate or greater capacity for reorganization of function.

Studies of aphasia following unilateral brain damage in left-handed subjects indicate that verbal functions are more often bilaterally represented in left-handers than in right-handers (Hecaen & Sauguet, 1971) and that functions are more diffusely represented within each hemisphere (Hecaen, DeAgostini, & Monzon-Montes, 1981). The estimates of left, right, and bilateral speech representation vary widely. Satz (1979) identifies a unilateral left-sided group (15%), a unilateral right-sided group (15%), and a bilateral group (70%). Segalowitz and Bryden (1983) estimate language lateralization to be 61, 20, and 19%, respectively, but Annett (1975) does not make provision for bilateral speech. Studies of right-handed patients show clear left hemisphere dominance for language, with only about 1% of the patients with lesions in the right hemisphere developing aphasia (Zangwill, 1960).

Sodium Amytal and Other Clinical Studies. Estimates of left hemisphere lateralization in right-handers range from 90 to 99%, using sodium amytal, and estimates of right hemisphere representation range from 1 to 10% (Harris & Carlson, 1988) with frequently reported figures being 96 and 4% (Rasmussen & Milner, 1975). Estimates of left hemisphere lateralization in left-handers range from 60 to 70% with the remaining being right hemisphere dominant or bilateral (Harris & Carlson, 1988). Rasmussen and Milner (1975) report 70, 15, and 15%, respectively. In a study of non-right-handed patients, Milner, Branch, and Rasmussen (1964) found that two-thirds of the patients with early left hemisphere damage were right hemisphere dominant for speech, whereas two-thirds of the patients without early damage were left hemisphere dominant for speech. This study provided evidence of a shift in speech dominance associated with a possible shift in manual preference as a result of early trauma to the left hemisphere. Similarly, Strauss and Wada (1983) found that patients with right hemisphere speech tended to show evidence of early left hemisphere dysfunction. In addition to handedness this study compared other measures of lateral preference (foot, eye, and ear) and found that if an individual displays left-sideness on all four indices of lateral preference, it is highly unlikely that speech is in the left hemisphere (3%). If an individual displays right-sideness on all four indices, it is highly unlikely that speech is in the right hemisphere (10%). Other combinations are considerably less predictive.

Findings from studies using electroconvulsive shock therapy are similar to those from sodium amytal with 94% of right-handers and 71% of left-handers having speech representation in the left hemisphere (Kopelman, 1982). Right hemisphere representation of speech is present in 4 and 21%, with estimates of bilateral speech being 2 and 8%, respectively.

Findings Using Noninvasive Techniques. Studies using the dichotic procedure typically find that right-handers recall significantly more verbal stimuli from the right ear than the left ear, whereas left-handers usually show smaller differences between the ears, often in the reversed direction (e.g., Curry & Rutherford, 1967). Studies using the tachistoscopic procedure have found smaller visual field advantages for left- than for right-handers (for reviews of findings with both techniques, see Segalowitz & Bryden, 1983). Several studies have shown a significant relationship between ear advantages on the dichotic procedure and handedness measures (e.g., Strauss, 1986).

Issues and Evaluation. Localizing language representation is difficult because language is comprised of multiple components that may be lateralized differently. Although the most common locus-of-dominance pattern among right-handers is the left hemisphere for handedness, speech output, and comprehension, in left-handers the locus of handedness may be separate from that for speech output and/or comprehension (Naeser & Borod, 1986). Clinical studies that do not distinguish between speech output and comprehension may consider left-handed patients bilateral for language functions while those that measure speech output only may consider similar patients left hemisphere dominant. Second, language tasks, and a person's responses to them, differ in the degree of right hemisphere involvement the tasks demand. Manual tasks differ from oral tasks in the amount of left hemisphere engagement they elicit, e.g., silent reading and reading aloud. The left hemisphere is clearly specialized for the articulatory muscles used in speaking (Sussman, 1971) and may obscure right hemisphere participation. Dichotic testing of commissurotomy subjects indicates more participation of the right hemisphere in language activities that do not require an oral response (Henninger-Pechstedt, 1989*a*). The use of oral, expressive speech in the sodium amytal procedure to deduce language representation is likely to underestimate the presence of language representation in the right hemisphere. Third, although left-handers show more bilateral representation of expressive speech than right-handers (Kimura, 1973), oral expression appears to be more consistently represented in the left hemisphere than other components of language. People differ in the amount of language representation in the right hemisphere (bilaterality) and there is more variability within left-handers.

Furthermore, investigators differ in what evidence they use to base their inference of function or deficit. Kinsbourne (1988) points out that some investigators have erroneously concluded that if a lesion of a hemisphere failed to cause a cognitive deficit, that domain was not represented in that hemisphere. After a reanalysis of the Hecaen case material (Bryden *et al.* 1983), in which he discarded this assumption, Kinsbourne concludes that 70% of non-right-handers have language represented bilaterally and that most of the remainder are left lateralized. In contrast, Hammond and Kaplan (1982) believe bilaterality in left-handers is overestimated because clinical samples generally exclude cases with unilateral brain damage without clinical symptoms.

In summary, approximately two-thirds of right-handers are strongly right-handed (Annett, 1972) with language unilaterally represented in the left hemisphere. Apparently two-thirds of left-handers have bilateral representation of language with left hemisphere dominance for oral expression. Approximately 15% (primarily brain damaged subjects) have language unilaterally represented in the right hemisphere and the remaining 15–30% have language unilaterally represented in the left hemisphere.

Laterality of Nonverbal Functions

Clinical studies comparing handedness groups on nonverbal functions suggest that these functions also are more bilaterally represented in left-handers. However, the pattern relating handedness to nonverbal functions is different from that obtained for language functions. In right-handers, visuospatial functions are not as dominantly lateralized to the right hemisphere as language functions are to the left hemisphere (Bryden & MacDonald, 1987). In left-handers, visuospatial processes are even less lateralized, about equally often to the left, right, or both hemispheres (Bryden *et al.*, 1983). Comparing right- and left-hemisphere lesion cases, Hecaen and Sauguet (1971) found fewer significant differences between the groups of left-handers than the groups of right-handers in visuospatial, perceptual, and constructional abilities. Similarly, Borod, Carper, Naeser, and Goodglass (1985) found that left-handed aphasics with left hemisphere lesions were more impaired than right-handed aphasics with left hemisphere lesions on tasks requiring visuoperceptual, constructional, and spatial organizational abilities. These results suggest that left-handers have more left hemisphere representation than right-handers for nonverbal functions, especially ones involving manipulation and assembly.

Left-handers with left hemisphere lesions often show deficits typically associated with right cerebral hemisphere lesions in right-handers, such as spatial disorientation and dressing apraxia (Hecaen & Ajuriaguerra, 1963, as cited by Hecaen & Sauguet, 1971), unilateral spatial agnosia and hemiasomatognosia (Hecaen & Sauguet, 1971), perception of faces and complex drawings (Tzavaras, Hecaen, & LeBras, 1971, as cited by Borod *et al.*, 1985), unilateral spatial agnosia, spatial (topographical) agnosia, and constructional apraxia (Hecaen *et al.*, 1981). However, on other nonverbal tasks, e.g., visual closure and maze learning (Newcombe & Ratcliff, 1973), this has not been the case. In some studies, performance has been moderated by the presence of familial sinistrality (e.g., Hecaen & Sauguet, 1971). There have been cases of reversed specialization with a left-hander with a right hemisphere lesion showing deficits in language functions but not in right hemisphere functions, e.g., melody recognition, visuospatial processing, constructional ability, dressing praxis, hemispace attention (Delis, Simpson, & Knight, 1983) and also a left-hander with a left hemisphere lesion showing severe hemispatial neglect, anosognosia, contralateral hypokinesia, aprosodia, and visual-spatial constructive difficulties with no evidence of accompanying aphasia (Dronkers & Knight, 1988). In sum, visuospatial functions are usually less lateralized in left-handers and, on occasion, they are reversed.

Consequences of Bilateral Representation

What would be the cognitive consequences of bilateral representation of speech? Bilateral representation of language or shifting of speech to the right hemisphere following damage to the left might compromise visual-spatial processing in the right hemisphere through "cognitive crowding" as both functions compete for neural tissue. Levy (1969) has postulated this competition hypothesis to explain differences in the patterns of verbal and spatial skill between normal right-handers with unilateral speech representation and normal left-handers who presumably have bilateral speech representation. In comparing intelligence test scores of right- and left-handed graduate students, she found that the two groups did not differ in verbal IQ but the left-handed subjects were significantly lower in performance IQ. Miller (1971) also found that right- and non-right-handed university students did not differ on a verbal intelligence test, but the right-handed students scored significantly higher on a spatial one. Lansdell (1969) examined discrepancies between verbal and performance IQs on the Wechsler–Bellevue intelligence scale in epilepsy patients with left-hemisphere lesions. He found that patients with early lesions showed decrements in Performance IQ whereas patients with lesions after 5 years of age showed decrements in Verbal IQ. He speculated that the early injury to the left hemisphere shifted language to the right hemisphere, thereby disrupting and displacing the visuospatial functions that otherwise would have developed there. Later injury would not result in a shift and thus produce the expected decrements in left hemisphere ability.

Although some investigators have found left-handers to be deficient in perceptual skills (Nebes, 1971), these results have not been reliable (Hardyck, 1977). Data from normal subjects suggest that trained left-handed musicians relative to trained right-handed musicians tend to be deficient in the right hemisphere in a complex melody recognition task, again suggesting cognitive crowding in the right hemisphere of left-handers (Henninger, 1989*b*.). On the other hand, other studies show enhanced musical (Deutsch, 1978) and spatial (Herrmann & van Dyke, 1978) skills in left-handers. Studies of discrimination of emotion show larger visual field differences in right-handers than in left-handers (Natale, Gur, & Gur, 1983).

Conclusions

Disparate findings suggest that variability within the left-handed population masks ability differences. This interpretation is supported by findings that the effects of handedness on spatial ability interact with sex and reasoning ability (Harshman, Hampson, & Berenbaum, 1983). Similarly, investigators have found differential verbal and spatial abilities in non-right-handers in science and nonscience courses (D'Amico & Kimura, 1987). These studies suggest that different subgroups have different cognitive and affective abilities and that until the measurement of subgroups is more developed, predicting these abilities in left-handers will be difficult.

Although left-handers are overrepresented in various fields using skills of the right hemisphere, there are many right-handers in these groups as well. A mediating factor may be hemisphericity, the preferred use of one hemisphere. Individuals with enhanced right hemisphere skills, regardless of which hemisphere is dominant for language, could be visually dominant (Peterson & Lansky, 1980). They may activate the right hemisphere preferentially and develop the skills of that hemisphere. Given the strong lateralization of function and unilateral left hemisphere representation of language in strongly right-handed people, it is likely that individuals with a right hemisphere preference would be more likely to be left-handed or at least would not be strongly right-handed.

In sum, the brain organization of left-handed people differs from that of right-handed people. Verbal and nonverbal functions are more bilaterally represented and representation within each hemisphere is more diffuse than in right-handers. However left-handers do not represent a homogeneous group. Being able to specify the nature of the handedness of any particular individual appears necessary to use handedness to predict cerebral organization.

Measuring Handedness

Handedness is not a simple unitary phenomenon. It is a continuum ranging from strong left-handedness across mixed handedness to strong right-handedness (Hardyck & Petrinovich, 1977). Handedness can refer to lateral preference or to lateral skill. They are not always the same. Inconsistent left-handers are likely to show superior dexterity in the right hand (Peters, 1990). It is often assumed that self-report of writing hand indicates handedness. Research indicates that this is not an adequate measure. Self-report of writing hand is usually accurate for right-handers, but it may misclassify approximately 40% of left-handers (e.g., Satz, Achenbach, & Fennell, 1967). Many manifest left-handers (people who appear to be left-handed because they write with their left hand) are "mixed" handers and do some manual activities with the left hand and others with the right. Left-handers who prefer their right hand for certain tasks are usually more skilled with their right hand for those tasks (Steenhuis & Bryden, 1988).

Writing hand is clearly influenced by environmental expectations, and the incidence of left-handedness for writing is influenced by the extent to which the culture is tolerant of left-handedness. In many cultures children are still pressured to write with the right hand. For example, a study of Chinese individuals showed that 18% had experienced frequent requests to change hand use from the left to the right and less than 1% used the left hand for writing (Teng, Lee, Yang, & Chang, 1976). Forcing a left-handed person to write with the right hand has consequences. Forced left-handers have been found to have significantly poorer mental rotation skills than either right- or left-handers, suggesting that linguistic activity compromised their spatial skills (Ardila,

Correa, Zuluaga, & Uribe, 1988). Evidence suggests differences in brain organization between individuals who switch back after they have finished their education as contrasted to those who do not switch back (Gloning, Gloning, Haub, & Quatember, 1969). A change in handedness may influence lateral organization of function. However, the corpus callosum of a forced right-hander is larger than that of a true right-hander (Witelson, 1989) indicating that forcing a handedness change does not change the basic anatomical structure.

The greatest obstacle to using handedness to predict lateralized function is the lack of consistency in how handedness is defined and measured. Some investigators distinguish only between right- and left-handers; others differentiate degrees of handedness (strong, weak). Others combine "mixed" and left-handed people into a single group and label it "non-right-handers." At present, terms such as *mixed, inconsistent, weak,* and *ambidextrous* are used almost interchangeably. However, future research may show important distinctions between these non-right-handers. For example, people who use one hand consistently for a task (mixed) regardless of which hand, are likely to differ from those who do not (inconsistent). Many studies do not give details of how handedness is defined. Few people use the category of ambidextrous, and those who do, vary in how they define it. Methods of assessment vary considerably. Some studies use only self-report of writing hand. Others use a preference questionnaire. Still others use a performance inventory or a combination of preference and performance measures. There is little agreement as to which items should be used on a questionnaire or which skills should be assessed to measure performance. Lastly, measurements are rarely repeated so there is little information regarding the reliability of the handedness assessment. Although most investigators agree that writing hand alone is inadequate, at present there is no consensual method of measuring handedness.

Preference Inventories

The most popular way to assess handedness is to ask a person which hand he or she prefers to use for a variety of unimanual tasks. Numerous inventories of this type are available. The most well known are Annett's hand preference questionnaire (Annett, 1970) and the Edinburgh Handedness Inventory (Oldfield, 1971), both of which have been standardized on large populations and have been retested for reliability. Another popular test that has also been retested for reliability is the handedness scale of Raczkowski, Kalat, and Nebes (1974). All three showed satisfactory reliability coefficients (0.80+). (See Appendix A for a description of the most popular questionnaires.) Neuropsychological batteries usually include a preference inventory, e.g., Reitan's Lateral Dominance Examination in the HRNB. Although degree of preference is noted, when inconsistency is present, writing hand alone is used as the index of handedness.

For testing handedness, items are wanted that reflect overlearned activities. The gross disparity between the two hands that manifest in well-established tasks is not displayed in unfamiliar tasks (Oldfield, 1971). One wants items that are reliable and valid. Some items such as "with which hand to you carry your book or book bag?" and "with which hand do you pick up the salt or pepper shaker?" are highly reliable (people will indicate the same hand on repeated testing), but they are not valid (people often do not use the hand they indicated when they actually perform the task) (Raczkowski *et al.*, 1974). The best items, in that they show consistency with other items, appear to be which hand you use to hammer a nail (Annett, 1970), which hand you use for writing, for drawing (Chapman & Chapman, 1987), for scissors, for throwing, and for using a toothbrush (Oldfield, 1971). These items have high validity (0.94+, Raczkowski *et al.*, 1974). Writing and drawing are highly correlated (Chapman & Chapman, 1987). The use of scissors is a good item in grading in the middle range of the left-handed range; the use of a toothbrush has an exceptionally sharp changeover in the middle of the right-handed range (Oldfield, 1971). If a quick, gross, and yet relatively accurate means of assessing handedness is wanted, asking a subject to describe him- or herself as one of the following: right-handed and strongly so; right-handed but only moderately so; left-handed but only moderately so; and left-handed and strongly so; may be adequate (Chapman & Chapman, 1987).

In general, left-handers are less certain about their hand preferences than right-handers (Raczkowski *et al.*, 1974), and left-handers are less likely to show a strong preference. More self-classified left-handers are likely to have poorly differentiated manual laterality. Some studies show smaller asymmetry between the two hands in left-handers; others do not. Group differences may be an artifact of the variable lateral preferences or the heterogeneity within the left-handed group.

Performance Measures

Inclusion of a behavioral measure of handedness for relating handedness to brain function is useful. Greater predictability of language lateralization can be obtained by combining knowledge of hand preference with measures of performance (Strauss & Wada, 1988). Greater reliability of hand preference is obtained when the subject knows that he or she will be asked to perform the task also (M. Peters, personal communication, June, 1989). Typically, subjects are required to make a simple unimanual movement and are timed at the task. The most common are a peg-moving task (Annett, 1985), a pencil–paper test in which subjects are asked to place dots in each of a number of small circles as fast as possible (Tapley & Bryden, 1985), and a pencil–paper test in which the subject places a mark in the center bull's eye of four concentric circles (Borod, Koff, & Caron, 1984). All three are reliable tests and correlate with measures of hand preference (Bryden & MacDonald, 1987). Performance tests that are typically used in a neuropsychological assessment may be used to measure handedness. Finger tapping with the index finger is a reliable measure and correlates with hand preference (Peters & Durding, 1979). Alternatively, many investigators ask the subject to perform the tasks that are on the preference questionnaires.

Theories of Handedness

The origin of handedness is of long-standing interest and controversy. The probability of two right-handed parents having a left-handed child is 0.02. It is 0.17 if one parent is left-handed and 0.46 if both are left-handed (Chamberlain, 1928, as cited in Annett, 1973). Although either a genetic model or an environmental model could account for these differences, an environmental model cannot account for the strong bias to the right. Moreover, parental handedness cannot play a major role since dissimilarity is more common than similarity; 54% of the children of two left-handed parents, and 72% of the children of left-handed mothers, are right-handed (Annett, 1973). Furthermore, anatomical asymmetries are present in the neonate that relate to hand dominance (LeMay & Culebras, 1972). Neonates display a variety of behavioral asymmetries such as the tonic neck reflex that correlate with handedness in the adult (Liederman & Coryell, 1982). Lastly, differences in degree of lateralization have been found within left- or right-handed populations as a function of the presence or absence of sinistrality in the subject's family (Zurif & Bryden, 1969) indicating that cerebral organization is not determined by hand usage. Although some investigators (e.g., Blau, 1946) believe that right-handedness is a learned response to a right-handed world and that left-handedness is a failure, for whatever reasons, to learn that response, the evidence supports a biological basis for handedness.

Genetic Theories

Three genetic models have been proposed to account for the association between handedness and language lateralization while accounting for crossed aphasias. The most popular model is that of Annett (1975). The essential features are that handedness is determined by three factors: accidental variation tending to make one side more efficient than the other for skilled activities, a right shift factor that shifted preference for one side to the right in human beings, and cultural pressures toward dextrality. The right shift is linked to a left hemisphere speech production factor in humans which incidentally also shifts handedness and is sex modified. The distribution to the right is shifted slightly further to the right in females than in males accounting for the greater proportion of right-handed females and the female advantage in the early stages of language acquisition. The shift depends on a single gene with two alleles, a dominant one producing a shift of control to the right or to the left hemisphere (*R*) and a recessive (*r*) one producing no shift. People who possess the dominant allele (either *RR* or *rr*) possess the right-shift factor and will tend to be right-handed and be left-hemispheric for language. In people who are homozygous recessive (*rr*), both handedness and language lateralization are determined by chance factors operating independently for each characteristic. Approximately 25% will show each handedness–language hemisphere (left–left, left–right, etc.) combination. In other words, there are genetic influences toward right- but not toward left-handedness (Annett, 1973). This model fits the quantitative data reasonably well (Bryden & MacDonald, 1987).

A second genetic theory, again postulating a single gene model with two alleles, is that of McManus (1985). He also ascribes to a right-shift and a chance factor. However, he considers the two alleles to be additive rather than dominant/recessive in the heterozygote. He extends his model to predict multiple dominance functions. His model is the most sophisticated and best available at present (Peters, personal communication, December 1989). A third genetic model is proposed by Levy and Nagylaki (1972). This model is no longer central but it is of interest in that it postulated a relationship between hand posture and motor representation, i.e., that ipsilateral hand control is marked by an inverted writing posture.

Members of monozygotic twin pairs frequently have opposite handedness and this has been used as an argument against a genetic basis. However, intrauterine influences on twins are different than those for singletons, possibly leading to a change in handedness in one twin. Also, the high incidence of mirror imaging in monozygotic pairs (25%) suggests that the splitting of the zygote may have occurred at a stage after bilateral symmetry is established with the result that one embryo will develop from what was to be the left half of the original embryo and one will develop from what was to be the right half (Springer & Deutsch, 1989). Causes of handedness in twins are likely to differ from the causes of handedness in singletons.

None of the genetic models deals well with bilateral representation of speech nor can any handle the reverse correlates of handedness that have been found recently with sex and reasoning ability. They do account for the distribution of handedness in families and provide a rationale for why handedness and language lateralization are not immutably linked.

Environmental Theories

Although the extreme environmentalist view has been discarded by most researchers, handedness can be modified by experience: intrauterine influences, accidents of nature, injuries, social pressure. Manifest handedness (which hand a person writes with) can be caused by one or a combination of these factors. Moreover, these factors may be linked. For example, people with a history of familial left-handedness, who thus presumably have a genetic basis for left-handedness, may be more vulnerable to intrauterine influences (Levy, 1976). Given the extent to which environmental factors can influence handedness, environmental factors must be considered as important as genetic factors in attempting to determine the nature of a person's handedness.

The strongest effect of the environment is to shift manual preference from the left to the right hemisphere. In the presence of some pathology, shifts away from right-sidedness occur because the physiological structures that support dextrality are altered by neurological insult. The majority of the people affected potentially would have been right-handed and are typically referred to as pathologically left-handed. If the trauma is extensive, both manual preference and language representation are shifted. In lesser cases, only the manual preference is affected. Recently, a theory has been proposed that links left-handedness to hormonal influences *in utero* (Geschwind & Behan, 1982). In a sense this theory suggests that all left-handedness is pathological; however, these hypothetical hormonal influences are genetically determined and, therefore, occur in natural left-handers.

Birth Order and Birth Stress. Bakan (1971) found an increased incidence of left-handedness among first- and later-born (fourth or higher) people and hypothesized that left-handedness is the most prevalent and benign condition resulting from birth stress. Methodological difficulties and the need for a large sample to assess increased incidence of left-handedness have made it difficult to test this hypothesis. A recent analysis of 23 studies that have examined the relationship between indicators of birth stress and lateral preference (Searleman, Porac, & Coren, 1989) suggest that Rh incompatibility, low birth weight, cesarean delivery, and breech delivery may be associated with increased non-right-handedness in males.

Hormonal Influences. Early brain damage leading to left-handedness may be caused by hormonal dysfunctioning *in utero* (Geschwind & Galaburda, 1985). Geschwind and Behan (1982) compared strongly right- and strongly left-handed individuals and found an increased incidence of immune disorders, migraine, and developmental learning disorders (dyslexia and stuttering) in left-handers and their right-handed first and second-degree relatives. Geschwind and his colleagues hypothesized that the raised frequency of the disorders was caused by testosterone (Geschwind & Galaburda, 1985). They hypothesized that excess testosterone or increased sensitivity to it during fetal development retards the normal migration of neurons to the left hemisphere and maturation of the immune system. They speculate that this slows development of both the left hemisphere and the thymus, leading to an increased rate of left-handedness and of susceptibility to immune disorders. It can cause abnormalities in the formation of the left hemisphere that disturb language functions, leading to learning disorders. The impairment that disturbs language may also cause the shift of handedness to the right hemisphere. The effect will usually be greater in males because the fetal testes secrete testosterone, and thus the greater frequency of left-handedness and of learning disabilities in males. The increased incidence of immune disorders and learning disabilities in right-handed relatives suggest a genetic basis for the effects of testosterone and immune responsiveness. The delayed growth of the left hemisphere may result in superior development of certain regions in the right hemisphere. This may lead to enhanced abilities of the right hemisphere, i.e., spatial or mathematical abilities (e.g., Kolata, 1983). Geschwind's theory of a syndrome linking prenatal hormonal influences, learning disabilities, immune disorders, and left- handedness is currently being tested by numerous investigators. Geschwind and Behan

(1982) believe that left-handedness is probably only one marker of anomalous dominance. Approximately 70% of the population has standard dominance (strong left hemisphere dominance for language and handedness). By contrast, 30% has anomalous dominance, i.e., some deviation from the standard pattern such as more nearly equal language abilities in both hemispheres, better language capacity in the right hemisphere, or manual skills other than strong right-handedness. The manifest left-handers probably constitute about one-third of those with anomalous dominance, but many of these with anomalous dominance are right-handers.

Pathological Left-handedness Syndrome. Whereas Bakan and Geschwind and their associates believe that virtually all left-handedness is pathological, Satz (1972) has postulated that manifest left-handers are comprised of natural left-handers (genetic or culturally determined) and pathological left-handers, those with early brain injury. It is the pathological left-handers who account for the raised incidence of left-handedness (17%) in clinical populations (mentally retarded or epileptic groups, e.g., Lucas, Rosenstein & Bigler, 1989). Early trauma to the left hemisphere has caused mental deficits and a shift in manual preference.

Satz, Orsini, Saslow, and Henry (1985) have identified a pattern of correlative changes associated with early brain injury in some left-handers and postulated a syndrome of pathological left-handedness. They believe the syndrome is caused by a lesion that is predominantly left-sided, or bilateral but asymmetric, that occurs before age 6. The pattern of changes includes any or all of the following features: a shift in manual preference, altered hemispheric speech dominance (right or bilateral), relatively preserved verbal cognitive functions, impaired visuospatial/constructional ability, a failure of the right side to develop fully resulting in right hemihypoplasia of the right upper and/or lower extremity, and sometimes, a unilateral sensory defect of the nonpreferred hand. The patient is unlikely to have left-handed family members. The most marked cognitive sign is the almost complete dissociation between performance on verbal–cognitive and visuospatial–constructional functions that appear on the WAIS. The dissociation is presumably due to the acquisition by the right hemisphere of skills normally performed by the left hemisphere which in turn displace the acquisition of normal right hemisphere skills. Bishop (1980) has proposed that the pathological left-hander ought to be less skillful with his right hand than his left hand to a greater degree than a natural left-hander and proposes that marked inferiority of the nonpreferred hand constitutes a unilateral "soft" neurological sign. She has found an increased incidence of left-handedness among children who are selected on the basis of increased clumsiness of the nonpreferred hand. She also found that the "target" children had a lower incidence of familial sinistrality than other left-handers and were impaired on cognitive tasks, supporting the hypothesis that their left-handedness resulted from early injury to the left hemisphere causing a shift in manual preference. These children, unlike the patients with greater severity of injury identified by Satz *et al.* (1985) who show normal language skills, showed impaired language skills suggesting that the injury encroached on left-hemisphere language zones with sufficient severity to cause right-hand clumsiness and a shift of hand control to the right hemisphere, but not with sufficient severity to force a shift of language function. These data support the assumption that the threshold for shifting hand preference is lower than the threshold for shifting language function. Other studies have found left-handedness in boys is more often a symptom of a pathological shift of handedness than is left-handedness in girls (Gordon, 1986). The existing evidence supports the position that some left-handedness is pathological in origin but the range of severity is considerable. Few individuals show the full pathological left-handedness syndrome. However, even mild CNS damage early in life may increase the probability of manual switch with or without other changes. Consequently, studies addressed to the association between handedness and other phenomena are confounded in that a proportion of the manifest left-handers will actually be natural right-handers. Measuring proficiency of the nonpreferred hand may be a helpful means of identifying these people (for a comprehensive review of pathological left-handedness, see Harris & Carlson, 1988).

Subject Variables Influencing Lateralized Cognitive Functions

Clearly handedness alone does not predict language lateralization, and the relationship between handedness and hemispheric asymmetries is more complex than originally believed. Other subject variables, acting independently or in conjunction with handedness, may provide greater predictability of hemispheric asymmetry of function (Searleman, Tweedy, & Springer, 1979). Subject variables proposed have been familial sinistrality (family history of left-handedness), hand posture during writing, and strength of handedness. Sex has also been found to interact with handedness. Results of studies with these variables have been contradictory. It is likely that each plays a role, but how important that variable is, and how it interacts with other variables, are currently matters of investigation.

Familial Sinistrality

A positive history of familial sinistrality (FS+) is defined as having at least one parent or sibling who is left-handed or ambidextrous, although not all investigators define it this way. Incidence of FS+ typically increases from right-handers to the ambidextrous to left-handers. The most likely effect of familial sinistrality would seem to be to decrease the degree of left-hemisphere dominance for language functions in both left- and right-handers. Evidence from a variety of clinical and experimental studies suggests that a positive history of familial sinistrality (FS+) is often associated with lessened left hemisphere dominance or bilateral representation of language (Hecaen & Sauguet, 1971; Zurif & Bryden, 1969). Other studies, however, have not found familial sinistrality to be relevant to language laterality (Briggs & Nebes, 1976), and still others have found familial sinistrality associated with more, rather than less, dependence upon the left hemisphere for language processing (e.g., Satz *et al.*, 1967).

Studies of spatial abilities also suggest a relationship between familial sinistrality and hemispheric specialization, but more research is necessary to clarify the findings. A positive history of familial sinistrality is associated with reduced hemispheric specialization for visuospatial processing but familial sinistrality interacts with sex: females without and males with a history of familial sinistrality show reduced specialization and this pattern correlates with increased spatial ability (Marino & McKeever 1982). Research with right-handed subjects shows the same interaction of familial sinistrality and sex, with FS− females and FS+ males being substantially less left hemisphere dominant for language, with greater spatial visualization ability (McKeever, Seitz, Hoff, & Marino, 1983). Reduced spatial ability has been found in children with familial left-handedness as contrasted with those without on the WISC block design and object assembly tests (Eme, Stone, & Izral, 1978). Finally, Casey, Brabeck, and Ludlow (1986) found differences between familial and nonfamilial non-right-handers suggesting that familially non-right-handed people have better spatial-visualization abilities than most people but more problems with left and right orientation.

The findings on familial sinistrality are unclear. In addition to the problem that familial sinistrality interacts with other variables is the problem of distinguishing FS− subjects who are pathological left-handers from those who are genotypic left-handers. Lastly, different means of measuring handedness, different tasks, and different subject populations compound the problem. However, the fact that the aphasia studies show bilateral representation of function primarily in familial left-handers and not in nonfamilial left-handers (Hecaen *et al.*, 1981) and that the prognosis for language recovery is improved if there is a history of familial sinistrality for both right- and left-handers (Luria, 1970, as cited by Searleman *et al.*, 1979) suggest that this variable is of relevance to the clinician. With further research, if both sex and familial sinistrality are taken into account, different ability groupings can be identified.

Hand Posture

Orientation of the hand relative to the line of writing has been proposed as a predictor of cerebral organization (Levy & Reid, 1976). The best estimates of inversion among left-handers are in the 40–51% range for males and in the 30–40% range for females (Weber & Bradshaw, 1981). Most right-handers (90–99%) use the noninverted position, with males being more likely to be inverters. Levy and Reid (1976) presented groups of left- and right-handers with normal or inverted writing postures with lateralized verbal (nonsense syllable) and visuospatial (dot location) tachistoscopic tests. The results suggested that subjects who write with an inverted posture (inverters) have language lateralized in the hemisphere ipsilateral to the writing hand, whereas subjects who write with a normal, noninverted posture (noninverters) have language lateralized in the hemisphere contralateral to the writing hand. Dichotic listening measures (Smith & Moscovitch, 1979) and sodium amytal testing (Strauss, Wada, & Kosaka, 1984) do not show differences related to hand posture. Differential involvement of the occipital lobe in these groups has been found, suggesting that hand posture distinguishes lateralized processing of visual print (Herron, Galin, Johnstone, & Ornstein, 1979). Reaction time studies have shown speed differences between left-handed inverters and noninverters (McKeever & Hoff, 1979) suggesting that inverters have a disorder of visuomotor integration (Levy & Wagner, 1984). These studies point out the importance of not treating language as a unitary process.

Hand posture is substantially related to familial sinistrality (McKeever, 1979) and its effects may interact with sex (Searleman, Porac, & Coren, 1984), making it unlikely that it will be a potent predictor of cerebral organization for language or visuospatial representation. Many studies have not found effects associated with hand posture (for a review, see Weber & Bradshaw, 1981), and many investigators do not consider it to be a useful variable. However, it may be a behavioral marker for a subgroup of left-handers. Since inverted left-handers have been found to have significantly lower spatial reasoning abilities than noninverters (Gregory, Alley, & Morris, 1980, as cited by Gregory & Paul, 1980) and an elevated probability of familial psychiatric problems (Cohen, 1978), it may be a marker for less than suboptimal adjustment in both psychological and neuropsychological areas. Whereas left-handed inverters and noninverters do not differ in their ear advantage on dichotic tests, right-handed inverters are more likely than noninverters to show a left ear advantage. Apparently inverted handwriting posture has a different basis in left-handers than in right-handers (Tapley & Bryden, 1983).

Strength of Handedness

Strength of handedness (how consistently one uses only one hand for manual activities) is a current area of active research. In general, strong or consistent handedness has been associated with more lateralized patterns of cerebral organization (e.g., Peters, 1990). Studies have found that strongly left-handed subjects have unilateral speech representation, either left (Dee, 1971) or right (Knox & Boone, 1970). Weak left-handers display variable or bilateral language representation (Dee, 1971). Strong handedness early in development (less than 1 year) has been associated with early brain damage to the ipsilateral hemisphere (Harris & Carlson, 1988).

Sex

Sex differences in brain organization (see Chapter 4) interact with handedness. In addition to the findings that familial sinistrality has opposite effects on spatial ability for the two sexes, these effects interact with reasoning ability. For subjects with above-median reasoning ability, the spatial scores of left-handed males are reduced but those of left-handed females are raised, relative to their right-handed counterparts; the opposite pattern is found for subjects with below-median reasoning ability (Harshman *et al.*, 1983). It is likely there are other cognitive abilities that may show similar interactions. Differences in callosal size between right- and non-right-handers have been found in males but not in females (Witelson, 1989). These results indicate that handedness does not index brain organization in the same way in the two sexes and suggest that the basis of lateralization differs in the two sexes. Investigations must differentiate between male and female right- and left-handers.

APPLICATION TO CLINICAL ASSESSMENT

Knowledge of handedness is useful in assessing the functional efficiency of the two cerebral hemispheres, in determining language lateralization in order to identify and assess deficits in verbal and nonverbal performance on standardized tests such as the WAIS in predicting outcome, and in recommending treatment.

Handedness Findings on Tests Used in Neuropsychological Assessment

Motor Performance Tests

Motor performance tasks that allow a comparison of the two sides of the body are typically included in neuropsychological test batteries to permit inferences about functional efficiency of the two hemispheres. It is generally accepted that a comparison of right- versus left-hand performance on basic motor tasks accounts for the influence of lateral preference since the preferred hand is expected to perform better than the nonpreferred hand. More complex motor tasks may show different patterns of performance because of the additional cognitive requirements of the task.

The Finger Tapping Test of the Halstead–Reitan Neuropsychological Battery (HRNB) is commonly used to assess simple motor skill. Finger tapping shows a larger difference between the dominant hands and nondominant hands for right-handers than for left-handers The nonpreferred hand of left-handers is faster than the nonpreferred hand of right-handers, where there is no significant difference between the preferred performance of both groups (Peters & Durding, 1979). Consistent right-handers have a significantly larger difference between the hands than consistent and mixed left-handers and tend to have a larger difference than mixed right-handers (Thompson, Heaton, Matthews, & Grant, 1987). Consistent left-handers are faster with the left hand; consistent right-handers are faster with the right hand; and mixed handers show less or no difference between the hands (Annett, 1975). Both speed and regularity of tapping discriminate well between preferred and nonpreferred hands of handedness groups, although differences in speed are more marked than in regularity (Peters & Durding, 1979).

On simple motor tasks such as the Finger Tapping Test, the preferred hand should perform about 10% better than the nonpreferred hand (Reitan & Wolfson, 1985). If preferred hand performance is worse than nonpreferred hand performance, it is a "strong" indication of damage to the dominant hemisphere. If the preferred hand is at least 20% better, it is a strong sign of damage to the nondominant hemisphere (Golden, 1978). However, the size of the expected difference differs for right- and left-handers. For example, one study comparing handedness groups found a mean difference between hands of 2.8 taps for the left-handers and 6.0 taps for the right-handers (Satz *et al.*, 1967). It should be noted that the finger tapping test also showed the fallibility of using self-report of writing hand alone for defining left-handedness. In the above study, only 51% of the self-reported left-handers demonstrated superior performance with the left hand; 87% of the right-handers demonstrated superior performance with the right hand.*

These results suggest bilaterality of representation for motor function in most left-handers and suggest modifying the percentage of difference used to infer damage if the patient is a mixed left- or right-hander. The recommended percentages are likely to miss damage in mixed left-handers and may overestimate it in consistent right-handers. Left/right differences in finger tapping performance have been found to be linearly related to hand preference (e.g., Peters & Durding, 1978) suggesting that linearly modifying the estimated differences is a valid means of modifying the recommended percentages for inferring damage. Bimanual tapping tasks also show reliable handedness differences with skill differences between the hands smaller for left-handers (Peters, 1985). These results suggest that finger tapping is a valid test of handedness.

Hand strength has also been used to infer functional efficiency of the two hemispheres and lateral preference. Consistent right-handers and mixed right-handers show a greater percent difference score than left-handers on the Smedley Hand Dynamometer test (Reitan & Wolfson, 1985; Thompson *et al.*,

*The finger tapping instrument, however, if asymmetrically designed, is likely to be biased against left-handers. A study by Rosenstein and Van Sickle (1991), comparing the Halstead-Reitan tapping instrument (which is asymmetrically designed) with the Western Psychological Services instrument (which is symmetrically designed), found that with the HR instrument, left-handers showed only a slightly higher tapping rate for their dominant, left hand. With the WPS instrument, the dominant-nondominant hand discrepancy was uniform for the left- and right-handers. Further research with a larger sample size and more trials per subject is needed to see whether symmetrically designed instruments produce results significantly different from asymmetrically designed instruments. Investigators should describe the design of the finger-tapping instrument used in their studies. Clinicians may need to take the design of the instrument they are using into account in making inferences based on tapping differences between the right and left hands.

1987). For example, a study comparing right- and left-handers found the functional difference between hands was 5.3 for the left-handers and 34.2 for the right-handers (Satz *et al.*, 1967). This test also showed the fallibility of using self-report of writing hand alone for handedness.

The Tactual Performance Test, a more complex motor task that measures spatial analysis, learning, problem-solving ability, and memory, utilizes first the preferred and then the nonpreferred hand. Because of the learning involved, the general guideline is that the nonpreferred hand is expected to perform about 30 to 40% faster on the second trial (Reitan & Wolfson, 1985). Satz and his associates (Satz *et al.*, 1985) have found this test to be sensitive to the visuospatial deficit in pathological left-handers. Pathological left-handers showed impaired scores for the initial hand (left) and even greater impairment for the right hand, which should have benefitted by transfer of training.

Although motor tests have been shown to be valid measures of handedness, one cannot necessarily infer language lateralization from motor skill. A dissociation between language and motor representation has been found in some left-handers (Heilman, Coyle, Gonyea, & Geschwind, 1973; Geschwind, 1975). Also, sex of the patient may need to be considered. The asymmetry in motor performance favoring the right hand is stronger in right-handed women than in right-handed men (Kimura, 1983). On the other hand, a multivariate analysis of performance of seizure patients on the HRNB examining the influence of sex, education, age, and socioeconomic status found that these variables did not differentially affect the dominant/nondominant hand ratio scores for finger tapping, grip strength, and tactual performance test scores of different handedness groups (Seidenberg, Gamache, Beck, Smith Giordani, Berent, Sackellares, & Boll, 1984). These results suggest that differences between handedness groups on these tests are small or that subgrouping is necessary to reveal reliable differences.

Intelligence Tests

Subtests of widely used intelligence scales have been associated with localized functions. The Verbal and Performance subscale IQs of the Wechsler Adult Intelligence Scale have been correlated to the biological integrity of the left and right cerebral hemisphere, respectively (Reitan, 1955). Recently, it has been shown that certain tests requiring greater conceptual ability such as problem solving are better measures of the whole brain, i.e., they require the intactness of both hemispheres (Reitan, Hom, & Wolfson, 1988). However, certain subtests of these two scales (tests of verbal and language skill tests as opposed to spatial and manipulatory skills) clearly differentiate between the two hemispheres.

Differences between handedness groups have been found on the WAIS tests of spatial organization (block design, object assembly), and tests of verbalizability (picture completion, picture arrangement) with left-handed aphasics with left hemisphere lesions showing more impairment than right-handed aphasics (Borod *et al.*, 1985). Similar findings were obtained on Parietal Lobe Battery tests of construction (drawings to copy, sticks to memory, sticks to copy, blocks to photo, blocks to model, addition/subtraction). These results indicate that left-handers have more left hemisphere representation than right-handers of nonverbal functions. As discussed earlier, in a study comparing WAIS scores of intellectually superior right- and left-handed males, Levy (1969) found that the left-handers showed a 25-point-lower Performance score than Verbal score and attributed it to bilateral representation of language and cognitive crowding of spatial functions. Lansdell (1969) found that pathological left-handedness results in lowered scores on either verbal or performance scale measures (Wechsler–Bellevue), depending upon whether the cerebral damage occurred before the age of 5 (higher verbal than nonverbal scores) or after (higher nonverbal than verbal scores). In sum, left-handers are likely to have bilateral representation of both verbal and nonverbal processes, making it potentially more difficult to identify cerebral damage from performance differences on the WAIS, WAIS-R, or similar tests. Large differences between verbal and performance measures may indicate current trauma, bilateral representation of function and cognitive crowding, or early damage to the left hemisphere.

Because of more diffuse representation of function in the brain, a left-hander may not show as severe a deficit from cerebral insult as a right-hander unless the damage is extensive. Because functions are more likely to be bilaterally represented, left-handers may be better candidates for rehabilitation and have a better prognosis for recovery. However, when deficits are extensive in a left-hander, it is likely that damage to the brain is greater and more global than in a right-hander.

Assessing Language Lateralization

Most right-handers are strongly so. The majority of left-handers are likely to write with their left hand but they are not strongly left-handed and they are likely to perform some other manual activity with the right hand. Those people who have strong handedness, right or left, are likely to have unilateral representation of language opposite their writing hand. Those with mixed handedness, even if it is in only one activity performed with the opposite hand, are likely to have bilateral representation or left hemisphere representation. The majority of people, right- and left-handed, are likely to have left hemisphere representation of oral speech. Pathological left-handers are likely to have bilateral or right hemisphere representation of language.

Subgroups within each handedness group make it difficult to determine language lateralization by writing hand alone. However, using other information about manual preference, motor skill, presence or absence of enhanced visuospatial skills, and results from a lateralized perceptual test such as a verbal dichotic test, it may be possible to infer language lateralization. Is it possible to identify which people belong to which subgroup? The following subgroups and how to differentiate them are proposed.

Natural Handedness

1. The strong left-hander: performs all manual activities with left hand, shows left-sided preference for foot, eye, and possibly ear. Left hand is superior to right hand by approximately 10% in finger tapping. Left ear advantage on dichotic test. Right hemisphere representation of speech.

2. The weak left-hander: left-handed for writing but does one or more other manual activities with the right hand. Small difference between hands favoring left hand in finger tapping. Familial sinistrality likely. If poor in visuospatial skills and small ear difference on dichotic test, bilateral representation of speech. If superior in visuospatial skills and right ear advantage on dichotic test, strongly lateralized with left hemisphere representation of language and right hemisphere representation of visuospatial processes.

3. Ambidextrous (mixed) hander: manual skill is approximately equivalent in both hands. Performs some skilled manual activities with one hand; others are performed with the other. Although skill in both hands may be similar, shows reliable preference for one hand or the other for a particular activity. It is speculated that ambidextrous-handers have bilateral representation of language.

4. The weak right-hander: writes and performs almost but not all other manual activities with the right hand; right hand superiority in finger tapping; small right ear advantage on verbal dichotic test. Familial sinistrality likely. Bilateral representation of language. Poor spatial skills.

5. The strong right-hander: performs all manual activities with right hand; right hand superiority in finger tapping; right ear advantage on verbal dichotic test. No familial sinistrality. Strongly lateralized with language represented in the left hemisphere and visuospatial processes represented in the right hemisphere.

Atypical Handedness

6. Pathological (mild prenatal trauma to left hemisphere) left-hander: cognitive deficits in verbal skills, learning disabilities. Left hand significantly better than right in finger tapping. Right hand performance lower than age norms. If trauma is strong, more serious cognitive deficits such as mental retardation. Familial sinistrality usually absent in milder cases; often present in stronger cases.

7. Ambiguous hander (pathological with early lesion to left hemisphere): changes hand preference on same task from one occasion to another. Incomplete language lateralization; bilateral representation. Cognitive deficits of the left hemisphere, autism, perhaps retardation, schizophrenia.

8. Conditional right- or left-hander (natural or at least no sign of left hemisphere damage; psychological trauma in early development): changes hand preference on same task from one occasion to another. Changes are predictable, may be voluntary, and are associated with personality or affective

state. Individual may manifest multiple personality disorder (see Henninger, submitted for publication). Left hemisphere or bilateral representation of language.

9. Pathological right-hander: these people are few and have not been investigated. Presumably they would show significantly better performance in the right hand in finger tapping with performance in the left hand lower than in their peers.

Testing Conditions

Accurate clinical assessment requires that the clinician attempt to elicit the best performance of which the client is capable. This may require advance preparation and modification of the test and testing environment for the left-handed client. For example, a written test in which the movement of the left hand would cover the response choices should be modified to enable the client to see the choices while writing. A finger-tapping instrument that is comfortable for positioning both the left and right hands should be used.

SUMMARY

This chapter discusses topics on laterality and handedness that at present appear to be most directly useful to clinicians: lateralized processing in the brain; how cognitive functions, particularly language and visuospatial abilities, are organized differently in different handedness groups; how handedness is measured; theories of handedness and the distinction between natural and pathological left-handedness; subject variables affecting handedness; and clinical applications of handedness. A summary of hypothesized subgroups with their respective language representation is presented.

Definitions of handedness vary and data on the incidence of handedness are extremely variable, depending on how handedness is measured. The etiology of a person's handedness is not obvious, and even when the nature of a person's handedness has been identified, it is difficult to determine which research findings apply. Nonetheless, identifying the source of a person's handedness and researching the relationships between handedness and brain function are well worth the effort. Knowing whether a person is naturally left-handed or whether his handedness is a result of brain damage is useful in completing a neuropsychological assessment. Understanding the relationships between handedness and lateralized functions would provide a behavioral marker for brain organization. If the genetic basis for handedness were to be discovered, it could indicate a genetic basis for cerebral dominance and provide a way to trace the evolution of hemispheric specialization.

The most salient difference in hemispheric specialization between right and non-right-handers is the presence of bilateral speech in non-right handers. Bilateral speech refers to the involvement of both hemispheres in speech production. It is important to differentiate representation of oral speech from the amount of bilateral representation of language function in general. It appears that few people have bilateral representation of oral speech but people have varying amounts of language represented in the right hemisphere and varying degrees of right hemisphere participation in speech activities. Since non-right-handers have language more diffusely represented over both hemispheres, it is likely that lowered performance on verbal tests in them does not reflect the same brain injury as the performance in a right-hander. However, until we have a better understanding of the role of the nondominant hemisphere in various language activities and of how to assess specific language functions noninvasively, differences between right- and left-handers, though likely to be present, are unlikely to be observed.

Researchers, e.g., Bryden, McManus, Peters, and others, are attempting to determine a model of handedness. Such a model will have to account for the overwhelming bias to the right in human beings and for the larger number of left-handed males than females. It will need to consider that left-handers and right-handers differ in the incidence of right hemisphere language representation. A theory will have to posit a factor(s) causing both handedness and language to be controlled by the same hemisphere in some cases and not in others.

This chapter presents findings suggesting that the bias to the right is genetic; that the increased incidence of left-handedness in males is due to an increased vulnerability of the male to intrauterine insults to the left hemisphere, perhaps due to hormonal influences; that the variability in right hemisphere language is primarily due to the development of bilateral language representation or incomplete lateralization in left-handers; that the high incidence of left hemisphere representation in both handedness groups is due to the use of oral speech as a measure of language; and that oral speech is lateralized to the left hemisphere in most people regardless of handedness. It suggests that much of the confusion in the handedness literature results from the fact that handedness alone is not an adequate marker of lateral specialization and that other subject variables, particularly sex, must be taken into account to adequately predict lateralized functioning. Researchers are working to clarify the nature of the brain organization of these subgroups.

APPENDIX A: HAND PREFERENCE INVENTORIES

The Annett questionnaire consists of 12 items, 6 of which are designated "primary" questions (writing, throwing, holding a racket, a match, a hammer, and a toothbrush). The other 6 items (use of scissors, threading a needle, hand at the top of a broom and at the top of a shovel, dealing cards, and unscrewing the lid of a jar) are designated "secondary." The latter require more involvement of the nondominant hand, i.e., holding the paper while one cuts. Subjects can be classified into one of six groups: consistent right-handers, inconsistent right-handers, right ambidexters, left ambidexters, inconsistent left-handers, and consistent left-handers. The groups have been validated against a test of manual speech, but ought not to be regarded as discrete but as parts on a continuum of manual preference and skill (Annett, 1970). In a retest study, 47% of subjects changed at least one response at retest, but only 16% were reclassified as a result (McMeekan & Lishman, 1975). Annett's questionnaire has been useful, and it has stimulated the development of others, e.g., Briggs and Nebes (1976). However, the scoring procedure is inadequate. It is difficult to ascertain precisely where an individual falls on the continuum and, therefore, which subgroups to assign him or her to. Also, a dichotomous response that does not allow for differences in strength of preference is used. Some investigators have used Annett's items but divide the subjects simply into right-handers and non-right-handers. A single non-right-handed response identifies the subject as a non-right-hander. Categorizing subjects in this way corresponds to differences in callosal size with subjects with a single non-right-handed response having larger callosi than subjects who respond consistently with the right hand (Witelson, 1989).

The Edinburgh Handedness Inventory (EHI) consists of ten items: writing, drawing, throwing, use of scissors, toothbrush, knife, spoon, broom (upper hand), striking a match, and opening a box. Subjects are instructed to indicate the strength of their hand preference for each item by putting two or one tick in the appropriate column, or one tick in each if they are indifferent about that item. The EHI provides a "Laterality Quotient" (LQ), which can range from +100 (totally right-handed) to −100 (totally left-handed). It is computed by adding all the +'s for each hand, subtracting the sum for the left from that for the right, dividing by the sum of both, and multiplying by 100. In a retest study, the absolute mean difference between first and second LQs was 10.95 (S.D. = 14.74) (McMeekan & Lishman, 1975). The EHI is useful in that it shows strength of preference and it results in a numerical score on a continuum which can then be correlated with other data. It has been used in many investigations and may be the best standard of comparison of findings from one study to another.

The inventory developed by Raczkowski *et al.* (1974) consists of 23 items. An abbreviated version of the 13 items showing the greatest reliability has been used to design a test with high reliability (Chapman & Chapman, 1987). The following items are included: draw, write, use bottle opener, throw, hammer, toothbrush, screwdriver, eraser, racket, scissors, match, stir, and shoulder on which you rest a bat before swinging. The same or similar versions of 10 of these items appear on the EHI; 8 appear on Annett's questionnaire. Items are scored "1" for right, "2" for either, or "3" for left. This scoring yields a total score that can range from 13 (completely right-handed) to 39 (completely left-handed). Again, cutting points for grouping subjects are arbitrary; these investigators used 13–17 for right-handed and 33–39 for left-handed with the remaining categorized as ambilateral. The abbreviated inventory is useful in that it consists of items with high reliability. The scoring procedure might be modified in the manner of the EHI to show strength of preference.

APPENDIX B: OUTLINE FOR CLINICIAN

A. Client's handedness: Right, left, or mixed? Weak or strong? Ambidextrous? Ambiguous?
   1. Decide how to measure:
      a. Self-report: Do you consider yourself to be strongly right-handed, moderately right-handed, moderately left-handed, strongly left-handed, or something else?
      b. Preference questionnaire; confirm with asking client to perform behaviors.
      c. Other behavioral measures: test both dominant and nondominant with tasks that are not reinforced environmentally; administer finger tapping test and/or bimanual task to both hands.
   2. Ask questions to clarify nature of handedness:
      a. Do you know when your handedness became established?
      b. Was your handedness ever changed?
      c. How skilled are you with your nondominant hand?
   3. Is client's handedness familial?
      a. Parents, siblings, grandparents, cousins.
      b. If subject is right-handed, it is still useful to know the extent of left-handedness in the family.
   4. Is there evidence suggesting that the client did not develop complete lateralization?
      a. Does client use right hand on some occasions and left on others for the same task?
      b. Was handedness unstable in elementary school years?
   5. Is there evidence suggesting that the client's handedness is pathological?
      a. Presence of prenatal complications.
      b. Evidence of trauma at birth, prolonged labor, anoxia, breach presentation.
      c. Early strong handedness.
      d. Clumsiness in nondominant hand.
      e. Learning disabilities during school years.
      f. Presence of autoimmune disorders in self and family.
      g. Membership in populations that typically show overrepresentation of left-handers: signs of autism, mental retardation.
      Note: Although it is possible to have pathological right-handedness, it is extremely uncommon and for the remaining questions, only pathological left-handedness will be considered. If the clinician suspects pathological right-handedness, the questions can be modified to investigate that possibility.
   6. If there is evidence suggesting pathological left-handedness, to which subgroup does the client belong?
      a. Does the left-handed client show cognitive deficits? If he or she shows significantly lessened motor skill in the nondominant hand and spatial

(performance) deficits relative to verbal abilities, this could suggest a possible early (before age 5) insult to the left hemisphere forcing the right hemisphere to subserve both verbal and nonverbal functions. If client shows reduced verbal abilities, this could be the result of later (after age 5) damage to the left hemisphere with the compromised left hemisphere continuing to subserve language functions. If motor skills are relatively similar for both hands and there is no evidence of brain damage, the client is likely to be a natural left-hander and the deficit in spatial skills is a result of bilateral representation of speech and cognitive crowding.

Lowered overall performance could reflect greater trauma to the left hemisphere and increased crowding in the right. Alternatively, it could reflect bilateral damage.

b. Is the client deficient or average in skills of the left hemisphere but shows enhanced right hemisphere skills? If so, this suggests enhanced development of the right hemisphere. If the deficiencies of the left hemisphere are fairly severe resulting in learning disabilities during the school years, one might suspect some structural compromising of the left hemisphere or corpus callosum. If left hemisphere skills are not notably low but simply lower than right hemisphere skills, the lower left hemisphere performance probably does not reflect a lesion.

B. Does the left-handed client have left, right, or bilateral speech representation?

1. Test or ask the client's footedness, eyedness, and earedness. If he or she is left dominant for hand, foot, eye, and ear, it is highly likely (97%) that he or she is right hemisphere dominant for speech. Other combinations are not highly predictive.
2. Administer a dichotic verbal test, preferably twice, and ask the client to report any strategy he or she used. Although many factors enter into the determination of an ear advantage, a left ear advantage suggests potential right hemisphere speech representation and possible dominance. A small ear difference (two-point difference in a test of 30 or more dichotic pairs in which performance is not at a ceiling in either one) indicates considerable involvement of the right hemisphere in the perception or processing of verbal material and may indicate right hemisphere speech representation also. A reported strategy of attending to the left ear does not necessarily alter this interpretation but may suggest repeated testing, controlling for attentional strategies by asking the subject to report information to one ear first. A large ear difference in opposite directions on repeated testing in the absence of a deliberate strategy suggests possible attentional lability or incomplete lateralization and may indicate callosal dysfunction. A large right ear advantage may indicate underutilization or unusually strong suppression of the right hemisphere in verbal processing and may also suggest atypical brain organization and possible dysfunction.

a. If the left-handed subject is left hemisphere dominant for speech, and has a history of familial sinistrality, it is likely that the left-handedness is a marker for enhanced right hemisphere skills. His or her primary abilities are those of the right hemisphere: manual skills related to visual-spatial processing, mathematical skills related to enhanced visuospatial comprehension or if they are verbal, they involve the sonority or affective connotation of words, not the more traditional semantic and functional uses. He or she is unlikely to be an accountant or lawyer and is more likely to be a mechanic, musician, engineer, surgeon, artist, athlete, dancer, poet, architect. If he or she is above average in intelligence, particularly performance IQ, but did not attain the educational level one might have expected for that level of intelligence, one might suspect that being in an educational system that reinforces verbal, sequential, nonmanual skills might have been non-reinforcing of this person's abilities and this person is right hemisphere dominant in his interests and a true left-hander.

b. Alternatively, if there is suggestion of prenatal or early trauma affecting the left hemisphere and there are associated learning disabilities, this subject's left hemisphere language may reflect that he or she is genotypically a right-hander. The early damage shifted handedness but not speech. If the handedness is weak and the client uses his or her right hand for manual skills requiring less dexterity, and if there is an absence of familial sinistrality, and if none of the abilities of the right hemisphere are enhanced, you can suspect that this person may not be genotypically a left hander.

3. Implications of speech representation
   a. If bilateral speech or left hemisphere representation with considerable right hemisphere involvement in verbal processing, he or she has a better prognosis for recovery.
   b. If he or she does not recover, suspect greater damage.
4. Examine interests/skills
   a. If evidence of reduced verbal skills relative to performance but both are within the normal range, suspect enhanced right hemisphere ability rather than left hemisphere injury and suggest pursuing other right hemisphere interests and abilities.
   b. If evidence of reduced spatial skills, with equivalent motor skills in both hands, suspect bilateral speech rather than injury to right hemisphere and teach verbal strategies for dealing with nonverbal problems.

ACKNOWLEDGMENTS. I thank Jennifer Dingman for her research assistance and Marcel Kinsbourne, Jameela Lares, and Michael Peters for their helpful comments on the manuscript.

REFERENCES

Annett, M. (1970). A classification of hand preference by association analysis. *British Journal of Psychology, 61,* 303–321.

Annett, M. (1972). The distribution of manual asymmetry. *British Journal of Psychology, 63,* 343–358.

Annett, M. (1973). Handedness in families. *Annals of Human Genetics, 37,* 93–105.

Annett, M. (1975). Hand preference and the laterality of cerebral speech. *Cortex, 11,* 305–328.

Annett, M. (1985). *Left, right, hand and brain: The right shift theory.* Hillsdale, N.J.: Erlbaum.

Ardila, A., Correa, P., Zuluaga, J., & Uribe, B. (1988). Spatial abilities in "forced" left-handers. *Developmental Neuropsychology, 4*(2), 147–150.

Bakan, P. (1971). Handedness and birth order. *Nature, 229,* 195.

Bakan, P. (1973). Left-handedness & alcoholism. *Perceptual and Motor Skills, 36,* 514.

Bates, E., O'Connell, B., Vaid, J., Sledge, P., & Oakes, S. (1986). Language and hand preference in early development. *Developmental Neuropsychology, 2*(1), 1–15.

Benton, A. L. (1965). The problem of cerebral dominance. *The Canadian Psychologist, 6a*(4), 332–348.

Bishop, D. V. M. (1980). Handedness, clumsiness and cognitive ability. *Developmental Medicine and Child Neurology, 22,* 569–579.

Blau, A. (1946). *The master hand.* New York: American Ortho-Psychiatric Association.

Borod, J. C., Koff, E., & Caron, H. S. (1984). The Target Test: A brief laterality measure of speed and accuracy. *Perceptual and Motor Skills, 58,* 743–748.

Borod, J. C., Carper, M., Naeser, M., & Goodglass, H. (1985). Left-handed and right-handed aphasics with left hemisphere lesions compared on nonverbal performance measures. *Cortex, 21,* 81–90.

Briggs, G. G., & Nebes, R. D. (1976). The effects of handedness, family history and sex on the performance of a dichotic listening task. *Neuropsychologia, 14,* 129–133.

Bryden, M. P. (1988). An overview of the dichotic listening procedure and its relation to cerebral organization. In K. Jugdahl (Ed.), *Handbook of dichotic listening* (pp. 1–44). New York: Wiley.

Bryden, M. P., & MacDonald, V. (1987). The measurement of handedness and its relation to neuropsychological issues. Unpublished manuscript, University of Waterloo.

Bryden, M. P., Hecaen, H., & DeAgostini, M. (1983). Patterns of cerebral organization. *Brain and Language, 20,* 249–262.

Casey, M. B., Brabeck, M. M., & Ludlow, L. H. (1986). Familial handedness and its relation to spatial ability following strategy instructions. *Intelligence, 10,* 389–406.

Chapman, L. J., & Chapman, J. P. (1987). The measurement of handedness. *Brain and Cognition, 6,* 175–183.

Cohen, D. B. (1978). Dark hair and light eyes in college students: A potential biologic marker for liability to psychopathology. *Journal of Abnormal Psychology, 87*(4), 455–458.

Corballis, M. C. (1980). Laterality and myth. *American Psychologist, 35*(3), 284–295.

Curry, F. K. W., & Rutherford, D. R. (1967). Recognition and recall of dichotically presented verbal stimuli by right- and left-handed persons. *Neuropsychologia, 5,* 119–126.

D'Amico, C. M., & Kimura, D. (1987). *Evidence for subgroups of adextrals based on speech lateralization and cognitive patterns* (Research Bulletin 664). London, Canada: University of Western Ontario, Department of Psychology.

Dawson, G. (1988). Cerebral lateralization in autism: Clues to its role in language and affective development. In D. L. Molfese & S. J. Segalowitz (Eds.), *Brain lateralization in children: Developmental implications* (pp. 437–461). New York: Guilford Press.

Dee, H. L. (1971). Auditory asymmetry and strength of manual preference. *Cortex, 7,* 236–245.

Delis, D., Simpson, G., & Knight, R. (1983). Reversed hemispheric organization in a left hander. *Neuropsychologia, 21, 1,* 13–24.

Deutsch, D. (1978). Pitch memory: An advantage for the left-handed. *Science, 199,* 559–560.

Dimond, S. (1972). *The double brain.* London: Churchill–Livingstone.

Dronkers, N. F., & Knight, R. T. (1988). Right-sided neglect in a left-hander: Evidence for reversed hemispheric specialization of attention capacity. *Neuropsychologia, 27*(5), 729–735.

Durost, W. N. (1934). The development of a battery of objective group tests of manual laterality with the results of their application to 1300 children. *Genetic Psychology Monographs, 16*, 223–336.

Eme, R., Stone, S., & Izral, R. (1978). Spatial deficit in familial left-handed children. *Perceptual and Motor Skills, 47*, 919–922.

Feehan, M., Stanton, W. R., McGee, R., Silva, P. A., & Moffitt, T. E. (1990). Is there an association between lateral preference and delinquent behavior? *Journal of Abnormal Psychology, 99*, 198–201.

Filskov, S. B., & Catanese, R. A. (1986). Effects of sex and handedness on neuropsychological testing. In S. B. Filskov & T. J. Bokk (eds.), *Handbook of clinical neuropsychology* (pp. 198–212). New York: Wiley.

Gabrielli, W. F., Jr., & Mednick, S. A. (1980). Sinistrality and delinquency. *Journal of Abnormal Psychology, 89*(5), 654–661.

Geschwind, N. (1975). The apraxias: Neural mechanisms of disorders of learned movement. *American Scientist, 63* 188–195.

Geschwind, N., & Behan, P. O. (1982). Left-handedness: Association with immune disease, migraine, and developmental learning disorder. *Proceedings of the National Academy of Sciences of the United States of America, 79*, 5097–5100.

Geschwind, N., & Galaburda, A. M. (1985). Cerebral lateralization. Biological mechanisms, associations and pathology. I: A hypothesis and a program for research. *Archives of Neurology, 42*, 428–459.

Gloning, I., Gloning, K., Haub, G., & Quatember, R. (1969). Comparison of verbal behavior in right-handed and non right-handed patients with anatomically verified lesion of one hemisphere. *Cortex, 5*, 43–52.

Gloning, K., & Quatember, R. (1966). Statistical evidence of neuropsychological syndromes in left-handed and ambidextrous patients. *Cortex, 2*, 484–488.

Golden, C. J. (1978). *Diagnosis and rehabilitation in clinical neuropsychology*. Springfield, Ill.: Thomas.

Golden, C. J., Hammeke, T. A. & Purisch, A. P. (1980). *The Luria–Nebraska Neuropsychological Battery manual*. Los Angeles: Western Psychological Services.

Gordon, N. (1986). Left-handedness and learning. *Developmental Medicine and Child Neurology, 28*(5), 656–661.

Gregory, R., & Paul, J. (1980). The effects of handedness and writing posture on neuropsychological test results. *Neuropsychologia, 18*, 231–235.

Hammond, G. R., & Kaplan, R. J. (1982). Language lateralization and handedness: Estimates based on clinical data. *Brain and Language, 16*, 348–351.

Hardyck, C. (1977). Handedness and part–whole relationships: A replication. *Cortex, 13*, 177–183.

Hardyck, C., & Petrinovich, L. F. (1977). Left-handedness. *Psychological Bulletin, 84*(3), 385–403.

Hardyck, C., Petrinovich, L. F., & Goldman, R. D. (1976). Left-handedness and cognitive deficit. *Cortex, 12*, 266–279.

Harris, L. J., & Carlson, D. F. (1988). Pathological left-handedness: An analysis of theories and evidence. In D. L. Molfese & S. J. Segalowitz (Eds.), *Brain lateralization in children: Developmental implications* (pp. 289–372). New York: Guilford Press.

Harshman, R. A., Hampson, E., & Berenbaum, S. A. (1983). Individual differences in cognitive abilities and brain organization. Part 1: Sex and handedness differences in ability. *Canadian Journal of Psychology, 37*(1), 144–192.

Hecaen, H., & Sauguet, J. (1971). Cerebral dominance in left-handed subjects. *Cortex, 7*, 19–48.

Hecaen, H., DeAgostini, M., & Monzon-Montes, A. (1981). Cerebral organization in left-handers. *Brain and Language, 12*, 261–284.

Heilman, K. M., Coyle, J. M., Gonyea, E. F., & Geschwind, N. (1973). Apraxia and agraphia in a left-hander. *Brain, 96*, 21–28.

Henninger-Pechstedt, P. (1989*a*). Commissurotomy subjects show lateralized difference between manual and oral responding. *Cortex, 25*(2), 325–329.

Henninger, P. (1989*b*). Right- and left-handed musicians show differential hemispheric responsiveness to musical training, *Caltech Biology Annual Report*, #410.

Henninger, P. (Submitted). Conditional handedness: Handedness changes in multiple personality disordered subject reflect shift in hemispheric dominance.

Herrmann, D. J., & van Dyke, K. A. (1978). Handedness and the mental rotation of perceived patterns. *Cortex, 14*, 521–529.
Herron, J., Galin, D., Johnstone, J., & Ornstein, R. E. (1979). Cerebral specialization, writing posture, and motor control of writing in left-handers. *Science, 205*, 1285–1289.
Ingram, D. (1975). Motor asymmetries in young children. *Neuropsychologia, 13*, 95–102.
Kimura, D. (1961*a*). Some effects of temporal-lobe damage on auditory perception. *Canadian Journal of Psychology, 15*(3), 156–165.
Kimura, D. (1961*b*.). Cerebral dominance and the perception of verbal stimuli. *Canadian Journal of Psychology, 15*(3), 166–171.
Kimura, D. (1973). Manual activity during speaking. II. Left-handers. *Neuropsychologia, 11*, 51–55.
Kimura, D. (1983). Sex differences in cerebral organization for speech and praxic functions. *Canadian Journal of Psychology, 37*, 19–35.
Kinsbourne, M. (1988). Sinistrality, brain organization, and cognitive deficits. In D. L. Molfese & S. J. Segalowitz (Eds.), *Brain lateralization in children: Developmental implications* (pp. 259–279). New York: Guilford Press.
Knox, A. W., & Boone, D. R. (1970). Auditory laterality and tested handedness. *Cortex, 6*, 164–173.
Kolata, G. (1983). Math genius may have hormonal basis. *Science, 222.*, 1312.
Kopelman, M. D. (1982). Speech dominance, handedness and electro-convulsions. *Psychological Medicine, 12*, 667–670.
Kramer, M. A., Albrecht, S., & Miller, R. A. (1985). Handedness and the laterality of breast cancer in women. *Nursing Research, 34*(6), 333–337.
Lansdell, H. (1969). Verbal and nonverbal factors in right-hemisphere speech: Relation to early neurological history. Journal of Comparative and Physiological Psychology, *69* 734–738.
LeMay, M., & Culebras, A. (1972). Human brain—morphologic differences in the hemispheres demonstrable by carotid arteriography. *New England Journal of Medicine., 287*, 168–170.
Levy, J. (1969). Possible basis for the evolution of lateral specialization of the human brain. *Nature, 224*, 614–615.
Levy, J. (1976). A review of evidence for a genetic component in the determination of handedness. *Behavior Genetics, 6*(4), 429–453.
Levy, J., & Nagylaki, T. (1972). A model for the genetics of handedness. *Genetics, 72*, 117–128.
Levy, J., & Reid, M. (1976). Variations in writing posture and cerebral organization. *Science, 194*, 337–339.
Levy, J., & Trevarthen, C. (1976). Meta-control of hemispheric function in human split-brain patients. *Journal of Experimental Psychology: Human Perception and Performance, 2*, 299–312.
Levy, J., & Wagner, N. (1984). Handwriting posture, visuomotor integration, and lateralized reaction-time parameters. *Human Neurobiology, 3*, 157–161.
Liederman, J., & Coryell, J. (1982). The origin of left hand preference: Pathological and nonpathological influences. *Neuropsychologia, 20*(6), 721–725.
Lucas, J. A., Rosenstein, L. D., & Bigler, E. D. (1989). Handedness and language among the mentally retarded: Implications for the model of pathological left-handedness and gender differences in hemispheric specialization. *Neuropsychologia, 27*(5), 713–723.
Luria, A. R. (1966). *Higher cortical functions in man*. New York: Basic Books.
Marino, M. F., & McKeever, W. F. (1982). The influence of sex and familial sinistrality on spatial laterality and spatial ability. Paper presented at the meeting of the International Neuropsychological Society, Pittsburgh.
McCreadie, R. G., Crorie, J., Barron, E. T., & Winslow, G. S. (1982). The Nithsdale Schizophrenia Survey: III. Handedness and tardive dyskinesia. *British Journal of Psychiatry, 140*, 591–594.
McKeekan, E. R. L., & Lishman, W. A. (1975). Retest reliabilities and interrelationship of the Annett hand preference questionnaire and the Edinburgh handedness inventory. *British Journal of Psychology, 66*(1), 53–59.
McKeever, W. F. (1979). Handwriting posture in left-handers: Sex, familial sinistrality and language laterality correlates. *Neuropsychologia, 17, 6*, 429–444.
McKeever, W. F., & Hoff, A. L. (1979). Evidence of a possible isolation of left hemisphere visual and motor areas in sinistrals employing an inverted hand posture. *Neuropsychologia, 17, 6*, 445–455.

McKeever, W. F., Seitz, K. S., Hoff, A. L., & Marino, M. F. (1983). Interacting sex and familial sinistrality characteristics influence both language lateralization and spatial ability in right-handers. *Neuropsychologia, 21*(6), 661–668.

McManus, I. C. (1985). Handedness, language dominance and aphasia: A genetic model. *Psychological Medicine*, Monograph Supplement #8, Cambridge University Press.

Mebert, C. J., & Michel, G. F. (1980). Handedness in artists. In J. Herron (Ed.), *Neuropsychology of left-handedness* (pp. 273–278). New York: Academic Press.

Miller, C. A. (1982). Degree of lateralization as a hierarchy of manual and cognitive skill levels. *Neuropsychologia, 20*(2), 155–162.

Miller, E. (1971). Handedness and pattern of human ability. *British Journal of Psychology, 62*, 111–112.

Milner, B. (1974). Hemispheric specialization: Scope and limits. In F. O. Schmitt & F. G. Worden (Eds.), *The neurosciences: Third study program* (pp. 75–89). Cambridge, Mass.: MIT Press.

Milner, B., Branch, C., & Rasmussen, T. (1964). Observations on cerebral dominance. In A. V. S. deReuck & M. O'Connor (Eds.), *Ciba Foundation symposium on disorders of language* (pp. 200–214). London: Churchill.

Myers, J. J. (1984). Right hemisphere language: Science or fiction? *American Psychologist, 39*(3), 315–320.

Naeser, M. A., & Borod, J. C. (1986). Aphasia in left-handers: Lesion site, lesion side, and hemispheric asymmetries on CT. *Neurology, 36*, 471–488.

Natale, M., Gur, R. E., & Gur, R. C. (1983). Hemispheric asymmetries in processing emotional expressions. *Neuropsychologia, 21*(5), 555–565.

Nebes, R. D. (1971). Handedness and the perception of part–whole relationships. *Cortex, 7*, 350–356.

Newcombe, F., & Ratcliff, G. (1973). Handedness, speech lateralization, and ability. *Neuropsychologia, 11, 4*, 339–407.

Oldfield, R. C. (1971). The assessment and analysis of handedness: The Edinburgh Inventory. *Neuropsychologia, 9*, 97–113.

Penfield, W., & Roberts, L. (1959). *Speech and brain mechanisms*. Princeton, N.J.: Princeton University Press.

Peters, M. (1985). Constraints in the performance of bimanual tasks and their expression in unskilled and skilled subjects. *The Quarterly Journal of Experimental Psychology, 37A*, 171–196.

Peters, M. (1990). Phenotype in normal left-handers: An understanding of phenotype is the basis for understanding mechanism and inheritance of handedness. In S. Coren (Ed.), *Left-handedness: Behavioral implications and anomalies* (pp. 167–192). Amsterdam: Elsevier.

Peters, M., & Durding, B. (1978). Handedness measured by fingertapping: A continuous variable. *Canadian Journal of Psychology, 32*, 257–261.

Peters, M., & Durding, B. (1979). Left-handers and right-handers compared on a motor task. *Journal of Motor Behavior, 11*, 103–111.

Peterson, J. M. (1979). Left-handedness: Differences between student artists and scientists. *Perceptual and Motor Skills, 48*, 961–962.

Peterson, J. M., & Lansky, L. M. (1974). Left-handedness among architects: Some facts and speculation. *Perceptual and Motor Skills, 38*, 547–550.

Peterson, J. M., & Lansky, L. M. (1980). Success in architecture: Handedness and visual thinking. *Perceptual and Motor Skills, 50*, 1139–1143.

Raczkowski, D., Kalat, J. W., & Nebes, R. (1974). Reliability and validity of some handedness questionnaire items. *Neuropsychologia, 12, 1*, 43–47.

Rasmussen, T., & Milner, B. (1975). Clinical and surgical studies of the cerebral speech areas in man. In K. J. Zulch, O. Creutzfeldt, & G. Galbraith (Eds.), *Otfrid Foerster symposium on cerebral localization* (pp. 238–257). Berlin: Springer.

Reitan, R. M. (1955). Investigation of the validity of Halstead's measures of biological intelligence. *Archives of Neurology and Psychiatry, 73*, 28–35.

Reitan, R. M., & Wolfson, D. (1985). *The Halstead–Reitan Neuropsychological Battery: Theory and clinical interpretation*, Tucson: Neuropsychology Press.

Reitan, R. M., Hom, J., & Wolfson, D. (1988). Verbal processing by the brain. *Journal of Clinical and Experimental Neuropsychology, 10*(1), 400–408.

Rosenstein, L. D., Van Sickle, L. F. (1991, February). Artificial depression of left-hand finger-tapping rates: A critical evaluation of the Halstead-Reitan Neuropsychological Finger Tapping test instrument. Poster presented at the meeting of the International Neuropsychological Society, Austin.

Satz, P. (1972). Pathological left-handedness: An explanatory model. *Cortex, 8,* 121–135.

Satz, P. (1979). A text of some models of hemispheric speech organization in the left- and right-handed. *Science, 203,* 1131–1133.

Satz, P. (1980). Incidence of aphasia in left-handers: A test of some hypothetical models of cerebral speech organization. In J. Herron (Ed.), *Neuropsychology of left-handedness* (pp. 189–197). New York: Academic Press.

Satz, P., Achenbach, K., & Fennell, E. (1967). Correlations between assessed manual laterality and predicted speech laterality in a normal population. *Neuropsychologia, 5, 4,* 295–310.

Satz, P., Orsini, D. L., Saslow, E., & Henry, R. (1985). The pathological left-handedness syndrome. *Brain and Cognition, 4,* 27–46.

Satz, P., Soper, H. V., & Orsini, D. (1988). Human hand preference: Three nondextral subtypes. In D. L. Molfese & S. J. Segalowitz (Eds.), *Brain lateralization in children: Developmental implications* (pp. 281–287). New York: Guilford Press.

Searleman, A., Tweedy, J., & Springer, S. P. (1979). Interrelationships among subject variables believed to predict cerebral organization. *Brain and Language, 7,* 267–276.

Searleman, A., Porac, C., & Coren, S. (1984). Writing hand posture and four indexes of lateral preference. *Brain and Cognition, 3,* 86–93.

Searleman, A., Porac, C., & Coren, S. (1989). Relationship between birth order, birth stress, and lateral preferences: A critical review. *Psychological Bulletin, 105*(3), 397–408.

Segalowitz, S. J., & Bryden, M. P. (1983). Individual differences in hemispheric representation of language. In S. J. Segalowitz (Ed.), *Language functions and brain organization* (pp. 341–372). New York: Academic Press.

Seidenberg, M., Gamache, M. P., Beck, N. C., Smith, M., Giordani, B., Berent, S., Sackellares, J. C., & Boll, T. J. (1984). Subject variables and performance on the Halstead neuropsychological test battery: A multivariate analysis. *Journal of Consulting and Clinical Psychology, 52*(4), 658–662.

Seltzer, B., Burres, M. S. K., & Sherwin, I. (1984). Left-handedness in early and late onset dementia. *Neurology, 34,* 367–369.

Serafetinides, E. A., Hoare, R. D., & Driver, M. V. (1965). Intracarotid sodium amylobarbitone and cerebral dominance for speech and consciousness. *Brain, 88,* 107–130.

Smith, L. C., & Moscovitch, M. (1979). Writing posture, hemispheric control of movement and cerebral dominance in individuals with inverted and noninverted hand postures during writing. *Neuropsychologia, 17, 6,* 637–644.

Sperry, R. W. (1974). Lateral specialization in the surgically separated hemispheres. In F. O. Schmitt & F. G. Worden (Eds.), *The neurosciences: Third study program* (Vol. 3, pp. 5–19). Cambridge, Mass.: MIT Press.

Springer, S. P., & Deutsch, G. (1989). *Left brain, right brain* (3rd ed.). San Francisco: Freeman.

Steenhuis, R. E., & Bryden, M. P. (1988, June). The relation between hand preference and hand performance. In M. Schwartz (Chair), *Handedness: Its measurement, performance and distribution in normal and problem populations.* Symposium conducted at the meeting of the Canadian Psychological Association, Montreal.

Strauss, E. (1986). Hand, foot, eye and ear preferences and performance on a dichotic listening test. *Cortex, 22,* 475–482.

Strauss, E., & Wada, J. (1983). Lateral preferences and cerebral speech dominance. *Cortex, 19,* 165–177.

Strauss, E., & Wada, J. (1988). Hand preference and proficiency and cerebral speech dominance determined by the carotid amytal test. *Journal of Clinical and Experimental Neuropsychology, 10*(2), 169–174.

Strauss, E., Wada, J., & Kosaka, B. (1984). Writing hand posture and cerebral dominance for speech. *Cortex, 20,* 143–147.

Sussman, H. M. (1971). The laterality effect in lingual–auditory tracking. *The Journal of the Acoustical Society of America, 496*(2), 1874–1880.

Tapley, S. M., & Bryden, M. P. (1983). Handwriting position and hemispheric asymmetry in right-handers. *Neuropsychologia, 21*(2), 129–138.

Tapley, S. M., & Bryden, M. P. (1985). A group test for the assessment of performance between the hands. *Neuropsychologia, 23*(2), 215–221.

Teng, E. L., Lee, P., Yang, K., & Chang, P. C. (1976). Handedness in a Chinese population: Biological, social and pathological factors. *Science, 193*, 1148–1150.

Thompson, L. L., Heaton, R. K., Matthews, C. G., & Grant, I. (1987). Comparison of preferred and nonpreferred hand performance on four neuropsychological motor tasks. *The Clinical Neuropsychologist, 1*(4), 324–334.

Weber, A. M., & Bradshaw, J. L. (1981). Levy and Reid's neurological model in relation to writing hand/posture: An evaluation. *Psychological Bulletin, 90*, 74–88.

Witelson, S. F. (1987). Neurobiological aspects of language in children. *Child Development, 58*, 653–688.

Witelson, S. F. (1989). Hand and sex differences in the isthmus and genu of the human corpus callosum: A postmortem morphological study. *Brain, 112*, 799–835.

Zaidel, E. (1976). Lexical organization in the right hemisphere. In P. A. Buser & A. Rougeul-Buser (Eds.), *Cerebral correlates of conscious experience* (pp. 177–197). Amsterdam: Elsevier.

Zangwill, O. (1960). *Cerebral dominance and its relation to psychological function*. Edinburgh: Oliver & Boyd.

Zurif, E. B., & Bryden, M. P. (1969). Familial handedness in left–right differences in auditory and visual perception. *Neuropsychologia, 7*, 179–187.

6

Socioeducational

ALFREDO ARDILA, MONICA ROSSELLI,
and FEGGY OSTROSKY-SOLIS

INTRODUCTION

Performance on neuropsychological tests can be influenced by different types of variables, some of which are internal (organic) and others, such as cultural and educational variables, are considered to be external. Culture can be defined as a historically transmitted pattern of meanings embodied in symbols, as a system of inherited conceptions expressed in symbolic forms by means of which individuals communicate, perpetuate, and develop their knowledge about and attitudes toward life (Geertz, 1973), or simply as the specific way of living of a human group. Education refers to the level of formal school training. Schooling is considered to fulfill the following fundamental aims which are roughly equivalent universally: (1) teaching broad-based generalized skills; (2) transmission in cultural knowledge ("scientific knowledge"); and (3) transmission in a large number of cultural norms (Jordan & Tharp, 1979). These fundamental aims would be similar regardless of locale, and thus schooling can be viewed as a transnational culture in itself.

Cultural background, and particularly educational level, can affect individual performance on psychological and neuropsychological tests. In this chapter, we analyze how cultural variables affect performance on different neuropsychological tests.

A central problem of neuropsychological evaluations has been distinguishing the effects of brain pathology from those resulting from the subject's membership in a different cultural group. This is particularly true when evaluating illiterate people, or when transferring assessment tests to a culture different

---

ALFREDO ARDILA and MONICA ROSSELLI • Instituto Colombiano de Neuropsicologia, Bogotá, Colombia. FEGGY OSTROSKY-SOLIS • Facultad de Psicologia, Universidad Nacional Autonoma de Mexico, Mexico City, Mexico.

HANDBOOK OF NEUROPSYCHOLOGICAL ASSESSMENT: A Biopsychosocial Perspective, edited by Antonio E. Puente and Robert J. McCaffrey. Plenum Press, New York, 1992.

from that in which they were originally developed. Moreover, research into cognitive functioning in different cultures and educational groups is important not only from a practical clinical point of view, but also because it can have important implications for our understanding of cerebral organization and the development of cognitive activity.

Cultural variables are important in the way children are raised and in which learning is acquired. Robinson (1974) observed that parents with a low socioeconomic level use more nonverbal strategies in their relationships with children, whereas parents with a higher educational level use verbal strategies more frequently. Bernstein (1974) points out that the language used by people with a low socioeconomic level is less fluent and has a simpler grammatical structure relying much more on emotional than logical strategies. Bruner, Olver, and Greenfield (1966) suggest that the linguistic ability of rural unschooled children relates to the immediate context of the referent, and that formal education facilitates the development of language into a fully symbolic tool.

Literacy, and schooling in general, is much more than the learning of a symbolic system to represent language in a written manner. Literacy represents the acquisition of a basic instrument used in interaction with other people and for obtaining information about the surrounding world. In our contemporary world, literacy is the basic conceptual instrument for obtaining knowledge. Reading and writing imply the possibility of access to a tremendous amount of established information. These two skills represent the acquisition of a new culture: the culture of literacy. Literacy, and the acquisition of academic training in general, might influence the brain organization not only of language but also of other cognitive abilities. However, reading and writing have only existed for four or five millenniums in the history of mankind but until two or so centuries ago, they were restricted to very small and selected groups. Even today, about one third of the world's population is illiterate, i.e., more than 1,500,000,000 people (UNICEF, 1985). Neuropsychological analysis of illiterate people is therefore a highly relevant task, especially when dealing with individuals from low socioeconomic or Third World countries.

THEORETICAL AND BASIC CULTURAL ISSUES

Research into cross-cultural cognitive psychology has shown that cultural background has very critical implications in terms of language, perception, memory, and logical reasoning (Laboratory of Comparative Human Cognition, 1983; Laurendeau-Bendavid, 1977). Specifically, cognitive activity is culture-dependent.

Perceptual abilities have been studied extensively in different cultures and across different school groups (e.g., Brislin, 1983; Segall, 1986). For example, perceptual performance in the use of three-dimensionality in drawings, recognition of schematized figures, and depth perception in pictures—elements of routine neuropsychological tests—vary according to cultural experience. It is important to point out that the use of perspective to represent distances was only introduced into Western painting some five centuries ago. Therefore, we cannot expect to find this ability in every culture and even less in individuals with no exposure to this concept. Similarly, recognizing schematized figures is an ability that requires training but it is an ability that is taken for granted. For example, Modiano, Maldonado, and Villasana (1982) showed an average error rate of 20% in Mexican Indian children in identifying color paintings and photographs of everyday objects.

The depth perception test using pictures by Hudson (1960) found that European children of approximately 12 years of age could perceive the pictures as three-dimensional. In contrast, three-dimensional perception was not found in Bantu or Ghanian children. Nonliterate Bantu, and also European laborers without this type of perceptual training, saw the pictures as flat, not three-dimensional. Deregowski (1980) has also highlighted the inability of African children to copy figures without rotating angles. Osuji (1982) observed difficulties in Nigerian school children in reproducing geometric patterns.

Differences in performance on the Bender-Gestalt and the Frostig Developmental Test of visual perception between black and white children from the same educational level have been reported by Amante, Van Houton, Grieve, Bader, and Margules (1977). These differences, according to the authors, were related to socioeconomic status and the parents' educational level. Mercer (1977) has shown that group differences in IQ among Anglo, black, and Chicano children are largely accounted for in terms of sociocultural variables. When these variables are sufficiently controlled, there are no differences.

Berry (1971, 1979) proposed that hunter societies with specific ecological demands usually present good visual discrimination and spatial skills. For instance, the Embedded Figures Test is better performed by cultural groups for whom hunting is important for survival. Berry emphasized that ecological demands and cultural practices are significantly related to the development of perceptual and cognitive skills. A good example of a specific culture-dependent cognitive skill was that reported by Gay and Cole (1967): When Kpelle farmers were contrasted with American working-class subjects, the former were found to be considerably more accurate in estimating the amount of rice in several bowls of different sizes.

Lantz (1979) showed that rural unschooled children performed better than schooled Indian or American children in coding and decoding culturally relevant objects, such as grain or seeds. Children without formal schooling are able to separate language symbols from the physical referent and to use these symbols for communicating accurately, but display of the ability depends upon the stimuli used (Laboratory of Comparative Human Cognition, 1983). Encoding and decoding information depends on the cultural salience of the stimuli used. It is consequently not enough to translate a test into the language of the examinee. The task must be meaningful in that particular culture.

Memory abilities are culture- and environment-dependent. Bartlett (1932) initially proposed that illiterates more frequently use procedures of rote learning: literate people prefer more active information integration procedures. However, Cole, Frankel, and Sharp (1971*a*) did not find evidence to support this hypothesis. Comparing Liberian Kpelle children with American children, they found that the latter recalled words better than objects. According to Cole and Scribner (1974), however, Kpelle subjects could recall objects better than spoken words. Similarly, illiterate subjects tend to do better in visual memory tasks than in verbal memory ones (Ardila, Rosselli, & Rosas, 1989). Klitch and Davidson (1983) found remembering visual experiences to be better in Aboriginal children than in rural Caucasian children. Memorizing is better when it relies on the coding system the subject has previously learned.

Cole, Frankel, and Sharp (1971) observed that when memorizing information, both literates and illiterates make use of their own groupings in order to structure recall. For instance, high school subjects rely almost exclusively on taxonomic categories while illiterate bush farmers make little use of this principle. This could explain differences in performing standard memory tasks. Cole and Scribner (1974) argue that cultural differences in memorizing do not consist in the presence or absence of mnemonic techniques in general, but in the utilization of specific techniques such as reorganization of the material to be recalled. People remember what is culturally relevant.

EDUCATIONAL LEVEL AND PERFORMANCE ON PSYCHOLOGICAL AND NEUROPSYCHOLOGICAL TESTS

An important correlation has been observed to exist between neuropsychological tests and measures of intelligence batteries such as the WAIS (Goldstein & Shelly, 1972; Reitan, 1956). Indeed, many of the tests used in routine neuropsychological assessment are the same as those given in psychometric intelligence evaluation. For instance, the Block Design Subtest is considered as a performance intelligence test and is also used as a basic test in assessing constructional abilities traditionally related to right parietal damage. Furthermore, intelligence scales are frequently used for neuropsychological purposes (Lezak, 1983), and many neuropsychological batteries include psychometric measures of intelligence. This is particularly true of the Wechsler Scales of Intelligence (e.g., WAIS-R).

A correlation of 0.70 between years of education and full IQ scale has been found (Matarazzo, 1972). Heaton, Grant, and Matthews (1986) obtained statistically significant correlations between level of education and scores on all WAIS subtests. Test performance was significantly associated with a high educational level. Moreover, when comparing the influence of different variables on intelligence batteries such as the WAIS, the subject's level of education has proven to have a more powerful effect on WAIS performance than age (Matarazzo, 1972). Studies have consistently shown that educational attainment is a particularly critical factor in verbal subjects (e.g., Ardila & Rosselli, 1988). Specifically, verbal abilities, as measured in psychometric intelligence tests, are more educationally dependent than nonverbal abilities.

Several studies have demonstrated a relationship between educational level and performance on various neuropsychological measures. Finlayson, Johnson, and Reitan (1977) used a series of psychological and neuropsychological tests to evaluate normal and brain-damaged adults. Their results showed that educational level significantly affects performance on neuropsychological tasks, particularly with normals. Although tests such as the Wechsler–Bellevue and the Halstead–Reitan Neuropsychological Battery (HRNB) distinguish normal and brain-damaged populations quite well, some subtests in the HRNB (e.g., Seashore Rhythm Test and Speech Sound Perception Test) and the majority of the Wechsler–Bellevue subtests (Information, Comprehension, Digit Span, Arithmetic, Similarities, and Vocabulary) show an overlap of low educational group scores in a normal population and higher educational group scores in a brain-damaged group. In other words, educational level can be as powerful a variable in the scores obtained on the Wechsler–Bellevue battery and in the HRNB as is brain damage.

Lecours, Mehler, Parente, Caldeira, Cary, Castro, Dehaout, Delgado, Gurd, Karmann, Jakubovitz, Osorio, Cabral, and Junqueira (1987, 1988) studied the relationships between brain damage and educational attainment with regard to both aphasic alteration in language and unilateral neglect. The authors emphasize the need to consider educational factors in neuropsychological evaluation in order to avoid the risk of over- or underestimating (Type I or II errors) the frequency of aphasia and other neuropsychological syndromes arising from brain damage. Neuropsychological sequelae of brain damage are not homogeneous across patients of varying educational levels.

Cornelius and Caspi (1987) observed that educational attainment has a significant relationship with performance on verbal meaning tests but is not systematically related to everyday problem-solving. Heaton, *et al.* (1986) compared performance on the HRNB for three different educational levels (9, 13, and 17 years of schooling on average) and for three age ranges (<40, 40–59, >60). The investigators found significant educational effects on all subtests; only some tests were related to age, particularly Psychomotor Speed, Conceptual Ability, Flexibility of Thinking, and Incidental Memory subtests. This relationship between educational level and neuropsychological performance has also been supported by Bornstein and Suga (1988).

Ostrosky, Canseco, Quintanar, Navarro, Meneses, and Ardila (1985) and Ostrosky, Quintanar, Meneses, Canseco, Navarro, and Ardila (1986) used a neuropsychological diagnostic battery on 109 subjects from two different socioeducational levels in Mexico City. The higher socioeducational group ($X = 14.96$ years) performed better on all sections of the battery (Motor Functions, Somatosensory Knowledge, Visuospatial Recognition, Auditory Knowledge and Language, Cognitive Processes, Oral Language, Reading, Writing and Calculations) than the low socioeducational group ($X = 7.06$ years). The differences were particularly notable in some areas. Using a factor analysis, the investigators found that the items more sensitive to socioeducational level are those that involve the use of complex conceptual aspects of language, as well as the organization of motor sequences and motor programming. This association between educational level, and language and motor abilities has been further confirmed (Rosselli, Ardila, and Rosas, 1990).

CLINICAL EVALUATION AND SOCIOEDUCATIONAL VARIABLES

The effects of socioeducational level on neuropsychological test performance have been well studied though not regularly considered in clinical practice. In this section, language, visuospatial, memory, and motor abilities will be addressed.

Language

It has been proposed that the brain organization of language is different in literates and illiterates (Cameron, Currier, & Haerer, 1971; Matute, 1988). Lecours *et al.* (1988) administered an aphasia screening test, comprising naming, repetition, word–picture matching, and sentence–picture matching tasks, to 188 unilateral stroke subjects. Subjects were either completely illiterate or had received at least four years of education. Repetition and matching tasks did not differentiate between groups. However, some degree of word-finding difficulty and reduction in speech output, as well as a sizeable production of phonemic paraphasia were observed more frequently in the illiterate group. These findings suggest that the cerebral representation of language might be different in illiterates and in educated subjects. Matute (1988) analyzed aphasia in illiterates and concluded that the severity of aphasia is significantly less in illiterates than in literate control subjects. This suggests that the left hemispheric specialization is more limited in illiterates. This suggestion is supported by Lecours *et al.* (1988) who proposed that left dominance for language does not change with the acquisition of reading and writing skills but cerebral asymmetry becomes more evident.

Many researchers have shown that the "verbal" subtests of the Wechsler Scales are the most sensitive to education. The relationship of education to scores on the verbal subtests of the WAIS, such as Vocabulary, Information, Similarities, and Comprehension, has been well established (Finlayson *et al.*, 1977; Heaton, *et al.*, 1986). Similar findings have been reported with aphasia assessment tests (Borod, Goodglass, & Kaplan, 1980). Rosselli, Ardila, Florez, and Castro (1990*a*) observed that all subtests of the Boston Diagnostic Aphasia Examination (Goodglass & Kaplan, 1972) were affected by educational level, except for Repetition of Words and Reciting. Educational level was observed to be a more important variable than age.

Ardila and Rosselli (1988) used a set of basic neuropsychological tests with a sample of normal completely illiterate and highly educated subjects. Two hundred neurologically intact, right-handed subjects were divided into groups according to three variables: (1) educational level (illiterates with no formal education and with illiterate parents versus professionals, or university students, with professional parents); (2) age (16–25, 26–35, 36–45, 46–55, and 56–65); and (3) sex (male versus female). The matched 2 × 5 × 2 design was obtained with ten subjects per cell. The results indicated that all language subtests (language comprehension, phonological discrimination, naming, repetition, and verbal fluency) were sensitive to educational level. Phonological discrimination and naming of figures were also sensitive to age, although age interacted with educational level. These results are supportive of previous reports. For example, in the HRNB, the Speech Sound Perception and Seashore Rhythm Test have been shown to be the most sensitive subtests relative to the subject's educational level (Finlayson *et al.*, 1977). Heaton *et al.* (1986) compared subjects of different educational levels (<12, 12–15, and >16 years of schooling). Statistically significant correlations were obtained between education and all HRNB measures. The Aphasia and the Speech Sound Perception subtests appeared to be the most sensitive to educational level.

Memory

Craik, Bynd, and Swason (1987) observed that differences in memory loss in aged subjects were related to educational attainment. Specifically, subjects with low educational attainment presented an earlier decline in memory abilities when compared with those with a high educational attainment. Ardila *et al.* (1989) studied neuropsychological performance of illiterates and found significant differences between educational groups on all but one memory subtest (digit retention, immediate memory for sentences, memory curve, logical memory, delayed recall of words, sentences, and paragraphs, visuospatial memory, and sequential memory). No group differences were noted on immediate memory of sentences. Age was a critical variable for digit retention, delayed memory of words, logical memory, delayed memory of paragraphs, and sequential memory, but this effect interacted with the subject's educational level. Sex differences were also found with digit and memory curve but, again, age and sex interacted with educational level. It is important to stress that one of the most widespread subtests for assessing immediate memory (digit span) is affected by educational attainment (Finlayson *et al.*, 1977; Heaton *et al.*, 1986; Ardila *et al.*, 1989).

Visuospatial Abilities

Even though the so-called performance subtests have been considered less sensitive to demographic variables like education (Matarazzo, 1972), visuospatial tasks also appear to be affected by the subject's educational level. For example, Benton, Levin, and Van Allen (1974) studied the influence of educational level on a geographical orientation task administered to patients with unilateral cerebral lesions. Educational background was related to performance level and interacted with diagnostic category. The less educated patients with brain damage differed more from their controls than did patients with a higher level of education. It has been reported that the right hemi-spatial neglect syndrome is more frequently found in low educational brain-damaged patients (Rosselli, Rosselli, Vergara, & Ardila, 1985). Also, one of the most used neuropsychological tests, the visuospatial subtest *block design*, has proved to be sensitive to educational level (Finlayson *et al.*, 1977; Heaton *et al.*, 1986).

Ardila *et al.* (1989) found that illiterate subjects display significant differences in tasks such as three-dimensional drawings and recognition of superimposed figures. All the visuospatial and constructional tasks used (copying of figures, telling time, recognition of superimposed figures, map recognition, and drawing a room plan) were found to be significantly different between educational groups (illiterates and professionals). The mistakes observed in figure copying were related to spatial disorganization and inadequate relationship among elements, as well as omission and absence of three-dimensionality. Differences were also found among age groups for the figure copying test, map recognition, and drawing a room plan. The best performances were noted for the younger groups but these differences interacted with educational level and were more evident among the various age groups of illiterate subjects. On the figure copying and telling time subtests, sex interacted with educational level. Specifically, in the illiterate group, men consistently outperformed women, while in the highly educated group there were no differences between sexes. Educational level interacted with socioeconomic status (Matarazzo, 1972). People from low socioeconomic status groups usually have low educational attainment. Further, positive correlations between socioeconomic status and the level of visuomotor development have been obtained by Amante *et al.* (1977).

Motor Abilities

Ostrosky *et al.* (1985, 1986) observed that low-education groups appear to have difficulties in performing fine movements, coordinated movements with both hands, carrying out sequences of movements, and reproducing hand positions. Using factor analysis, the author found a "motor factor" that accounted for a significant percentage of the variance between educational groups. Rosselli *et al.* (1990*a*) observed that, in illiterate people, all the praxic ability subtests (buccofacial praxis, ideomotor and ideational praxis, finger alternating movements, meaningless movements, cancellation tests, coordinating movements with both hands, and motor impersistence) were significantly different between educational groups. Cancellation, hand coordinated movements, and performance of buccofacial movement tests were sensitive to age, although age interacted with educational level. Thus, for motor abilities, educational level is a more significant variable than age, and when age differences do appear, they tend to interact with the educational level (Ardila & Rosselli, 1989).

In a similar study, the Trial Making Test–Part B appeared to be affected by education (Finlayson *et al.*, 1977), accounting for about 20% of the variance among the three educational groups studied (> 12, 12–15, >16 years of schooling) (Heaton *et al.*, 1986).

CONCLUSIONS

Cognitive abilities, as measured by neuropsychological tests, are not "natural" abilities unaffected by socioeconomic and educational variables. On the contrary, they represent highly trained skills that are culture- and education-dependent.

Culture makes specific demands on the individual. Some aspects of the surrounding world are particularly relevant. There are things that should be learned and memorized. Padilla (1979) has emphasized that to adapt a test to a culture does not mean simply translating the instrument since it is also necessary to adapt it to the specific demands existing in that culture. For instance, some of the questions included in the WAIS do not seem to be meaningful in the Latin American culture. Neuropsychological tests are not usually so strongly culturally biased as are intelligence tests, but nevertheless cultural background and educational level in particular have a significant influence.

Olmedo (1981) stresses that the evaluation of other cultural groups must take into account: (1) the social, political, and socioeconomic realities facing these groups today: (2) the relevance of educational opportunities to those realities; and (3) the significance of linguistic and cultural factors to both educational opportunities and socioeconomic realities.

Cross-cultural studies have shown that although people belonging to different cultural groups tend to score lower on our routine psychological and neuropsychological tests, this cannot be simply taken to mean that they have lower verbal, memory, perceptual, or motor abilities. This would be a misleading and naive interpretation. Hence, two basic points should be emphasized:

(1) Performance on psychometric tests can represent an unusual, culturally nonrelevant task. Testing situations are completely unusual in other cultural environments or in illiterate people. They just do not understand the reason for being asked apparently silly nonsensical questions such as "Repeat after me: /pa/, /ba/," or "try to assemble a figure with these cubes exactly like this model." They often respond with surprise and embarrassment. Highly educated people in a psychometric-oriented society are much more used to testing situations.

(2) Adaptative abilities are not necessarily equivalent in different cultural groups. Rural children do better in calculating the number of grains or seed in a bowl, but not in recognizing superimposed figures. A "smart" child living in the Amazonian jungle is the one particularly skilled in fishing. In developed societies, it is the one who never fails a subject at school. This only means that we do not possess adequate tests for measuring abilities of every cultural group. Neuropsychologists have been trying to measure people belonging to other cultural groups, with different adaptative demands, using tests developed for

urban, Western, middle-class, literate people. We just do not have good enough tests for evaluating illiterates or for evaluating people belonging to different cultures.

If we compare people with regard to cognitive abilities, those with many years of cognitive training will outperform those with no formal training in them. This only means that cognitive abilities are learned. This should be a basic assumption in neuropsychological assessment. Studies reviewed in this chapter have shown that cultural and educational variables are more important than age as factors in the interpretation of neuropsychological test performance. This is particularly true for verbal abilities. Usually, changes in performing neuropsychological tests across ages are also culture-dependent. Clinical neuropsychological evaluations of other cultural groups have to take into account their specific cultural characteristics. While we develop adequate evaluation instruments and appropriate norms, neuropsychological assessment has to rely more on the understanding of the cultural idiosyncracies and the clinical ability of the examiner than on the raw score obtained from psychometric tests.

REFERENCES

Amante, D., Van Houton, V. W., Grieve, J. H., Bader, C. A., & Margules, P. H. (1977). Neuropsychological deficit, ethnicity, and socioeconomic status. *Journal of Consulting and Clinical Psychology, 45*, 524–535.

Ardila, A., & Rosselli, M. (1988). Sociocultural effects on language abilities. Eighth meeting of the National Academy of Neuropsychologists, Orlando.

Ardila, A., & Rosselli, M. (1989). Neuropsychological characteristics of normal aging. *Developmental Neuropsychology, 5*, 307–320.

Ardila, A., Rosselli, M., & Rosas, P. (1989). Neuropsychological assessment in illiterates: Visuospatial and memory abilities. *Brain and Cognition, 11*, 147–166.

Bartlett, F. C. (1932). *Remembering*. London: Cambridge University Press.

Benton, A. L., Levin, H. H., & Van Allen, W. V. (1974). Geographic orientation in patients with unilateral brain disease. *Neuropsychologia, 12*, 183–191.

Bernstein, B. (1974). Language and roles. In R. Huxley & E. Ingram (Eds.), *Language acquisition: Models and methods*. New York: Academic Press.

Berry J. W. (1971). Ecological and cultural factors in spatial perceptual development. *Canadian Journal of Behavioral Science, 3*, 324–336.

Berry, J. W. (1979). Culture and cognitive style. In A. J. Marsella, R. G. Tharp, & T. J. Ciborowski (Eds.), *Perspectives in cross-cultural psychology* (pp. 117–135). New York: Academic Press.

Bornstein, R. A., & Suga, L. J. (1988). Educational level and neuropsychological performance in healthy elderly subjects. *Developmental Neuropsychology, 4*, 17–22.

Borod, J. C., Goodglass, H., & Kaplan, E. (1980). Normative data on the Boston Diagnostic Aphasia Examination and the Boston Naming Test. *Journal of Clinical Psychology, 2*, 209–215.

Brislin, R. W. (1983). Cross-cultural research in psychology. *Annual Review of Psychology, 34*, 363–400.

Bruner, J., Oliver, R., & Greenfield, P. (1966). *Studies in cognitive growth*. New York: Wiley.

Cameron, R. F., Currier, R. D., & Haerer, A. F. (1971). Aphasia and literacy. *British Journal of Disorders of Communication, 6*, 161–163.

Cole, M., & Scribner, S. (1974). *Culture and thought*. New York: Wiley.

Cole, M., Frankel, F., & Sharp, D. W. (1971). The development of free recall learning in children. *Developmental Psychology, 4*, 109–123.

Cornelius, S. W., & Caspi, A. (1987). Everyday problem solving in adulthood and old age. *Psychology and Aging, 2*, 144–153.

Craik, F. M., Bynd, M., & Swason, J. M. (1987). Patterns of memory loss in three elderly samples. *Psychology and Aging, 2*, 79–86.

Deregowski, J. B. (1980). *Illusions, patterns, and pictures: A cross-cultural perspective*. New York: Academic Press.

Finlayson, M. A., Johnson, K. A., & Reitan, R. M. (1977). Relationship of level of education to neuropsychological measures in brain-damaged and non-brain damaged adults. *Journal of Consulting and Clinical Psychology, 45*, 536–542.

Gay, J., & Cole, M. (1967). *The new mathematics and the old culture*. New York: Holt, Rinehart & Winston.

Geertz, C. (1973). *The interpretation of culture*. New York: Basic Books.

Goldstein, G., & Shelly, C. H. (1972). Statistical and normative studies of the Halstead Neuropsychological Test Battery relevant to neuropsychiatric setting. *Perceptual and Motor Skills, 34*, 603–620.

Goodglass, H., & Kaplan, E. (1972). *Assessment of aphasia and related disorders*. Philadelphia: Lea & Febiger.

Heaton, R. K., Grant, I., & Matthews, C. (1986). Differences in neuropsychological test performance associated with age, education, and sex. In I. Grant & K. M. Adams (Eds.), *Neuropsychological assessment in neuropsychiatric disorders* (pp. 108–120). New York: Oxford University Press.

Hudson, W. (1960). Pictorial depth perception in subcultural groups in Africa. *Journal of Social Psychology, 52*, 183–208.

Jordan, C., & Tharp, R. G. (1979). Culture and education. In A. J. Marsella, R. G. Tharp, & T. J. Ciborowski (Eds.), *Perspectives in cross-cultural psychology* (pp. 265–285). New York: Academic Press.

Klitch, L. Z., & Davidson, R. G. (1983). A cultural difference in visual memory: on le voit, on ne le voit plus. *International Journal of Psychology, 18*, 189–201.

Laboratory of Comparative Human Cognition. (1983). Culture and cognitive development. In P. Mussen (Ed.), *Handbook of child psychology* (Vol. 1, pp. 342–397). New York: Wiley.

Lantz D. (1979). A cross-cultural comparison of communication abilities: Some effects of age, schooling and culture. *International Journal of Psychology, 14*, 171–183.

Laurendeau-Bendavid, M. (1977). Culture, schooling and cognitive development: A comparative study of children in French Canada and Rwanda. In P. R. Dasen (Ed.), *Piagetian psychology: Cross-cultural contributions*. New York: Gardner.

Lecours, A. R., Mehler, J., Parente, M. A., Caldeira, A., Cary, L., Castro, M. J., Dehaout, F., Delgado, R., Gurd, J., Karmann, D., Jakubovitz, R., Osorio, Z., Cabral, L. S., & Junqueira, M. (1987). Illiteracy and brain damage: 1. Aphasia testing in culturally contrasted populations (control subjects). *Neuropsychologia, 25*, 231–245.

Lecours, A. R., Mehler, J., Parente, M. A., Caldeira, A., Cary, L., Castro, M. J., Dehaout, F., Delgado, R., Gurd, J., Karmann, D., Jakubovitz, R., Osorio, Z., Cabral, L. S., & Junqueira, M. (1988). Illiteracy and brain damage 3. A contribution to the study of speech and language disorders in illiterates with unilateral brain damage (initial testing). *Neuropsychologia, 26*, 575–589.

Lezak, M. D. (1983). *Neuropsychological assessment* (2nd ed.). New York: Oxford University Press.

Matarazzo, J. D. (1972). *Wechsler's measurement and appraisal of adult intelligence*. Baltimore: Williams & Wilkins.

Matute, E. (1988). El aprendizaje de la lectoescritura y la especializacion hemisferica para el lenguaje. In A. Ardila & F. Ostrosky (Eds.), *Lenguaje oral y escrito*. Mexico: Trillas.

Mercer, J. R. (1977). Identifying the gifted Chicano children. In J. L. Martinez (Ed.), *The Chicano psychology*. New York: Academic Press.

Modiano, N., Maldonado, L. M., & Villasana, S. (1982). Accurate perception of color illustrations: Rates of comprehension in Mexican Indian children. *Journal of Cross-Cultural Psychology, 13*, 490–495.

Olmedo, E. L. (1981). Testing linguistic minorities. *American Psychologist, 36*, 1078–1085.

Ostrosky, F., Canseco, E., Quintanar, L., Navarro, E., Meneses, S., & Ardila, A. (1985). Sociocultural effects in neuropsychological assessment. *International Journal of Neuroscience, 27*, 53–66.

Ostrosky, F., Quintanar, L., Meneses, S., Canseco, E., Navarro, E., & Ardila, A. (1986). Actividad cognoscitiva y nivel sociocultura. *La Revista de Investigacion Clinica* (Mexico), *38*, 37–42.

Osuji, O. N. (1982). Constructing complex geometric patterns: A study of age and ability among Igbo children of eastern Nigeria. *Journal of Cross-Cultural Psychology*, *13*, 481–499.

Padilla, A. M. (1979). Critical factors in the testing of Hispanic Americans: A review and some suggestions for the future. In R. W. Tyler & S. H. White (Eds.), *Testing, teaching and learning: Report of a conference on testing*. Washington, D.C.: National Institute of Education.

Reitan, R. M. (1956). Investigation of relationships between "psychometric" and "biological" intelligence. *The Journal of Nervous and Mental Disease*, *123*, 536–541.

Robinson, W. P. (1974). Social factors and language development in primary school children. In R. Huxley & E. Ingram (Eds.), *Language acquisition: Models and methods*. New York: Academic Press.

Rosselli, M., Rosselli, A., Vergara, I., & Ardila, A. (1985). Topography of the hemi-inattention syndrome. *International Journal of Neuroscience*, *27*, 165–172.

Rosselli, M., Ardila, A., Florez, A., & Castro, C. (1990*a*). Normative data on the Boston Diagnostic Aphasia Examination in a Spanish-speaking population. *Journal of Clinical and Experimental Neuropsychology*, *12*, 313–322.

Rosselli, M., Ardila, A., & Rosas, P. (1990*b*). Neuropsychological assessment in illiterates II: Language and praxic abilities. *Brain and Cognition*, *12*, 281–296.

Segall, M. H. (1986). Culture and behavior: Psychology in global perspective. *Annual Review of Psychology*, *37*, 523–564.

UNICEF. (1985). *Estado mundial de la infancia*. Mexico: Siglo XXI-UNICEF.

7

Bilingualism

SONIA MANUEL-DUPONT, ALFREDO ARDILA, MONICA ROSSELLI, AND ANTONIO E. PUENTE

Approximately half of the world's population is bilingual or multilingual at some level of proficiency. Despite these numbers, there is little agreement among researchers concerning the cerebral representations and/or functions of multiple languages in any one individual. The reason for this lack of agreement is basically the dearth of systematically collected data available on both normal and brain-damaged multilingual language users (Paradis, 1987).

While several authors have produced excellent reviews of available historical data, theories, and experimental evidence (Albert & Obler, 1978; Vaid & Lambert, 1979; Vaid & Genesee, 1980; Ojemann & Whitaker, 1978; Vaid, 1986; Paradis, 1987, 1989; Solin, 1989; Zatorre, 1989), these overviews have best served as a means of demonstrating conflicting evidence and raising new issues rather than answering basic questions.

The purpose of this chapter will not be to answer these questions but to review arguments suggesting that multilinguals should be treated and tested as a very distinct population from monolinguals and to present some interesting linguistic performance data by Spanish–English-speaking Cuban Americans on Spanish and English versions of the Bilingual Aphasia Test (Paradis, 1987).

Among the many different issues discussed by authors of the previously cited reviews, it is clear that the most important finding is that bilinguals do not form a homogeneous group. They vary along a number of dimensions including:

1. Sociolinguistic background/support for bilingualism
2. Types of bilingualism
3. Degree of proficiency/communicative competence

SONIA MANUEL-DUPONT • Departments of Communicative Disorders and English, Utah State University, Logan, Utah 84322-1000. ALFREDO ARDILA and MONICA ROSSELLI • Instituto Columbiano de Neuropsicologia, Bogotá, Colombia. ANTONIO E. PUENTE • Department of Psychology, University of North Carolina at Wilmington, Wilmington, North Carolina 28403-3297.

HANDBOOK OF NEUROPSYCHOLOGICAL ASSESSMENT: A Biopsychosocial Perspective, edited by Antonio E. Puente and Robert J. McCaffrey. Plenum Press, New York, 1992.

4. Age and sequence of language acquisition
5. Method of acquisition
6. Language-specific factors
7. Anatomical dimensions

THEORETICAL AND NEUROBIOLOGICAL ISSUES

Sociolinguistic Background and Support for Bilingualism

For our purposes, the most critical issue arising from all the studies that have been conducted on bilinguals is understanding not only the location and behavior of the second language in the brain, but also the bilingual speaker's attitude toward second language acquisition and retention in reference to his/her social milieu.

Given the state of affairs for the latter issue, Miller (1984) argues that until recently the academic world has labored under various misconceptions involving bilingualism that have clouded the issue of when, how, and why bilingualism occurs. In particular, he cites linguists and psychologists who have simplistically treated bilinguals as humans with two languages in their brains without attention to the use and function of any one individual's bilingualism.

This oversight reduces the study of bilingualism to one of anatomical properties and functions which ignores the status and function of both languages in the individual's context. The relative status of one language in relation to the other is usually the consequence of complex historical and social interactions which may involve any or all of the following: the community's tie to religious heritage, cultural and political legacies, trade relations or economic trends, and demographic characteristics. In areas where bilingualism is politically and socially encouraged, a different set of learning expectations and individual speaker participation in the learning process will occur relative to areas in which there is active suppression of a language, strict adherence to cultural and social norms and economic constraints placed on bilingual individuals. The speaker who learns two languages in the latter situation will have vastly different needs, motives, and perceptions than the first, some determined by social norms and ideals, while others are determined by individual needs and expectations. In addition to the role of cultural and societal influences on the acquisition of two languages, bilingualism itself is rarely the compartmentalization of one language from the other. Miller (1984) notes that the exchanges between bilinguals are commonly typified by utterances that are not analyzable by reference to one grammar of either language. Rather, the utterances contain features of both languages triggered by individual preference to express concepts in one particular language over another. These preferences can be triggered by topic selection, place of interaction, type of interlocutors, status of in-group/out-group member interchange, and/or the speaker's willingness to comply with or deny the linguistic conventions that would normally operate in the presence of any of these factors. This type of "language-mixing" is called code-switching. As a normal linguistic process, it has been grossly misunderstood by researchers, not the least of whom are those purporting to analyze the linguistic behavior of bilingual aphasic individuals.

Types of Bilingualism

Perhaps the misunderstanding of language-mixing has arisen from the blind application of Weinrich's (1953) early research on the three types of bilingualism. According to Paradis (1978), Weinrich discovered three types of bilingualism in his extensive review of bilingual literature. Type A (coordinate bilingualism) is characterized by separate signs (sound images and meaning units) for each language. This means that this type of bilingual speaker has two sets of meaning units and two sets of corresponding sound images or words (one for each language). Type B (compound bilingualism) is characterized by one unit of meaning with two units of sound images (one for each language). Thus, this type of bilingual speaker draws upon one merged set of meanings from the two languages, but has the capability of expressing himself/herself with the sound images (words) from both languages. The final category, Type C (subordinate bilingualism), is characterized by the meaning unit of the mother tongue with the corresponding sound image in the mother tongue and an equivalent unit of expression in the second language. Like the compound bilingual, the subordinate bilingual has only one set of meaning units and two sets of sound images. Unlike the compound bilingual, the subordinate bilingual draws from only the mother tongue units and has the sound images of the second language as rough translation quasi-equivalents of the mother tongue units.

Given the differing roles of the meaning units and sound images in these three types of bilinguals, Paradis (1977, 1978) notes that only the coordinate bilingual could function as a native speaker of each language, drawing the appropriate sound image from the appropriate meaning unit of each language. The compound bilingual would not function as a native speaker of either language, since his/her units of meaning would represent a merging of content from both languages disallowing for appropriate retrieval from either language's sound images to meaning units. In a similar fashion, despite having native speaker abilities in the mother tongue, the subordinate bilingual would not speak his/her second language like a native speaker as it would be filtered through the meaning units of the mother tongue. While this model provides an analysis of three very different types of bilingual speakers, and is widely accepted by psychologists and neuropsychologists engaging in bilingual research (see Paradis, 1977, 1985; Albert & Obler, 1978; Vaid & Genesee, 1980), most researchers have misinterpreted Weinrich's types as mutually exclusive. Bilingual speakers have been treated as being purely coordinate, compound, or subordinate with no regard for actual language usage. This misinterpretation has caused further misunderstanding as researchers have chosen to lump compound and subordinate bilinguals together thus arriving at a coordinate versus compound (or native speaker-like versus non-native speaker-like) dichotomy.

Degree of Proficiency/Communicative Competence

The important distinctions obscured by this dichotomy include the degree and type of language competence exhibited by each of these kinds of individuals. Canale and Swain (1980) and Canale (1981) have argued that communicative competence is an essential part of actual communication. This competence includes knowledge about the language and other aspects of communication in addition to the skill that underlies actual communication in a systematic and necessary way. Given this interpretation, if a speaker is a "competent" or "proficient" speaker of a language, one must look at not only his/her grammatical knowledge and skills, but also his/her sociolinguistic, discourse, and strategic competencies. These additional competencies include knowing not only when and where to speak but which language or combination of language features (i.e., code-switching) is appropriate for the situation, knowing how to connect a series of utterances to form a meaningful conversation, and being able to compensate for breakdowns in communication. Thus, an understanding of an individual's degree of proficiency in any language must take the sociocultural setting into account as well as the behavior of the individual to judge if the linguistic behavior has adequately met the constraints of the communicative situation.

To further complicate the issue of communicative competence, one must measure the linguistic abilities of bilinguals in relation to the cultural and societal demands of the current environmental situation. As stated earlier, the community in which the multilingual child or adult acquires his/her languages will greatly influence the degree of competence and usage of each language. One such influence will be on the spheres of knowledge a speaker will be required to acquire in each language. It is indeed a rare situation in which one individual is required to express the entire content of his/her knowledge in both languages. A far more common situation is for experiences, ideas, spheres of knowledge, etc. to be language-specific. It is indeed not unusual for a person to learn all work-related jargon, scientific language, or argot in one language but not the other, or to learn the vocabulary of a particular setting or event (i.e., religious prayers, hymns, songs, oaths, etc.) in one language but not another.

Judging degree of language proficiency in a bilingual, therefore, is a much more complicated task than it is in a monolingual. To adequately assess a bilingual's linguistic skills, the examiner must know which languages correlate with which spheres of knowledge and which sociocultural situations. To simply blindly test all spheres of knowledge in both languages is to guarantee that gaps will be produced. Once these gaps are found, it is an extremely difficult and time-consuming task to separate naturally occurring, socially appropriate gaps from deficiencies caused by insult or injury to the brain.

Age and Sequence of Language Acquisition

To separate the naturally occurring gaps from the injury-related gaps, one of the first areas of inquiry should concern the age and sequence of language acquisition of each of the languages. Lamendella (1977) and Whitaker (1978) (as cited in Vaid and Genesee, 1980) have noted that if two languages of a bilingual are acquired successively rather than simultaneously, one might expect some differences in their underlying neural organization insofar as the maturational state of the brain differs during the time of the acquisition of the first language versus the second. They postulate that the effect of these two factors—neurological age and cognitive maturity—should give rise to a pattern of hemispheric involvement more closely resembling that of monolinguals of the same age the earlier the second language is acquired. It will differ from that of monolinguals the later the second language is acquired. These differences, often referred to as simultaneous versus sequential or successive bilingualism (Miller, 1984), have ramifications for the actual language learning process.

Method of Acquisition

It has been postulated by several researchers that the strategies used by language learners in the beginning stages of second language acquisition are more compatible with the linguistic capabilities of the right hemisphere than the left (Galloway, 1979). Vaid and Genesee (1980) note that this argument has been supported by research demonstrating that the early utterances of the second language learners tend to be highly contextualized (Scarcella, 1979), and that speech comprehension relies more on content than on function words, prosodic rather than phonetic features, and pragmatic rather than syntactic information (McLaughlin, 1978). These findings led several researchers to further postulate that right hemisphere processing would be more evident in the initial than final stages of second language acquisition (Krashen & Galloway, 1978; Silverberg, Bentin, Gaziel, Obler, & Albert, 1979).

Vaid and Genesee (1980) have reviewed nearly 20 studies attempting to support this theory using dichotic listening and tachistoscopic procedures. While the majority provide evidence that the left hemisphere is dominant for language functioning, the majority failed to show greater right hemisphere involvement in the earlier stages of second language acquisition. Some studies showed equivalent left hemisphere involvement in the first and second languages of nonproficient bilinguals (Albert & Obler, 1978; Gordon, 1980; Piazza & Zatorre, 1981) while others showed greater left hemisphere participation in the less proficient as compared to the more proficient language (Rogers, TenHouten, Kaplan, & Gardiner, 1977). Vaid and Genesee concluded that there was little evidence that right involvement was more likely in the beginning than in the advanced stages of second language acquisition. Rather they postulated that right hemisphere participation was more likely the later the second language was acquired relative to the first, and the more informal the exposure to the second language.

Krashen (1977) defines informal language learning—language acquisition—as that which is acquired in naturalistic communication settings where the user's attention is directed more to the content than the form of linguistic utterances. Formal language acquisition—language learning—on the other hand, is characterized by emphasis on rule isolation and error correction which makes the learner aware of the language as an abstract, rule-governed system.

Lamendella (1977) proposed that language acquisition and language learning have different neural representations with respect to the involvement of the limbic system. He argued that when a second language is acquired in a natural environment, it is better integrated into the individual's communication hierarchy with greater participation of the limbic structures. When it is learned in a formal setting through rule learning, it is more like any other subject matter than involves mainly neocortical structures.

In discussing limbic system involvement, Paradis (1985) has argued that while the limbic system is involved in the learning process in several critical ways from establishment of neurofunctional mechanisms to attain automatic fluent production of speech to the provision of empathy and integrative attitudes, this involvement will vary with the age of the learner, the degree of emotional involvement of the learner, the motivation to learn the second language, and the relative prestige of the two languages in addition to the learning situation—informal versus formal.

Given these different learning experiences, Vaid and Genesee (1980) proposed a model to best account for the relationship between age, stage and manner of acquisition, and the participation of each hemisphere in the learning process. They proposed that the right hemisphere involvement will be more likely the later the second language is learned relative to the first, the more informal the exposure to the second language, and possibly the earlier the stage of language acquisition. In contrast, left hemisphere involvement will be more likely the earlier the second language is learned relative to the first, the more formal the exposure to the second language, and the more advanced the stage of acquisition. In addition, the more similar the conditions of the first and second language acquisition, the greater is the likelihood that bilinguals will show comparable patterns of hemispheric involvement in processing their two languages. Conversely, the less similar the conditions of language acquisition, the greater is the likelihood of dissimilar patterns of hemisphere involvement.

Language-Specific Factors

While the model of Vaid and Genesee accounts for many different variations in the language learning/acquiring process, there is yet another factor that may affect hemisphere involvement. Vaid and Genesee (1980) argue that different languages may require different perceptual/cognitive processes which may depend on intra- or interhemispherically distinct cortical systems. The areas of language-specific factors they address include differences in language-related thought patterns, visual field preferences, characteristics of vowels, tonality, and direction of script.

Several researchers have suggested that languages that elicit appositional versus propositional modes of thinking should yield differential patterns of hemisphere involvement (Hynd & Scott, 1980). However, EEG alpha wave activity testing and dichotic listening tests have not consistently demonstrated this difference (see Vaid and Genesee, 1980, for a review). Further, there are many problems associated with the theoretical assumptions that languages differ in the degree to which they serve as instruments for appositional versus propositional thought. Visual field asymmetries in the processing of verbal material have been subject to several interpretations (Vaid and Genesee, 1980). The two areas that have received the most attention include a cerebral laterality effect and a scanning effect that accounts for visual field preferences in terms of directional postexposural scanning mechanisms that develop from reading habits (Heron, 1957). Most experimental studies involve tachistoscopic measurements comparing left-to-right versus right-to-left visual modalities. Some studies have indicated the presence of a scanning effect (LVF preference under unilateral presentation for languages read from right to left), while others have demonstrated an overriding cerebral laterality effect (RVF superiority) especially under conditions where the scanning effects are minimized, as when words are presented vertically for shorter exposure durations or with a central fixation control. In addition, it has been suggested that proficiency and order of language learning may reinforce certain scanning effects (Vaid and Genesee, 1980).

For the third factor it has been proposed by a number of researchers that vowels of different languages will be processed in different hemispheres. Tsunoda (1971) has suggested that this difference is due to the fact that listeners will perceive vowels more analytically in languages in which they often form meaningful words as compared to languages in which consonants are more salient. The former rely more on left hemisphere processing. The outcome of several experiments testing this theory are equivocable.

A fourth factor has been postulated suggesting that when tonal changes carry changes in meaning, tones will be processed more efficiently in the left hemisphere. There is supporting evidence from Thai–English studies (Van Lancker & Fromkin, 1978), Chinese–English studies (Naeser & Chan, 1980), and Vietnamese–French studies (Hecaen, Mazars, Rannier, Goldblum, & Merienne, 1971). But Benson, Smith, and Arreaga (1974) indicate that the difference merges only when the tones are presented in a linguistic context.

For the fifth factor, the sound–symbol correspondence of different writing systems has been tested in bilingual aphasics to determine if site of lesion has a greater effect on phonetic or ideographic orthographies. It was found that lesions in the temporal cortex have been associated with greater impairment of reading and/or writing of scripts that are phonetically based (de Agostini, 1977; Hinshelwood, 1902; Luria, 1960; Peuser & Leischner, 1980; Sasanuma & Fujimura, 1971) while lesions in the posterior occipito-parietal cortical areas have been associated with greater impairment in reading and/or writing of scripts with an ideographic or irregular phonetic basis (Lyman, Kwan & Chao, 1938; Newcombe in Critchley, 1974; Sasanuma, 1975).

Anatomical Dimensions

Specifically involved in the discussions of these dimensions is the question of where the second language is found in the bilingual's brain. Paradis (1985, p. 12) offers the following summary of possible sites for the second language (L2) of a bilingual:

1. L2 is in the right hemisphere.
2. L2 is represented bilaterally.
3. L2 is less lateralized than the first language (L1), and although both are subserved by the left hemisphere, there is relatively greater participation of the right hemisphere for L2.
4. Both languages are less lateralized.
5. Both languages are equally lateralized to the left and there is no difference between bilinguals and monolinguals.

The first option is closely tied to the language-specific effect hypothesis, which argues that structures of certain languages lend themselves to more right hemisphere participation than other languages. The second hypothesis is tied to the age hypothesis, which argues that languages acquired after a particular point in time will involve more right hemisphere participation than languages acquired earlier. The third alternative involves the second language hypothesis, which states that a second language acquired after a first has been learned will find more right hemisphere participation than the first did. The fourth possibility involves the stage hypothesis, which argues that the right hemisphere will be more involved in the language acquisition process in the beginning stages than in the end. Finally, the fifth option involves the bilingual type hypothesis according to which coordinate bilinguals keep their two languages separate, and store them in different ways, with a greater involvement of the right hemisphere for one of the languages.

Paradis notes that within these five theories are direct contradictions. The stage hypothesis predicts that as the second language becomes more nativelike, it will gradually shift to the left hemisphere, while the bilingual type hypothesis predicts that the more nativelike the two languages are, the more separate they are to be kept, thus the greater the possibility of right hemisphere participation for the second language.

While there have been numerous proponents and opponents of each of these theories, most agree that these models are too simplistic to answer neuroanatomical questions. In addition, Paradis (1987) notes that available data support neither theories postulating that multiple languages have completely separate neurophysiological representations nor ones postulating completely merged representations. In attempting to account for the available data (1987, p. 9), he argues convincingly that "bilinguals have two subsets of neural connections, one for each language . . . while at the same time they possess one larger set from which they are able to draw elements of either language at any time." This hypothesis successfully accounts for data that indicate that some elements of both languages are undifferentiated in their representation while others, because they normally occur in mutually exclusive environmental contexts, are stored separately and subserved by a different network of neural connectors. This theory again supports the argument that each individual bilingual speaker will have a neuroanatomical configuration for language that best represents his/her sociocultural speaking environments as well as his/her linguistic and educational past experiences.

At this point, it is tempting to postulate that since no two individuals will have identical linguistic and educational experiences nor identical sociocultural environments, attempts to determine language characteristics of a specific group of multilingual speakers would be futile. To determine if it would be possible to find shared language characteristics among a group of bilingual speakers, Spanish and English versions of the Bilingual Aphasia Test (BAT) were given to a small group of bilingual (Paradis & Ardila, 1989*a*,*b*) Cuban-Americans residing in Miami, Florida.

SPANISH–ENGLISH BILINGUAL APHASIA TEST RESULTS

As Paradis (1987) and others have noted, the single greatest hindrance to understanding the neuroanatomical constructs of multiple languages in an individual is the dearth of systematically collected data on both normal and brain-damaged individuals. To this end the BAT (Paradis, 1989) was chosen as an instrument to describe the linguistic performance of a group of non-brain-damaged Spanish–English bilinguals.

The BAT (Paradis, 1987, p. 19) was designed to cover in a nonexhaustive manner a number of language structures (phonemic, phonological, morphological, syntactic, lexical, semantic) and some language usage characteristics (comprehension, repetition, judgment, propositionizing, reading, and writing) in most modalities (auditory, visual, oral, and digitomanual) with the word, sentence, and paragraph as units of analysis. The BAT is a test of language performance that excludes nonlinguistic means of communication and language-mixing as communicative strategies. The Spanish and English versions of the BAT have been administered to other non-brain-damaged controls "to ensure that every fluent speaker of each language met criterion on each section" (Paradis, 1987, p. 43).

There are three sections on the BAT. Part A contains 50 questions on the history of bilingualism. Part B is a test of a specific language with sections on spontaneous speech, verbal comprehension, pointing, commands, verbal auditory discrimination, syntactic comprehension, semantic categories, synonyms, antonyms, grammaticality judgment, semantic acceptability, repetition, series, verbal fluency, naming, sentence construction, semantic opposites, derivational morphology, morphological opposites, description, mental arithmetic, listening comprehension, reading words aloud, reading sentences aloud, reading a paragraph for comprehension, copying, dictation, reading comprehension for words and sentences, and spontaneous writing.

A special section, Part C, evaluates the ability to translate and the recognition of grammaticality errors resulting from grammar interference between both languages. This section requires the subject to recognize words, translate words and sentences, and make grammaticality judgments.

This particular test was chosen because of its breadth and depth of evaluation procedures. The purpose of using this test was to probe the linguistic characteristics of normal Cuban-American Spanish–English bilinguals.

Sociocultural Background

While Cuban immigration to the United States dates back to the 19th century, the most recent immigrant waves in the early 1960s and 1980s have had the strongest influence on southern Florida communities in Dade County (Diaz, 1983). The Cuban wars of independence from 1868 to 1895 fostered the first waves of immigrants who settled mainly in the Tampa and Key West areas. These immigrants established the tobacco industry in southern Florida, eventually constituting a significant portion of the labor force. After the wars of independence, scores of other immigrants moved to the United States for better economic opportunities. Due to the proximity of Florida to Cuba, many of these immigrants traveled back and forth bringing knowledge of American technology to Cuba while providing a strong link with Cuban religious, political and linguistic institutions for Cubans living in the United States.

With the establishment of the Castro regime in the 1960s another wave of skilled, professional white-collar workers left Cuba. These immigrants represented a largely educated, middle-class group accustomed to an urban-professional standard of living. However, by the late 1960s and early 1970s a larger group of students, children, housewives, and older persons from lower socioeconomic strata were being airlifted into the United States (Diaz, 1983). These groups were not as accustomed to an urban life-style and often had few transferable job skills. Finally the last large wave of immigration occurred in the summer of 1980 when 125,000 Cubans immigrated to the United States by private and chartered boat (Diaz, 1983). This last group was largely male, with a median age in the low 30s and with lower educational and skill levels than previous immigrants had had. This last group of immigrants spoke little or no English and had little familiarity with the American way of life.

As a result of these different waves of immigration in the 1990s we find that the current generation of Cuban-Americans, born in the United States, account for almost 20% of the Cuban community (Diaz, 1983) and that one in every five Cubans has attended an American school. Despite this exposure to the U.S.

educational system and the use of English as the medium of instruction, it is still the case that Cubans overwhelmingly prefer to speak Spanish at home. While English language usage is found in the work force, at school, and with print and electronic media, even many Cuban college graduates choose to speak Spanish over English in many social situations. This Spanish language usage does not appear to be fostered through formal instruction—over 80% of Cuban children attend the Dade public school system. It is nourished through the Spanish media and a "ghetto economy" system of stores and businesses, owned and operated by Cubans, which precludes the use of English (Diaz, 1983).

While Cubans can be found at every socioeconomic level and in every profession, the largest populations are found in Miami, Sweetwater, and Hialeah and there is a dearth of Cuban professionals in many white-collar professions, particularly education.

Recent surveys in the Cuban communities of Dade County show that learning English ranks among the most important needs felt by this group (Diaz, 1983). At the same time, many Cubans maintain strong cultural (and linguistic) ties with their native homeland because the large, strong Cuban communities in the United States make them feel "at home" in Dade County but not in other American communities. In addition, many feel that their immigration is only temporary and that they will eventually return to Cuba.

Linguistically, one finds that many Cuban children are taught to read and write in Spanish before attending English-medium schools. Technical subjects such as science, math, and literature are generally known in English but not Spanish. Despite this technical knowledge in English, many children experience some word finding difficulties, and difficulties exist with the use and understanding of complex syntax. Code-switching and borrowing phenomena are evident. Some examples include:

- I think *que de todas maneras voy a enviar la* letter
- When I was testing the patient, *comenzo a protestar*
- *Muchos libros en la* library *estan* reserved
- Yard →/jarda/
- Gang → /ganga/
- Key West → /kajo weso/

Interestingly, the Spanish-speaking second generation often uses English as a base language when speaking among themselves. This may be due to two reasons: they know English better than Spanish (Spanish is only spoken in the home), and they have a stronger identification with the Anglo culture than with the Hispanic culture. As such, language often becomes a source of family conflict. Sometimes, parents are forced to speak English with their children or they may force their children to speak Spanish to them. Sometimes schoolchildren use English to confuse parents and grandparents, making family communication a difficult task.

Because of this interesting mixture of English and Spanish linguistic and cultural traditions in this group, it was felt that this group would make an excellent test group to determine language usage patterns in a bilingual population.

Method

Subjects

A sample of 14 subjects (7 males, 7 females) was selected. All of them were born in Cuba, and arrived in the United States during early childhood as native Spanish speakers. They began using English when they started school (average age 4.8; S.D. 0.77; range 4–5), but they continued using Spanish at home. At the time of testing the average age was 25.46 (S.D. 5.3; range 17–35). All of the subjects were students or professionals with an average educational level of 14.5 (S.D. 2.65; range 11–19) and without any history of neurological or psychiatric pathology.

Procedure

The BAT English version (Paradis, Hummel, & Libben, 1988), Spanish version (Paradis & Ardila, 1989*a*), and English/Spanish bilingualism section (Paradis & Ardila, 1989*b*) were given individually to each subject in two sessions. The order of evaluation (English–Spanish, or Spanish–English) was balanced. All of the subjects were nonpaid volunteers, and were informed about the purpose of the testing.

Research Question

Since the BAT has been designed to allow all non-brain-damaged subjects to reach criterion on most subtests, it was assumed that this group of subjects would not perform significantly differently on the English versus the Spanish version of this test.

Results

Table 7.1 shows the means and standard deviations for each subsection of the Spanish and English versions of the BAT. As can be seen, there were few statistically significant results between the languages. The few significant differences included sentence construction, number of words, morphological opposites, and reading.

In another measure, it is interesting to note that in the Spanish version of the test the mean scores for these subjects were below the error range expected for normal subjects for repetition, series, semantic opposites, derivational morphology, mental arithmetic, and dictation. In the English version, scores were lower than the expected error range for derivational morphology and morphological opposites.

TABLE 7.1. Means and Standard Deviations Found for the Different Subtests of the BAT for Spanish and English[a]

		Spanish		English			
Section	Max.	Mean	S.D.	Mean	S.D.	t	p
Pointing	(10)	10.00	0.00	0.00	0.00	—	—
Commands	(30)	29.35	1.64	30.00	0.00	1.44	NS
Auditory Disc	(18)	17.64	0.84	17.89	0.83	−1.00	NS
Syntactic Com	(87)	85.00	1.41	85.14	1.40	0.33	NS
Semant Cat	(5)	5.00	0.00	4.93	0.27	−1.00	NS
Synonyms	(5)	4.57	0.94	4.85	0.36	1.00	NS
Antonyms	(10)	9.21	0.89	9.42	0.75	0.90	NS
Gram Judgm	(10)	9.93	0.76	9.79	0.42	−1.00	NS
Sem Accept	(10)	9.64	0.63	9.71	0.82	0.32	NS
Repetition	(67)	64.85*	1.75	65.21	1.76	0.47	NS
Series	(3)	2.78*	0.42	3.00	0.00	1.88	NS
Fluency		24.00	7.28	28.26	7.77	1.54	NS
Naming	(20)	20.00	0.00	20.00	0.00	—	—
Sentence Const	(15)	14.14	0.77	14.79	0.58	−2.39	0.03
Number Words		58.14	3.03	48.86	2.41	3.51	0.004
Semantic Oppos	(10)	8.78*	0.89	9.36	0.93	1.66	NS
Deriv Morphol	(10)	7.14*	1.70	7.71*	1.49	1.00	NS
Morphol Oppos	(10)	8.43	1.40	7.43*	1.70	2.46	0.03
Ment Arithmet	(15)	12.93*	1.90	13.21	1.58	−1.17	NS
List Compreh	(5)	4.64	0.50	4.57	0.94	−0.23	NS
Reading	(26)	24.40	1.55	25.43	0.65	2.01	0.06
Copying	(5)	5.00	0.00	5.00	0.00	—	—
Dictation	(10)	8.85*	2.03	9.71	0.46	1.46	NS
Read Comp	(20)	19.42	0.93	19.21	1.31	−1.15	NS

[a]Maximum score for each subtest is shown in parentheses. t-test values and level of significance of the differences are also shown.
*The mean error is below the error range for normal subjects.

In the spontaneous writing portion (Part B) of both versions of the BAT, patterns such as number of words, number of errors, and types of errors were measured. The mean number of words used in the written description in Spanish was 64.35 (S.D. 24.12; range 25–104); in English, 93.00 (S.D. 30.49; range 52–168). The average number of errors in Spanish was 4.78 (S.D. 3.64; range 0–15); in English, 0.64 (S.D. 1.1; range 0–4). All of the writing errors in English were substitution spelling errors. In Spanish, besides orthographic errors, additions, omissions, and substitutions were frequently found (errors in accent marks were not considered).

In the Spanish writing sample, 10 of the 14 subjects demonstrated problems with number agreement between articles, nouns, adjectives, and verbs. The BAT labels these errors paragrammatisms. Borrowing from English was clearly evident in the alphabetic renderings of some words (e.g., telefono → telephono; diferente → differente).

Organizational patterns in the Spanish texts often showed some influence from English with numerous paragrammatical errors:

> *Hoy es un dia bonito* (n → n) *para trabaja* (trabajar). *A mi me gusto* (gusta) *medicina mucho* (word-order error) *porque puedo ayudar a los enfermo* ("s" omission; concordance error). *Como hoy esta el dia feo, es en* (un) *dia bueno para estar aqui en el trabajo. Medicina* (article omission) *te deja ayudar a los que necessita* (necesitan) *ayudar* (ayuda) (the whole sentence is agrammatical). *Como enfermero tu puedar* (puedes) *asuer* (hacer) *muchas cosas differente* (diferentes).

It is interesting to note that there were no instances of Spanish language interference in the English tests and few instances of paragrammatism in the English texts.

On Part C of the BAT, the translation portion of the exam, mean errors in translation from English to Spanish (5%) and Spanish to English (6%) were nearly equivalent. There were no significant differences between scores on word recognition, translation of words, and translation of sentences for the two versions of this test.

There were significant differences, however, between scores for grammaticality judgments for the two versions. On the Spanish-to-English test the mean score was 11.46 (S.D. 1.39) and on the English-to-Spanish test, 14.54 (S.D. 1.85) (see Table 7.2).

Discussion

On the three sections of tests given to these subjects, the BAT English version, the BAT Spanish version, and the Spanish/English bilingualism test, it is clear that these Cuban-American bilinguals offer a unique linguistic performance pattern. They do not use their two languages as "ideal or perfectly balanced" bilinguals (Bloomfield, 1953). Instead they demonstrate strengths and weaknesses directly tied to their linguistic and educational heritages.

In answer to the research question, these subjects do perform significantly differently in some areas of linguistic skills.

They have poorer performance in Spanish sentence construction, number of words, morphological opposites, and reading because they have learned

TABLE 7.2. Spanish/English Bilingualism[a]

		Spanish-to-English		English-to-Spanish			
Section	Max.	Mean	S.D.	Mean	S.D.	t	p
Word recogn	(5)	4.93	0.26	4.93	0.26	0.00	NS
Trans words	(10)	9.31	1.03	9.38	0.96	0.23	NS
Trans sent	(18)	16.92	1.44	17.15	1.40	0.79	NS
Gram judgm	(16)	11.46	1.39	14.54	1.85	5.18	0.001

[a]Spanish-to-English and English-to-Spanish translation in the first three sections, and grammaticality judgments in the fourth section.

primary literary skills in English in school. This is also reflected in the fewer words, more errors, and the strong English influence on spelling seen in the Spanish writing sample. Other academically related language skills that were weaker in Spanish included repetition, series, semantic opposites, mental arithmetic, and dictation. All of these areas may be partially described as pertaining more readily to the English-dominated world of academic study than the Spanish-dominated world of home and family communications.

The possible influence of academic training in English is also seen in results for Part C, the translation section of the exam. While subjects showed virtually equivalent abilities in isolated translating tasks, there were significant differences in their abilities to judge grammaticality in English and Spanish.

Again it is not surprising that these bilinguals would demonstrate fewer problems judging English grammaticality errors than Spanish. These judgments are very academically oriented exercises that would have been learned and practiced in an English-dominated academic content. These bilinguals would have developed a greater "sphere of knowledge" and greater linguistic analytical skills in the language in which these skills were learned—English at school. This trend is also seen in the spontaneous writing sample (Part B of the BAT) where subjects who are more accustomed to formal writing tasks in English exhibit typical patterns (paragrammatisms) found in written language samples of primarily oral language users.

Since these subjects are more accustomed to speaking in both languages but writing formally only in English, more oral language patterns are found in Spanish writing samples. These patterns include concordance errors, spelling words phonetically as they sound, incorrect tense and aspect designations on verbs, and other inflectional errors. Overall, these bilingual subjects do not demonstrate equivalent linguistic skills in both languages in all areas of language aptitude and production.

SUMMARY

Today we live in a world where half of the population is bilingual or multilingual. While we have formally recognized that bilingualism exists, we continue to struggle to understand how bilinguals use and store their languages. Research from many sources points very conclusively to the fact that bilinguals can be considered neither to be like monolinguals nor to form a homogeneous group themselves. To fully understand the linguistic capacity and performance of any bilingual speaker, it is necessary to collect extensive information on that person's sociolinguistic background, his or her educational experiences, the methods of language acquisition, and the opportunities for usage of each language.

In the actual assessment process it is critical that the subject be tested in all applicable languages with instruments that are linguistically functionally equivalent, not mere translations of each other.

With the Cuban-American bilingual data collected in this study, it is clear that this small test group did not perform as was predicted by error norms on either the Spanish or English version of the BAT. Certain sociocultural constraints and academic training in English left these individuals with distinct strengths and weaknesses in each language that should be considered normal for this group of bilingual speakers.

What this finding suggests is a need to collect baseline data on large populations of normal bilingual speakers to establish basic trends in language usage for each group of speakers. It is not enough to norm a Spanish version of the BAT on one group of (e.g., Mexican-American) bilingual speakers. These trends may not be applicable to other Spanish–English bilingual groups.

Until we can work together as Paradis (1987) has suggested to *systematically* collect and analyze speakers, we will continue to struggle in our understanding of their language use and capacities.

Summary Highlights

1. Multilinguals do not demonstrate the same linguistic performance patterns as monolinguals.
2. Multilinguals do not form a homogeneous group themselves. While certain linguistic parameters may be shared by groups of multilingual speakers, each individual will have language usage patterns and preferences that will diverge from the group.
3. The degree of functional independence between the languages of a multilingual is dependent on the social constraints of language usage, the socioeconomic status and setting of the linguistic interchange, the educational methodology and level of attainment of the speaker, the age of the speaker when learning each language, the sequence of acquisition, the structure of each language, and the attitude of the speaker toward each language and its usage.
4. Multilinguals must be tested in each of their languages with instruments that are linguistically equivalent.
5. Each cultural/ethnic/social group of multilingual speakers is more likely to have a different pattern of strengths and weaknesses in each of their languages than a similar cultural/ethnic/social group. Language usage patterns should be determined for each group.
6. The home environment will produce language usage patterns that are different from academic environments. Language tests that require academic analytical skills will favor the languages most often used in academic settings.

ACKNOWLEDGMENTS. We express our gratitude to Jesus Abilio Rodriguez for his support in collecting the data of this research, and to Dr. Michel Paradis for his encouragement, support, and very valuable suggestions in manuscript preparation.

REFERENCES

Albert, M. L., & Obler, L. K. (1978). *The bilingual brain*. New York: Academic Press.
Benson, P., Smith, T., & Arreaga, L. (1974). Lateralization of linguistic tone—Evidence from Cantonese. *Bis Report*, Los Angeles: UCLA, pp. 19–20.
Bloomfield, L. (1953). *Language*. New York: Holt, Rinehart, & Winston.
Canale, M. (1981). From communicative competence to communicative language pedagogy. In J. C. Richards & R. Schmidt (Eds.), *Language and communication*. Clevedon, Avon, England: Multilingual Matters (pp. 1–47).
Canale, M., & Swain, M. (1980). Theoretical bases of communicative approaches to second language teaching and testing. *Applied Linguistics*, *1*(1), 1–47.
Critchley, M. (1974). Aphasia in polyglots and bilinguals. *Brain and Language*, *1*, 15–27.
de Agostini, M. (1977). A propos de l'agraphie des aphasiques sensoriels: Etude comparative Italien-Français. *Languages*, *47*, 120–130.
Diaz, G. (1983). Dade Cuban immigrants: Integration patterns and special education needs. In R. Samuda & S. Woods (Eds.), *Perspectives in immigrant and minority education* (pp. 128–136). Washington, D.C.: University Press of America.
Galloway, L. (1979). The cerebral organization of language in bilinguals and second language learners: Clinical and experimental evidence. Unpublished doctoral dissertation, UCLA.
Gordon, H. W. (1980). Cerebral organization in bilinguals. *Brain and Language*, *9*, 255–268.
Hecaen, H., Mazars, G., Rannier, A., Goldblum, M., & Merienne, L. (1971). Aphasie croissee chez un sujet droitier bilingue (Vietnamien-français). *Revue Neurologique*, *124*, 319–323.
Heron, W. (1957). Perception as a function of retinal locus and attention. *American Journal of Psychology*, *70*, 38–48.
Hinshelwood, J. (1902). Four cases of word blindness. *Lancet*, *1*, 358–363.
Hynd, G., & Scott, S. (1980). Propositional and appositional modes of thought and differential cerebral speech lateralization in Navajo Indian and Anglo children. *Child Development*, *51*, 909–911.
Krashen, S. (1977). The monitor model for adult second language performance. In M. Burt, H. Dulay, & M. Finocchiaro (Eds.), *Viewpoints on English as a second language* (pp. 6–47). New York: Regents.
Krashen, S., & Galloway, L. (1978). The neurological correlates of language acquisition: Current research. *SPEAQ Journal*, *2*, 21–35.
Lamendella, J. (1977). General principles of neurofunctional organization and their manifestations in primary and nonprimary language acquisition. *Language Learning*, *27*, 155–196.
Lurai, A. (1960). Differences between disturbance of speech and writing in Russian and in French. *International Journal of Slavic Linguistic Poetics*, *3*, 13–22.
Lyman, R., Kwan, S., & Chao, W. (1938). Left-occipital-parietal brain tumor with observations on alexia and agraphia in Chinese and English. *Chinese Medical Journal*, *54*, 491–516.
McLaughlin, B. (1978). *Second language acquisition in childhood*. Hillsdale, N.J.: Erlbaum.
Miller, N. (1984). *Bilingualism and language disability*. San Diego: College-Hill Press.
Naeser, M., & Chan, S. (1980). Case study of a Chinese aphasic with the Boston Diagnostic Aphasia Exam. *Neuropsychologia*, *18*, 389–410.
Ojemann, G. A., & Whitaker, H. A., (1978). The bilingual brain. *Archives of Neurology*, *35*, 409–412.
Paradis, M. (1977). Bilingualism and aphasia. In H. A. Whitaker & H. Whitaker (Eds.), *Studies in Neurolinguistics*, *3* (pp. 65–121). New York: Academic Press.
Paradis, M. (Ed.). (1978). *Aspects of bilingualism*. Columbia, S.C.: Hornbeam Press.
Paradis, M. (1985). On the representation of two languages in one brain. *Language Sciences*, *7*(1), 1–39.
Paradis, M. (1987). *The assessment of bilingual aphasia*. Hillsdale, N.J.: Erlbaum.
Paradis, M. (1989). Bilingual and polyglot aphasia. In F. Boller & J. Grafman (Eds.), *Handbook of neuropsychology* (Vol. 2, pp. 117–140). Amsterdam: Elsevier.
Paradis, M. (1989). La lateralizacion cerebral diferencial en los bilingues: Basta, por favor! *Invesigaciones Psicologicas*, *7*, 95–106.

Paradis, M., & Ardila, A. (1989*a*). *Prueba de afasia para bilingues*. Hillsdale, N.J.: Erlbaum.
Paradis, M., & Ardila, A. (1989*b*). *Bilingual aphasia test. Part C. Bilinguismo Espanol/Ingles*. Hillsdale, N.J.: Erlbaum.
Paradis, M., Hummel, K., & Libben, G. (1988). *The bilingual aphasia test (English version)*. Hillsdale, N.J.: Erlbaum.
Peuser, G., & Leischner, A. (1980). Impairments of phonetic script in an aphasic. In M. Paradis (Ed.), *Readings on aphasia in bilinguals and polyglots*. Montreal: Didier.
Piazza, D., & Zatorre, R. (1981). Right ear advantage for dichotic listening in bilingual children. Unpublished manuscript, Brown University.
Rogers, L., TenHouten, W., Kaplan, C., & Gardiner, M. (1977). Hemispheric specialization of language: An EEG study of bilingual Hopi children. *International Journal of Neurological Sciences, 8*, 1–6.
Sasanuma, S. (1975). Kana and Kanji processing in Japanese aphasics. *Brain and Language, 2* 369–383.
Sasanuma, S., & Fujimura, O. (1971). Selective impairment of phonetic and nonphonetic transcription of words in Japanese aphasic patients: Kana vs. Kanji in visual recognition and writing. *Cortex, 7*, 1–18.
Scarcella, R. (1979). "Watch Up!" A study of verbal routines in adult second language performance. *Working Papers in Bilingualism, 19*, 79–88.
Silverberg, R., Bentin, S., Gaziel, T., Obler, L., & Albert, M. (1979). Shift of visual field preference for English words in native Hebrew speakers. *Brain and Language, 8*, 184–190.
Solin, D. (1989). The systematic misrepresentation of bilingual crossed aphasia data and its consequences. *Brain and Language, 36*, 92–116.
Tsunoda, T. (1971). The difference of the cerebral dominance of vowel sounds among different languages. *Journal of Auditory Research, 11*, 305–314.
Vaid, J. (Ed.). (1986). *Language processing in bilinguals: Psycholinguistic and neuropsychological perspective*. Hillsdale, N.J.: Erlbaum.
Vaid, J., & Genesee F. (1980). Neuropsychological approaches to bilingualism: A critical review. *Canadian Journal of Psychology, 34*, 417–445.
Vaid, J., & Lambert, W. (1979). Differential cerebral involvement in the cognitive functioning of bilinguals. *Brain and Language, 8*, 92–110.
Van Lancker, D., & Fromkin, V. (1978). Cerebral dominance for pitch contrasts in tone language speakers in musically untrained and trained English speakers. *Journal of Phonetics, 6*, 19–23.
Weinrich, U. (1953). *Languages in contact*. New York: New York Linguistics Circle.
Whitaker, H. A. (1978). Bilingualism: A neurolinguistics perspective. In W. C. Ritchie (Ed.), *Second language acquisition and research: Issues and implications* (pp. 21–32). New York: Academic Press.
Zatorre, R. J. (1989). On the representation of multiple languages in the brain: Old problems and new directions. *Brain and Language, 36*, 127–147.

II

Psychopathological Factors

Introduction

Part II examines various psychopathological factors as they are likely to impact on both basic research and also on the interpretation of neuropsychological assessment profiles in clinical settings. To date, there have been three major psychopathological disorders that have been evaluated extensively from a neuropsychological perspective; these include the anxiety, depressive, and schizophrenic disorders. In part, this reflects the strong biological basis associated with each of these disorders as well as the acceptance of biological etiologies and treatment for them. Moreover, clinical neuropsychology is in a unique position to contribute to the examination of these various conditions from an interdisciplinary perspective encompassing both biological and behavioral variables.

The chapter on anxiety disorders by Orsillo and McCaffrey provides an extensive review of the neurological, neuroimaging, and neuropsychological literature associated with various anxiety-based disorders. Additionally, serious methodological limitations on the part of investigators in this area are highlighted. The chapter on depressive disorders by Newman and Sweet provides an in-depth evaluation of the potential confounds in neuropsychological interpretation secondary to underlying depressive disorders. Finally, the chapter on schizophrenic disorders by Walker *et al.* provides an up-to-date review of the literature with a discussion of important hypotheses that remain to be evaluated.

In addition to addressing the major types of psychopathology, this section also focuses on pseudoneurological and somatic disorders as well as the detection of deception and malingering. The chapter by Horton provides an overview of the role of neuropsychology in the differential diagnosis of pseudoneurological disorders from actual neurological disorders and also reviews the literature on psychosomatic disorders. The issues of deliberate deception and the detection of malingering are reviewed by Binder. These two chapters are useful in terms not only of routine clinical neuropsychological assessment but also of forensic neuropsychology.

8

Anxiety Disorders

SUSAN M. ORSILLO and ROBERT J. McCAFFREY

INTRODUCTION

Anxiety disorders are far more prevalent than any other mental health disorder in the United States, including depression and substance abuse (Barlow, 1988). Despite this fact, neuropsychological investigations of anxiety-based disorders in humans are only beginning to be undertaken. This reflects, in part, the changing conceptualization of the nature of anxiety disorders and the ongoing efforts to refine further their diagnostic classification system (viz., *Diagnostic and Statistical Manual of Mental Disorders–IV*). The absence of a unified conceptual framework and the ongoing development of a diagnostic classification system have imposed serious limitations on an examination of the human neuropsychological aspects of the anxiety disorders.

The inclusion of a chapter focusing on anxiety and its disorders in the present text was based on two major factors. Given that anxiety-based disorders are the most prevalent of the mental health disorders, practitioners may be faced with the task of partialing out the neuropsychological effects due to either known or presumed CNS dysfunction from those that are present due to an anxiety disorder. The other major consideration was that the research in this area reflects the use of multifaceted neuropsychological assessment techniques and state-of-the-art technology. In this regard, research into the neuropsychology of anxiety-based disorders may serve as a model for the evaluation of other mental health disorders.

Throughout this discussion, the reader should keep several points in mind. First, conflicting findings may reflect methodological differences between studies. In contrast, ongoing changes in both the conceptualization and diagnosis of the anxiety disorders also serve as a significant source of variance. This

---

SUSAN M. ORSILLO and ROBERT J. McCAFFREY • Department of Psychology, The University at Albany, State University of New York, Albany, New York 12222.

HANDBOOK OF NEUROPSYCHOLOGICAL ASSESSMENT: A Biopsychosocial Perspective, edited by Antonio E. Puente and Robert J. McCaffrey. Plenum Press, New York, 1992.

is especially important given the revisions of the *Diagnostic and Statistical Manual of Mental Disorders* (American Psychiatric Association, 1952, 1968, 1980, 1987) and the impending release of DSM-IV in 1992.

The primary focus of this chapter will be on the neuropsychological correlates of the anxiety disorders as they are outlined in the DSM-III-R (American Psychiatric Association, 1987). Nonclinical forms of anxiety and anxiety stemming from trauma to the central nervous system will also be reviewed. Before discussing the state-of-the-art techniques that have been used to assess anxiety disorders as they are presently classified, however, it is important to review the historical bases for studying anxiety. The next section includes a review of the major contributions to this area from a biological and theoretical perspective.

HISTORICAL OVERVIEW OF THE BIOLOGICAL BASES OF ANXIETY

Many studies have been directed at discovering the neuronal mechanisms of anxiety. Animal models developed from ablation, lesioning, and stimulation studies, in addition to anti-anxiety drug trials in humans have contributed to a significant body of literature that suggests that specific brain structures and neurotransmitter systems are associated with the emotion of anxiety. Although a complete review of the neurobiology of anxiety is beyond the scope of this chapter, a brief survey of the studies that have been influential in this area is included below.

CNS Structures

The limbic system has been defined as including the hypothalamus, hippocampus, amygdala, cingulum, septum, and other medial structures of the brain that form a ring around the inner border of the cortical mantle (Taylor & Arnow, 1988; Kuhar, 1986). Emotional expression is often ascribed to the limbic system, primarily because of its involvement in somatic and autonomic activities (Garoutte, 1987). Several experiments in the area of behavioral–anatomical research have used lesion or ablation procedures to test the hypothesis that the limbic system is involved in the mediation of anxiety. In one such study, Horel, Keating, and Misantone (1975) demonstrated that both removal of the bilateral temporal neocortex in one group of monkeys, and the bilateral destruction of the amygdyla in another, resulted in an avoidance of novel stimuli and hypoemotionality.

Further experimental support for the involvement of limbic structures in anxiety has been provided by LeDoux, Thompson, Iadelcola, Tucker, and Reis (1983). Local cerebral blood flow was measured in rats by quantitative autoradiography during the processing of environmental stimuli. Presentation of a neutral tone produced increased blood flow in the rat's auditory pathway. However, when the rat had been previously conditioned to fear the tone, blood flow additionally increased in the hypothalamus and amygdala.

The role of the locus coeruleus in anxiety disorders has also received considerable attention. It has been proposed that the locus coeruleus serves as a relay center for alarm. Taylor and Arnow (1988) suggested that pathways from the locus coeruleus affect many of the physiological responses to pain and fear, and that other pathways to and from the cerebral cortex may provide cognitive feedback such as appraisal of the meaning of these stimuli.

Some support for the hypothesis that the locus coeruleus mediates the expression of anxiety has been evidenced from animal studies. Low-intensity stimulation of electrodes placed in the locus coeruleus of monkeys has been found to produce an alerting response manifested by widening of the peripheral fissures and increased body movements (Redmond, Huang, Snyder, & Maas, 1976). In a follow-up study, Redmond and Huang (1979) demonstrated that an increase in the intensity of stimulation to the locus coeruleus produced a terror reaction, characterized by chewing, mouth and tongue movements, grinding of the teeth, scratching, hair pulling, hand wringing, and spasmodic single body jerks. This reaction, they reported, closely resembled the fear response that the monkey displays when exposed to overwhelming threat in the wilderness.

Contradictory results were found in an investigation of the role of the locus coeruleus in mediating anxiety responses in rats (File, Deakin, Longden, & Crow, 1979). These investigators found that bilaterally lesioning the locus coeruleus in rats did not impair their responses to anxiety-producing stimuli, such as a home cage intruder. File *et al.* (1979) suggested that although the locus coeruleus does not appear to be involved in anxiety mechanisms, it may be involved in the control of some components of agonistic behavior.

The role of the frontal lobes in anxiety is perhaps best illustrated by the psychosurgical procedures performed to alleviate severe, chronic, and unremitting anxiety disorders. Modified bimedial leucotomy, a procedure that destroys the tissue in the supraorbital region, has been shown to improve severe agoraphobia and obsessive–compulsive neurosis and to maintain that improvement for several years follow-up (Marks, Birley, & Gelder, 1966, Tan, Marks, & Marset, 1971).

Although several neuroanatomical structures appear to be involved in the expression of anxiety, a more comprehensive approach suggests that it is important to consider the neurotransmitter systems involved in brain function. For instance, it is difficult to ascribe the mediation of anxiety to the locus coeruleus without investigating the role of the noradrenergic neurotransmitter system. Several neurotransmitter systems have recently been studied in relation to anxiety. The noradrenergic, serotonergic, and GABAergic neurotransmitter systems are all considered below.

Neurotransmitter Systems

Based on a review of several animal studies, Charney and Redmond (1983) reported that hyperactivity of the noradrenergic system may be associated with some anxiety states in humans. It has been suggested that anxiety, manifested as panic disorder, may be a result of abnormal regulation of noradrenergic function. To test this hypothesis, the effects of yohimbine, an α-adrenergic antagonist that increases the rate of firing in the locus coeruleus, were studied in healthy subjects and patients with panic disorder (Charney, Heninger, & Breier, 1984). Patients experiencing frequent panic attacks were found to have a significantly greater plasma methoxy-4-hydroxyphenylglycol (MHPG, a norepinephrine metabolite) response to yohimbine than healthy subjects and patients with less frequent attacks. Further, patients reported experiencing a reaction to the yohimbine injection that was similar to a naturally occurring panic attack.

The investigators concluded that patients with panic disorder have increased sensitivity to augmented noradrenergic function in anxiety associated with panic. Charney *et al.* (1984) further suggested that impaired presynaptic noradrenergic neuronal regulation may be the cause of this low threshold.

In a later study, Charney and Heninger (1986) administered clonidine hydrochloride, an α_2-adrenergic receptor agonist that decreases noradrenergic function, to patients diagnosed as agoraphobic with panic attacks. Clonidine produced significantly greater decreases in plasma MHPG levels in these patients as compared to controls. Charney and his colleagues suggested that these results may be indicative of an abnormality in either the regulatory inputs to the noradrenergic receptor, the inputs to noradrenergic neurons, or dysfunction in the α_2-adrenergic receptor effect or coupling mechanism or the intracellular effector system.

Another neurotransmitter system that has recently been studied in relation to anxiety is the serotonergic. Serotonergic neurons are found in nine clusters of cells lying in the midline of the pons and upper brain stem that innervate the hypothalamus, thalamus, limbic system, neocortex, cerebellum, and spinal cord (Kolb & Wishaw, 1985).

Considerable research suggests that serotonin may be involved in the expression of anxiety. As the noradrenergic system has been linked specifically to panic disorder, abnormal regulation of serotonergic function is most often hypothesized to be related to obsessive–compulsive disorder. Pharmacological evidence for the involvement of serotonin in the expression of obsessive–compulsive disorder comes from trials proving the therapeutic efficacy of chlorimipramine (a potent serotonin reuptake blocker) and L-tryptophan (a precursor of serotonin) in the treatment of obsessive–compulsive disorders (Yaryura-Tobia, Neziroglu, & Bhagavan, 1979). The success of amitriptyline hydrochloride, which inhibits the uptake of both serotonin and norepinephrine, in the treatment of anxiety further implicates the involvement of the serotonergic system in the expression of anxiety (Hoehn-Saric, 1982). Partial support for the hypothesis that decreased serotonergic function is linked to the neurophysiology of obsessive–compulsive disorder has also been found by Charney, Goodman, Price, Woods, Rasmussen, and Heninger (1988).

A final neurotransmitter that has received considerable attention in research investigating the neurobiology of anxiety is γ-aminobutyric acid (GABA). The interest in this inhibitory neurotransmitter comes from research that evidenced the therapeutic efficacy of benzodiazepines, a class of potent anxiolytic drugs, in the treatment of panic disorder (Noyes, Anderson, Clancy, Crowe, Slyren, Ghoreim, & Hinrich, 1984). The therapeutic action of benzodiazepines has been found to be connected with their ability to facilitate transmission in GABA synapses (Haefely, Kulcsar, Mohler, Pieri, Polc, & Schaffner, 1975; Costa, Guidotti, & Mao, 1975). The establishment of this link between benzodiazepines and GABA functioning led investigators to explore the role of this neurotransmitter in the expression of anxiety.

Costa (1985) developed a model to investigate the neurobiology of anxiety based on the ability of benzodiazepines to regulate GABAergic transmission. Briefly, Costa's model postulates that the function of some GABAergic synapses, possibly located in the septum and the amygdaloid nuclei, is related to an endogenous mechanism that regulates anxiety.

Although much of the evidence connecting neurotransmitter systems to the expression of various anxiety disorders is compelling, there is still some controversy surrounding this area of research. The basic assumption of research in this area is that examining the mechanism of action of anxiolytic drugs will offer insight into the underlying neuronal substrates of anxiety. However, it has been argued that this premise is incorrect. Reiman (1987) noted that many therapeutic agents in medicine work by compensating for underlying abnormalities rather than by correcting them. Thus, he argues, studying the neuropharmacology of psychotropic medication leads to a better understanding of the therapeutic action of the drugs rather than an understanding of the underlying neurological basis of the disorder. Further, the research implicating one area of the brain or one neurotransmitter system fails to capture the complexity of anxiety disorders. Several more complex models of anxiety have been developed by personality theorists, animal learning proponents, and neurobiologists to address these limitations. Two of the more influential models are discussed below.

THEORETICAL MODELS OF ANXIETY

Gray's Behavioral Inhibition System

The behavioral inhibition system proposed by Jeffrey Gray (1982, 1985*a*,*b*, 1988) has received a great deal of attention specifically for its attempt to link the pharmacological, neuroanatomical, neurophysiological, and behavioral aspects of anxiety into one theory. Gray's theory is based heavily on the behavioral manifestations of antianxiety drugs, specifically benzodiazepines, barbiturates, and alcohol, in a wide variety of species.

Gray's theory suggests that a "behavioral inhibition system" (BIS) exists and that the basic activity in this system constitutes anxiety. The principal task of the BIS is to compare actual environmental cues to expected stimuli. If a match is made, then the BIS does not override other CNS functions. If the stimuli are discordant or if the preelicited stimuli are aversive, however, the BIS is activated and subsequently the execution of the ongoing motor program is inhibited, and a series of precautional consequences occur, such as a "tagging" of the discordant stimuli for further review. This process is designed to help the organism deal with the stimulus and be better prepared for future contact.

Gray suggests that three basic types of stimuli act upon the BIS: punishment, the omission of an expected reward, and novel stimuli. Antianxiety drugs act on the system by counteracting the behavioral change produced by these stimuli, specifically, inhibiting ongoing behavior, increasing attention to the environment (especially novel stimuli), and increasing level of arousal. Thus, Gray describes anxiety as a central state elicited by threats of punishment, frustration or failure and novelty of uncertainty.

Gray suggests that the BIS couched in terms of stimulus inputs and response outputs offers a behavioral analysis of anxiety. Conversely, identifying the brain structures that constitute the BIS moves toward a more cognitive analysis of anxiety. The BIS, according to Gray, has its neuronal basis in the septohippocampal system and interconnected structures. The theory allots functions to each of the areas in the system as well as to the ascending noradrenergic afferents to these areas.

Each of the neuronal substrates plays an intricate role in the expression of anxiety. The main *comparator* function is held to take place in the subicular area, the origin of major efferents from the hippocampal formation. *Predictions* as to the "expected" state of the world are held to be generated by the Papez circuit. *Long-term storage* of stimulus–stimulus regularities derived from classical conditioning, of response–stimulus regularities derived from instrumental conditioning is in the temporal lobe. The prefrontal cortex is presumed to be involved in making *predictions* regarding what will happen next.

As stated before, the primary function of the BIS is to suppress behavior that threatens to produce pain or nonreward. Gray suggests that the system can then only be useful if some other system is producing behavior that needs to be suppressed. He proposes that there are two major motivational systems that fulfill this function. The first is the "reward system" that Gray proposes mediates approach and active avoidance behavior in response to stimuli associated with reward or the omission of anticipated punishment. The second motivational system is the fight/flight system that responds to unconditioned pain and nonreward.

Cloninger's Model

Cloninger (1987) also presented a general theory of anxiety based on heritable personality traits and their neurobiological bases. The theory proposes that three independent dimensions of personality exist as patterns of response to specific types of environmental stimuli.

The first dimension, novelty seeking, is similar to Gray's behavioral activation or motivating system. It is characterized by an irritable tendency toward frequent exploratory activity and intense excitement in response to novel stimuli. Chronic anxiety in this dimension would present as global uneasiness or alarm without cues, frequent bodily pains due to a low pain and sensation threshold, a low sedation threshold, and slow fatigability. Cloninger suggests that there is evidence that this dimension is correlated with low basal dopaminergic activity.

The second dimension, harm avoidance, is similar to Gray's behavioral inhibition system. Those with this trait would be expected to respond intensely to aversive stimuli and to learn to avoid punishment, novelty, and nonreward passively. Chronic anxiety is characterized by frequent anticipatory worries based on specific cues, high pain and sedation thresholds, and easy fatigability. Cloninger suggests this trait is associated with increased serotonergic activity in the system.

The final dimension Cloninger proposes is labeled reward dependence. This trait is characterized by an intense response to reward and relief, and a tendency to learn to maintain rewarded behavior. Chronic anxiety or frustration would result in agitated dysphoria, overeating, and increased sexual activity. As this trait is correlated with low basal noradrenergic activity, chronic anxiety in this dimension results in noradrenergic hyperactivity.

Both of these models attempt to take a broad-based approach to understanding the neurobiological and psychological mechanism of anxiety by incorporating neurological, neurochemical, and behavioral data. Much of the research done thus far, upon which these theories are based, has been limited to animal populations. Unfortunately, it is often difficult to extrapolate the fear and/or aggressive behaviors in animals to clinical anxiety disorders in humans. There have, however, been several recent attempts to assess the neuropsychological/neurological aspects of clinical anxiety in humans. Electrophysiological recording (electroencephalogram and evoked potentials), neuroimaging techniques (magnetic resonance imaging, computerized axial tomography, and positron emission tomography), and neuropsychological assessment have all been employed to investigate a variety of anxiety disorders in humans. The following is a review of the major findings using these techniques in the areas of panic disorder, generalized anxiety disorder, obsessive–compulsive disorder, posttraumatic stress disorder, simple phobia, and atypical anxiety disorders. For the most part, each section will also include a discussion of clinical applications of these findings to assessment.

PANIC DISORDER

Panic disorder has recently received a great deal of attention regarding the possibility of an underlying neurological anomaly or genetic marker for the development of the disorder. Panic disorder is a fairly prevalent anxiety disorder. Preliminary data from the epidemiologic catchment area (ECA) study survey, sponsored by the National Institute of Mental Health, suggested that the prevalence of panic disorder in the population is between 0.6 and 1.9% (Myers, Weissman, Tischler, Holzer, Leaf, Orvaschel, Anthony, Boyd, Burke, Kramer, & Stoltzman, 1984).

Panic disorder is defined in the DSM-III-R (American Psychiatric Association, 1987) as a condition marked by one or more discrete periods of intense fear or discomfort, which occur unexpectedly and are accompanied by several physical and cognitive symptoms such as dyspnea, dizziness, trembling, palpitations, and fear of going crazy, which occur unexpectedly. This disorder may occur with or without the presence of agoraphobia. Agoraphobia refers to a condition in which the individual experiences a fear of being in situations from which escape may be embarrassing or help may not be available. As a result of this fear, agoraphobics often restrict their life-style by either enduring agoraphobic situations while experiencing great distress, by traveling only in the company of a companion, or in the most extreme cases by becoming housebound. In clinical settings, patients with panic disorder often present with agoraphobia. An important methodological issue in research done with panic-disordered patients is the presence or absence of a codiagnosis of agoraphobia. Not all of the literature reviewed in this section provides information on this potentially important distinction. As such, the results of the studies reviewed below must be considered with this point in mind.

Several features of panic disorder lend support for a genetic contribution. The morbidity risk for panic or probable panic disorder has been found to be much higher for first-degree relatives of probands with panic disorder (24.7%) than in the general population (Crowe, Noyes, Pauls, & Slymen, 1983). Studies comparing the prevalence rate of panic disorder in monozygotic versus dizygotic twins also lend support for a genetic transmission of the disorder. Torgensen (1983) reported that probands diagnosed with either panic disorder or agoraphobia with panic had a 31% cotwin diagnosis of "anxiety disorder with panic attack" for monozygotic twins as opposed to 0% for dizygotic twins.

There have also been several lines of research that have implicated a biological basis for panic disorder. There is a large body of literature, as discussed earlier, in support of a pharmacological treatment for panic disorder which is often taken as evidence for a biological basis for the disorder. Also, several biological challenges, such as sodium lactate infusion or inhalation of carbon dioxide, have been found to precipitate panic attacks in patients who are diagnosed with panic disorder but not in normal controls, suggesting the presence of an underlying biological anomaly.

In addition to the genetic and biological aspects of panic disorder, several lines of research have been directed at investigating the neurological/neuropsychological concomitants. Evoked potentials and brain imaging techniques, in addition to clinical neuropsychological assessment investigations have been used to assess panic disorder.

Electrophysiological Recordings

Evoked Potentials

Evoked potentials consist of a short train of large slow waves recorded from the scalp and largely reflect the activities of the dendrites (Goodwin, 1989).

Hillgard and Kutas (1983) provide an excellent and comprehensive discussion of these electrophysiological correlates of cognitive processing. Yeudall, Schopflocher, Sussman, Barabash, Warneke, Gill, Otto, Howarth, and Termansen (1983) examined central nervous functioning in individuals suffering from chronic panic attacks with and without agoraphobia using auditory brain-stem evoked potential recordings. A preliminary analysis of the evoked potential data revealed that 62.5% of the subjects had a compromised left hemisphere caudal brain-stem functioning relative to the right hemisphere. At the level of the rostral brain-stem, 82.25% of the patients showed a greater left than right compromise in functioning. When brain-stem evoked potential readings from both sides were combined for interpretation, all the subjects evidenced some compromised brain-stem functioning. These results were predicted by Yeudall and his colleagues based on the autonomic symptomatology that is pathognomonic to the disorder.

Yeudall *et al.* (1983) proposed a brain stem–diencephalic hierarchical overactivation model of panic attacks. Rather than implicating cortical structures, Yeudall *et al.* suggest that this dysfunction is localized to the brain stem and midbrain diencephalic areas of the brain. The spontaneous nature of panic attacks, the associated autonomic symptomatology, and the extreme fear that is typically followed by a flight reaction are all cited as evidence against significant cortical involvement. Based on the progression of symptoms that occurs during a panic attack, Yeudall *et al.* proposed a hierarchical progression of abnormal activation of brain-stem functioning. It is suggested that initially an overactivation of specific nuclei located in the brain stem that are involved in the control of respiration (nucleus solitarius), heart rate (nucleus ambiguus), bronchial constriction (nucleus ambiguus), and balance (vestibular nucleus) would occur. This activation would then be followed by overactivation of midbrain limbic structures (posterior hypothalamic nuclei, mesial temporal lobe, amygdala, hippocampus, and orbital frontal lobes).

Although evoked potential recording is a promising starting point for understanding the neuropsychology of panic, it has limited utility. Recent advances in neuroimaging technologies have provided a more detailed analysis of the neurobiology of panic disorders.

Neuroimaging

Positron Emission Tomography (PET)

PET has been shown to be a relatively safe brain imaging technique that provides quantitative regional measurements of biochemical and physiological processes (Raichle, 1983). PET scans document changes in regional blood flow which have been demonstrated to be associated with changes in local neuronal activity. Most of the PET imaging work with panic disorder patients has been conducted by Reiman and his colleagues.

In the first of a series of studies, Reiman, Raichle, Butler, Herscovitch, and Robins (1984) identified a discrete brain abnormality in panickers as compared to controls. A lower left-to-right ratio for cerebral blood flow was revealed in the parahippocampal gyrus of patients with panic disorder by a scan done during a resting state. The other areas of the brain chosen to be measured because of their supposed role in mediating symptoms of anxiety did not produce abnormal results. Since the scans were done while the subject was in a resting state as opposed to during a panic attack, the authors postulated that the asymmetry represented a vulnerability to experience panic attacks.

In a replication, Reiman, Raichle, Robins, Butler, Herscovitch, Fox, and Perlmutter (1986) confirmed their original findings. In addition, patients with a panic disorder who evidenced parahippocampal gyrus cerebral blood flow asymmetry also showed a significantly lower ratio of left-to-right parahippocampal blood volume and metabolic rate for oxygen as compared to normal controls and an abnormally high whole brain metabolism.

In a theoretical review of these findings, Reiman (1987) offered several hypotheses to explain the occurrence of PET scan abnormalities in patients with panic disorder. One possibility he suggested was that the abnormality represented a persistent genetic marker for panic disorder. Conversely, Reiman concluded it is possible that the blood flow and metabolism abnormalities may have represented nothing more than the presence of state anxiety (i.e., anxiety secondary to the PET scan procedures).

There has also been speculation regarding the cause of the abnormality. One explanation proposed by Reiman was that the abnormality reflected an asymmetry in the cellular processes innervating the parahippocampal gyrus. This hypothesis, Reiman stated, could be investigated further by using magnetic resonance imaging. A second hypothesis is that the asymmetry may have represented an increase in the permeability of the blood–brain barrier in the parahippocampal area. Lastly, Reiman suggested that patients with panic disorder may be characterized by increased neuronal activity in the parahippocampal area with concomitant increases in blood flow. All of these hypotheses may be investigated in future studies.

It is interesting to note how the results of the PET scan studies lend converging evidence to previous hypotheses regarding the neurological processes underlying panic disorder. Projections to and from the parahippocampal area originate from and extend to many regions of the brain suspected to be involved in the expression of anxiety. For example, projections to the parahippocampus arise in the hippocampus and locus coeruleus, and projections from the parahippocampal area innervate the hypothalamus, septum, amygdala, hippocampal region, and posterior cingulate gyrus (Nieuwenhuys, Vooad, & Van-Huitzen, 1981). All of these areas as discussed earlier have been implicated in the expression of anxiety.

Reiman (1987) also applied his findings to the theory of the neuropsychology of anxiety espoused by Gray. As noted earlier, Gray's 1982 theory suggested the involvement of the afferent and efferent connections of the hippocampus in the neurobiology of anxiety. Gray suggested that the septohippocampal system is responsible for comparing environmental cues to expected stimuli. As noted by Reiman (1987), Gray hypothesized that by activating the noradrenergic or serotonergic projections to the hippocampus, the sensitivity of the hippocampal area to environmental cues would increase resulting in the behavioral manifestation of anxiety. Thus, the findings from the imaging studies lend support to Gray's theory.

There are some difficulties with these studies, however. In both of the Reiman studies, patients diagnosed with panic disorder were subdivided into two groups: those who responded positively to sodium lactate infusion and those who responded negatively. Only those patients who responded positively to sodium lactate infusion showed brain abnormalities on PET scan imaging while panic-disordered patients who did not respond to sodium lactate infusion did not significantly differ from non-panic-disordered controls on most measures.

Infusion of sodium lactate, in addition to other biological challenges such as carbon dioxide inhalation, caffeine intoxication, and administration of yohimbine, has been found to induce panic in patients who spontaneously experience panic attacks (Pitts & McClure, 1967; Gorma, Askanazi, Liebowitz, Fyer, Stein, Kinney, & Klein, 1984; Charney, Heninger, & Jatlow, 1985; Charney *et al.*, 1984). Liebowitz, Gorman, Fyer, Levitt, Dillon, Levy, Appleby, Anderson, Palij, Davies, and Klein (1985) found that although not all patients diagnosed with panic disorder responded to sodium lactate infusion by panicking, none of the controls did. There has been some controversy over the issue of provocation of panic attacks. Barlow (1988) suggested that one of the major difficulties precluding the interpretation of sodium lactate infusion studies lies in the issue of defining panic in terms of essential versus nonessential aspects of a panic attack. In other words, panic attacks experienced in the laboratory may not be qualitatively the same as spontaneously occurring panic attacks. Ehlers, Margraf, and Roth (1986) used psychometrically sound scales to assess the panic symptoms of panic-disordered patients, as well as recording psychophysiological variables. In this study, laboratory-induced panic attacks were rated to be similar to naturally occurring panic attacks in 70% of the panic-disordered patients. Unfortunately, not all investigators have used such detailed methodological procedures monitoring the occurrence of panic attacks.

It is unclear upon what basis Reiman classified the groups in his studies as positive and negative responders. Clearly, additional work is needed in defining the artificiality or authenticity of experimentally induced panic attacks before the results of Reiman's work can be considered to be diagnostic. Thus, caution should be exercised before accepting Reiman's interpretation that there exist two subgroups of panic-disordered patients that are distinguishable by sodium lactate infusion response and the ratio of parahippocampal blood flow on PET scan.

Another controversial aspect of the Reiman studies is the conclusion that the PET scan abnormalities may reflect an underlying genetic vulnerability to panic disorder. In an extensive review, Barlow (1988) reported that a factor common to all laboratory-based anxiety procedures is that a high level of apprehension or high state anxiety seems to be a consistent predictor of positive panic responders. Unfortunately, Reiman and his colleagues failed to record systematically this important variable in their earlier studies. This may well have influenced their findings as anticipatory anxiety has been shown to produce changes in regional blood flow.

The most recent PET imaging study done by Reiman, Fusselman, Fox, and Raichle (1989*a*) evaluated the role of anticipatory anxiety in a group of healthy volunteers. Subjects were studied before, during, and after the administration of an electric shock. Both subjective [S-Anxiety scale of the State–Trait Anxiety Inventory (STAI) (Spielberger, 1983)] and physiological (heart rate and electrodermal activity) measures of state anxiety were taken from subjects to ensure that subjects were indeed experiencing anticipatory anxiety. Significant increases in each of the measurements of state anxiety were evidenced during anticipation of the shock by every subject. PET scanning during this period revealed significant increases in regional blood flow in the bilateral temporal poles.

Reiman *et al.* (1989*a*) concluded that panic disorder and nonclinical anticipatory anxiety seem to share a common neuronal pathway involving the temporal poles. However, they maintained that panic disorder is distinguishable from nonclinical forms of anxiety by the presence of a regional brain blood flow abnormality in the parahippocampal area in the nonpanic state.

Regardless of the presence of a persistent genetic marker for panic disorder, there does appear to be evidence that changes occur during the panic attacks themselves, when they are experimentally induced. Stewart, Devous, Rush, Lane, and Bonte (1988) performed PET scans on five normal controls and ten patients with panic disorder at rest and after sodium lactate infusion. The preinfusion scan did not include a visualization of the parahippocampal area; therefore, Reiman's (1987) finding of an anomaly in that area in panic-disordered patients could not be replicated. During the infusion, 60% of the patients and one of the controls responded with a panic attack. PET scanning evidenced a significantly greater increase in blood flow bilaterally in the occipital area for patients who panicked as compared to all other subjects. Further, a nonsignificant trend for decreased left frontal blood flow during the panic attack was observed.

The infusion of sodium lactate also produced changes in the patients who did not panic and in the controls. Total left hemispheric blood flow was significantly increased for all subjects who did not experience a panic attack compared to those patients who did. There was also a trend for increased total right hemispheric blood flow in nonpanicking subjects. Stewart *et al.* (1988) postulated that this increased blood flow, independent of anxiety state, may have been secondary to a sodium lactate-induced increase in serum bicarbonate, increased plasma volume, or to a lessor degree, hemodilution.

Stewart *et al.* (1988) suggested two mechanisms that may account for the finding that patients who experienced lactate-induced panic showed a minimal increase or decrease in total cerebral flood flow. They proposed that patients with a vulnerability to lactate-induced panic may have a higher baseline cerebral blood flow and/or cerebral vasoconstriction of such a magnitude that it may mediate the lactate-induced increase in blood flow.

Reiman, Raichle, Robins, Mintun, Fusselman, Fox, Price, and Hackman (1989*b*) also collected PET measurements of regional blood flow to assess local neuronal activity in patients with panic disorder and normal controls before and during the infusion of sodium lactate. Subjects were divided for analysis into three groups: normal controls, patients diagnosed with panic disorder who responded to sodium lactate infusion, and panic-disordered patients who did not respond to the challenge. Sixteen of the twenty-four patients and eleven of the normal controls were subjects included in the previous Reiman *et al.* (1986) report on the nonpanic state prior to lactate infusion. Seven of the patients and three of the controls experienced significant interscan head movement and were eliminated from subsequent data analysis. The results indicated that all three groups experienced a significant increase in number of anxiety symptoms, heart rate, and arterial pH level and a significant reduction in hematocrit when infused with sodium lactate. The group of patients who responded to the infusion differed from the remaining two groups in that they experienced a significant increase in number of anxiety symptoms, systolic blood pressure, and a decrease in arterial PCO_2.

Results of the PET scan analysis were based on change scores. It is unclear whether the groups were significantly different in regard to blood flow activity prior to lactate infusion. Significant blood flow increases were identified in the group of patient responders bilaterally in the temporal poles, in or near the superior colliculus, and in or near the left anterior cerebellar vermis. Lactate infusion was not associated with significant increases or decreases in regional blood flow in the nonpanicking patients and control subjects. Post hoc analysis with *t* tests (uncorrected for multiple comparisons) revealed that healthy controls had consistent increases in blood flow activity near the bilateral superior colliculi and the left anterior cerebellar vermis. The main finding that sodium lactate-induced panic attacks are associated with increased bilateral flow in the temporal lobes is comparable with many other findings implicating the temporal lobe as an anatomical structure involved in the experience of anxiety.

There were, however, several methodological obstacles in this study. As was noted by Stewart *et al.* (1988), and acknowledged by Reiman, hyperventilation may result in a reduction of arterial PCO_2 which is known to be associated with a decrease in whole brain blood flow. Thus, the change in blood flow may be an artifact of hyperventilation. Also, in light of the difficulties discussed earlier in regard to the authenticity of laboratory-induced panic attacks, it remains unclear whether these results are generalizable to spontaneously occurring panic attacks.

In summary, there is relatively conclusive evidence that changes in cerebral blood flow occur during a sodium lactate-induced panic attack and that during the infusion, cerebral blood flow patterns differ between panic-disordered patients and nonresponders. What remains unclear is whether or not these patterns reflect a neuronal abnormality. The contribution of the somatic symptomatology accompanying panic disorder, such as hyperventilation and possibly increased vigilance and scanning, needs to be established independent of the contribution of the actual emotional or cognitive components in future studies. Although definitive conclusions cannot be made from these studies, there is some evidence that the right temporal/medial and the brain stem areas may be involved with the expression of panic disorder. Prospective studies utilizing brain imaging techniques may be useful when supplemented with behavioral data.

Neuropsychological Assessment

Neuropsychological assessment has also been applied to the investigation of patients with panic disorder. In the study discussed earlier, Yeudall *et al.* (1983) also examined CNS functioning using neuropsychological measures. The test battery included both the Halstead–Reitan Neuropsychology Battery and the Wechsler Adult Intelligence Scale. Analysis of these neuropsychological variables for a group of panic attack subjects was compared to a normative data base and a cluster analysis was performed to determine homogeneity of the neuropsychological profiles.

A Hotelling's T^2 analysis revealed that on 13 of the neuropsychological tests administered, panic-disordered patients' scores differed significantly from the norms. Nine of the thirteen variables were found to be significant by the T^2 analysis: Wepman–Jones Aphasia Test, Speech Sounds Perception Test, Trail Making Part B, Raven's Colored Progressive Matrices, Oral Word Fluency, WAIS Verbal IQ. These data were interpreted as reflecting dysfunction of the left (hemisphere dominant for language) cerebral hemisphere. An ideographic analysis of these data revealed that 43% of the panic-disordered patients showed some evidence of cortical dysfunction with a predominant left hemisphere involvement.

Yeudall *et al.* (1983) proposed a model of panic based on their evoked potential findings as discussed earlier. Given the results of the neuropsychological testing, they also proposed a neurological basis for the development of agoraphobia. Eighty-two percent of the individuals diagnosed as panic disorder with agoraphobia were in the only cluster of patients who evidenced significant neuropsychological deficits on tests that implicated left hemisphere frontotemporal lobe dysfunction. Yeudall *et al.* (1983) suggested that given this dominant hemisphere dysfunction, patients with agoraphobia may have difficulties cognitively mediating their physiological arousal. Yeudall suggested that this decrease in ability to control the autonomic panic symptoms using cortical processes would cause these individuals to experience more frequent and intense panic attack symptoms. This process would then make the patient with agoraphobia more vulnerable to avoidance learning and more susceptible to the fear of experiencing the fear associated with panic attacks.

These findings by Yeudall and his colleagues contradict the results of the neuroimaging studies in that dysfunction was evidenced in the left rather than the right hemisphere. This difference in findings may be attributable to differences between the two populations in regard to the presence of a codiagnosis of agoraphobia. Future studies should include a more rigorous classification criterion in selecting subject groups. Further, handedness must be assessed to clarify these hemispheric differences.

Applications to Clinical Assessment

The role of neurological factors in the presentation of panic disorder is controversial and incompletely understood (Ghardirian, Gauthier, & Bertrand, 1986). Several organic factors manifest behavioral expression of anxiety and may often, therefore, be overlooked by both physicians and clinicians. It has been suggested that once a psychiatric disorder is suspected, practitioners are likely to miss the presence of organicity as they may inaccurately ascribe signs and symptoms to anxiety (Dietch, 1984). It has been shown that one-sixth of psychiatric referrals, done by nonpsychiatric physicians, were actually suffering from a major medical illness that went undiagnosed by the referring physician (Koranyi, 1979). In order for the clinician to make an accurate assessment, it is important to review some cases of neurological dysfunction masked by panic symptomatology.

One example of a patient with anxiety attacks who initially presented to the office of a psychiatrist but who ultimately was treated successfully with neurosurgery was reported by Ghardirian *et al.* (1986). A 69-year-old woman with no previous psychiatric illness presented with frequent anxiety attacks that had been occurring for the past 2 years. Her anxiety persisted over time and she began to behave as if she were experiencing periods of depersonalization and derealization. A seizure sent her to the emergency room where a computerized axial tomography (CAT) scan revealed a right temporal lobe meningioma. Following removal of the tumor, the anxiety attacks ceased, and this remission was monitored at 8 months follow-up.

Dietch (1984) also reported a case involving a 55-year-old woman presenting with anxiety attacks, who was later diagnosed as having neurological involvement. In this case, a left-sided fronto-parietal glioblastoma multiform was evidenced by EEG and computer tomography. This finding is difficult to interpret given the strong support that the temporal lobe is the area involved in the expression of anxiety. An interesting note from this study is that even though the panic attacks were organically induced, the patient still developed agoraphobia which abated following removal of the tumor.

Another area of interest for clinicians is the similarity between the symptomatic expression of periods of the fear/arousal spells induced by seizure and idiopathic panic attacks. It has been suggested that this similarity in symptomatology may represent a common neural mechanism for the two disorders (Weilburg, Bear, & Sachs, 1987). A review of the research in this area is important both to understand the possible neuronal mechanism underlying the expression of anxiety and to assist the practitioner in selecting the treatment of choice for the patient.

Roth (1959) first proposed that there existed a new form of neurotic illness, which he termed the phobic–anxiety–depersonalization syndrome. In addition to the symptoms of anxiety and depersonalization, Roth reported that 40% of patients also showed features characteristic of temporal lobe dysfunction. The symptomatology included a "deja vu" phenomenon, metamorphopsia, panoramic memory, obsessional, hysterical, depressive features, and vasomotor disturbance. Although EEG activity did not differ significantly between patients and normal controls, there was some evidence for neurotransmitter differences between the groups.

Brodsky, Zuniga, Casenas, Ernstoff, and Sachdev (1983) furthered the theory that a subclass of anxiety disorders may be associated with an epileptic process. They proposed that in addition to expressing the notable symptomatology Roth reported, this class of patients was unusually refractory to antianxiety agents and frequently exhibited paradoxical reactions to the major psychotropic drugs. Brodsky *et al.* (1983) proposed that this anxiety disorder subtype is a manifestation of abnormal neuronal firing that can be demonstrated only through 24-hr sleep deprivation EEG recording, and that the symptomatology should be refractory to the use of anticonvulsant medication. All ten cases evaluated by Brodsky *et al.* (1983), initially diagnosed as borderline schizophrenic, traumatic neurotic, and paranoid schizophrenic, were successfully treated with anticonvulsants resulting in a clinical improvement that was maintained at 3–4 years follow-up.

In a more recent case report, Weilburg *et al.* (1987) presented three cases in which panic attacks and seizures coexisted. They suggest that panic symptoms may arise, in some atypical cases, from epileptic-ictal or interictal neuronal activation of temporo-limbic structures. The three cases reported by Weilburg *et al.* (1987) are representative of three different ways that panic disorders and seizure disorders may occur together. These include: (1) panic attacks representing the aura of an underlying complex, partial seizure; (2) panic attacks resulting from interictal behavior change; and (3) panic attacks and seizures coexisting independently.

In the first case, the patient reported attacks of "funny dizziness," which were diagnosed as a panic–anxiety syndrome. Imipramine therapy, however, worsened her symptomatology and psychotherapy was unsuccessful. Afraid of experiencing the "spells" in public, the patient confined herself to home.

Although the patient's symptoms seemed characteristic of panic disorder with agoraphobia, neuropsychological evaluation including CAT scan and EEG revealed temporo-parietal dysfunction. Further, phenytoin, when maintained, resolved the panic and agoraphobic symptomatology.

In the second case, the patient initially experienced complex partial seizures at a very early age, consistent with her family history of epilepsy. Unlike the patient in Case 1 who most likely developed panic attacks in conjunction with the onset of epilepsy, this patient began to experience panic states approximately 6 years after her first seizure while on phenytoin. These panic states ultimately led the patient to develop agoraphobia. Weilburg *et al.* (1987) suggested that the development of this patient's anxiety symptoms secondary to her seizure disorder may be explained by the development of a secondary epileptic focus possibly resulting from kindling. They proposed that ictal discharges from this secondary focus may then cause another class of seizures characterized by fear and autonomic arousal.

Another possibility discussed to explain the delayed onset of panic attacks is that a patient with a temporal lobe focus develops limbic pathways from sensory association cortices through a hyperactive amygdala to the hypothalamus. Weilburg and his colleagues suggested that the increased arousal resulting from the development of connections could possibly pair with previously neutral stimuli leading to development of agoraphobia.

Case 3 was a patient with a history of panic attacks that had developed in her early childhood. At the age of 20, the patient experienced a single generalized tonic clonic convulsion without any associated aura. It was determined in this case that the patient was suffering from both disorders without any clear etiological interrelationships. Both anticonvulsants and anxiolytics were needed to dissipate the patient's symptomatology.

Edlund, Swann, and Clothier (1987) also described a series of patients presenting with atypical panic attacks and temporal EEG abnormalities. Many of these patients responded to alprazolam or carbamazepine, tricyclics generally used to lower seizure threshold in patients with organic involvement.

Thus, it appears that panic disorder and epilepsy may share some common neurological mechanisms, specifically involvement of the temporal areas. Further studies directed at investigating the two disorders may lead to a more complete understanding of the neurological factors associated with the expression of fear. Clinically, it is important to professionals treating patients with these symptoms to be able to distinguish the two. Several guidelines exist to help the practitioner in diagnosing idiopathic versus organic manifestation of panic attacks. Table 8.1 lists important features on the organic presentation of panic attacks drawn from the clinical literature (Dietch, 1984; Ghardirian *et al.*, 1986; Edlund *et al.*, 1987; Weilburg *et al.*, 1987).

TABLE 8.1. Factors Commonly Associated with a Specific Physical Cause for Symptoms of Panic Disorder

No history of psychiatric disorder
Initial age of onset > 35
Atypical or fluctuating symptoms
Variations in severity of panic attacks
Visual illusions or hallucinations
No familial occurrence of any anxiety disorder
Severe derealization
Severe autonomic symptoms
Increased irritability or overt aggression immediately before or after the panic attacks
Abnormal EEG (specifically in the temporal lobe if epilepsy is suggested)
A worsening or lack of change after treatment via anxiolytics
A positive response to anticonvulsant medication

GENERALIZED ANXIETY DISORDER

Generalized anxiety disorder (GAD) is defined in the DSM-III-R as a condition marked by unrealistic or excessive anxiety and worry about two or more circumstances for a period of 6 months or longer. Symptoms of motor tension, autonomic hyperactivity and vigilance and scanning are often present when the individual is anxious (American Psychiatric Association, 1987). The DSM-III (American Psychiatric Association, 1980) criterion for GAD was more vague, requiring only that individuals be excessively nervous for a 1-month period. Unfortunately, this definition produced a great deal of confusion among clinicians and investigators, which led to difficulties in obtaining reliable diagnoses (Barlow, 1988). Because of this confusion, estimates of the prevalence of GAD are few, and often conflictual. The available studies estimate the prevalence rate to be approximately 2.4 to 6.4% of the population and make GAD the most frequently reported anxiety disorder (Anderson, Noyes, & Crowe, 1984; Weissman, 1985).

Most likely as a result of the historical difficulties with the classification of GAD, very little information exists concerning possible underlying neurological mechanisms of the disorder. Evidence for a familial or genetic transmission of GAD is inconclusive. Early studies examining the familial and genetic transmission of all anxiety disorders often used the term *anxiety neurosis* to define clinical anxiety without distinguishing between panic and generalized anxiety (Barlow, 1988). In other cases, GAD was conceptualized as a residual subcategory of the anxiety disorders. There is support for a genetic predisposition to develop an anxiety disorder. Barlow (1988) hypothesized that what may be transmitted is a psychological vulnerability to develop one of the anxiety disorders given the occurrence of particular stressors. Unfortunately, it is difficult to determine if GAD as defined in DSM-III-R has a genetic basis. Methodologically sound studies directed at testing this hypothesis using consistent operational definitions of GAD are needed.

Electrophysiological Recordings

Electroencephalogram

Few studies have examined the possible neurological substrates of GAD. The leading hypothesis is that patients with GAD may experience a diminution of attention to external stimuli. Findings from EEG and brain imaging investigations have contributed to this theory.

An early study by Siciliani and his colleagues evaluated the correlations between levels of anxiety and alpha activity in a group of chronic moderate anxiety patients (Siciliani, Schiavon, & Tansella, 1975). Twenty male neurotic inpatients underwent a clinic interview with a psychiatrist to determine their anxiety level on the Hamilton Rating Scale for Anxiety States (RSAS; Hamilton, 1959). Three Hamilton scores were obtained: total score, psychic anxiety factor, and somatic anxiety factor. Patients were then assessed via EEG to determine their level of alpha activity (frequency and percent time) and fast activity.

An analysis of the EEG data revealed no significant asymmetry. Average alpha percent time in the total sample was, however, reported to be very low (19.84%) relative to what has been reported to be normal in the literature. Further, the three Hamilton anxiety factors showed a consistent trend to correlate positively with alpha index and negatively with alpha frequency.

In the second phase of the study, patients were treated with either 80 mg per day of temazepam, a diazepam metabolite that has been shown to have anxiolytic properties, or placebo for a period of 2 weeks. Patients underwent clinical interviews and EEG assessment at weeks 1 and 2 of treatment. After temazepam treatment, patients showed a decrease in anxiety (RSAS total and psychic scores) which was found to be significantly correlated with an increase in alpha index. Siciliani *et al.* (1975) concluded that alpha index may be a valid measure for detecting the presence of severity of anxiety in this population. These results are not that surprising given that alpha is associated with states of decreased arousal.

The effects of the anxiolytic clorazepate on patients diagnosed with GAD were investigated via EEG power spectral estimate mapping of left hemisphere only (Buchsbaum, Hazlett, Sicotte, Stein, & Zetin, 1985). Initially, baseline EEG and anxiety levels were obtained from 20 patients with a diagnosis of GAD and 10 healthy controls. Anxiety levels were measured using the Hamilton Anxiety Scale and the State–Trait Anxiety Inventory. EEG analysis revealed differences between the GAD patients and the controls. Specifically, GAD patients were found to have less delta and alpha activity relative to controls while beta levels were similar. These differences were found to be most prominent over the temporal lobe.

The second phase of the study was a double-blind placebo-controlled trial of clorazepate (Tranxene). Two hours after drug/placebo administration, the Hamilton and STAI scales were repeated and the EEG was recorded. The dosage of clorazepate was then increased to 22.5 mg/day for 14 days and control patients received matching placebo. On days 7 and 14 of drug/placebo usage, the anxiety scales were readministered and the EEG recorded. The results from this phase of the study differed from those of the first phase in that the temporal region was not the area of greatest drug effect. Instead, EEG changes following clorazepate treatment were heterogeneous across the 16 electrode recording sites. Delta activity, typically associated with drowsiness, was found to be decreased primarily in the posterior frontal and parietal cortex. Conversely, beta activity, associated with activation, increased following treatment at these same sites. Alpha activity was decreased posttreatment most frequently at the occipital recording sites.

Buchsbaum *et al.* also evaluated individual differences in response to drug treatment. Increases in beta activity were found to correlate with improvement posttreatment on the Hamilton item that assesses intellectual functioning. This finding supports the hypothesis that GAD patients have a cognitive deficit that may preclude them from using visual imagery or cognitive processes to cope with anxiety. While this is an interesting hypothesis, further research is warranted.

Buchsbaum *et al.* (1985) also found that a relatively low alpha level at baseline was a predictor for improvement on most of the Hamilton ratings. This finding is inconsistent with that of Siciliani *et al.* (1975) that patients with anxiety had lower levels of alpha activity than controls at pretreatment. Additional work in this area needs to be conducted in order to sort out these conflicting findings.

EEG activity recording has also been used to assess cortical changes in normals and patients with GAD in response to visual stimuli (Grillon & Buchsbaum, 1987). In this study, 19 GAD patients and 11 controls rested for 10 min while their EEG was recorded during the last 30-sec period. During the second phase, a series of ten 4-sec white light stimuli were presented with interstimulus intervals of 30 to 60 sec.

No difference was found at rest between the GAD patients and the normal controls, on any of the five EEG wavebands recorded. These findings contradict the results of Buchsbaum *et al.* (1985) but are congruent with those of Nowack and Marczynski (1981). Grillon and Buchsbaum suggested that their earlier finding of a difference between the groups could be attributed to small procedural variations in the rest durations used, the recording sequence, and patients' familiarity with the laboratory setting.

The EEG reactivity to visual stimuli, however, did differ quantitatively and qualitatively between GAD patients and normal controls. Normal controls showed greater responsivity in the parieto-occipital regions while the GAD patients demonstrated greater responsivity in the centro-parietal region. Further visual stimulation was associated with a decrease in beta I activity in controls and an increase in GAD patients. Beta I was defined in this study as the activity computed by summing adjacent values 13.3–19.9 cycles per second.

Grillon and Buchsbaum (1987) proposed that the GAD patients' diminished ability to suppress alpha activity when presented with visual stimuli may be due to an inability to suppress internal processes in the presence of external events. Grillon and Buchsbaum also suggested that it is possible that physiological arousal could be a major contributory factor to that internal interference. They interpreted the finding of increased beta activity in GAD patients during stimulation as evidence for this increase in levels of physiological arousal.

Neuroimaging

PET

PET scans have been used to investigate the effects of the benzodiazepine/clorazepate on the regional glucose metabolic rate in GAD patients (Buchsbaum, Wu, Haier, Hazlett, Ball, Katz, Sokolski, Lagunas-Solar, & Langer, 1987). Eighteen patients underwent a PET scan before and after a 21-day double-blind placebo-controlled study of clorazepate. During the scannings, patients were administered the degraded stimulus continuous performance test (CPT). The test consists of single digits presented for 40 msec at a rate of one every second. The digits were blurred such that they were barely recognizable. Patients were told that they should respond each time they detected the digit zero, and that they would be given feedback about their performance via colored flashing lights (e.g., green means performance is average). The lights were actually changed every 2 min according to a random series and were independent of the subject's actual performance.

When clorazepate was administered to the GAD patients, the PET scanning revealed a decrease in regional glucose metabolic rates primarily in the occipital and frontal cortex. This finding is consistent with the Buchsbaum *et al.* (1985) study discussed above that found the magnitude of anxiety reduction to be correlated with a reduction of alpha activity in the occipital area. This decrease was greater in the right hemisphere than the left. Conversely, an increase in metabolic rate was found in the subcortical structures, specifically the basal ganglia and the thalamus.

A significant correlation was found between relative metabolic rate and benzodiazepine receptor density. For example, the occipital cortex, an area that displayed a large decrease in metabolic rate, was found to have a relatively high receptor density. Therefore, Buchsbaum *et al.* (1987) suggested that benzodiazepines seem to facilitate GABA's inhibitory function specifically by decreasing metabolic rate.

From the studies reviewed above, there does not seem to be any evidence for a neuronal abnormality in GAD patients that distinguishes them from normals at a baseline assessment. The findings that suggest that this population may experience an information processing deficit, however, have important implications for future work. It would be interesting to test the hypothesis that GAD patients undergo a diminution of attention to an external stimulus using clinical neuropsychological assessment. Also, normative data for GAD patients need to be established on standardized neuropsychological tests. Finally, it would be interesting to pursue the divergent findings of whether or not there is a baseline difference on PET scan imaging between GAD patients and controls. Perhaps a more sensitive technique than EEG, such as the PET scan, could be used on medication-free GAD patients.

OBSESSIVE–COMPULSIVE DISORDER

There has been considerable controversy in the literature regarding the possible neurological basis of obsessive–compulsive disorder (OCD). Though previously considered to be a relatively rare and uncommon anxiety disorder, recent reports have suggested that the 6-month prevalence rate for the disorder in the population is between 1.3 and 2.09% (Myers *et al.*, 1984). OCD is defined in the DSM-III-R (American Psychiatric Association, 1987) as a condition marked by recurrent obsessions or compulsions sufficiently severe to cause marked distress, be time-consuming or significantly interfere with the person's normal routine, occupational functioning, or usual social activities and/or relationships with others. Obsessions are defined as persistent ideas, thoughts, impulses, or images reexperienced as intrusive and senseless. Compulsions are repetitive, purposeful, and intentional behaviors performed in response to obsessions according to certain rules or in a stereotyped fashion.

Several features of OCD suggest a familial contribution. Insel, Hoover, and Murphy (1983*b*) interviewed 27 OCD patients regarding the presence of obsessive–compulsive symptoms in their families. None of the subjects reported any symptoms in their biological parents, although one subject reported that their son engaged in compulsive checking behavior. When 10 of the patients' biological parents were given the Leighton Obsessional Inventory, however, the results indicated that 3 parents scored greater than two standard deviations above the mean. Although there were discrepancies between the self-report and "other" report aspects of this study, the results do suggest the possibility of a familial transmission for OCD-like behavior.

The genetic basis of OCD has also been studied. Rinieris, Stefanis, Rabavilas, and Vaidakis (1978) examined the ABO blood types of patients diagnosed with obsessive–compulsive neurosis. Blood type analysis revealed that patients with obsessive–compulsive neurosis had a significantly higher incidence of phenotype A ($p < 0.001$) and a significantly lower incidence of type O ($p < 0.01$) than the general population.

Finally, twin studies have been used to investigate the genetic nature of OCD. Carey and Gottesman (1981) reported a high concordance rate for OCD in monozygotic (MZ) twins. Concordance rates for twins receiving psychiatric or general practitioner treatment for obsessional symptoms were 33% for MZ twins and 7% for dizygotic twins. For obsessional symptoms or features with or without concomitant treatment, the rates reported were 87% for MZ twins and 47% for DZ twins. Thus, evidence exists for a genetic predisposition to OCD or obsessional symptomatology.

There has also been a recent proliferation of work directed toward the neurological/neuropsychological aspects of OCD. In this section, we will examine the findings from several studies using EEG, evoked potentials, neuropsychological testing, and brain imaging techniques directed at more fully understanding the neuropsychology of OCD.

Electrophysiological Recordings

Evoked Potentials

Average evoked potentials were collected from a group of patients and matched nonpsychiatric controls using three types of visual stimulation tasks (Ciesielski, Beech, & Gordon, 1981). This study, along with a follow-up (Beech, Ciesielski, & Gordon, 1983), analyzed the N220 and P350 components of evoked potential waveforms and concluded that OCD patients had significantly shorter evoked potential latencies and lower peak amplitudes as compared to controls. These differences were found to be positively correlated with task complexity.

These findings partially support a theory proposed by Beech (1971) that obsessive–compulsives have an exaggerated reaction to relatively low levels of stimulation. Beech (1971) hypothesized that obsessional patients are characterized by a tendency toward an exaggerated state of generalized arousal. Beech further suggested that there is some critical level of heightened arousal that inherently produces an incrementation or augmentation of that arousal rather than the expected habituation. Beech proposed that this potentiation effect can also arise during the period of recuperation from an "arousal" response to a stimulus. In this case, Beech predicted that a prolonged state of "vulnerability" would exist. This state of heightened arousal and slow recuperation may also be accompanied by substantial spontaneous fluctuations in arousal which could result in increased susceptibility to vicarious forward and backward conditioning. Discriminable cues in the environment may then become associated with the state of heightened arousal.

More recent studies have been directed toward using evoked potential recording to differentiate between patients with OCD and other psychological disorders. Shagass, Roemer, Straumanis, and Josiassen (1984*a*) obtained evoked potential data from three groups: obsessive–compulsive patients, nonpatient controls and patients diagnosed with other neuroses. The results suggested that the OCD group showed a higher N60 amplitude of somatosensory evoked potential than did either of the control groups. This finding had previously been observed only in chronic schizophrenics and in some patients with epilepsy (Shagass, Roemer, Straumanis, & Amadeo, 1979; Williamson, Allison, Goff, & Mattson, 1977). Shagass *et al.* (1984*a*) concluded that OCD patients and chronic schizophrenics seemed to share a common anomaly, and thus a direct comparison of the two groups was needed to ascertain the extent of somatosensory evoked potential similarity or difference between these two groups.

In an attempt to investigate the possibility of whether a similarity exists between OCD and schizophrenia, Shagass, Roemer, Straumanis, and Josiassen (1984*b*) compared the somatosensory evoked potentials of obsessive–compulsives with neurotics, nonpatients, chronic schizophrenics, "other" schizophrenics, latent schizophrenics, and major depressives. Shagass *et al.* (1984*b*) discussed their findings in relation to current theories of OCD and cerebral dysfunction. They suggested that their finding of high-amplitude N60 in OCD patients may be a result of an underlying epileptic focus.

The finding that left median nerve shocks for SEP (LSEP) 90 contralateral factor scores were lower and right median nerve shocks for SEP (RSEP) 90 contralateral scores higher in OCD patients is suggestive of a relative increase in RSEP responses. This finding along with the finding that N130 anterior factor scores were higher in OCD patients supports the premise of left frontal dysfunction with inhibitory deficits proposed by Flor-Henry, Yeudall, Koles, and Howarth (1979).

Further, Shagass *et al.* (1984*b*) found that OCD patients could be reliably discriminated from all other groups based on 11 evoked potential factors. The 11 factors included three peaks of the somatosensory evoked potential N60, P90, N130 × left versus right × 14 leads. The only group that could not be reliably distinguished from OCD was major depression. This finding was not unexpected given that OCD and major depression often occur concurrently.

The efficacy of the evoked potential method of discerning the presence of OCD from other disorders in these studies lends substantial support to the theory that an underlying neurological anomaly exists. These results, obtained in an adult population, have not, however, been entirely replicated with an adolescent population.

Visual and auditory evoked potentials were collected from nine adolescents with OCD and a group of matched controls by Rapoport, Elkins, Langer, Sceery, Buchsbaum, Gillon, Murphy, Zahn, Lake, Ludlow, and Mendelson (1981). Evoked potentials revealed very few significant differences between OCD patients and controls. While the measure of visual evoked potential augmenting (for P100 component, Cz lead) differed significantly between the two groups, values were within normal limits. No other significant differences in evoked potentials were obtained. The OCD patients did, however, show a trend for shorter latencies and less decrease in latency with increasing stimulus intensity for the N120 and P200 components.

Electroencephalogram

EEG

Several studies have attempted to investigate the EEG activity of OCD patients. Sleep EEG patterns of three obsessional neurotics with waking EEG abnormalities, but no indication of epilepsy, were studied by Epstein and Bailine (1971). Sleep EEGs revealed an abnormality of theta waves and spiking localized to the temporal region. Epstein and Bailine reported that this EEG pattern is similar to the patterns elicited by patients with temporal lobe epileptic disorder. Thus, these findings lend evidence to the hypothesis discussed earlier that implicated the temporal area in the genesis of anxiety, as well as lending evidence to the similarity between temporal lobe epilepsy and the anxiety disorders.

A later study analyzed the EEG characteristics of 10 OCD patients and 23 normals at rest and while performing cognitive tasks (Flor-Henry *et al.*, 1979). The Vocabulary subtest of the WAIS was chosen because it is designed to tap dominant hemispheric functioning while the Block Design subtest was used to assess nondominant hemispheric functioning. A comparison of the two groups revealed no significant differences in the EEG between normals and OCD patients except for a reduced left temporal variability found in the eyes-closed condition for the 13- to 50-Hz band and an increase in the average log right–left coefficient variations (13–20 Hz) parietally for the eyes-open condition.

In a more recent study, however, only two of eight adult OCD patients revealed EEG abnormalities (Insel, Donnelly, Lalakea, Alterman, & Murphy, 1983*a*). One patient's EEG revealed nonspecific intermittent left temporal sharp wave activity. This patient later experienced a generalized seizure following a syncopal episode in response to venipuncture. The other patient with abnormal

EEG showed left hemisphere bursts of rhythmic theta activity; no epileptiform activity was evident on a second recording done with nasopharyngeal electrodes. Neither of these two patients showed impaired performance on any of the neuropsychological variables (specific results discussed below). EEG examination did reveal an increase in theta activity in 5 of the other 18 patients; however, this increase was not localized and was interpreted as "nonspecific" and within normal limits.

The sleep EEGs (5 patients) and awake-only EEGs (7 patients) of 12 patients diagnosed with severe OCD were evaluated by Jenike and Brotman (1984). The results revealed that one third of the patients had EEG abnormalities over the temporal lobes, again consistent with the presenting EEG of temporal lobe epileptics. Although each of these patients was given a trial of antiseizure medication, only one subject responded positively to treatment.

Jenike and Brotman (1984) suggested that temporal lobe abnormalities may be reversed by anticonvulsant medication if the abnormality is detected earlier in the course of the illness. Long-standing temporal lobe seizures, however, have been proposed to cause irreversible damage to brain structures (Jenike, 1984). Jenike and Brotman recommended that if obsessive–compulsive symptomatology presents after the age of 35, and EEG or CAT scan should be done routinely to rule out temporal lobe seizures.

Adolescent OCD patients have also been studied using EEG. Rapoport *et al.* (1981) reported that 8 of the 9 adolescent OCD patients they obtained routine EEGs from were normal; the exception was one boy whose EEG revealed "diffuse nonlocalized slowing."

Mild EEG abnormalities were also only found in 3 of the 17 adolescent OCD patients studied by Behar, Rapoport, Berg, Denkla, Mann, Cox, Fedio, Zahn, and Wolfman (1984). An additional EEG was read as irregular with diffuse theta activity, and 5 were interpreted as normal with intermittent slow activity. Although these results differ from those presented above, it is important to note that both populations were comprised by adolescents.

Thus, research employing electrophysiological assessment of adults diagnosed with OCD has revealed abnormal activity in the temporal region. Adolescent populations, however, do not consistently show these abnormalities. These contradictory findings could suggest chronological variability within the course of OCD or they may represent error within these assessment techniques. Further, more advanced technology has offered new ways to investigate cerebral abnormalities using brain imaging. These methods will be discussed below.

Neuroimaging

Computerized Transaxial Tomography (CT)

CT scanning has played an important role in the assessment of OCD. This technique provides a three-dimensional representation of the brain constructed by the pooling of data obtained from several X rays (Goodwin, 1989).

Eighteen OCD patients were studied with CT scans to determine if structural anomalies were present (Insel, *et al.*, 1983*a*). The OCD patients were compared to age- and gender-matched nonpsychiatric patients with normal neurological exams. CT scans did not reveal a significant difference in ventricular brain ratio (VBR) between patients and controls. Further, no correlation between VBR and deficiencies on the Halstead–Reitan Neuropsychological Battery (results reported below) was found. Finally, OCD patients did not show CT evidence of overall cortical atrophy.

A similar study of Behar *et al.* (1984) investigated the brain structures of 17 OCD patients versus those of a group of controls. Patients were found to have a higher than expected brain ventricular enlargement. Ventricular size did not correlate with sex, age of onset, duration of OCD, previous drug treatment, height, IQ, severity of obsessions or depression, Leyton Inventory Scores, neuropsychological performance (discussed in more detail below), neurolinguistic scores, history of birth trauma, or head trauma. Behar *et al.* suggested that a possible explanation for the lack of correlation between VBR and neuropsychological performance is that the tests that were chosen tapped primarily the anterior frontal lobe functions, whereas the ventricular measurement differences were mainly contributed to from posterior brain regions. There was, however, some indication that patients who had rituals without associated thoughts were more likely to have enlarged ventricles; unfortunately, the sample size in the study was too small to permit definitive conclusions.

There were several methodological problems with the Behar *et al.* study that require consideration. First, 15 of the 17 patients had had more than one episode of major depression. Thus, the study is confounded since it is not clear whether the ventricular brain enlargement was due to OCD, depression, both, or neither. Another problem involves the selection of the control group. The CT scans were obtained from local hospitals and were of individuals referred for headache, possible arteriovenous malfunction, seizures, and traumas. Although the investigators excluded those read as clinically questionable, the controls had been referred for suspected pathology. Finally, correlations between the CT scans and neuropsychological performance in the control group were not possible because separate groups were evaluated, one for the CT scanning and one for the testing.

It is difficult to draw any conclusions from these two CT-scanning studies, given their contradictory results. CT scanning is, however, limited in its ability to assess the neurological processes involved in OCD.

Although Insel *et al.* (1983*a*) did not find a localized neuropsychological dysfunction, they did not propose that their study negated the possibility of the presence of such an anomaly. Moreover, they suggested that new techniques for imaging cerebral glucose metabolism or cerebral blood flow may yield a clearer map of neuropsychological functioning in the disorder.

The next section will review two studies that have used PET scanning to assess the presence or absence of abnormalities in glucose metabolism and blood flow activity in OCD patients.

PET

The global and local cerebral metabolic rates for glucose (LCMRGlc) were studied in OCD patients using PET scans to determine the nature of any possible underlying CNS abnormalities (Baxter, Phelps, Mazziotta, Guze, Schwartz, & Selin, 1987). The results were compared with those obtained from patients with major depressive disorder, unipolar type and a group of normal controls with no DSM-III Axis I diagnosis. The patients with depression and OCD did not differ in levels of anxiety or tension as measured by the Breif Psychiatric Rating Scale (Overall & Gorham, 1962) or depression as measured by the Hamilton Depression Scale (Hamilton, 1967).

The OCD patients revealed significantly higher LCMRGlc values for both hemispheres relative to the depressed controls. The metabolic rates in the OCD patients were also significantly higher in the left orbital gyrus and bilaterally in the caudate nuclei compared to both controls and depressed patients. LCMRGlc in the right orbital gyrus was also higher in OCD patients than in depressed patients, but the results failed to reach statistical significance. Baxter *et al.* (1987) also performed statistical analysis of metabolic ratios. The metabolic rate for the left LCMRGlc orbital gyrus/LCMRGlc hemisphere was significantly elevated for OCD patients compared to the other two groups.

A second phase of this study involved the treatment of a group of 10 patients with trazodone hydrochloride with or without a monoamine oxidase inhibitor. The results of the drug trial revealed that although the mean LCMRGlc for both hemispheres, the caudate nuclei, and the orbital gyri decreased after treatment, these changes were not statistically significant. Furthermore, these measures also decreased in two patients who did not respond to treatment. The only significant change that did occur in the group that responded to treatment was a uniform increase bilaterally for the LCMRGlc caudate nucleus/LCMRGlc hemisphere ratio, which was at a normal level in the premedication baseline PET scan. Baxter *et al.* (1987) concluded that although there were similarities between patients with unipolar depression and those with OCD on the Hamilton Depression Scale, the Brief Psychiatric Rating Scale, and the presence of obsessional thoughts, the two disorders are distinct and most likely mediated by different cerebral structures and processes.

Baxter *et al.* (1987) present a theory regarding the neurobiological processes underlying OCD based on two findings. The first is the evidence from their study that OCD, with or without secondary depression, is characterized by high levels of activity in cortical areas such as the orbital gyri. The theory also draws from animal work suggesting that one function of the caudate nucleus is that it allows animals to switch from one behavioral response to a more appropriate one given a stimulus in the environment (Rosvold, 1968). Baxter and his colleagues proposed that in OCD patients, the caudate nucleus is no longer able to operate adequately given the increase in functional activity in the cortical region. This dysfunction of the caudate nucleus is proposed to result in the perseverative symptomatology associated with OCD as lesions to the caudate nucleus in animals result in a perseverative interference in switching behaviors (Alexander, DeLong, & Strick, 1986). It would follow from this that after successful treatment, the caudate nucleus would reestablish its processing capacities through an increase in metabolic rate relative to the structures with which it interacts. This increase in the ratio of metabolic rate for the caudate nucleus as compared to the rate of the entire hemisphere was evidenced in the Baxter *et al.* (1987) study.

The authors further predict that the metabolic changes demonstrated in this study are not limited to pharamacological intervention. It is suggested that other treatment modalities such as behavioral modification would result in the same functional changes in the same neuroanatomical regions. Future studies should be aimed at testing this intriguing hypothesis.

The results of the Baxter *et al.* (1987) study lend support to the theory that the orbital gyri, or more broadly the frontal areas and the caudate nucleus or the basal ganglia, are indeed involved in OCD. Empirical support for this interpretation is found in the research literature. Mettler (1955) suggested that the basal ganglia are involved in the shifting of attention and that damage to this system may result in a loss of mobility in the shift of attention from one source of sensory input to another. Further, he hypothesized that the symptomatology of perseveration may be due to disturbances of striatal function with unbalance in the sensory systems. More recently, Laplane, Baulac, Widlocher, and Dubois (1984) suggested in a case report that patients with bilateral lesions of the basal ganglia exhibited stereotyped behavior that strongly resembled the compulsive-behavior exemplary of OCD. Schneider (1984) also implicated the basal ganglia in the development of OCD. He suggested that the basal ganglia act as a sensory information gating station, to maintain the normal flow of afferent information to both ascending and descending structures. Dysfunction of this system producing unmodulated afferent information may then lead to inappropriate behavioral responses.

The Baxter *et al.* (1987) study is interesting and offers several hypotheses regarding the neurobiological basis of OCD. However, the authors have conceded that the sample was biased because the sexes were not evenly represented in the sample, most of the patients had concurrent major depression, some of the patients were on medication, and finally, handedness was not controlled across groups (Baxter, Schwartz, Mazziotta, Phelps, Pahl, Guze, & Fairbanks, 1988).

Given these limitations, Baxter *et al.* (1988) replicated their initial study using drug-free, nondepressed, right-handed patients compared with right-handed sex- and age-matched controls. The results of this methodologically sound study confirmed the earlier findings that OCD patients had significantly higher glucose metabolic rates than controls in the whole cerebral hemisphere, the heads of the caudate nuclei, and the orbital gyri. The orbital gyrus–hemisphere ratio was also found to be higher, bilaterally, in OCD patients. In the earlier study, this increased ratio was found only for the left hemisphere of OCD patients. Differing demographic profiles for the two studies are suggested to be responsible for this small difference in results.

Neuropsychological Assessment

The neuropsychological characteristics of OCD patients have also been examined. Flor-Henry *et al.* (1979) administered a neuropsychological battery based on Reitan's (1959) including the Wechsler Adult Intelligence Scale to 11 patients with a diagnosis of primary obsessional syndrome and a group of 11 subjects matched for age, education, and IQ abstracted from the Department of Neuropsychology control data file stored on magnetic tape. The Wepman–Jones Aphasia Test, Seashore Speech Sounds Perception Test, Trail Making Part B, and Oral Word Fluency were included to investigate dominant hemisphere dysfunction according to Flor-Henry *et al.* (1979, p. 121). The Trail Making Part A, Memory for Designs, Raven's Colored Progressive Matrices, Symbol Gestalt, Halstead Category, Organic Integrity, and Seashore Rhythm were also administered to determine any nondominant hemisphere dysfunction.

A clinical profile analysis of each patient evidenced three patterns of dysfunction. Ten of the eleven patients showed bilateral frontal dysfunction, left hemisphere greater than right. Three patients showed bilateral temporal left greater than right, two patients right greater than left and two patients showed bilateral parietal dysfunction left greater than right. Comparisons between the OCD and normal control group were also done. Patients with OCD were found to be significantly impaired on the Wepman–Jones Aphasia Screening test, Purdue Pegboard (both hands), Colored Progressive Matrices, Symbol Gestalt, Halstead Category, Minute Estimation, Tactual Performance Test (all forms), and Seashore Rhythm Test. The two WAIS subtests that showed significant impairment in the obsessionals, Digit Span and Digit Symbol, are two of the WAIS subtests that consistently correlate highly with frontal lobe dysfunction. A great deal of individual case variation was found regarding deficits on these tests which precluded the meaningfulness of computing average effects.

The results of the group data, however, were interpreted by Flor-Henry *et al.* (1979) as suggestive of dysfunction in the frontal area of the dominant hemisphere and bilaterally in the temporal area in OCD patients. Unfortunately, there are some limitations in this study that preclude any definitive interpretations. For example, the two subtests of the WAIS that evidenced the most deficits in performance have been shown to be negatively influenced by anxiety (Matarazzo, 1972). Flor-Henry's findings may have been influenced by an enhanced state anxiety, which may occur simply as a result of the testing environment. Another shortcoming in this study involves the disadvantages of using archival data for a control group. Most notably, cohort differences cannot be accounted for.

A more recent study using neuropsychological testing to assess the cognitive abilities of 18 OCD patients also did not include a control group (Insel *et al.*, 1983*a*). Patients in this study were administered the Wechsler Adult Intelligence Scale and the Halstead–Reitan Neuropsychological Test Battery. Overall impairment was not evidenced on the Halstead–Reitan, although one subtest, the Tactual Performance Test, evidenced consistent deficits in performance. Patients did not show the impairment on the Digit Span and Digit Symbol subtests of the

WAIS as seen in the Flor-Henry *et al.* (1979) study. In fact, no single WAIS subtest was consistently low across the subjects. There was, however, some evidence that the OCD patients were generally impaired on the performance subtests. Specifically, 50% of the patients had a scaled score of less than 8 on at least one of three performance subtests: picture arrangement, object assembly, and digit symbol. More evidence for a deficit in general performance abilities is that in 50% of the patients, raw verbal scores exceeded performance scores by at least 15 points.

Insel *et al.* (1983*a*) concluded that the abnormalities shown by the OCD subjects on the Tactual Performance Test and the performance subtests of the WAIS were suggestive of right hemisphere dysfunction. This finding is contradictory to the Flor-Henry *et al.* (1979) finding that OCD was associated with left or dominant hemisphere dysfunction. They also conceded that the presence of depression, obsessional slowness, and fear of contamination from some of the testing apparatus severely confounds this conclusion. Indeed, in these studies it is difficult, if not impossible, to discern the cognitive behavioral manifestations of OCD from an organic abnormality, depression, or state-anxiety.

CNS dysfunction, as measured by neuropsychological test performance, has also been studied in adolescents. Sixteen adolescents with OCD and 16 matched controls were administered the following neuropsychological tests: Money's Road Map Test of Directional Sense, to assess frontal lobe abilities, the Stylus Maze Learning Task, sensitive to right frontal and temporal lobe functioning, Rey Word List Learning, Rey-Osterrieth Complex Figure Test, thought to be sensitive to frontal and parietal dysfunction especially in the right hemisphere, dihaptic (tactual) testing reaction time, and the two-flash threshold tasks (Behar *et al.*, 1984).

The results of this study suggested that patients showed significant deficits as compared to controls on the Stylus Maze Learning Task. Patients also performed significantly poorer than controls on the Money Road Map Test. OCD adolescents did not differ significantly on the remaining tests. Behavioral observations, however, suggested that all OCD adolescents observed during copy sequences adopted an "immature" approach to copying on the Rey–Osterrieth Complex Figure. Because reaction time, two-flash threshold, and decision times did not significantly differ between patients and controls, Behar *et al.* (1984) point out that their findings do not lend support for the hyperattentional hypothesis of OCD proposed by Beech (1971).

Rapoport *et al.* (1981) also reported no difference between their adolescent OCD patients and controls in sustained attention and reaction time tasks. No significant differences in either autonomic arousal, responsivity, or habituation to stimuli were found. Another interesting finding of the Rapoport *et al.* (1981) study was that although the WISC-R was administered, none of the patients scored significantly lower on the Digit Span or Symbol Digit subscales.

Neuropsychological assessment has found some support for bilateral frontal and temporal involvement in OCD. Between studies, however, there is great variability in the specific areas implicated; most notably, emphasis on the importance of left versus right hemispheric changes drastically from study to study. Again there is some suggestion that the brain regions involved may differ depending on the age of the population (adults versus adolescents). The limited number of studies and lack of replication, however, make it impossible to draw definite conclusions.

Insel *et al.* (1983*a*) suggested that the discrepancies in results between their findings and those of Flor-Henry *et al.* were attributable to a difference in the age, sex, education, and severity of illness between the two samples. Further, they suggested that future studies should address the presence of secondary depression which is commonly associated with OCD. Both of these studies also lacked an active control group. Further, state anxiety and handedness are also important variables that need to be assessed and controlled for. Clearly, more work needs to be done in the neuropsychological investigation of OCD.

Applications to Clinical Assessment

Some controversy exists over whether OCD is best conceptualized as a neurological or a psychological disorder. The contribution of both of these is incompletely understood, yet knowledge in this area has important assessment and treatment implications for clinicians.

A starting point to understand the nature of OCD is to examine etiological factors. Several investigators have examined birth history as an important aspect in the development of OCD.

Capstick and Seldrup (1977) compared the birth history of 33 patients with obsessional neuroses to a group of psychological patients matched for age, sex, source, and period of referral, who had never exhibited any obsessional symptoms. The results suggested that 11 of the 33 patients with obsessional symptoms had an abnormal birth history, as compared to only 2 of the control patients. The following are some examples of the categories of abnormal birth history: breach, forceps, pelvic abnormality, 3-day labor, and upper motor neuron lesion.

Using the ritual classification system developed by Capstick and Seldrup (1973), the quality of the rituals of the 9 obsessional patients with abnormal birth history were then compared with those of the 22 obsessional patients who gave a normal birth history. The results indicated that patients in the abnormal birth group always showed bizarre rituals and none showed purely normal rituals that characterized the normal birth group. Also, the patients in the abnormal birth group who reported a history of both obsessions and depression, indicated that obsessions occurred first, followed by depression, whereas in the normal birth group, 39% of the patients with both symptoms, developed obsessions during the course of a depression. Finally, the abnormal group tended to have a longer history before seeking treatment; 55% reported a history of 10 years or more as compared to 19% of the normal birth group.

It is not established that any brain damage occurred in the abnormal birth group. While Capstick and Seldrup conceded that the patients could have suffered minimal organic brain damage, they argued that psychological factors, such as the anxiety the newborn suffers being separated from the mother, were most likely the main contributors to the development of the disorder.

There have been several other studies examining the "organic theory" or the correlation of neurological illness and OCD. In a study similar to the Capstick and Seldrup study, Grimshaw (1964) found that 20 of 103 obsessional patients, as compared to 8 of 105 controls, reported a history of neurological illness, including encephalitis, Sydenham's chorea, convulsions during infancy, and epilepsy. OCD onset has also been reported to occur after the development of epileptic seizures (Kettl & Marks, 1986).

These studies present some evidence for a neurological factor in the presentation of OCD. Another growing area of research, developed to gain a better understanding of the disorder, involves studying the similarities between OCD and Gilles de la Tourette syndrome (GTS). An increased prevalence of OCD in Tourette patients and their biological relatives, and similarities between both disorders in onset patterns, symptomatology, and treatment approaches have led investigators to study GTS in order to better understand the etiology of OCD (Nee, Caine, Polinsky, Eldridge, & Ebert, 1980; Cummings & Frankel, 1985). The evidence, however, remains inconclusive.

POSTTRAUMATIC STRESS DISORDER

According to DSM-III-R, the diagnosis of a posttraumatic stress disorder (PTSD) is made when a person experiences an event that is outside the range of normal human experience and that is markedly distressing. Persistent symptoms are increased arousal, avoidance of stimuli associated with the trauma or numbing of general responsiveness, and reexperiencing the trauma through either recurrent and intrusive distressing recollections, distressing dreams, dissociative episodes, or intense psychological distress when exposed to events that symbolize or resemble aspects of a traumatic event.

To date, the majority of the research conducted on PTSD has been confined to combat veterans (Figley, 1978). While there have been a few studies evaluating PTSD in noncombat situations (McCaffrey & Fairbank, 1985; McCaffrey, Hickling, & Marazzo, 1989), these studies represent only a small population of the total literature on the topic.

Neuropsychological Hypothesis of PTSD

In a recent review of the human psychophysiological literature of PTSD and the literature on conditioned fears in animals, Kolb (1987) postulated that the symptoms of PTSD in veterans are the result of changes in the CNS. Specifically, the symptoms of PTSD are presumed to be the result of changes in the agonistic neural system that impair cortical control of hindbrain structures involved with the expression of aggressive behavior, sleep–wake cycles, and dream functions.

The hypothesized cortical neuronal and synaptic changes in PTSD are presumed to occur as a consequence of excessive and prolonged sensitizing stimulation present during combat conditions.

To date, we are unaware of any direct test of Kolb's hypothesis from a clinical neuropsychological perspective. Given that the proposed etiological mechanism for PTSD involves alterations in CNS functioning, clinical neuropsychological assessment of veterans with and without a diagnosis of PTSD might provide a test of the Kolb hypothesis.

Neuropsychological Assessment

The diagnostic criteria for a PTSD include persistent symptoms of increased arousal: difficulty falling or staying asleep, irritability or outbursts of anger, difficulty concentrating, hypervigilance, exaggerated startle response, and increased physiologic reactivity to events that symbolize or resemble an aspect of the traumatic event(s). As noted above, several investigators (see Kolb, 1987) believe that the behavioral manifestation of a PTSD reflects underlying alterations in CNS activity. As such, the relationship between alterations in CNS activity and their behavioral correlates might be of diagnostic utility for the clinician working with this population.

A review of the few pertinent studies involving the effects of PTSD on neuropsychological test performance reveals that the studies have been confined exclusively to combat-related forms of PTSD. In one of the earliest reports, Dalton, Pederson, Blom, and Besyner (1986) evaluated a group of 22 combat veterans who were undergoing inpatient treatment in a stress disorders treatment unit connected with a VA Medical Center. The neuropsychological assessment battery consisted of the WAIS-R, time to completion and number of errors on the Trail Making Test (Parts A and B), the Temporal Orientation Test, the Serial Digit Learning Test, the Stroop Word Test (word, color, color–word, and interference), the Conceptual Quotient of the Shipley–Hartford, and the Controlled Oral Word Association Test. The performance of the PTSD patients was compared to available norms for all of the assessment instruments in the neuropsychological battery. The poorest performance in the PTSD group was obtained in the Digit Span and Digit Symbol, subtests of the WAIS-R that have been shown to be sensitive to the presence of anxiety (Golden, 1979).

In a follow-up study, Dalton, Pederson, and Ryan (1989) evaluated 100 combat veterans who were seeking inpatient treatment in a stress disorders treatment unit. The purpose of this study was to develop a set of norms for this particular population and also to attempt to replicate the earlier findings. The neuropsychological assessment battery in the follow-up study consisted of the WAIS-R, the Rey Auditory Learning Test, the Temporal Orientation Test, the Conceptual Quotient of the Shipley–Hartford, time and errors on the Trail Making Test (Parts A and B), the Serial Digit Learning Test, the Benton Visual Retention Test, and the Stroop Word Test (word, color, color–word, and interference). As in the previous study, the performance of the PTSD patients was compared to available normative data and not to a control of veterans without a diagnosis of PTSD. The results of this study revealed a very slight decrement on the Digit Span and Digit Symbol subtests of the WAIS-R. The authors reported a slight decrement in PTSD patients' performance on the Benton Visual Retention Test relative to available norms. In addition, the PTSD patients' performance on the Stroop Test was slightly impaired relative to norms. Based on both the preliminary study and the follow-up study, Dalton and his colleagues concluded that the neuropsychological assessment of combat-related patients with a PTSD appears comparable to a mild or moderate anxiety disorder.

A pilot study by Everly and Horton (1988) hypothesized that PTSD patients would show evidence of short-term memory problems with no impairment of long-term memory functions. In this study, 14 patients diagnosed with PTSD were evaluated using the Weschler Memory Scale and the Peterson Memory Paradigm. An analysis of long-term memory data revealed no significant departures from normative data. On the other hand, the short-term memory data revealed deviations from the normative data. While the results of this pilot study are clearly not definitive, the authors conclude that they provide partial support for the hypotheses of Kolb (1987) and Everly (1985, 1987).

The only remaining published data on the neuropsychological correlates of PTSD are from the Wechsler Memory Scale–Revised (Wechsler, 1987, p. 80). As part of a more global evaluation of several clinical groups, a group of 19 PTSD patients were administered the Weschler Memory Scale–Revised. The mean performance on the five indexes were General Memory 85.0, Attention/Concentration 89.2, Verbal Memory 89.4, Visual Memory 82.3, and Delayed Recall 85.6. Whether or not these data reflect the presence of memory dysfunction in PTSD patients is difficult to evaluate since a control group of combat veterans with no diagnosis of PTSD matched on age and education was not included. It is interesting to note, however, that the average of the Verbal and Visual Memory indexes was 85.8 compared to the delayed recall index of 85.6. These data fail to support the hypothesis tested by Everly and Horton (1988) that PTSD patients would show greater deficits in short-term memory relative to long-term memory.

The studies reviewed in this section reveal that Vietnam veterans with a diagnosis of PTSD are clearly not severely impaired on any of the neuropsychological instruments compared to available normative data. The studies by Dalton *et al.* (1986, 1989) reveal that the performance of patients with a PTSD is only slightly impaired on the Digit Span and Digit Symbol subtests of the WAIS-R and the Benton Visual Retention Test. The data presented on the Wechsler Memory Scale–Revised (Wechsler, 1987) were overall within one standard deviation of the mean, suggesting only mild impairment. Even this modest support of Kolb's hypothesis must be interpreted cautiously since the veterans with a diagnosis of PTSD were not compared to an appropriate control group of veterans without a diagnosis of PTSD.

To date, the research into the neuropsychological correlates of PTSD has focused exclusively on veteran populations with diagnosed PTSD. Whether or not non-combat-related forms of PTSD are the same or different in terms of neuropsychological test performance remains an empirical issue. A recent study by McCaffrey and Fairbank (1985) found that non-combat-related forms of PTSD tended to exhibit lower psychophysiological arousal to trauma-relevant stimuli compared to that reported for combat-related forms of PTSD (Malloy, Fairbank, & Keane, 1983). The psychological characteristics of non-combat-related forms of PTSD have recently been reported to differ from those of veterans with combat-related forms of PTSD (McCaffrey, Hickling, & Marazzo, 1989). In addition, the studies involving neuropsychological correlates of PTSD are all based on studies that did not employ control groups of veterans without a diagnosis of PTSD. Rather, the studies reported to date have used available normative data from multiple sources. The absence of an appropriate control condition is a serious methodological limitation since factors other than PTSD may be involved in subtle neuropsychological differences among veteran populations. For example, the possibility of a traumatic brain injury, exposure to various toxic substances, and also a history of substance abuse may, in and of themselves, be responsible for the subtle differences noted among the veteran groups with a diagnosis of PTSD. Finally, it should be noted that while DSM-III-R (American Psychiatric Association, 1987) has deleted memory impairment as one of the criteria of a PTSD, the data presented for the Wechsler Memory Scale–Revised reveal that the PTSD population was approximately 0.6 to 1.0 S.D. below the mean of the standardization sample. Whether or not the apparent memory-related problems in the PTSD population as cited by Wechsler (1987) reflect the influence of PTSD *per se* or the presence of the other factors noted above remains unclear.

SIMPLE PHOBIA

Neuroimaging

PET

The hypothesis that anxiety should be correlated with cerebral blood flow in the brain regions thought to be involved in the expression of anxiety was investigated by Mountz, Modell, Wilson, Curtis, Lee, Schmaltz, and Kohl (1989). A total of seven patients with a DSM-III diagnosis of simple phobia–animal subtype underwent five PET scans in a rest–fear–rest–fear–rest paradigm where the fear condition was exposure to the animal. Eight controls were also evaluated in a similar manner. The patients with the simple phobia demonstrated increased state anxiety to the phobic stimulus, as indexed by the Spielberger State–Trait Anxiety Inventory and the Subjective Units of the Stress Scale. The phobic group also demonstrated significantly lower absolute and local regional cerebral blood flow during the fear PET scans than during the rest PET scans. When hypocapnia secondary to anxiety-induced hyperventilation was controlled for, however, all of the cerebral blood flow differences between the two groups were insignificant. The failure to obtain a correlation between anxiety and cerebral blood flow in this study suggests either that blood flow changes induced by state anxiety are not measurable by current PET scanning technology or that no correlation exists. Whether or not previous PET scanning research on panic disorder, general anxiety disorder, and obsessive–compulsive disorder patients reflects the underlying pathophysiology of the disorder and not state-anxiety changes is unclear since hypocapnia is not consistently controlled for in this type of research.

ATYPICAL ANXIETY DISORDERS

Within the DSM-III-R classification of anxiety disorders, there exists the category of anxiety disorders not otherwise specified. This category is used for disorders in which there is prominent anxiety of phobic avoidance that are not classifiable as specific anxiety disorders or an adjustment disorder with anxious mood. One such disorder that has recently been investigated focuses on space phobia. In a number of publications, Marks (1969, 1981; Marks & Bebbington, 1976) briefly described a disorder that he termed "pseudoagoraphobia" or "space phobia." According to Marks, the primary complaint is a fear of falling when perceiving space without nearby support. Marks has reported that the patient requires visual boundaries rather than physical support to walk or drive across open spaces. In severe forms of the disorder, the patient may be unable to cross a room except on hands and knees. Marks has noted that space phobia differs from agoraphobia inasmuch as the former has a later age of onset, only rarely involves accompanying depression, nonsituational or panic, is frequently associated with diverse signs of brain stem, cervical, or labyrinthine pathology and/or cardiovascular disorder, and does not respond to *in vivo* exposure treatment. Apart from the descriptions by Marks and his colleagues, there has been only one other report of this disorder in the literature.

In an attempt to evaluate the possible interrelationship between psychological and neuropsychological factors involved in disorder of space phobia, McCaffrey, Rapee, Gansler, and Barlow (1990) presented both an in-depth psychological and a neuropsychological evaluation of two cases of space phobia. The results of the psychological evaluation revealed both patients to be excessively demanding, dependent, and having an almost inordinate need for attention and affection. Performance on the State–Trait Anxiety Inventory (Spielberger, Gorsuch, & Luschene, 1970) were considerably above normal and in the range often reported for individuals diagnosed with an anxiety disorder. Evaluation using various phobic measures reveals that the patients were most similar to agoraphobics but not consistently so.

Due to the nature of the symptoms associated with space phobia, a number of neuropsychological assessment instruments designed to provide data on the patients' neuropsychological functioning, and in particular on visual spatial functioning, were administered. Each of the patients showed deficits on the Block Design Subtests of the WAIS-R, Speech Sounds Perception Subtest of the HRNB, problems copying the Rey–Osterrieth Complex Figure, and deficits on sensory–perceptual examination suggestive of right hemisphere dysfunction.

The results of these two cases were interpreted by the authors as suggestive of an interaction between neuropsychological and psychological factors in the presentation of this atypical-anxiety space disorder. While one of the patients was known to have suffered from a cerebral vascular accident a number of years prior to the assessment, the other patient was consistently found to be neurologically intact by several local neurologists and specialists in major medical centers. McCaffrey *et al.* (1990) speculate that both the psychological and neuropsychological abnormalities are important in the development and maintenance of this disorder in an interactive fashion. Certainly, additional work on this patient population and other atypical anxiety disorders is warranted.

Although there has been multifaceted assessment of the clinical anxiety disorders, clearly more research is needed before we fully understand the contribution of neurological factors. One of the major issues precluding the interpretation of many of the studies discussed thus far is the contribution of state anxiety. In many of the studies reviewed, state anxiety at the time of the assessment was not measured or controlled for, rendering the results unclear. It is impossible to conclude that deficits during neuropsychological assessment or the abnormalities evidenced by brain imaging represent any underlying genetic neurological anomaly without knowing the effects of state anxiety on these assessment techniques. The following section reviews studies that have attempted to measure the impact of state anxiety independent of trait anxiety. Understanding these effects is a first step needed to clarify the interpretation of research with clinical populations.

THE IMPACT OF STATE–TRAIT ANXIETY ON NEUROPSYCHOLOGICAL TEST PERFORMANCE

The interpretation of neuropsychological test performance assumes that the patient has provided his or her best level of performance. It is incumbent upon the evaluator to determine the role, if any, of other factors that may have affected an individual patient's performance. The present discussion will focus exclusively on the role of various forms of state and trait anxiety as they impact on neuropsychological performance in college students. While the Wechsler Intelligence Scales are often incorporated in neuropsychological assessment batteries, a detailed discussion of the relationship between various forms of state and trait anxiety and subject performance on the Wechsler Intelligence Scales is beyond the scope of this chapter. Interested readers are referred to the excellent presentation by Matarazzo (1972) for a discussion of the impact of anxiety on WAIS performance.

A review of the sparse literature revealed four studies, which are summarized in Table 8.2. Buckelew and Hannay (1986) found that subjects who were high on A-state performed more poorly relative to those who were low on A-state on the Block Design subtest of the WAIS and the Simple Word Fluency task. The study by King, Hannay, Masek, and Burns (1978) evaluated the performance of college students on the formboard and the Finger Oscillation Test. The results indicated significant correlations between high A-trait scores and impaired performance for women but not men on the Finger Oscillation Test and the formboard test (preferred hand and both hands). The authors note, however, that only a few of the subjects in their sample had clinically elevated anxiety scores and that anxiety seemed to be generally more prevalent among the females than among the males.

The study by Chavez, Trautt, Brandon, and Steyaert (1983) evaluated the relationship between test anxiety as indexed by the Test Anxiety Scale (Sarason, 1972) and performance on the Digit Symbol and Digit Span subtests of the WAIS, the Trail Making Test (Parts A and B), and the Finger Oscillation Test. Test anxiety did not significantly affect subjects' performance on any of the neuropsychological tests.

Finally, Martin and Franzen (1989) attempted to induce anxiety in a sample of college students and to evaluate their performance on several neuropsychological tests. Unfortunately, the anxiety manipulation failed and no definitive statements regarding this study can be made.

The impact of state–trait anxiety on neuropsychological test performance is far from clear. The studies reviewed in this section indicate that additional research is necessary to evaluate more fully and delineate the role of state versus trait anxiety as a factor in clinical neuropsychological assessment.

ANXIETY ARISING FROM TRAUMA TO THE CENTRAL NERVOUS SYSTEM

While cognitive deficits following a traumatic brain injury (TBI) have been shown to improve with the passage of time, the emotional recovery of patients who have sustained a TBI may or may not parallel the recovery in cognitive functions. In fact, emotional functioning may actually deteriorate (Prigatano, 1987). In terms of changes in anxiety, Lezak (1983) reports that patients may experience an increased or decreased level of anxiety relative to their premorbid state. Patients who show an increased level of anxiety following trauma to the CNS may be responding to focal neurological deficits, particularly those with a focus in the temporal lobe (Mulder & Daly, 1952). On the other hand, patients may begin experiencing an increased level of anxiety post-TBI due to their increased "awareness" of their impairment in neuropsychological and physical functioning (e.g., Novack, Daniel, & Long, 1984). Fordyce, Rouche, and Prigatano (1983) evaluated patients who were either 6 months or less postinjury or more than 6 months postinjury. Based on the findings from the Minnesota Multiphasic Personality Inventory and the Katz Adjustment Scale, the patients

TABLE 8.2. Summary of Neuropsychological Studies of State–Trait Anxiety in College Students

Study	Subjects	Group Factor	Neuropsychological tests	Anxiety manipulation	Outcome
Buckelew & Hannay (1986)	College students 60 male 60 female	(1) STAI (Trait) (2) Marlow–Crowne Social Desirability Scale	Digit Symbol (WAIS) Word Fluency (NCCEA) Simple Word Fluency Block Design (WAIS) Finger Oscillation Test *Ss* rated State Anxiety after each test	—	High A-State anxious *Ss* had poorer performance than low A-State on Block Design and Simple Word Fluency
Chavez, Trautt, Brandon, & Steyaert (1983)	College students 28 male 28 female	Text Anxiety Scale (Sarason, 1972)	Digit Symbol (WAIS) Digit Span (WAIS) Trait Making Test (Parts A & B) Finger Oscillation Test	—	Test anxiety had no effect on the performance on any of the measures
King, Hannay, Masek, & Burns (1978)	College students 30 male 30 female	STAI	Form Board Finger Oscillation Test	—	High A-Trait had a significant deleterious effect on the women's performance on the FOT and FB (preferred hand and both hands)
Martin & Franzen (1989)	College students 19 male 37 female	Random assignment to anxiety or neutral condition	Randt Memory Test Knox Cube Tapping Test Stroop Word and Color Test Finger Oscillation Test	(A) Anxiety condition "official-looking" electronic equipment with a neuroanatomy chart in test room and verbal instructions (B) Neutral condition	Anxiety manipulation did not work as indexed by pre–post STAI scores. Results meaningless

who were more than 6 months postinjury were more anxious and depressed, confused, and more socially withdrawn compared to patients who were less than 6 months postinjury. Interestingly, Fordyce, Roueche, and Prigatano (1983) found that the differences in emotional functioning appeared to be independent of the level of neuropsychological impairment and the duration of coma. The differences in terms of emotional functioning were attributed to both the patients' premorbid personality and their increased awareness of residual deficits and accompanying problems in social adjustments, which may not be as salient to patients who are in the acute stages of recovery. While the duration of coma has been shown to be an indicator of the level of severity of the injury and also a predictor of recovery of function (Strub & Black, 1988), the duration of coma was not found to relate to group differences in emotional functioning by Fordyce *et al.* (1983).

The distinction between clinically significant versus non-clinically significant emotional disorders was evaluated by Oddy, Coughlan, Tyerman, and Jenkins (1985). They reported that approximately 25% of the survivors of TBI suffered from increased levels of anxiety or tension but that only 10% displayed a level of anxiety or depression that would be considered clinically significant. Thus, a distinction must be made between the presence of anxiety that is clinically significant versus anxiety that would not fit any of the diagnostic categories in DSM-III-R. For example, Daniel, Haban, Hutcherson, Bolter, and Long (1985) found that 10 of 11 patients who sustained accidental, high-voltage, electrical injuries reported an increased level of anxiety and depression. MMPI profiles were obtained for 9 of the 11, and 6 of these revealed *t* scores greater than 70 on the Pt subscale. In no case, however, did Daniel *et al.* (1985) indicate that any of their patients met the criteria for a DSM-III-R anxiety disorder.

McKeon, McGuffin, and Robinson (1984*a*) reported the development of an OCD in four cases following a TBI. Three were obtained from a consecutive series of 25 patients who were participating in an investigation of the relationship between life events and the onset of obsessive–compulsive neurosis (McKeon, Roa, & Mann, 1984*b*). In all four cases, the development of the OCD began within 25 hr of the head injury. McKeon *et al.* (1984*a*) reported that only one of the four cases had a premorbid personality, described as mildly obsessional. Thus, the time frame in terms of the onset of an anxiety-based disorder must be carefully considered along with premorbid personality characteristics.

A recent report by Davidoff, Kessler, Laibstain, and Mark (1988) indicated the importance of differential diagnosis in patients who have sustained a TBI in regard to the symptoms of the postconcussion syndrome versus the symptoms associated with a PTSD. While there is a considerable degree of overlap between the somatic, cognitive, and affective/behavioral symptoms of postconcussion syndrome and a PTSD, in our own work on patients who have a period of posttraumatic amnesia, any sequelae are most likely attributable to postconcussion syndrome and not PTSD. This distinction is based on the fact that the diagnosis of a PTSD necessitates the recollection of the traumatic event, which presumably a patient with posttraumatic amnesia would not have.

In addition to anxiety disorders arising from environmental trauma to the CNS, there are reports of anxiety disorders being the result of a cerebral tumor. Blackman and Wheeler (1987) report the case of a 12-year-old boy who was diagnosed as having overanxious disorder of childhood and school phobia that was refractory to antidepressant medication and psychotherapy. He was later diagnosed as having a choroid plexus papilloma of the fourth ventricle. The anxiety symptoms abated following neurosurgical interventions.

In summary, anxiety resulting from CNS trauma may be due to focal neurological deficits, may reflect subclinical levels, or may actually present as a DSM-III-R anxiety disorder.

SUMMARY AND CONCLUSIONS

At the present time, it would be premature to attempt to integrate the results of the studies reported in this chapter into a single unifying theoretical perspective on the neuropsychology of anxiety disorders. One factor that is consistently reported is the involvement of the temporal lobe area. Clinical reports have also suggested that temporal lobe epilepsy and trauma to the temporal area result in symptoms similar to those accompanying the anxiety disorders. There are some exceptions to this general finding, most notably the research by Yeudall *et al.* (1983) and Flor-Henry *et al.* (1979), which reported both left frontal and left temporal dysfunction in panic disorder and OCD patients. One possible explanation for these differential results is that these studies employed neuropsychological tests that assess intelligence, verbal abilities, and attention rather than visual and verbal memory. The findings from electrophysiological and brain-imaging assessment techniques suggest that future studies should utilize memory tasks to confirm the presence or absence of temporal lobe dysfunction.

Another factor that may contribute to the contradictory results reported in this chapter is the use of the *Diagnostic and Statistical Manual of Mental Disorders* to classify subjects. As mentioned earlier, with the major revisions that have occurred over the past 20 years, several categories of the anxiety disorders have changed dramatically. A further problem with the classification in the panic disorder literature is that many investigators fail to specify whether the subjects' diagnosis is panic disorder with or without agoraphobia.

Another area of contradiction in this literature is the importance of left versus right hemisphere in the expression of anxiety. One explanation for these differential findings may be that different anxiety disorders, depending on their symptomatology, may involve different functions and subsequently different hemispheres. Unfortunately, because many investigators failed to assess or report subjects' handedness, it is impossible to make definitive conclusions regarding the importance of each hemisphere.

Another major issue that may have confounded many of the studies reviewed is the role of state versus trait anxiety. The findings by Mountz *et al.*

(1989) in their investigation of simply phobia certainly suggest that PET scan can be influenced greatly by hyperventilation, a correlate of state anxiety. Given this, all of the brain imaging studies reviewed in this section must be interpreted cautiously. State anxiety may also influence the neuropsychological performance of patients and, therefore, should be assessed and controlled for in future studies.

Finally, for the majority of the anxiety-based disorders, there has been a limited application of neuropsychological assessment as a correlate of the underlying anxiety disorder. There have also been very few studies utilizing CT scan and MRI scan technology compared to studies utilizing PET scans. This may, in part, reflect an underlying assumption that the presence of anxiety disorders reflects more of a functional change in the CNS rather than a structural change. Certainly what is needed is a stronger interdisciplinary approach across electrophysiological, neuroimaging, and neuropsychological assessment modalities in order to further elucidate the neuropsychological basis of the anxiety disorders.

REFERENCES

Alexander, G. E., DeLong, M. R., & Strick, P. L. (1986). Parallel organization of functionally segregated circuits linking basal ganglia and cortex. *Annual Review of Neuroscience, 9*, 357–381.

American Psychiatric Association. (1952). *Diagnostic and statistical manual of mental disorders* (1st ed.). Washington, D.C.: Author.

American Psychiatric Association. (1968). *Diagnostic and statistical manual of mental disorders* (2nd ed.). Washington, D.C.: Author.

American Psychiatric Association. (1980). *Diagnostic and statistical manual of mental disorders* (3rd ed.). Washington, D.C.: Author.

American Psychiatric Association. (1987). *Diagnostic and statistical manual of mental disorders* (3rd ed. rev.). Washington, D.C.: Author.

Anderson, D. J., Noyes, J., Jr., & Crowe, R. R. (1984). A comparison of panic disorder and generalized anxiety disorder. *American Journal of Psychiatry, 141*, 572–575.

Barlow, D. H. (1988). *Anxiety and its disorders: The nature and treatment of anxiety and panic*. New York: Guilford Press.

Baxter, L. R., Phelps, M. E., Mazziotta, J. C., Guze, B. H., Schwartz, J. M., & Selin, C. E. (1987). Local cerebral glucose metabolic rates in obsessive–compulsive disorder. A comparison with rates in unipolar depression and normal controls. *Archives of General Psychiatry, 44*, 211–218.

Baxter, L. R., Schwartz, J. M., Mazziotta, J. C., Phelps, M. E., Pahl, J. J., Guze, B. H., & Fairbanks, L. (1988). Cerebral glucose metabolic rates in nondepressed patients with obsessive–compulsive disorder. *American Journal of Psychiatry, 145*, 1560–1563.

Beech, H. R. (1971). Ritualistic activity in obsessional patients. *Journal of Psychosomatic Research, 15*, 417–422.

Beech, H. R., Ciesielski, K. T., & Gordon, P. K. (1983). Further observations of evoked potentials in obsessional patients. *British Journal of Psychiatry, 142*, 605–609.

Behar, D., Rapoport, J. L., Berg, C. J., Denkla, M. B., Mann, L., Cox, D., Fedio, B., Zahn, T., & Wolfman, M. G. (1984). Computerized tomography and neuropsychological test measures in adolescents with obsessive–compulsive disorder. *American Journal of Psychiatry, 141*, 363–369.

Blackman, M., & Wheeler, G. H. T. (1987). A case of mistaken identity: A fourth ventricular tumor presenting as school phobia in a 12 year old boy. *Canadian Journal of Psychiatry, 32*, 584–587.

Brodsky, L., Zuniga, J. S., Casenas, E. R., Ernstoff, R., & Sachdev, H. S. (1983). Refractory anxiety: A masked epileptiform disorder? *The Psychological Journal of the University of Ottawa, 8*, 42–45.

Buchsbaum, M. S., Hazlett, E., Sicotte, N., Stein, M., Wu, J., & Zetin, M. (1985). Topographic EEG changes with benzodiazepine administration in generalized anxiety disorder. *Biological Psychiatry, 20,* 832–842.

Buchsbaum, M. S., Wu, J., Haier, R., Hazlett, E., Ball, R., Katz, M., Sokolski, K., Lagunas-Solar, M., & Langer, D. (1987). Positron emission tomography assessment of effects of benzodiazepines on regional glucose metabolic rate in patients with anxiety disorders. *Life Sciences, 40,* 2392–2400.

Buckelew, S. P., & Hannay, H. J. (1986). Relationships among anxiety, defensiveness, sex, task difficulty, and performance on various neuropsychological tasks. *Perceptual and Motor Skills, 63,* 711–718.

Capstick, N., & Seldrup, J. (1973). Phenomenological aspects of obsessional patients treatment with clomipramine. *British Journal of Psychiatry, 112,* 517.

Capstick, N., & Seldrup, J. (1977). Obsessional states: A study in the relationship between abnormalities occurring at the time of birth and the subsequent development of obsessional symptoms. *Acta Psychiatrica Scandinavica, 56,* 427–431.

Carey, G., & Gottesman, I. I. (1981). Twin and family studies of anxiety, phobic and obsessive disorders. In D. F. Klein & J. Rabkin (Eds.), *Anxiety: New research and changing concepts* (pp. 117–135). New York: Raven Press.

Charney, D. S., & Heninger, G. R. (1986). Abnormal regulation of noradrenergic function in panic disorders: Effects of clonidine in healthy subjects and patients with agoraphobia and panic disorder. *Archives of General Psychiatry, 43,* 1042–1054.

Charney, D. S., & Redmond, D. E. (1983). Neurobiological mechanisms in human anxiety: Evidence supporting central noradrenergic hyperactivity. *Neuropharmacology, 22,* 1531–1536.

Charney, D. S., Heninger, G. R., & Breier, A. (1984). Noradrenergic function in panic anxiety: Effects of yohimbine in healthy subjects and patients with agoraphobia and panic disorder. *Archives of General Psychiatry, 41,* 751–763.

Charney, D. S., Heninger, G. R., & Jatlow, P. I. (1985). Increased anxiogenic effects of caffeine in panic disorder. *Archives of General Psychiatry, 42,* 233–243.

Charney, D. S., Goodman, W. K., Price, L. H., Woods, W., Rasmussen, S. A., & Heninger, G. R. (1988). Serotonin function in obsessive–compulsive disorder: A comparison of the effects of tryptophan and chlorophenylpiperazine in patients and healthy subjects. *Archives of General Psychiatry, 45,* 177–185.

Chavez, E. L., Trautt, G. M., Brandon, A., & Steyaert, J. (1983). Effects of test anxiety and sex of subject on neuropsychological test performance: Finger Tapping, Trail Making, Digit Span and Digit Symbol tests. *Perceptual and Motor Skills, 56,* 923–929.

Ciesielski, K. T., Beech, H. R., & Gordon, P. K. (1981). Some electrophysiological observations in obsessional states. *British Journal of Psychiatry, 37,* 1350–1357.

Cloninger, R. C. (1987). A systematic method for clinical description and classification of personality variants: A proposal. *Archives of General Psychiatry, 44,* 573–588.

Costa, E. (1985). Benzodiazepine/GABA interactions: A model to investigate the neurobiology of anxiety. In A. H. Tuma & J. Maser (Eds.), *Anxiety and the anxiety disorders* (pp. 27–52). Hillsdale, N.J.: Erlbaum.

Costa, E., Guidotti, A., & Mao, C. C. (1975). Evidence for involvement of GABA in the action of benzodiazepines: Studies on rat cerebellum. *Advances in Biochemical psychopharmacology, 14,* 113–130.

Crowe, R. R., Noyes, R., Pauls, D. L., & Slymen, D. (1983). A family study of panic disorder. *Archives of General Psychiatry, 40,* 1065–1069.

Cummings, J. L., & Frankel, M. (1985). Gilles de la Tourette syndrome and the neurological basis of obsessions and compulsions. *Biological Psychiatry 20,* 1117–1126.

Dalton, J. E., Pederson, S. L., Blom, B. E., & Besyner, J. K. (1986). Neuropsychological screening for Vietnam veterans with PTSD. *VA Practitioner, July,* 37–47.

Dalton, J. E., Pederson, S. L., & Ryan, J. J. (1989). Effects of post traumatic stress disorder on neuropsychological test performance. *International Journal of Clinical Neuropsychology, 11,* 121–124.

Daniel, M., Haban, G. F., Hutcherson, W. L., Bolter, J., & Long, C. (1985). Neuropsychological and emotional consequences of accidental, high-voltage electrical shock. *The International Journal of Clinical Neuropsychology, 7,* 102–106.

Davidoff, D. A., Kessler, H. R., Laibstain, D. F., & Mark, V. H. (1988). Neurobehavioral sequelae of minor head injury: A consideration of post-concussive syndrome versus post-traumatic stress disorder. *Cognitive Rehabilitation, 6,* 8–13.

Dietch, J. T. (1984). Cerebral tumor presenting with panic attacks. *Psychosomatics, 25,* 861–863.

Edlund, M. J., Swann, A. C., & Clothier, J. (1987). Patients with panic attacks and abnormal EEG results. *American Journal of Psychiatry, 144,* 508–509.

Ehlers, A., Margraf, A., & Roth, W. T. (1986). Experimental induction of panic attacks. In I. Hand & H. V. Wittchen (Eds.), *Panic and phobias: Empirical evidence of theoretical models and long term effects of behavioral treatments,* (pp. 53–66). Berlin: Springer-Verlag.

Epstein, A. W., & Bailine, S. H. (1971). Sleep and dream studies in obsessional neurosis with particular reference to epileptic state. *Biological Psychiatry, 3,* 149–158.

Everly, G. S. (1985, Nov.). Biological foundations of psychiatric sequelae in trauma and stress-related disorders of arousal. Paper presented to the Eighth National Trauma Symposium, University of Maryland School of Medicine, Baltimore.

Everly, G. S. (1987, Oct.). PTSD: A reformation and integration of findings. Paper presented to the Third Annual Meeting of the Society for Traumatic Stress Studies, Baltimore.

Everly, G. S., & Horton, A. M. (1988). Cognitive impairment and post-traumatic stress disorder (PTSD): A neuropsychological perspective. *Bulletin of the National Academy of Neuropsychology, 5,* 1–2.

Figley, C. R. (Ed.). (1978). *Stress disorders among Vietnam veterans.* New York: Brunner–Mazel.

File, S. E., Deakin, J. F. W., Longden, A., & Crow, T. J. (1979). An investigation of the role of the locus coeruleus in anxiety and agonistic behavior. *Brain Research, 169,* 411–420.

Flor-Henry, P., Yeudall, L. T., Koles, Z. J., & Howarth, B. G. (1979). Neuropsychological and power spectral EEG investigations of the obsessive–compulsive syndrome. *Biological Psychiatry, 14,* 119–130.

Fordyce, D. J., Roueche, J. R., & Prigatano, G. P. (1983). Enhanced emotional reactions in chronic head trauma patients. *Journal of Neurology, Neurosurgery, and Psychiatry, 46,* 620–624.

Garoutte, B. (1987). *Survey of functional neuroanatomy.* Greenbrae, Calif.: Jones Medical Publications.

Ghardirian, A. M., Gauthier, S., & Bertrand, S. (1986). Anxiety attacks in a patient with a right temporal lobe meningioma. *Journal of Clinical Psychiatry, 47,* 270–271.

Golden, C. J. (1979). *Clinical interpretation of objective psychological tests.* New York: Grune & Stratton.

Goodwin, D. M. (1989). *A dictionary of neuropsychology.* Berlin: Springer-Verlag.

Gorman, J. M., Askanazi, J., Liebowitz, M. R., Fyer, A. J., Stein, J., Kinney, J. M., & Klein, D. F. (1984). Response to hyperventilation in a group of patients with panic disorder. *American Journal of Psychiatry, 141,* 857–861.

Gray, J. A. (1982). Precis of the neuropsychology of anxiety: An enquiry into the functions of the septo-hippocampal system. *The Behavioral and Brain Sciences, 5,* 469–534.

Gray, J. A. (1985*a*). Issues in the neuropsychology of anxiety. In A. H. Tuma & J. Maser (Eds.), *Anxiety and the anxiety disorders* (pp. 5–25). Hilldale, N.J.: Erlbaum.

Gray, J. A. (1985*b*). A whole and its parts: Behavior, the brain, cognition and emotion. *Bulletin of the British Psychological Society, 38,* 99–112.

Gray, J. A. (1988). The neuropsychological basis of anxiety. In C. G. Last & M. Hersen (Eds.), *Handbook of anxiety disorders.* Elmsford, N.Y.: Pergamon Press.

Grillon, C., & Buchsbaum, M. S. (1987). EEG topography of response to visual stimuli in generalized anxiety disorder. *Electroencephalography and Clinical Neurophysiology, 66,* 337–348.

Grimshaw, L. (1964). Obsessional disorder and neurological illness. *Journal of Neurology, Neurosurgery and Psychiatry, 27,* 229–231.

Haefely, W., Kulcsar, A., Mohler, H., Pieri, L., Polc, P., & Schaffner, R. (1975). Possible involvement of GABA in the central action of benzodiazepines. *Advances in Biochemical Psychopharmacology, 14,* 131–151.

Hamilton, M. (1959). The assessment of anxiety states by rating. *British Journal of Medical Psychology, 32,* 50–55.

Hamilton, M. (1967). Development of a rating scale for primary depressive illness. *British Journal of Social Psychology, 6,* 278–296.

Hillgard, S. A., & Kutas, M. (1983). Electrophysiology of cognitive processing. *Annual Review of Psychology, 34*, 33–61.

Hoehn-Saric, R. (1982). Neurotransmitters in anxiety. *Archives of General Psychiatry, 39*, 735–742.

Horel, J. A., Keating, E. G., & Misantone, L. J. (1975). Partial Kluver–Bucy syndrome produced by destroying temporal neocortical amygdala. *Brain Research, 94*, 349–359.

Insel, T. R., Donnelly, E. F., Lalakea, M. L., Alterman, I. S., & Murphy, D. L. (1983*a*). Neurological and neuropsychological studies of patients with obsessive–compulsive disorder. *Biological Psychiatry, 18*, 741–751.

Insel, T. R., Hoover, C., & Murphy, D. L. (1983*b*). Parents of patients with obsessive–compulsive disorder. *Psychological Medicine, 13*, 807–811.

Jenike, M. A. (1984). Obsessive–compulsive disorder: A question of a neurologic lesion. *Comprehensive Psychiatry, 25*, 298–304.

Jenike, M. A., & Brotman, A. W. (1984). The EEG in obsessive–compulsive disorder. *Journal of Clinical Psychiatry, 45*, 122–124.

Kettl, P. A., & Marks, I. M. (1986). Neurological factors in obsessive compulsive disorder: Two case reports and a review of the literature. *British Journal of Psychiatry, 149*, 315–319.

King, G. D., Hannay, H. J., Masek, B. J., & Burns, J. W. (1978). Effects of anxiety and sex on neuropsychological tests. *Journal of Consulting and Clinical Psychology, 46*, 375–376.

Kolb, B., & Wishaw, I. Q. (1985). *Fundamentals of human neuropsychology*. San Francisco: Freeman.

Kolb, L. C. (1987). A neuropsychological hypothesis explaining posttraumatic stress disorders. *American Journal of Psychiatry, 144*, 989–995.

Koranyi, E. K. (1979). Morbidity and rate of undiagnosed physical illness in a psychiatric clinic population. *Archives of General Psychiatry, 36*, 414–419.

Kuhar, M. J. (1986). Neuroanatomical substrates of anxiety: A brief survey. *Trends in Neurosciences, 9*, 301–311.

Laplane, D., Baulac, M., Widlocher, D., & Dubois, B. (1984). Pure psychic akinesia with bilateral lesions of basal ganglia. *Journal of Neurology, Neurosurgery, and Psychiatry, 47*, 377–385.

LeDoux, J. E., Thompson, M. E., Iadelcola, C., Tucker, L. W., & Reis, D. J. (1983). Local cerebral blood flow increases during auditory and emotional processing in the conscious rat. *Science, 221*, 576–578.

Lezak, M. D. (1983). *Neuropsychological assessments* (2nd ed.). New York: Oxford University Press.

Liebowitz, M. R., Gorman, J. M., Fyer, A. J., Levitt, M., Dillon, D., Levy, G., Appleby, I. L., Anderson, S., Palij, J., Davies, S. O., & Klein, D. F. (1985). Lactate provocation of panic attacks. II. Biochemical and psychological findings. *Archives of General Psychiatry, 42*, 709–719.

Malloy, P. F., Fairbank, J. A., & Keane, T. M. (1983). Validation of a multimethod assessment of posttraumatic stress disorders in Vietnam veterans. *Journal of Consulting and Clinical Psychiatry, 51*, 488–494.

Marks, I. M. (1969). *Fears and phobias*. London: Heineman.

Marks, I. M. (1981). Space "phobia": A pseudoagoraphobic syndrome. *Journal of Neurology, Neurosurgery, and Psychiatry, 44*, 387–391.

Marks, I. M., & Bebbington, P. (1976). Space phobia: Syndrome or agoraphobic variant? *British Medical Journal, 2*, 345–347.

Marks, I. M., Birley, J. L. T., & Gelder, M. G. (1966). Modified leucotomy in severe agoraphobia: A controlled serial inquiry. *British Journal of Psychiatry, 112*, 757–769.

Martin, N. J., & Franzen, M. D. (1989). The effect of anxiety on neuropsychological function. *International Journal of Clinical Neuropsychology, 11*, 1–8.

Matarazzo, J. D. (1972). *Wechsler's measurement and appraisal of adult intelligence* (5th ed.). New York: Oxford University Press.

McCaffrey, R. J., & Fairbank, J. A., (1985). Behavioral assessment and treatment of accident related post-traumatic stress disorder: Two case studies. *Behavior Therapy, 16*, 406–416.

McCaffrey, R. J., Hickling, E. J., & Marazzo, M. J. (1989). Civilian-related posttraumatic stress disorder: Assessment-related issues. *Journal of Clinical Psychology, 45*, 72–76.

McCaffrey, R. J., Rapee, R. M., Gansler, D. A., & Barlow, D. H. (1990). Interaction of neuropsychological and psychological factors in two cases of "space phobia." *Journal of Behavior Therapy and Experimental Psychiatry, 21*, 113–120.

McKeon, J. P., McGuffin, P., & Robinson, P. (1984*a*). Obsessive–compulsive neurosis following head injury: A report of four cases. *British Journal of Psychiatry, 144,* 190–192.

McKeon, J. P., Roa, B., & Mann, A. (1984*b*). Life events and personality traits in obsessive–compulsive neurosis. *British Journal of Psychiatry, 144,* 185–189.

Mettler, F. A. (1955). Perceptual capacity. Functions of the corpus striatum and schizophrenia. *Psychiatric Quarterly, 29,* 89–111.

Mountz, J. M., Modell, J. G., Wilson, M. W., Curtis, G. C., Lee, Y. L., Schmaltz, S., & Kohl, D. E. (1989). Positron emission tomographic evaluation of cerebral blood flow during state anxiety in simple phobia. *Archives of General Psychiatry, 46,* 501–504.

Mulder, D. W., & Daly, D. (1952). Psychiatric symptoms associated with lesions of the temporal lobe. *Journal of the American Medical Association, 150,* 173–176.

Myers, J. K., Weissman, M. M., Tischler, G. L., Holzer, C. E., III, Leaf, P. J., Orvaschel, H., Anthony, J. C., Boyd, J. H., Burke, J. D., Jr., Kramer, M., & Stoltzman, R. (1984). Six month prevalence of psychiatric disorders in three communities. *Archives of General Psychiatry, 41,* 959–967.

Nee, L. E., Caine, E. D., Polinsky, R. J., Eldridge, R., & Ebert, M. H. (1980). Gilles de la Tourette syndrome: Clinical and family study of 50 cases. *Annals of Neurology, 7,* 41–49.

Nieuwenhuys, R., Vooad, J., & VanHuitzen, C. (1981). *The human central nervous system, a synopsis and atlas* (2nd ed.). Berlin: Springer-Verlag.

Novack, T. A., Daniel, M. S., & Long, C. J. (1984). Factors related to emotional adjustment following head injury. *The International Journal of Clinical Neuropsychology, 6,* 139–142.

Nowak, S. M., & Marczynski, T. J. (1981). Trait anxiety is reflected in EEG alpha response to stress. *Electroencephalography and Clinical Neurophysiology, 52,* 175–191.

Noyes, R., Jr., Anderson, D. J., Clancy, J., Crowe, R. R., Slyren, D. J., Ghoreim, M. M., & Hinrich, J. V. (1984). Diazepam and propanolol in panic disorder and agoraphobia. *Archives of General Psychiatry, 41,* 287–292.

Oddy, M., Coughlan, T., Tyerman, A., & Jenkins, D. (1985). Social adjustment after closed head injury: A further follow-up seven years after injury. *Journal of Neurology, Neurosurgery, and Psychiatry, 48,* 564–568.

Overall, J. E., & Gorham, D. R. (1962). The Brief Psychiatric Rating Scale. *Psychological Reports, 10,* 799–812.

Pitts, F. N., & McClure, J. N. (1967). Lactate metabolism in anxiety neurosis. *New England Journal of Medicine, 277,* 1329–1336.

Prigatano, G. P. (1987). Personality and psychosocial consequences after brain injury. In: M. Meir, L. Dillard, & A. Benton (Eds.), *Neuropsychological rehabilitation* (pp. 355–378). London: Churchill Livingstone.

Raichle, M. E. (1983). Positron emission tomography. *Annual Review of Neuroscience, 6,* 249–267.

Rapoport, J., Elkins, R., Langer, D. H., Sceery, W., Buchsbaum, M. S., Gillon, J. C., Murphy, D. L., Zahn, T. P., Lake, R., Ludlow, C., & Mendelson, W. (1981). Childhood obsessive–compulsive disorder. *American Journal of Psychiatry, 138,* 1545–1554.

Redmond, D. E., & Huang, Y. H. (1979). New evidence for a locus coeruleus–norepinephrine connection with anxiety. *Life Sciences, 25,* 2149–2162.

Redmond, D. E., Huang, Y. H., Snyder, D. R., & Maas, J. W. (1976). Behavioral effects of stimulation of the nucleus locus coeruleus in the stump-tailed monkey. *Brain Research, 116,* 502–510.

Reiman, E. M. (1987). The study of panic disorder using positron emission tomography. *Psychiatric Developments, 1,* 63–78.

Reiman, E. M., Raichle, M. E., Butler, F. K., Herscovitch, P., & Robins, E. (1984). A focal brain abnormality in panic disorder, a severe form of anxiety. *Nature, 310,* 683–685.

Reiman, E. M., Raichle, M. E., Robins, E., Butler, F. K., Herscovitch, P., Fox, P., & Perlmutter, J. (1986). The application of positron emission tomography to see the study of panic disorder. *American Journal of Psychiatry, 143,* 469–477.

Reiman, E. M., Fusselman, M. J., Fox, P. T., & Raichle, M. E. (1989*a*). Neuroanatomical correlates of anticipatory anxiety. *Science, 24,* 1071–1073.

Reiman, E. M., Raichle, M. E., Robins, E., Mintun, M. A., Fusselman, M. J., Fox, P. I., Price, J. L., & Hackman, K. A. (1989*b*). Neuroanatomical correlates of a lactate induced anxiety attack. *Archives of General Psychiatry, 46,* 493–500.

Reitan, R. M. (1959). *The effects of brain lesions on adaptive abilities in human beings*. Indianapolis Mimeographic Reproduction.

Rinieris, P. M., Stefanis, C. N., Rabavilas, A. D., & Vaidakis, N. W. (1978). Obsessive–compulsive neurosis anancastic symptomatology and ABO blood types. *Acta Psychiatrica Scandinavica, 57*, 377–381.

Rosvold, H. E. (1968). The prefrontal cortex and caudate nucleus: A system for effecting correction in response mechanisms. In C. Rupp (Ed.), *Mind as a tissue* (pp. 21–38). New York: Harper & Row.

Roth, M. (1959). The phobic anxiety–depersonalization syndrome (abridged). *Proceedings of the Royal Society of Medicine, 21*, 587–595.

Sarason, I. G. (1972). Experimental approaches to test anxiety: Attention and the uses of information. In C. D. Spielberger (Ed.)., *Anxiety: Current trends in theory and research* (pp. 383–403). New York: Academic Press.

Schneider, J. S. (1984). Basal ganglia role in behaviors: Importance of sensory gating and its relevance to psychiatry. *Biological Psychiatry, 19*, 1693–1701.

Shagass, C., Roemer, R. A., Straumanis, J. J., & Amadeo, M. (1979). Spatial distribution of sensory evoked potentials in psychiatric disorders. In E. Callaway & D. Lehmann (Eds.), *Human evoked potential: Applications and problems* (pp. 347–362). New York: Plenum Press.

Shagass, C., Roemer, R. A., Straumanis, J. J., & Josiassen, R. C. (1984*a*). Evoked potentials in obsessive–compulsive disorder. *Advanced Biological Psychiatry, 15*, 69–75.

Shagass, C., Roemer, R. A., Straumanis, J. J., & Josiassen, R. C. (1984*b*). Distinctive somatosensory evoked potential features in obsessive–compulsive disorder. *Biological Psychiatry, 19*, 1507–1524.

Siciliani, O., Schiavon, M., & Tansella, M. (1975). Anxiety and EEG alpha activity in neurotic patients: Baseline correlations and changes during a double-blind trial with Temazepam. *Acta Psychiatrica Scandinavica, 52*, 116–131.

Spielberger, C. D. (1983). *Manual for the State-Trait Anxiety Inventory* (STAI Form Y). Available from Consulting Psychologists Press, Palo Alto, Calif.).

Spielberger, C. D., Gorsuch, R. W., & Luschene, R. E. (1970). *State Trait Anxiety Inventory*. Palo Alto, Calif.: Consulting Psychologists Press.

Stewart, R. S., Devous, M. D., Rush, A. J., Lane, L., & Bonte, F. J. (1988). Cerebral blood flow changes during sodium-lactate-induced panic attacks. *American Journal of Psychiatry, 145*, 442–449.

Strub, R. L., & Black, F. W. (1988). *Neurobehavioral disorders: A clinical approach*. Philadelphia: Davis.

Tan, E., Marks, I. M., & Marset, P. (1971). Bimedial leucotomy in obsessive–compulsive neurosis: A controlled *serial* enquiry. *British Journal of Psychiatry, 118*, 155–164.

Taylor, C. B., & Arnow, B. (1988). *The nature and treatment of anxiety disorders*. New York: Free Press.

Torgensen, S. (1983). Genetic factors in anxiety disorders. *Archives of General Psychiatry, 40*, 1085–1089.

Wechsler, D. (1987). *Wechsler Memory Scale—Revised*. New York: Psychological Corporation.

Weilburg, J. B., Bear, D. M., & Sachs, G. (1987). Three patients with concomitant panic attacks and seizure disorder: Possible clues to the neurology of anxiety. *American Journal of Psychiatry, 144*, 1053–1056.

Weissman, M. M. (1985). The epidemiology of anxiety disorders: Rates, risks, and familial patterns. In A. H. Tuma & J. D. Maser (Eds.), *Anxiety and the anxiety disorders* (pp. 275–296). Hillsdale, N.J.: Erlbaum.

Williamson, P. D., Allison, T., Goff, W. R., & Mattson, R. H. (1977). Evoked potential abnormalities in epilepsy: The E-wave. *Electroencephalography and Clinical Neurophysiology, 4*, 729–730.

Yaryura-Tobias, J. A., Neziroglu, F., & Bhagavan, H. N. (1979). Obsessive–compulsive disorders: A serotonergic hypothesis. In B. Saletu, P. Bener, & L. Hollister (Eds.), *Neuro-psychopharmacology Proceedings of the 11th Congress of the Collegium Internationale Neuro-Psychopharmacologium* (pp. 117–126). Elmsford, N.Y.: Pergamon Press.

Yeudall, L. T., Schopflocher, D., Sussman, P. S., Barabash, W., Warneke, L. B., Gill, D., Otto, W., Howarth, B., & Termansen, P. E. (1983). Panic attack syndrome with and without agoraphobia: Neuropsychological and evoked potential correlates. In P. Flor-Henry & J. Gruzelier (Eds.), *Laterality and psychopathology* (pp. 195–216). Amsterdam: Elsevier.

9

Depressive Disorders

PETER J. NEWMAN and JERRY J. SWEET

INTRODUCTION

Until recently, the "conventional wisdom" within the field of neuropsychology was that depression had little or no impact upon neuropsychological test performance. In many of the currently influential neuropsychology textbooks, depression is either not dealt with (e.g., Golden, 1981) or is dismissed as an insignificant variable. For example, Reitan and Wolfson (1985) state that "a severe and clinically significant degree of depression . . . usually seem[s] to be irrelevant to interpretation of neuropsychological test findings." There has been a growing body of research in recent years, however, that clearly challenges this long-held belief. Studies with ability tests and neuropsychological measures with psychiatric populations have been accumulating and growing interest in this area has recently spawned a flurry of research showing that depression can have a significant impact upon neuropsychological test performance.

Neurologically impaired individuals struggle with depression at some time in their illness, either in response to loss of function and self-esteem or as a result of damage to brain structures responsible for mediating emotion (e.g., Reifler, Larson, & Hanley, 1982; Robinson, Starr, Kubos, & Price, 1983). Among psychiatric populations, depression is the most frequently occurring emotional disorder (e.g., Lipkin, 1985; Weissman & Boyd, 1985). Since depression is ubiquitous in the clinical populations with which neuropsychologists work, its potential for confounding test performance needs to be addressed and steps taken to identify its effects on neuropsychological measures. The purpose of this chapter will be to review the general research in the area of depressive deficits. We will attempt to: outline the types of deficits seen in depressed and

PETER J. NEWMAN • Illinois State Psychiatric Institute, Chicago, Illinois 60612-4397. JERRY J. SWEET • Evanston Hospital and Northwestern University, Evanston, Illinois 60201.

HANDBOOK OF NEUROPSYCHOLOGICAL ASSESSMENT: A Biopsychosocial Perspective, edited by Antonio E. Puente and Robert J. McCaffrey. Plenum Press, New York, 1992.

pseudodemented patients, clarify the relative influence of such variables as severity and subtype of depression, consider the neurobiological substrates for these deficits, discuss four neurological conditions in which depression is common, and provide case examples that illustrate the diverse clinical presentation of depression on neuropsychological measures.

HISTORICAL FOUNDATIONS

The term *psychological deficits* was first coined by Hunt and Cofer (1944) to describe the impaired performance of psychiatric patients on intellectual and laboratory tasks. Although specific interest in depressive deficits was never great, the accumulating fragmentary and often inconsistent findings clearly documented the frequently striking impact of depression upon test performance (Miller, 1975). Perhaps the greatest impetus for research into depressive deficits was the need for neuropsychologists to validate their measures with psychiatric populations. Much of this research initially focused upon the use of these tests with schizophrenic patients, since their striking cognitive disturbance could so obviously influence test performance. The much less conspicuous depressive symptoms did not attract as much research attention. Of the many studies investigating the accuracy of neuropsychological tests in diagnosing psychiatric patients, only 5 of the 94 published between 1960 and 1975 examined affective disorders (Heaton, Baade, & Johnson, 1978). Of the 14 additional studies of this type published between 1975 and 1978, only 2 were concerned with depressive disorders (Heaton & Crowley, 1981). Until recently, there has been no systematic research to explore the specific impact of depression upon neuropsychological test performance. The growing awareness of the significance of this area is attested to by the burgeoning number of studies published in the past several years.

By and large, studies of the effects of depression upon neuropsychological test performance have made use of clinically depressed samples and have compared these samples with normal, brian-damaged, schizophrenic, and mixed psychiatric controls. Several studies have also examined the effects of depression in medically ill or brain-damaged subjects. The depressed subjects have been variously defined as meeting DSM-III or RDC criteria for the depressive syndrome, or as exceeding some cutoff on standardized depression measures (e.g., Hamilton Depression Rating Scale, Beck Depression Inventory, Schedule for Affective Disorders and Schizophrenia). Severity of depression has ranged from mildly depressed college students to severely depressed psychiatric inpatients. The subjects have primarily been adults, although both children and the elderly have also been studied. While a significant literature exists with regard to laboratory studies of experimentally induced depression (e.g., Singer & Salovey, 1988), the present chapter will be concerned only with clinical depression.

Methodological Issues

In his review of the literature on depressive deficits, Miller (1975) noted several important methodological problems. He observed that the tremendous variety of tests employed in the already published studies, the frequently inadequate specification of diagnoses, and the use of differing diagnostic criteria have all made the comparison of findings across studies nearly impossible. He also noted that few studies directly compared the performance of different types of depressives on the same task. His emphasis on the need for standardization of diagnostic criteria and neuropsychological measures, as well as the need for greater methodological rigor, was well taken. Nearly 15 years later, Miller's criticisms still seem appropriate.

A more specific consideration of the methodological deficiencies seen in individual studies in this area has been provided by Heaton *et al.* (1978). Eight frequently observed problems that obscure the findings in the studies were reviewed. Almost all of the studies reviewed failed to adequately deal with three or more of these eight important criteria. Heaton *et al.* noted the common failure of researchers: (1) to clearly indicate that their subjects were representative of any specific clinical population; (2) to mention whether neurological clinical exams or laboratory procedures had been performed on the so-called "functional" psychiatric patients to rule out brain dysfunction; (3) to use clearly specified diagnostic criteria in establishing the psychiatric diagnoses and to mention the credentials and level of training of the clinicians making the evaluations; (4) to indicate whether or not the initial or the discharge diagnosis was used in subject selection; (5) to make reference to whether neurological diagnoses, when made, were done by a qualified physician using appropriate clinical and laboratory procedures; (6) to report or control for chronicity and to mention whether the subject groups were comparable with regard to age and education; (7) to report or control for somatic treatments used; and (8) to recognize and avoid the confound involved in using IQ tests to match subjects on level of intellectual functioning, since these tests are sensitive to brain pathology as well.

While, overall, the level of research has significantly improved since the publication of these reviews, there still continues to be problems that frequently render the findings of neuropsychological studies of depression uninterpretable. The adoption of *Diagnostic and Statistical Manual–Revised* (DSM-III-R) (American Psychiatric Association, 1987) and the widespread use of the Research Diagnostic Criteria (RDC) (Spitzer, Endicott, & Robins, 1978) have resulted in a tremendous improvement in the reliability of diagnoses within and across studies. It is therefore troublesome that several recent studies have utilized other criteria for assigning subjects to the depression group. For example, some studies have used measures such as the BDI and MMPI to define their depressives, even though there is inconsistent evidence to suggest that severity of depression, as measured by these instruments, correlates with severity of deficits in test performance. As will be discussed later, there is substantial evidence to show that the presence of a diagnosable depressive disorder is strongly related to impaired neuropsychological test findings.

Neuropsychological Effects of Depression

The effects of depression upon neuropsychological test performance can range from the striking and extreme, as seen in the severe deficits of patients with depressive pseudodementia, to the very subtle and minimal impairments seen in patients suffering from mild to moderate depressions. As will be seen, it appears that there is a continuum of severity of deficits between these two extremes, while the types of deficits remain essentially the same. In the following section, the pseudodementia syndrome will be described as an example of the most extreme manifestation of depressive deficits. This will be followed by a review of the literature on depressive deficits in general, with the goals of (1) clarifying the types of deficits frequently seen in depression, (2) identifying those measures that may be most useful in discriminating depression from other disorders, and (3) discussing the impact on test performance of several important variables such as depressive subtype and severity.

Pseudodementia

The term *pseudodementia* has been attributed to Madden, Luhan, Kaplan, and Manfredi (1952), who first described the phenomenon in a discussion of nondementing psychoses in the elderly. The term was initially used to refer to patients who presented with both depression *and* dementialike symptoms. It has become widely recognized, however, that pseudodementia can occur in association with a variety of diverse psychiatric disorders in addition to depression (e.g., Caine, 1981; McAllister, 1983), and, even though most often seen in the elderly, is not limited to the elderly (e.g., Friedman & Lipowski, 1981). Thus, as the term is currently used, pseudodementia is a condition in which patients of any age present with dementialike symptoms when the complaints and appearance suggestive of a pathologically diminished level of abilities actually are due to psychiatric disorder. Wells (1979) has described the condition as ". . . a caricature or burlesque, not an imitation, of dementia." However, as noted by McAllister (1985), pseudodementia is not a homogeneous syndrome; in some patients the clinical picture is a "caricature," while in others the cognitive impairment is quite similar to that seen in true dementia. Pulling together a number of salient features, Caine's (1981) criteria-based definition may be the most practical: (1) intellectual impairment in patients with a primary psychiatric disorder, (2) intellectual abnormalities that at least partially resemble true brain-based cognitive deficit, (3) reversibility of the dementia, and (4) no identifiable neuropathological disorder.

The clinical problem presented by pseudodementia stems from the difficulty in clearly establishing the correct diagnosis. Very different treatment implications are associated with each diagnosis. Despite tremendous technological advances in neuroimaging and bioassay methods, there are still no specific anatomical or other objective referents of dementia. Diagnosis of dementia has remained a clinical judgment based largely on patient history, observed and measurable behavioral and cognitive changes, and congruity of medical tests of brain integrity. If a psychiatric patient is incorrectly diagnosed as being demented, then important potentially beneficial treatment may be withheld from the patient. Conversely, a demented patient may be given treatment inappropriately for a psychiatric condition that may place unrealistic expectations on the patient, perhaps even creating an environment that produces depression, while preventing the patient and family from dealing with the important issues and implications associated with the diagnosis of dementia.

Various investigators have attempted to determine how often diagnostic errors are made with regard either to demented patients being diagnosed incorrectly as suffering from psychiatric disorder, or to psychiatric patients being diagnosed incorrectly as demented. Studies that have retrospectively followed up on patients originally diagnosed as having dementia have reported a range of incorrect diagnoses of 8 to 35%, with these patients ultimately receiving psychiatric diagnoses (e.g., Haward, 1977; Kendell, 1974; Marsden & Harrison, 1972; Nott & Fleminger, 1975; Ron, Toone, Garralda, & Lishman, 1979). A wide range also has been reported in studies that have investigated the reverse circumstance, the diagnosis of depression that actually turns out to be dementia. In these studies the number of mistaken diagnoses has been between 3 and 30% (e.g., Kendell, 1974; Gustafson, 1975; Liston, 1977; Zeigler, 1954).

Of course, such studies should *not* suggest that clinicians should consider these conditions to be mutually exclusive; depression and pseudodementia can, and do, occur in patients with actual brain dysfunction (e.g., Feinberg & Goodman, 1984). In such cases, the deficits caused by the brain disorder may be exacerbated, and conversely, with treatment for emotional disorder the patient's overall neuropsychological presentation may be significantly improved. Based on a study of geriatric outpatients, Reifler *et al.* (1982) estimated that cognitive impairment and depression may coexist 20 to 25% of the time. In reviewing a number of studies reporting coexistence of depression and dementia in the elderly, as well as the prevalence of each condition in the elderly, Teri and Reifler (1987) estimated that between 1 and 4% of all individuals over 65 years of age suffer depression and dementia simultaneously. This figure compares to an estimated 9% of all persons over age 65 suffering from depression (Gallagher & Thompson, 1983) and an estimated 10% of all persons over age 65 suffering from dementia (Zarit & Zarit, 1983). While these data on the elderly serve to illustrate the point that depression and dementia primarily caused by Alzheimer's disease often coexist, this phenomenon is not limited to the elderly or to a particular etiology; such can be the case for younger individuals with other brain disorders as well.

As mentioned earlier, depression is not the only emotional or psychiatric disturbance known to cause pseudodementia. The variety of case reports and clinical observations in the literature (Caine, 1981; McAllister, 1983; Koenigsberg, 1984; McEvoy & Wells, 1979), as well as clinical experience of the present authors, suggest that disorders that result in emotional states and behavioral responses related to passivity, helplessness, avoidance, and anxiety (including somatic anxiety/hypochondriasis) can also cause pseudodementia. It should not be surprising, then, to see pseudodementia in patients with personality disorders, such as, but not limited to, the histrionic, borderline, dependent, passive–aggressive, self-defeating, and obsessive–compulsive types. Additionally, anxiety disorders and some psychotic states can produce pseudodementia (Madden *et al.*, 1952).

Numerous clinicians have described the variable features that often distinguish between depression and dementia. A compilation of these features is presented in Table 9.1.

Types of Deficits Seen in Depressive Disorders

Findings of deficits in clinically depressed individuals appear to cluster around three major areas of impairment: psychomotor speed, motivation and attention (sustained effort and concentration), and memory and learning. Indeed, this clustering seems appropriate since these areas encompass the major symptoms of the depressive syndrome.

Psychomotor Retardation. Slowed motor and mental functioning are among the most consistent findings in the literature on depression (e.g., Nelson & Charney, 1981) and are included among diagnostic criteria for several depressive subtypes (DSM-III-R, RDC). As would be expected, the effects of psychomotor slowing have been seen in studies examining depressives' performance on a variety of timed neuropsychological tests (Blackburn, 1975; Miller, 1975; Newman & Sweet, 1986; Rush, Weissenburger, Vinson, & Giles, 1983; Shipley, Kupfer, Spiker, Shaw, Coble, Neil, & Cofsky, 1981; Weckowicz, Nutter, Cruise, Yonge, & Cairns, 1978). Some investigators have posited slowed mental and motor speed to be the cause of all depressive deficits (Weckowicz *et al.*, 1978), although findings of cognitive deficits on measures presumably not affected by speed of performance have led others to disagree (e.g., Abrams & Taylor, 1987).

The impact of psychomotor retardation upon test performance has led to some controversy over the interpretation of certain test findings in depression. For example, based upon the research showing that depressives tend to do poorly on tasks of visuospatial functioning [such as the Trailmaking Test and the Tactual Performance Test (e.g., Gray, Dean, Rattan, & Cramer, 1987)], some investigators have concluded that depression is associated with right parietal lobe brain impairment (Abrams & Taylor, 1987). Since these and many other such tests of visuospatial abilities are also timed, however, it remains unclear whether poor performance in depressives is simply an "artifact" of the psychomotor retardation commonly seen in depression, or whether it is due to underlying right hemisphere impairment.

TABLE 9.1. Features That May Distinguish Depression from Dementia[a]

Feature	Primary depression	Primary dementia
General features	Family aware of illness	Family often unaware of illness
	Onset more acute and can be dated	Insidious onset, only vaguely dated
	Symptoms of short duration	Symptoms of long duration
	Rapid progression	Slow progression
	Family history of affective disorder	Possible family history of dementia
Patient's history	Past history of depression	No history of depression
	Seeks help with complaints of memory loss	Few complaints of memory loss
	Complaints given in great detail	Vague, nonspecific complaints
	Cognitive deficits emphasized	Cognitive deficits concealed
	Failings highlighted by patient	Accomplishments highlighted by patient
Mental state observations	History consistent and sequential	Inconsistent history with poor temporal sequencing
	Patient makes little effort on tasks	Patient struggles with tasks
	Patient readily gives up on tasks	Efforts sustained and may use cue, aids, notes, or evasions
	Subjective distress common	Unconcerned attitude common
	Affective symptoms pervasive	Affect may be shallow or labile
	Complaints greater than observed dysfunction	Observed dysfunction greater than complaints
Cognitive testing	"I don't know" answers typical	Frequent "near-miss" answers
	"Don't know" answers in orientation	Orientation tests poor
	Recent and remote memory loss are equal	Recent memory worse than remote memory
	Poor memory for specific periods common	No gaps in memory
	Concentration worse than general knowledge and memory testing	Memory and general knowledge worse than concentration
	Test performance may be highly variable	More consistently poor performance
	No typical WAIS pattern	WAIS performance scores worse than verbal scores
Neurological examination	No primitive, frontal release reflexes	Primitive frontal lobe reflexes may be present
	No dyspraxias or agnosias	Dyspraxias and agnosias common
	No language difficulties and will correct word intrusions	Word finding problems common and may demonstrate word intrusions
	Cerebral CAT scan normal	CAT scan usually abnormal with increased ventricular size

[a]Modified from McLean (1978) with permission.

Motivational and Attentional Deficits. It is reasonable to expect that lack of energy, low motivation, negative self-assessment, and poor attention and concentration—all cardinal symptoms of depression—might significantly affect neuropsychological test performance. Indeed, clinical reports emphasizing the frequent difficulty in engaging depressed patients in testing and seeking appropriate levels of motivation may be found in the literature (e.g., Heaton & Heaton, 1981; Lezak, 1983).

The meaning and significance of reduced motivation for depressives' test performance have been viewed from several different perspectives. Depressive deficits may, for example, be seen as being artifacts of the reduced concentration and attention so common to depressive disorders. In a similar vein, some have speculated that depressives do more poorly on ability tests because they use more conservative response strategies (Hale & Strickland, 1976). The role of depression in enhancing fatigue effects, particularly in the elderly, and thereby reducing performance levels has also been explored (Kennely, Hayslip, & Richardson, 1985). Still others have focused on depressives' tendency to negatively self-evaluate, highlighting the impact of learned helplessness and negative self-perception in affecting test performance (Marcopulos, 1987; Popkin, Gallagher, Thompson, & Moore, 1982; West, Boatwright, & Schlester, 1984; Williams, Little, Scates, & Blockman, 1987). This latter view asserts that elderly depressed patients, in particular, may complain of deficits, even though their performance is strictly normal. Support for the role of reduced motivation is also offered by studies finding that reaction times of depressives improve when they are given positive feedback about their performance and when they are instructed to relax before proceeding, whereas the reaction times of brain-damaged patients do not improve with such feedback (Adams, Craig, & Parsons, 1986).

The most comprehensive examination of these motivational deficits has been offered by Cohen, Weingartner, Smallberg, Pickar, and Murphy (1982) who assert that the neuropsychological impairments seen in depressives are the result of a neurochemically mediated deficit in a "central motivational state." According to this viewpoint, depressed individuals do more poorly on tasks requiring increasing levels of sustained effort and concentration, and, therefore, perform better on minimally demanding tasks.

Memory and Learning. Memory functioning in depression has been perhaps the most extensively studied of all the areas and is probably the most documented of the depressive deficits. It has frequently been found that patients suffering from depression do more poorly than normals on memory tasks, although they do not do as poorly as brain-damaged (e.g., Kopelman, 1986) or schizophrenic subjects (Malec, 1978). Similarly, studies of memory performance during and after episodes of depression consistently reveal significantly more memory deficits while depressed, with return to normal levels of memory functioning following remission of the depressive symptoms (Frith, Stevens, Johnstone, Deakin, Lawler, & Crow, 1983; Johansen, Gustafson, & Risberg,

1985; Staton, Wilson, & Brumback, 1981; Sternberg & Jarvik, 1976; Sweet, 1983). Deficits have been found on virtually every standardized memory test in clinical use, including the Wechsler Memory Scale (e.g., Stromgren, 1977), the Wechsler Memory Scale–Revised (e.g., Wechsler, 1987), the Benton Visual Retention Test (e.g., Zung & Krugman, 1968), Paired Associates (Kopelman, 1986), and a variety of smaller and less widely known measures of immediate and delayed memory (e.g., Cronholm and Ottoson, 1961), serial-learning and free recall (e.g., Miller, 1975), short-term memory (e.g., Sternberg & Jarvik, 1976), and recognition memory (e.g., Watts, Morris, & MacLeod, 1987), to name just a few. As noted earlier, the memory deficits for depressives are rarely as severe as for brain-damaged subjects (e.g., Kopelman, 1986), although they are often significant and can pose potential problems for differential diagnosis (Newman & Sweet, 1986), especially among the elderly (e.g., Teri & Reifler, 1987).

Findings of memory deficits have by no means been conclusive, however, as a number of studies have failed to discover them in clinically depressed samples (e.g., Gass & Russell, 1986). In fact, one interesting line of research with elderly depressed individuals has found that depressives negatively assess their abilities and report deficits even when none actually exist (e.g., Popkin *et al.*, 1982). Typically, these studies examine the self-assessments of memory impairment in addition to actual measures of memory functioning.

Since the neuropsychologist is most frequently confronted with the task of differentiating depression (sometimes in the form of pseudodementia) from dementia, the remainder of this section will explore what is currently known about features of memory functioning that may be used to discriminate between these two groups. Research suggests that four types of memory/learning tasks may be useful: incidental versus intentional learning (Hart, Kwentus, Wade, & Hamer, 1987), recognition versus recall memory (Calev & Erwin, 1985), easy versus hard paired associate learning (Kopelman, 1986), and recall for random versus related word lists (Weingartner & Silberman, 1982).

Incidental versus intentional learning. Depressives have been found to do more poorly when they are directed to learn or remember new information (intentional learning) as opposed to when the new information is learned incidentally. Incidental learning is by its nature a relatively effortless task, since the subject is not asked to try to remember that material. Hart *et al.* (1987) followed the administration of the Digit Symbol subtest of the WAIS-R by asking their elderly subjects to remember the symbols associated with each of the numbers. It was found that although both DAT and depressed patients were comparable in their slowed performance on the Digit Symbol test, the depressives revealed significantly better incidental memory than the DAT patients, recalling more of the symbols and correctly pairing them with the numbers. The depressives also did significantly worse than normals. None of the DAT patients in this study recalled more than two of the ten pairs of symbols and numbers. The poor performance of the DAT patients on both the Digit Symbol subtest and the test of incidental memory was interpreted as being due to brain impairment preventing new learning. Slowed functioning on the Digit Symbol test, but better performance on the relatively easier incidental memory measure, was taken to reflect a general deficit in motivational state wherein depressives do better on tasks requiring less sustained effortful processing.

The mild to moderate impairment of depressives on measures of incidental memory from the Halstead–Reitan Battery (TPT Location and Memory scores) (Gray *et al.*, 1987) indicates that depressives do worse than normals. Demented patients have poorer recall of the shapes and their relative positions on the TPT formboard. Further research will be needed to validate the usefulness of incidental memory tests in differential diagnosis with depressed patients.

Recognition versus recall. Calev and Erwin (1985) examined the performance of depressives, normals, and DAT patients on both recall and recognition tasks. They found that normals performed equally well on both the recall and the recognition tests, while the DAT subjects did equally poorly on both, performing in the significantly impaired range. Depressives, on the other hand, did poorly on only the recall test. Two explanations were offered for these findings. One explanation was along the lines of the one proposed by Hart *et al.* above (e.g., that the recognition task required significantly less effort than the recall task). Whereas the DAT patients' poor performance on both tasks was seen as being due to brain damage, the poor performance of the depressives was hypothesized to be related to motivational factors. Calev and Erwin offered another interesting interpretation of the findings, that the depressives' poorer performance on recall tasks may be due to an underlying associative disturbance that led to a reduction in the clustering of free recall information. Presumably, depressives do not do as well as normals on the recall task because they are less able to organize the words meaningfully to assist recall. When structure is provided, as it is during the recognition task, they are able to do better.

Other investigators, in contrast, have found deficits in recognition memory in depressed individuals (e.g., Watts *et al.*, 1987), although the severity of the impairments relative to neurologically impaired patients was not evaluated. When compared to brain-damaged subjects, depressives have been found to exhibit significantly better word recognition memory, although their performance was significantly worse than normal controls (Coughlan & Hollows, 1984). There were no group differences between depressed, normal, and brain-damaged subjects, however, on a facial recognition task. Further research will clearly be needed to validate the clinical effectiveness of these measures in differentiating depressed from neurological patients.

Easy versus hard paired associate learning. The ability of depressives' memory performance to benefit from external structure has also been reported for paired associate learning tasks (Kopelman, 1986). Kopelman found that normal, depressed, and Korsakoff patients all did equally well in learning very easy word pairs, while only the DAT patients, because of their very impaired learning ability, did poorly on this simple task. For the more difficult word pairs, however, the depressives and Korsakoff patients did not do as well as the normals, although none did as poorly as the DAT patients. The findings that the depressives did better on the easy versus hard word pairs, while the DATs did poorly on both, are consistent with the interpretation given by Calev and Erwin (1985) for performance on recognition versus recall tasks. Again, the depressives appear to do better remembering related word pairs, but do more poorly when they must provide their own strategies for pairing unrelated words.

Recall for related versus unrelated word lists. Weingartner and Silberman (1982) believe that the form of the learning and memory impairment in dementia patients is quite different from that seen in depressed patients. They have found that depressives do better at remembering semantically related word lists (e.g., lists of words having to do with animals or vegetables) than lists of unrelated words, whereas patients in the early stages of progressive dementia do equally poorly on both kinds of tasks. The difficulty of depressives in learning the unrelated words was presumed to be due to their difficulty imposing organization on a task that lacked easily discernible internal structure. The inherent structure provided by the semantically related word list was enough to help them overcome this difficulty. The dementing patients, on the other hand, were not able to make use of the organizational or semantic relational properties as an aid in encoding the information and, as a result, showed no improvement in learning or memory with increased organization. The finding that depressives, but not DAT patients, can make better use of cognitive organizational strategies to facilitate memory has been reported by other investigators as well (Adams *et al.*, 1986).

Miscellaneous Deficits. There is also preliminary research suggesting that performance on vocabulary tests and on productive naming tests may be helpful in discriminating depressed from dementing patients, although more research will be needed to validate these findings.

Productive naming. When compared to dementia patients, depressives have been found to be able to name a greater number of words that are related to each other, either by starting with the same letter (i.e., "say as many words as you can beginning with the letter c") or by being part of a larger category of information (e.g., types of flowers or parts of a house) (Weingartner, Cohen, Martello, & Gerdt, 1981). In fact, depressives and normals appear to do better at listing words that are related to categories than words beginning with a certain letter, while progressive dementia patients show a reversed pattern (better at words starting with same letter than semantically related words). Hart, Kwentus, Taylor, and Hamer (1988) partially replicated these findings in that the Animal Naming test, but not the Controlled Oral Word Association Test, differentiated the DAT patients from the depressives, with the depressives doing significantly better than the DATs on the Animal Naming test.

Vocabulary test performance. Qualitative differences in vocabulary performance have been found between depressed and dementing patients (Houlihan, Abrahams, La Rue, & Jarvik, 1985). When asked to define words, patients with Alzheimer's disease gave poor explanations as definitions more often and gave superior synonyms as definitions less often than depressed patients. The use of a qualitative vocabulary scoring system, such as the one used in this study, may be of help in more precisely identifying the language disturbance that is characteristic of and specific to the dementing illnesses.

Impact of Subtype of Depression

There is considerable heterogeneity in the manifestation, course, and presumed etiology of major depressive disorders. The RDC and the DSM-III-R have brought into greater focus some of the prominent characteristics of the different forms of affective disorders. Several of the subtype distinctions made by the RDC include primary–secondary, endogenous–nonendogenous, psychotic–nonpsychotic, unipolar–bipolar, agitated–nonagitated, and retarded–nonretarded. Substantial clinical and research validation exists for these subtypings. In addition, biological subtypings are also being developed based upon response to the dexamethasone suppression test (e.g., Silberman, Weingartner, Targum, & Barnes, 1985) and other biological markers.

Research into the effects of depression on neuropsychological test performance has also explored subtype differences, although the findings have not been entirely consistent across studies and no theoretical rationale for the subtype differences has yet been offered. Endogenous depressives, for example, have been reported to perform more poorly than nonendogenous depressed patients on a battery of neuropsychological measures (Rush *et al.*, 1983). Several studies have found that bipolar depressives make more errors on the Category Test (Savard, Rey, & Post, 1980) and perform more slowly on tests of mental and motor speed (Blackburn, 1975) when compared to unipolar depressed patients. Other studies, however, have not always found such deficits for either ill (Newman & Silverstein, 1987) or recovered bipolars (Kerry, McDermott, & Orme, 1983), and have even suggested that when bipolars do exhibit more severe deficits, those impairments may be related more to long-term neuroleptic treatment than to subtype diagnosis (Mukherjee, Shukla, & Rosen, 1984).

Given the well-known susceptibility of neuropsychological measures to schizophrenia (Malec, 1978), it would seem likely that the psychotic–nonpsychotic depressive subtype distinction might also be meaningful. In fact, several studies have found that the presence of psychotic features contributes significantly to poor test performance (Newman & Silverstein, 1987; Shipley *et al.*, 1981). In addition, it appears that psychosis in depression affects the severity of the neuropsychological deficits but not the type of deficits (Fromm-Auch, 1983; Fromm & Schopflocher, 1984).

It is understandable that subtype differences have not been more thoroughly explored, given the early stage of research into depressive deficits. In the future, there will certainly be more research attention paid to such subtype differences in neuropsychological test performance. In light of the well-documented influence of depressive psychomotor retardation on test performance (e.g., Weckowicz *et al.*, 1978), it might also be reasonable to predict that the retarded–nonretarded subtype diagnosis might provide differentiation on neuropsychological performance.

Impact of Severity of Depression

Miller (1975) initially suggested that severity of depression would be the crucial variable mediating performance in tests of ability. Subsequent findings have not supported this contention. Some studies have found a correlation between severity of depression and neuropsychological test performance (e.g., Goulet Fisher, Sweet, & Pfaelzer-Smith, 1986; Sternberg & Jarvik, 1976), while others have not (e.g., Coughlan & Hollows, 1984; Newman & Sweet, 1986; Shipley *et al.*, 1981). While it is clear that patients with more severe forms of depressive diagnoses perform more poorly as a group than less disturbed patients (severely disturbed inpatients versus mildly to moderately depressed outpatients), the impact of actual depression severity on test performance is not well understood and needs further examination.

Since diagnosis of any depressive disorder, as opposed to severity of depression, has been found to be more consistently related to neuropsychological impairment, it would seem to be unwise to assign patients to a depression or control group on the basis of their scores on depression inventories alone (e.g., Gass & Russell, 1986). Similarly, it would be premature to conclude that because severity of depression does not correlate with impairment on a neuropsychological measure, then that measure must be unaffected by depression (e.g., Heinrichs, 1987).

Summary

Research clearly indicates that depression can have a significant impact on neuropsychological test performance and can lead to confusion with regard to the interpretation of test findings. Depressive deficits have been found on tasks requiring psychomotor speed, sustained effort and concentration, and memory and learning for relatively demanding material. Certain specific types of neuropsychological tasks appear to be of potential use in discriminating depression from dementia, although further research is clearly needed. There does not appear to be a direct correlation between severity of depression and test performance, and deficits are not always apparent in depressed individuals. As yet, the role of subtype of depression in test performance is unclear, although diagnostic subtypes based on symptoms of psychomotor retardation or psychosis would appear to be the most affected.

THEORETICAL AND BASIC NEUROBIOLOGICAL ISSUES

The preceding sections have had more of a descriptive focus, with little attention paid to the presumed underlying mechanisms that may be responsible for depressive deficits. The next section will attempt to orient the reader to the current and emerging issues in the neurobiology of depression. To begin with, four neurological disorders that frequently present with depression will be discussed to clarify the possible neurological foundations for that disorder. A more general discussion of the current theoretical explanations for depression will follow.

Depression and Neurological Disorders

Depression has often been observed concomitantly with a variety of medical illnesses and neurological disorders. For the present discussion, when the depression is observed in a medical patient as a function of the direct effects of the illness on the brain itself, we can refer to this depression as *brain-based*. These direct effects may occur via metabolic, electrical, toxic, and/or structural abnormalities within the brain. When it occurs in a medical patient as a secondary effect of the illness, not as a direct effect on the brain, but rather because of social and life-style changes caused by the illness, this may be referred to as *reactive* depression (even though still mediated by the brain and perhaps resulting in measurable physiological changes within the brain). While a clinically useful distinction, and one based on etiology, it does not seem possible at present to distinguish between these two conditions on the basis of neuropsychological testing alone.

There simply is not enough controlled research available on this topic. Thus, the discussion that follows is based solely on the literature pertaining to some of the more common neurological disorders known, or suspected, to cause brain-based affective disturbance. The reader may wish to refer to Tarter, Van Thiel, and Edwards (1988) for a description of various medical conditions (e.g., endocrine disorders, organ tumors, organ failure, hypoxemia) that can cause depression.

Parkinson's Disease

Numerous investigators have described the presence of depression in patients with Parkinson's disease as a common part of the clinical presentation (e.g., Brown & Wilson, 1972). Parkinson's disease typically involves degeneration of the basal ganglia, particularly the substantia nigra, and disruption of the dopaminergic neurotransmitter system in the brain. Prominent features of the disorder, such as tremor, rigidity, and slowed movement, occur early in the course of the disease. Eventually, significant neuropsychological deficits will occur in many patients, with at least mild dementia in approximately 50% of Parkinson's patients (Mortimer, Christensen, & Webster, 1985), and severe dementia in 10 to 20% (Strub & Black, 1981).

As a common part of the clinical presentation, depression has been a focus of study in Parkinson's disease patients in recent years. In reviewing some of this literature, Mayeux (1983) reports a prevalence of depression of 37–50% in Parkinson's disease patients, with 10–15% experiencing depression *before* the onset of the more prominent motoric symptoms. While reactive depression to such a potentially debilitating disorder might be expected, the depressive symptoms have not been consistently related to degree of disability, and are instead commonly believed to represent an endogenous depression caused by dopamine depletion (Strub & Black, 1981). Most investigators note the strong clinical response of Parkinson's disease patients to antidepressant medication as support for the neurotransmitter-related endogenous depression hypothesis. Also supporting this hypothesis is the finding that Parkinson's disease patients show a significantly greater degree of depression than patients suffering from other physically disabling disorders (Mayeux, 1983).

However, Mayeux (1983) has acknowledged the multifactorial realities of Parkinson's disease by stating:

> It is reasonable to conclude that Parkinson's disease may predispose patients to depression. In some, this may represent a reaction to the disability inherent to the disease, while in others altered monoamine metabolism or medications may be a contributing or causal factor. [p. 144]

Multiple Sclerosis

Multiple sclerosis (MS), like Parkinson's disease, is a neurological disorder that is both chronic and disabling. Typically a disease of young and middle-aged adults, the course of the illness can vary dramatically, from extended years of remission between relapses which cause slow deterioration in function, with a relatively normal life span, to a rapid, unremitting progressive course resulting in paralysis, dementia, and death. The hallmark of the disease is a discrete localized lesion of demyelination, called a plaque, within the white matter of the central nervous system. Clinical presentation, although quite variable, frequently includes: ocular disturbance (including diplopia and nystagmus), muscle weakness, spasticity and hyperreflexia, intention tremor, bladder disturbance, gait ataxia, dysarthria, and paresthesias, and is subject to change across time (Peyser & Poser, 1986). Within the brain, the periventricular white matter and superior frontal gyrus appear to be preferential sites for plaque formation (e.g., Brownell & Hughes, 1962; Lumsden, 1970; Barnard & Triggs, 1974). Strub and Black (1981) have suggested that the frontal white matter lesions surrounding the anterior horns of the lateral ventricles can effectively act as a cingulotomy or frontal leukotomy by severing limbic fibers that normally connect the cingulate to the frontal lobes.

While studies of MS patients have often focused exclusively on demonstrating that intellectual and cognitive deficits exist in greater frequency than represented in the medical literature (e.g., Beatty & Gange, 1977; Marsh, 1980; Heaton, Nelson, Thompson, Burks, & Franklin, 1985), clinical and scientific interest in mood and personality disturbance associated with MS date to the early history of both psychiatry (Charcot, 1877) and American neuropsychology (Ross & Reitan, 1955). In a review of the medical and neuropsychological literature on MS, Peyser and Poser (1986) have noted that: some investigators believe depression to be an equal or more prevalent finding than the more often cited euphoria among MS patients (e.g., Baretz & Stephenson, 1981); depression can be the initial presenting symptom in MS (e.g., Goodstein & Ferrell, 1977; Matthews, 1979; Whitlock & Siskind, 1980); and depression among MS patients is more frequent than among some other medically disabled groups [e.g., degenerative cerebellar, motor neuron, and muscular diseases (Whitlock & Siskind, 1980); temporal lobe epilepsy (Schiffer & Babigian, 1984)]. While the latter two points have been cited as support for a brain-based etiology of depression, observations of the fear and uncertainty associated with the diagnosis, the frequent significant disability, and the inconsistency between depression and cognitive deficit have been used to support a reactive etiology (Peyser & Poser, 1986). In an effort to clarify this point, Schiffer, Caine, Bamford, and Levy (1983) compared depressive episodes in patients with predominantly cerebral involvement to those with predominantly spinal cord and cerebellar involvement. The findings suggest that despite similar Kurtzke disability ratings, duration of illness, and performance on mental status exam and brief neuropsychological testing, the patients with cerebral involvement had significantly more major depressive episodes. Both groups reported some depressive episodes in response to stressful events in relationships or at work brought on by the disease. Following a similar study, Rabins, Brooks, O'Donnell, Pearlson, Moberg, Jubelt, Coyle, Dalos, and Folstein (1986) concluded that while depression in MS patients appeared partly determined by brain involvement of the disease, it also represented an emotional reaction to the disorder.

In his review of the MS literature, Rao (1986), in keeping with the brain-based hypothesis, has noted the similarity of MS dementia to that of "subcortical dementias," such as that associated with Parkinson's disease. As Rao notes, intact language, poor memory retrieval with relatively intact encoding, impaired complex reasoning despite relatively preserved general intellect, decreased cognitive efficiency, personality disturbance, apathy, and depression can be features of an MS dementia consistent with the controversial concept of "subcortical dementia," as opposed to a "cortical dementia," like Alzheimer's disease. As with Parkinson's disease, the present state of knowledge suggests a moderate viewpoint that both brain-based and reactive factors play a role in the depression observed in MS patients, with a great deal of individual variability in the effects of these different factors from one patient to another.

Head Injury

Patients suffering from head injury have attracted much attention from neuropsychologists and various other health professionals in recent years. Among the many possible sequelae that can be seen in head-injured populations, depression is one of the more common findings (McKinlay, Brooks, Martinage, & Marshall, 1981; Varney, Martzke, & Roberts, 1987). While much discussion has focused on the multiple factors (i.e., genuine cognitive or emotional deficit/syndrome caused either directly by brain dysfunction or secondarily through psychological reaction, compensation, litigation, malingering) that motivate self-reported complaints following head injury, particularly when minor in nature, few investigators or clinicians today would question the notion that a majority of the often observed emotional sequelae to head injury are significant and genuine (McMordie, 1988). Varney *et al.* (1987) found that twice as many closed head injury patients suffer major depression as patients suffering from low back injury (77 versus 38%). As noted by Atteberry-Bennett, Barth, Loyd, and Lawrence, (1986), the etiology of head injury-related depression has been discussed as due either to physiological effects of the brain dysfunction or, alternatively, to the patient's perception of loss of cognitive–behavioral functioning that make life goals less attainable. McMordie (1988) recently reported on survey data from neurosurgeons and neuropsychologists that suggest that 62 and 65%, respectively, believe that emotional factors aggravate or have an effect upon postconcussion symptoms. However, both groups also highly endorse "organic" factors as the *chief* cause of postconcussion symptoms (55 versus 72%). In discussing the possibility that depression after brain injury may have a neurochemical basis, Prigatano (1987) has noted the absence of any literature concerning abnormal serum cortisol levels among traumatically brain-injured patients, whereas as many as 50% of CVA patients have been shown to have abnormal dexamethasone tests.

While immediate physiological abnormalities such as edema, decreased cerebral blood flow, and increased intracranial pressure can cause depressive symptoms (Lishman, 1968), these factors are typically short-lived. More persistent emotional symptoms may be attributable to structural and electrophysiological abnormalities, lowered arousal level due to reticular activating system dysfunction, or even to less-than-optimal functioning of remaining neurons which have only partial capabilities. [The interested reader may wish to refer to Levin, Benton, and Grossman (1982), Levin, Grafman, and Eisenberg (1987), or Reitan and Wolfson (1985) for a discussion of the complex pathophysiology of closed head injury.] With regard to depression and other emotional sequelae to traumatic brain injury, the findings of damage or dysfunction in the frontotemporal regions (e.g., Bigler, 1988, Chapter 4), diffuse white matter (representing axonal strain or shearing; e.g., Gennarelli, 1986), limbic system, and neurotransmitter systems are thought to be particularly relevant. Varney *et al.* (1987) point out that approximately half of head-injured patients who suffer major depression do not do so until 4 months after injury. Observations of a sometimes sizable delay between time of injury and onset of affective and other posttraumatic disturbances have typically been interpreted as indicative of a reactive or psychological problem (Alves, Colohan, O'Leary, Rimel, & Jane, 1986). In addition, numerous investigators have documented the significant psychological/emotional problems that head injury creates for the relatives of the victim, suggesting that there is a much broader context within which additional secondary factors can contribute to depression (Livingston, 1987; Livingston & Brooks, 1988; Rees, 1988; McCaffrey, Pollock, & Burns, 1987).

In summary, findings such as these point out the need to consider both brain-based aspects of depression and reactive aspects of depression in victims of head injury, as well as the reactive difficulties of the family of the victim, as all three could play a role.

Stroke

A relatively large literature exists concerning the diverse emotional changes that can accompany stroke. Poststroke depression occurs in 30–60% of patients (Robinson *et al.* 1983), with increased severity and frequency 6 months to 2 years poststroke (Robinson & Price, 1982). Much of this literature has attempted to determine the relationship between location of the vascular lesion and the type of emotional disorder present. While not in complete agreement, some general conclusions concerning the influence of *inter-* and *intra*hemispheric involvement in depression among stroke patients have been sought and discussed by a number of neuroscientists (e.g., Benson & Geschwind, 1975; Gainotti, 1972; Heilman & Satz, 1983; Kinsbourne, 1988).

Among the most agreed-upon findings to date are the *catastrophic reaction* and *indifference reaction*, as well as the *graded location effect* (cf. Finset, 1988; Starkstein & Robinson, 1988). Essentially, the findings of investigators such as Gainotti (1972) strongly suggest that left hemisphere stroke patients exhibit a much different emotional response than right hemisphere stroke patients. In general, left hemisphere stroke is more likely to be associated with catastrophic reaction, while right hemisphere stroke is more likely to be associated with indifference. The term *catastrophic reaction* was first used by Goldstein (1942), and referred to an explosive outpouring of emotion beginning with anxiety and leading to serious depression. In elaborating experiential (reactive) explanations of depression in left hemisphere stroke patients, other investigators have noted the greater awareness of cognitive and motor deficits, and the possibility that because of impaired language ability, patients rely more heavily on "nonpropositional affective systems" (i.e., speech intonation and facial expression) resulting in a predominance of right hemisphere "negative" emotion (Heilman, Watson, & Bowers, 1983, p. 60). Related to these points, some investigators have found depression to be associated with aphasia in left hemisphere patients, while others have not. Kinsbourne (1988) has noted three possible explanations for depression occurring in a patient with a left frontal lesion: (1) the patient cannot plan, (2) the patient feels helpless and hopeless because he cannot plan, and/or (3) a different part of the brain (presumably in the right hemisphere) that mediates negative emotion has been released from inhibition. Kinsbourne goes on to state, "Theorists by and large tend to invoke a neurologizing (disinhibition) explanation and perhaps insufficiently consider the compensatory activity" (p. 146).

The indifference reaction seen in right hemisphere patients includes anosognosia, indifference and apathy, inappropriate jocularity, undue cheerfulness, and minimization (e.g., Finset, 1988; Gainotti, 1972; Starkstein & Robinson, 1988). Since the right hemisphere appears to be involved with the perception and expression of emotion (Bryden & Ley, 1983; Ross, 1981), and has also been implicated with respect to awareness of deficits (Gainotti, 1972), one could postulate that the usual clinical signs of depression may be less apparent in these patients because they are not as aware of their problems and cannot perceive and express their emotions as well. In other words, there may be limited ability in right hemisphere patients to experience depression in a normal manner. Ruckdeschel-Hibbard, Gordon, and Diller (1986) have suggested that indifference in right hemisphere patients may actually reflect affect communication deficits, rather than the individual's subjective state.

However, the situation is made more complex by the observations that not all left hemisphere patients exhibit depression, not all right hemisphere patients exhibit indifference, and some studies have not supported the stereotypes of catastrophic and indifference reactions when left and right hemisphere patients have been compared. Such observations have led Robinson and others to investigate intrahemispheric lesion location as a means of understanding the varied emotional concomitants of stroke (as summarized in Starkstein & Robinson, 1988). These investigations have led to the relatively consistent finding of a graded location effect within the hemispheres, such that more prominent indications of depression are associated both with more anterior lesions within the left hemisphere and with more posterior lesions within the right hemisphere. Within the left hemisphere, this has been hypothesized to occur as a result of the locus of disruption of noradrenergic transmitter pathways that arise from the brain stem and travel anteriorly to the frontal cortex and then pass posteriorly through the cortex. Lesions closer to the frontal pole would presumably interrupt the transmitter pathway more "upstream," thereby causing greater disruption to the noradrenergic concentrations "downstream" (Starkstein & Robinson, 1988). Finset (described in Finset, 1988) has found that an added dimension to the posterior positioning of the right hemisphere lesion may be the depth of the lesion, with deeper posterior lesions associated with greater depression. Finset also emphasizes that the depression seen in right hemisphere patients is less severe and qualitatively different than in left hemisphere patients and may, instead of obvious depressive thought content and significant anxiety, consist of "generally lowered mood with less specific depressive symptomatology and often with a certain degree of inertia and lack of initiative. . ." (p. 57).

In addition to the psychological (reactive) explanations of depression mentioned above (and elaborated in Kinsbourne, 1988), various physiological explanations have been posited for depression in both left and right hemisphere patients. One of the more prominent hypotheses concerns the possibility that disruption of anterior "biogenic amine pathways" may bring about the observed depression of anterior left hemisphere patients, as well as the unusual indifference reaction of anterior right hemisphere patients (Robinson, Kubos, Starr, Rao, & Price, 1984). Effective treatment of many poststroke depressions with tricyclic antidepressants appears to lend support to this hypothesis.

In summarizing the various hypotheses regarding poststroke depression,

Robinson *et al.* (1984) note that significant correlations between depression and both severity of impairment and severity of impairment of activities of daily living suggest a reactive psychological basis. The time of onset of depression appearing well after the stroke for a number of patients would also seem to suggest a reactive basis. Robinson *et al.* note, however, that several findings favor a neural or brain-based etiology: (1) the relationship between proximity of the vascular lesion to severity of depression; (2) the strength of this association accounting for 50 to 70% of the variance, while relationships of depression to severity of impairment account for only 10 to 20%; (3) the syndromelike presentation of depressive symptoms among anterior left hemisphere patients, and (4) the lack of a consistent specific impairment (against which to react) in post-stroke patients who become depressed.

Theoretical Issues

Initial efforts at understanding the neurological basis of depression focused upon attempts at localizing parts of the brain responsible for this emotion and for depressive disorders. A growing body of clinical and research findings seemed at first to implicate the right hemisphere of the brain as being responsible for mediating emotion. Right hemisphere dysfunction was seen as being the cause of depression (Flor-Henry, 1979). Subsequent developments of this theoretical approach, however, also began to emphasize the importance of the *interaction* between the hemispheres, and particularly the frontal lobes, as being vitally important in regulating mood through reciprocal inhibition and activation (Flor-Henry, 1984). Recent advances have broadened consideration from this *inter*hemispheric (left versus right) emphasis to take into account findings of *intra*hemispheric variables. More recent research has also begun to implicate deep or subcortical versus cortical structures in the experience and expression of depression. The next section will briefly describe the current understanding in each of these areas. Space does not allow discussion of the numerous biochemical hypotheses of depression.

Interhemispheric Variables

Flor-Henry (1983) has advanced an explanation of affective disturbance based upon a cumulative body of research identifying each of the cerebral hemispheres with differing functions in the experience and control of emotion. Flor-Henry reviewed studies of psychiatric surgery, unilateral lesions, hemispheric activation, EEG, evoked potentials, epilepsy, monotic and dichotic listening, and PET scans to support his hypotheses that different emotions are lateralized in the brain and that changes in hemispheric organization are associated with pathological disturbances of mood. The overwhelming evidence provided suggested that right hemisphere dysfunction was related to depression, and pointed to the roles of each of the hemispheres in inhibiting the other. Although the neural substrate for emotion in general was seen as being largely nondominant, Flor-Henry saw the regulation of emotion as being a function of the interaction of the two hemispheres through transcallosal neural inhibition. When the dominant hemisphere is no longer controlled by the nondominant hemisphere, the reaction is anger, paranoid mood, or euphoria. On the other hand, the failure of the dominant hemisphere to adequately control the nondominant hemisphere results in the release of the emotional-catastrophic reaction, dysphoric emotions, or sadness. According to this model, the release of emotions may be caused either by activation of the ipsilateral hemisphere or through loss of contralateral inhibition. Flor-Henry's approach emphasizes the importance of the relative balance between right and left hemisphere activation. "When the balance of relative right/left hemispheric activation is altered to an abnormal state of left hemispheric preponderance, the induced emotion is of euphoria; when it is shifted to excessive right hemispheric preponderance, sadness or dysphoric emotionality emerges" (Flor-Henry, 1983).

Of interest with regard to laterality studies are the findings of two studies that investigated patients with lateralized parkinsonism and did not find any differences in level of depression related to either left hemisphere or right hemisphere parkinsonism (Barber, Tomer, Sroka, & Myslobodsky, 1985; Spicer, Roberts, & LeWitt, 1988).

Intrahemispheric Variables

As noted in the section on depression and neurological disorders, more recent studies have suggested that discussion of the right and left hemispheres as influencing emotion is too simplistic. In keeping with the trend in the neurosciences away from a "naive localizationalism" (Kinsbourne, 1988) and in part because of increasingly sophisticated research methodologies, newer theories have tried to take into account as well intrahemispheric activation and inhibition, and the role of neurotransmitter pathways in the brain.

As discussed earlier, it has become clear that within each of the hemispheres there is a graded location effect. Within the left hemisphere, the closer a lesion is to the frontal pole, the greater the depression. The opposite holds true for the right hemisphere where more intense depression is associated with the more posterior the lesion (Finset, 1988). Furthermore, the quality of the depressive symptoms is quite different for the left-frontal versus right-posterior depressions, with the former expressing the more severe depressive symptoms and greater anxiety characteristic of clinical depression and the right-posterior patients exhibiting more of a diffusely depressed mood without the complaints of severe depression. As noted above in the section on strokes, the locus of disruption of noradrenergic transmitter pathways may account for the graded location effect seen in stroke patients.

Tucker (1988) advances a quadrant model of cortical representation of emotion, essentially elaborating upon the role of interhemispheric functioning in emotion. According to this model, emotional stability is achieved not only through a balance between the right and left hemispheres, but also through a balance between the anterior and posterior regions of the brain. The anterior brain is seen as providing a regulatory function, while the posterior part of the brain is seen as specializing in a representative function, representing information about the environmental context of emotion. Substantial reciprocity is hypothesized between the anterior and posterior systems within each hemisphere, such that increased frontal activation would presumably lead to decreased activation in the posterior regions. Indeed, research findings of increased right frontal lobe EEG activation in depressives (Schaffer, Davidson, & Saron, 1983) is consistent with the repeated findings of depressives doing poorly on visuospatial tasks. That is, in depression, an activated right frontal lobe may inhibit the right posterior functions that are responsible for visuospatial functioning.

Cortical versus Subcortical Variables

In light of some of the earlier noted findings of depression in neurological disorders (e.g., Parkinson's disease) caused by damage to subcortical structures, it is clear that this dimension needs further attention. In work with brain-damaged patients, severity of depression has been found to vary as a function of the depth of the lesion (Finset, 1988). In addition, some investigators (e.g., Cummings & Benson, 1984; Cummings, 1986) have described a distinctive clinical syndrome, subcortical dementia, that is associated with damage to subcortical structures or subcortical neurotransmitter systems. This syndrome is characterized by slowed cognitive processes, memory impairment, difficulty with complex intellectual tasks, visuospatial problems, and prominent mood disturbance. Although the concept of subcortical dementia has been challenged (Whitehouse, 1986), the striking similarity between these symptoms and the depressive deficits described earlier would suggest an important role of subcortical structures in depression.

There is a clear lack of research in this area, perhaps as a result of the inability of past research technologies to adequately investigate this part of the brain. With new advances in brain imaging, there is the hope that this important area will be explored more thoroughly.

APPLICATION TO CLINICAL ASSESSMENT

As has been described earlier in this chapter, the effects of depression on neuropsychological measures are not uniform and not entirely predictable. Until recently, the number of empirical studies on this topic was quite small, and still does not come close to approximating the vast literature on neuropsychological effects of schizophrenia. To illustrate the diverse and complex presentations of depression on neuropsychological functioning, discussion of a number of clinical cases will follow. Both typical (easy) and unusual (difficult) cases will be included for consideration.

Clinical Cases

Typical Dementia Cases

Case #1. The first typical dementia case is that of a right-handed 56-year-old Caucasian male attorney. The attorney was referred by his family physician who, along with family members, friends, and colleagues, had observed a significance decline in his memory and cognitive abilities. Decreased reading comprehension was noted to have begun 10 years earlier shortly after the death of his father. The patient underwent brief antidepressant therapy successfully at that time. However, the perception of decreased reading comprehension continued. Friends, family, and colleagues had noticed forgetfulness and occasional confusion within the last year. As a senior law partner, the patient had delegated more and more responsibility, and was now avoiding cases involving courtroom litigation. Detailed questioning of the patient and his wife and brother-in-law revealed similar decline in functioning among several siblings and other immediate relatives.

The patient and his wife agreed strongly that there had been no signs of depression in his mood or behavior. Interview information and observations of the patient during formal testing failed to elicit any evidence of depression. The results of a neuropsychological screening battery, extended from the Wysocki and Sweet (1985) screening battery, are presented in Table 9.2.

The pattern of test results does *not* appear consistent with that of depressed patients, and instead is consistent with a diagnosis of early Alzheimer's-like dementia (in view of family history, possibly the familial type). In particular, there is no evidence of slowness of responses, basic sensory motor and language functions are intact, and memory for complex, semantic information is significantly worse than for complex figural information, whereas the opposite is observed in some depressed patients. More suggestive of dementia, learning and memory (both recall and recognition) are impaired, both verbal and nonverbal reasoning are moderately impaired, there is decreased cognitive efficiency and evidence of selective vulnerability to cognitive interference. Along with the probable diagnosis, recommendation was made for complete neurological work-up since none had yet been performed, and we wanted to be sure that treatable dementias were ruled out. Approximately 10 months later, patient #1 underwent a comprehensive work-up at another medical center, which confirmed our earlier diagnosis and his downhill course.

Case #2. The second typical dementia case is that of a right-handed 80-year-old Caucasian female. The patient is a retired secretary with a high school diploma who was referred by her neurologist in order to assist in ruling out pseudodementia. The patient's daughter had noticed a decline in cognitive functioning over the last 6 months, beginning with word-finding difficulties in normal conversation. Memory had declined significantly, and she was no longer able to handle her own finances or even her shopping. Examples of memory

TABLE 9.2. Case #1—Age 56, Education 19, Sex M, Handedness R, Vocation Attorney

	Raw Score	Russell Ratings
Tapping		
Dominant	55.7	0
Non-Dominant	47.2	1
Trailmaking Test		
Part A	27″	1
Part B	82″	1
Spatial Relations	2	1
Wechsler Memory Scale		
Semantic Immediate	5	5
Semantic Delayed	1	5
Figural Immediate	9	2
Figural Delayed	6	3
Associate Learning	[Easy/Hard: 4/0, 3/1, 4/1]	
Digit Span	[Forward 7/Backward 5]	
Orientation	[Oriented × 3]	
Digit Symbol	[Scaled Score 3; Age Corrected 6]	

	Raw Score	T-Score
Stroop Color Word Test		
Word	101	47
Color	67	41
Color–Word	28	33
LNNB Pathognomonic Scale		
Critical level 53	11	41
Shipley Institute of Living Scale		
Vocabulary	36	62
Abstraction	16	50
Abs. Quot.		78

Rey Auditory Verbal Learning Test
Trials 1–5 5,5,5,7,7
Interference 3
Immed. Recall 4; Immed. Recog. 14 (3 false positives)
Delayed Recall 0; Delayed Recog. 0
MAE Controlled Oral Word Association Test
Raw Score 45 Percentile Rank 77–89
WAIS-R—*Scaled Score*
Sim. 9 B.D. 8
Category Test
91 errors
Grip Strength
Rt. hand 43.5 kg; Lt. hand 39 kg

impairment included forgetting who her son-in-law was, and on occasion forgetting who her grandchildren were. Concern regarding the patient's ability to maintain an independent residence was expressed. There was no history of psychiatric disorder.

Patient #2 was well-dressed and well-groomed at the time of the evaluation.

She exhibited socially appropriate behaviors and gave the impression of having been a dignified and refined lady. While word-finding difficulties were evident in the conversation, she remained quite articulate. Upon interview, the patient denied having any problems, stating that she had no reason to be tested. However, she was unable to provide accurate responses to basic questions regarding her personal and family history (e.g., education, occupation, year of husband's death, number of grandchildren, names and ages of grandchildren, daughter's age, daughter's education, number of years daughter married, her own phone number). Signs of depression were denied by the patient and her daughter, and no overt indications of depression were observed during formal testing. Responses to failure during testing, ranged from emotionally distant statements indicating her daughter could "check on that," to surprise and frustration, both at being asked to perform and at being unable to.

The results of a partial neuropsychological screening battery are presented in Table 9.3. Low stamina and the patient's frustration did not allow the completion of all planned measures. The available data suggest impairments in naming, verbal and nonverbal memory, cognitive flexibility, cognitive efficiency, and verbal reasoning, with preservation of basic writing, spelling, and constructional skills. Without any indication of depression in overt behavior or in descriptions by the patient or daughter, or in the test data (see Table 1 for listing of depressive signs), the testing results were viewed as confirming the presence of a dementing process. Since subsequent neuroradiological assessment ruled out alternative etiologies, the neurologist assumed the process to be Alzheimer's disease.

Memory Complaints Caused by Depression

Far more common than pseudodementia, in our clinical experience, are patients referred because of memory complaints caused by depression. These individuals are often middle-aged or young elderly outpatients experiencing concentration problems because of depression, which is often *mistakenly* attributed to "early Alzheimer's." A fairly detailed description of the often relatively minor concentration and forgetting examples experienced in day-to-day life can usually be elicited without difficulty from these patients (i.e., they often *remember* and *concentrate* on these problems). Actual neuropsychological performance typically shows inconsistent mild abnormalities or normal functioning.

Case #3. Patient #3 is a 44-year-old Caucasian male referred by his internist because of concentration and memory complaints. The complaints dated back 5 years, and consisted primarily of difficulty recalling facts. While acutely aware of the problem himself, he admitted that his co-workers experience his problems as only an occasional annoyance. Low energy level was also reported. Upon questioning, he noted that his wife had described him as a "Type A." He also reported past problems with both headaches and ulcers.

Results of an extended neuropsychological screening battery are presented

TABLE 9.3. Case #2—Age 80, Education 12, Sex F, Handedness R, Vocation Housewife

	Raw Score	Russell Ratings
Tapping		
Dominant	37	3
Non-Dominant	37.6	2
Trailmaking Test		
Part A	65″	4
Part B	Discontinued	5
Spatial Relations	1	0
Wechsler Memory Scale		
Semantic Immediate	4.5	5
Semantic Delayed	1	5
Figural Immediate	4	4
Figural Delayed	2	4
Associate Learning	[Easy/hard: 2/0, 4/0, 4/0]	
Digit Span	[Forward 8/Backward 4]	
Orientation	[Oriented to person, place, & year/month]	
Digit Symbol	[Scaled Score 4; Age Corrected 8]	
Immediate Recall	[Symbols 1; Pairs 0]	
	Raw Score	**T-Score**
Stroop Color Word Test		
Word	89	40
Color	44	26
Color–Word	15	20
Shipley Institute of Living Scale		
Vocabulary	29.5	53
Abstraction	8	44
Abs. Quot.		85
MAE Controlled Oral Word Association Test		
Raw Score 26 Percentile Rank 12		
MAE Visual Naming Test		
Raw Score 26 Percentile Rank 0		

in Table 9.4. Test data indicate that patient #3 performed variably, but essentially within normal limits on most measures. The pattern of performance, the fact that tasks requiring effortful concentration were performed more poorly, self-report of concentration difficulties and loss of energy, exaggerated complaints, endorsement of dysphoric moods and feelings on several checklists, and his behavioral manifestations of depression (including increased response latencies, sighing, and constricted affect) led to the conclusion that the patient's complaints were actually a manifestation of his significant clinical depression. Psychological intervention was recommended.

Case #4. Referred by her internist because of memory complaints, Case #4 is a 65-year-old right-handed Caucasian female who lives alone. Memory complaints were unusual and inconsistent (e.g., recalling a story of having

TABLE 9.4. Case #3—Age 44, Education 19, Sex M, Handedness R, Vocation Electrical Engineer

	Raw Score	Russell Ratings
Tapping		
Dominant	58.4	0
Non-Dominant	61.2	0
Trailmaking Test		
Part A	41″	2
Part B	91″	2
Spatial Relations	2	1
Wechsler Memory Scale		
Semantic Immediate	29	0
Semantic Delayed	26.5	0
Figural Immediate	13	0
Figural Delayed	13	0
Associate Learning	[Easy/hard: 6/0, 6/3, 6/4]	
Digit Span	[Forward 6/Backward 4]	
Orientation	[Oriented × 3]	
Digit Symbol	[Scaled Score 8; Age Corrected 10]	
Immediate Recall	[Symbols 8; Pairs 8]	
Stroop Color Word Test		
Word	90	41
Color	58	35
Color–Word	35	40
	Raw Score	**T-Score**
LNNB Pathognomonic Scale		
Critical level 52	6	33
Shipley Institute of Living Scale		
Vocabulary	37	60
Abstraction	38	67
Abs. Quot.		109
California Verbal Learning Test		
List A (1–5): 5,8,11,12,9		
List B 6		
Immed. Recall 6; Immed. Cued Recall 12		
Delayed Recall 10; Delayed Cue Recall 12		
Delayed Recog. 15		
MAE Controlled Oral Word Association Test		
Raw Score 32 Percentile Rank 25–75		
MAE Visual Naming Test		
Raw Score 50 Percentile Rank 27		
Category Test		
33 errors		
Grip Strength		
Rt. hand 40 kg; Lt. hand 46 kg		
Beck Depression inventory		
Raw Score 10		
POMS Depression Scale		
Raw Score 3 T-Score 37		

failed to recognize that she had left money at work in great detail). She had left her job as a word processor three to four weeks earlier because of work-related stress. She had two years of business college, and additional college courses. Psychiatric history includes inpatient hospitalizations, outpatient therapy, and pharmacological treatment for depression some years ago. Presently there are days when she feels depressed and doesn't get out of bed. Recently, she has been stressed by caring for sick, elderly parents and has been isolating herself socially.

Data from an extended neuropsychological screening battery are presented in Table 9.5. As is readily evident, much of the neuropsychological test performance of this patient was within normal limits. In fact, her performance was above average in several domains, including verbal learning as well as immediate and long-term memory. The perceived deficits reported by patient #4 most likely represent emotionally based, rather than brain-based impairment. Notable are the patient's previous history of depression, current behavioral indicators of depression (decreased activity, social withdrawal, sad affect), a pattern of test performance characteristic of patients with problems of a psychiatric nature, significant life stressors, and self-deprecating comments about her own test performance. Psychological intervention was recommended.

Dementialike Symptoms Due to Depression (Pseudodementia)

Case #5. This 45-year-old right-handed Caucasian female was referred as a psychiatric inpatient to help rule out pseudodementia. In addition to a 6-month history of depression, culminating with several suicide attempts prior to admission, she had exhibited seizurelike behavior while hospitalized. She complained vaguely of concentration and memory disturbance.

The neuropsychological data presented in Table 9.6 suggest some specific mild difficulties with complex verbal memory and incidental memory for symbols which is not consistent with the remainder of the test data, which in most cases is within normal limits. During testing she yawned frequently and appeared tired, and also depreciated her learning abilities. She was able to reliably report her own history. A conclusion of major depression without significant brain dysfunction was felt to be supported when the patient responded extremely well to antidepressant therapy and was able to be discharged to normal daily routine without further cognitive complaints.

Case #6. Case #6 is a 42-year-old right-handed Caucasian female referred as a psychiatric inpatient. This patient had a previous diagnosis of bipolar disorder and had been treated with medications for many years. She expressed concern that she may have damaged herself by taking medications for years without supervision. Included among depressive symptomatology were complaints of poor concentration and memory disturbance.

Patient #6 was reluctant to undergo formal testing, and even after she reluctantly agreed to do so, continued to display passive–aggressive-type

TABLE 9.5. Case #4—Age 65, Education 14+, Sex F, Handedness R, Vocation Word Processing

	Raw Score	Russell Ratings
Tapping		
Dominant	50	1
Non-Dominant	39	2
Trailmaking Test		
Part A	53″	3
Part B	88″	2
Spatial Relations	3	1
Wechsler Memory Scale		
Semantic Immediate	19	2
Semantic Delayed	14.5	2
Figural Immediate	10	1
Figural Delayed	9	1
Digit Symbol	[Scaled Score 7; Age Corrected 12]	
Immediate Recall	[Symbols 7; Pairs 6]	
	Raw Score	**T-Score**
Stroop Color Word Test		
Word	114	53
Color	73	45
Color–Word	56	61
LNNB Pathognomonic Scale		
Critical level 62	11	41
Shipley Institute of Living Scale		
Vocabulary	36	64
Abstraction	20	56
Abs. Quot.		93
California Verbal Learning Test		
List A (1–5): 12,10,14,13,16		
List B 7		
Immed. Recall 12; Immed. Cued Recall 13		
Delayed Recall 12; Delayed Cue Recall 12		
Delayed Recog. 16		
MAE Controlled Oral Word Association Test		
Raw Score 41 Percentile Rank 25–75		
MAE Visual Naming Test		
Raw Score 50 Percentile Rank 27		
Beck Depression Inventory		
Raw Score 6		

behaviors. She expressed frustration and was impatient with herself when tasks were experienced as difficult. Her response latencies were often very long, and she appeared to labor over some tasks, while giving up too quickly in response to others. Most of the time she appeared ambivalent and confused about how to respond (e.g., after protracted completion of the MMPI, she insisted that she be allowed to take it again because she had "misrepresented" herself). As can be

TABLE 9.6. Case #5—Age 45, Education 17, Sex F, Handedness R, Vocation Homemaker

	Raw Score	Russell Ratings
Tapping		
Dominant	50	1
Non-Dominant	46.4	0
Trailmaking Test		
Part A	33″	1
Part B	47″	0
Spatial Relations	3	1
Wechsler Memory Scale		
Semantic Immediate	17.5	2/3
Semantic Delayed	10	3
Figural Immediate	13	0
Figural Delayed	12	0
Associate Learning	[Easy/hard: 6/0, 6/0, 6/2]	
Digit Span	[Forward 6/Backward 7]	
Orientation	[Oriented × 3]	
Digit Symbol	[Scaled Score 8; Age Corrected 10]	
Immediate Recall	[Symbols 5; Pairs 2]	
	Raw Score	**T-Score**
Stroop Color Word Test		
Word	107	49
Color	74	46
Color–Word	44	49
LNNB Pathognomonic Scale		
Critical level 55	10	40
Shipley Institute of Living Scale		
Vocabulary	36	59
Abstraction	30	60
Abs. Quot.		98
Rey Auditory Verbal Learning Test		
Trials 1–5: 6,8,11,11,12		
Interference 7		
Immed. Recall 8; Immed. Recog. 14 (1 false positive)		
Delayed Recall 8; Delayed Recog. 15		
MAE Controlled Oral Word Association Test		
Raw Score 52 Percentile Rank 89		
Beck Depression Inventory		
Raw Score 27		
MMPI		
Depression Scale [T-Score 87]		
Welsh code: *278″613′40-9/5:# KF/L:		

seen in Table 9.7, neuropsychological performance was in many cases impaired from the standpoint of traditional cutoffs and decision rules. Intact incidental and recognition memory appeared inconsistent with other test data. Clinical impressions based on observations of the patient and collateral sources of information, strongly suggested that the patient's psychological needs were being met by maintaining a passive and debilitated presentation. Thus, a diagnosis of pseudodementia was given. Subsequent feedback regarding the patient's behavior following a very lengthy hospitalization indicated that her significant depression was alleviated to a large extent and she was able to return to a normal daily routine, including successful return to gainful employment without complaints or observations suggesting cognitive impairment.

Depressionlike Symptoms Due to Dementia

Case #7. Referred as an outpatient by her psychotherapist because of complaints of cognitive difficulties intermixed with severe depressive symptomatology, patient #7 is a 31-year-old right-handed female with a college education. She was on leave from work, having recently been demoted because of "poor work performance and poor attitude." The patient was extremely difficult to test, in that she displayed a very high level of anxiety, was tearful and broke down emotionally as soon as she was asked to perform, demonstrated inappropriate laughter during personality tests, complained often of fatigue even during initial portions of the neuropsychological testing, refused to respond to a number of projective stimuli, and after completing the neuropsychological screening measures became offended by the projective testing and left the office. She completed the tests at a later date.

Overall, the patient's behavior was suggestive of a very fragile, possibly psychotic individual whose self-reported history of prior accomplishments academically was difficult to trust. Despite the wide range of performance, including significant impairments, evident in the data presented in Table 9.8, the patient's poorly organized and out-of-control behavior was thought to be so disruptive as to prevent a valid indication of her neuropsychological abilities, especially in the absence of clear pathognomonic signs. In other words, the testing was considered invalid. While a CT scan of the brain near the time of testing was normal, an MRI approximately 9 months later revealed severe atrophy of the frontal lobe and significant thinning of the corpus callosum. At the time of the MRI, cognitive abilities had also deteriorated dramatically (retesting was not carried out), to the point that she was no longer able even to write a check. Diagnosis was eventually determined to be Pick's disease with serious psychiatric symptoms attributed to extreme thinning of the corpus callosum.

Depression with Secondary Dementia

Case #8. Patient #8 was referred as a psychiatric inpatient to aid in differentiating dementia from pseudodementia. The patient had presented with

TABLE 9.7. Case #6—Age 42, Education 12, Sex F, Handedness R, Vocation Clerk

	Raw Score	Russell Ratings
Tapping		
Dominant	42.6	2
Non-Dominant	44.2	1
Trailmaking Test		
Part A	53″	3
Part B	240″	4
Spatial Relations	4	2
Wechsler Memory Scale		
Semantic Immediate	13	4
Semantic Delayed	8	4
Figural Immediate	5.5	3
Figural Delayed	4.5	3
Associate Learning	[Easy/hard: 4/0, 6/0, 6/0]	
Digit Span	[Forward 5/Backward 5]	
Orientation	[Oriented × 3]	
Digit Symbol	[Scaled Score 7; Age Corrected 9]	
Immediate Recall	[Symbols 9; Pairs 7]	

	Raw Score	T-Score
Stroop Color Word Test		
Word	84	38
Color	74	46
Color–Word	26	31
LNNB Pathognomonic Scale		
Critical level 60	26	65

Rey Auditory Verbal Learning Test
- Trials 1–5: 3,4,6,3,9
- Interference 4
- Immed. Recall 9; Immed. Recog. 15
- Delayed Recall 9 (3 intrusions); Delayed Recog. 14

MAE Controlled Oral Word Association Test
- Raw Score 33 Percentile Rank 25–75

MAE Visual Naming Test
- Raw Score 50 Percentile Rank 27

WAIS-R—Scaled Scores (Age Corrected)

Inf.	6 (6)	Pic Com.	5 (6)
Dig. Sp.	8 (9)	Pic. Arr.	6 (7)
Voc.	8 (8)	B.D.	5 (6)
Arith.	3 (4)	O.A.	5 (6)
Comp.	5 (5)	Dig. Sym.	7 (9)
Sim.	7 (6)		

IQ 80; PIQ 79; FSIQ 79

Beck Depression Inventory
- Raw Score 18

MMPI
- Depression Scale [T-Score 69]
- Welsh code: *″4′2387 69-10/:5# K/LF:

TABLE 9.8. Case #7—Age 31, Education 16, Sex F, Handedness R, Vocation Unknown

	Raw Score	Russell Ratings
Tapping		
Dominant	49.6	1
Non-Dominant	37.4	2
Trailmaking Test		
Part A	68″ (1 error)	4
Part B	discontinued	5
Spatial Relations	2	1
Wechsler Memory Scale		
Semantic Immediate	7.5	5
Semantic Delayed	3.0	5
Figural Immediate	3.0	4
Figural Delayed	0	5
Associate Learning	[Easy/hard: 3/0, 4/0, 4/0]	
Digit Span	[Forward 5/Backward 3]	
Orientation	[Oriented × 3]	
Digit Symbol	[Scaled Score 2; Age Corrected 2]	
Immediate Recall	[Symbols 5; Pairs 4]	

	Raw Score	T-Score
Stroop Color Word Test		
Word	38	<20
Color	24	<20
Color–Word	8	<20
LNNB Pathognomonic Scale		
Critical level 52	15	48
Shipley Institute of Living Scale		
Vocabulary	46	25
Abstraction	6	32
Abs. Quot.		82
Rey Auditory Verbal Learning Test		
Trials 1–5: 5,4,4,3,5		
Interference 0		
Immed. Recall 2; Immed. Recog. 5 (8 false positives)		
Delayed Recall 2; Delayed Recog. 7 (15 false positives)		
MAE Controlled Oral Word Association Test		
Raw Score 14 Percentile Rank <1		
MAE Visual Naming Test		
Raw Score 48 Percentile Rank 18		
Beck Depression Inventory		
Raw Score 8		

a history of forgetting, increased confusion, an inability to dress herself, and significant depressive symptomatology. The patient noted that her present problems began approximately 2 years ago, which she associated with the death of her husband (hospital records indicate that he actually died 7 years earlier). In a paradoxical manner, she noted a gradual onset of memory problems, but denied that the difficulties had gotten worse across time. She is a right-handed Caucasian female with a 10th grade education. She had worked in various unskilled factory positions.

Because of concerns that the data obtained from the patient at the initial time of testing were not representative of her optimal performance, especially given some indications of a psychiatric pattern in the test results, some of the measures were readministered 2 days later. An examination of Table 9.9, along with Fig. 9.1, shows the dramatic changes over a very brief period of time during which there was no change in her medical or neurological status. In addition to data shown in Fig. 9.1, readministration of Trails A resulted in improvement from 190″ to 93″. It was felt that in addition to genuine brain-based deficits, the patient's primary difficulty was depression that when treated would improve her level of functioning considerably, although not to premorbid levels. A CT scan

TABLE 9.9. Case #8—Age 75, Education 10, Sex F, Handedness R, Vocation Unknown

	Raw Score	Russell Ratings
Tapping		
Dominant	35.2	3
Non-Dominant	33.8	2
Wechsler Memory Scale		
Semantic Immediate	11	4
Semantic Delayed	5	4
Figural Immediate	1	5
Figural Delayed	0	5
Trailmaking Test		
Part A	190″	5
Part B	Discontinued	5
Spatial Relations	10	5
Digit Symbol	[Scaled Score 1; Age Corrected 3]	
	Raw Score	T-Score
Stroop Color Word Test		
Word	36	23
Color	18	<20
Color–Word	0	0
LNNB Pathognomonic Scale		
Critical level 73	42	92
Shipley Institute of Living Scale		
Vocabulary	17	31
Abstraction	4	40
Abs. Quot.		106
MAE Controlled Oral Word Association Test		
Raw Score 26 Percentile Rank 12		
MAE Visual Naming Test		
Raw Score 48 Percentile Rank 18		
Beck Depression Inventory		
Raw Score 33		

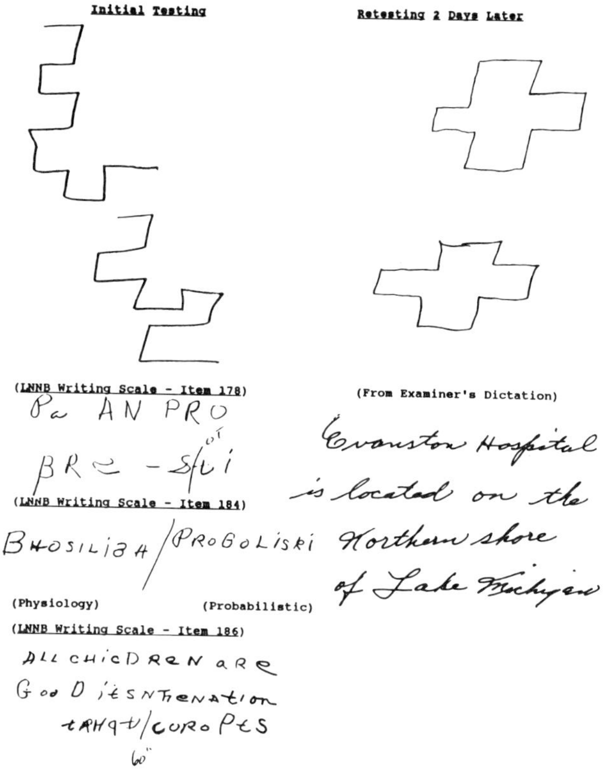

FIGURE 9.1. Writing samples for case #8 at initial testing and at retesting 2 days later.

during her admission indicated a single old subcortical infarct. Consistent with cases reported by Fogel and Sparadeo (1985) and Sweet (1983), such individuals are seen as having focal cognitive deficits exacerbated by depression.

Case #9. Case #9 was referred while a psychiatric inpatient because of possible dementia with depression. This right-handed, 88-year-old Caucasian female had a high school education. The patient's family had become concerned about memory deficit and their observations of behavior and conditions in her home suggesting that it may not be safe for her to continue living alone. She reported a gradual decline in memory, "but nothing unusual." No symptoms of depression could be elicited, nor were any signs of depression evident during the evaluation. On the basis of her clinical presentation and the test data presented in Table 9.10, patient #9 was thought to be demented. Independent observations of the attending psychiatrist led him to the same conclusion. Nursing home placement was recommended.

Approximately 15 months later, upon request of the family, the patient's internist referred her for reevaluation. Placement into an active, structured, and

TABLE 9.10. Case #9—Age 88, Education 12, Sex F, Handedness R, Vocation Unknown

	First admin.		Second admin.	
	Raw Score	Russell Ratings	Raw Score	Russell Ratings
Tapping				
Dominant	24	4	27	4
Non-Dominant	20.2	4	20	4
Trailmaking Test				
Part A	173″	5	87″	5
Part B	dc'd	5	dc'd	5
Spatial Relations	4	2	1	0
Wechsler Memory Scale				
Semantic Immediate	4.5	5	14	3
Semantic Delayed	4.5	5	6	4
Figural Immediate	2.5	4	4	4
Figural Delayed	0	5	4	3

	First admin.	Second admin.
Associate Learning		
Easy/hard:	5/0, 6/0, 6/1	5/1,5/1,6/2
Digit Span		
Forward/Backward:	5/4	6/3
Orientation		
Oriented	Day incorrect	×3
Rey Auditory Verbal Learning Test		
Trials 1–5:	2,5,7,9,6	4,4,6,8,8
Interference	3	4
Immed. Recall	6	5
Immed. Recog.	7 (2 false pos.)	9 (4 false pos.)
Delayed Recall	3	0
Delayed Recog	13 (10 false pos.)	9 (10 false pos.)
LNNB Pathognomonic Scale		
Critical level 69	77	58
MAE Controlled Oral Word Association Test		
Raw Score	27	30
Percentile Rank	12–22	12–22
MAE Visual Naming Test		
Raw Score	n/a	46
Percentile Rank	n/a	12
Beck Depression Inventory		
Raw Score	n/a	1
Digital Symbol		
Scaled Score	1	3
Age Corrected	4	7
Immediate Recall		
Symbols	n/a	6
Pairs	n/a	1

continued

TABLE 9.10. *Continued*

	First admin.		Second admin.	
	Raw Score	T-Score	Raw Score	T-Score
Stroop Color Word Test				
Word	43	<20	65	28
Color	dc'd	dc'd	37	20
Color–Word	dc'd	dc'd	26	30
Shipley Institute of Living Scale				
Vocabulary	dc'd	dc'd	22	39
Abstraction	dc'd	dc'd	6	42
Abs. Quot.		dc'd		93

stimulating nursing home environment had apparently brought about a dramatic return of the patient's old sociable personality style, which according to the family had not been evident in 15 years. Despite some continued memory problems, the patient was happy and her family was no longer worried. In fact, they now sought reassurance that their mother was not going to be suffering a decline because of degenerative dementia. Data from retesting showing improvement were presented in Table 10. In retrospect, the reported and observed changes strongly suggested that an atypical (asymptomatic) depression had been the primary problem, with a mild dementia being secondary.

Dementia with Secondary Depression

Case #10. Patient #10 was initially referred by her neurosurgeon for psychological counseling because of difficulties in coping. The 69-year-old right-handed Caucasian female had suffered a fall 18 months earlier, and also described a serious "relapse" recently. Only an old infarct, unrelated to the fall, had been identified on CT 18 months earlier. An MRI report from another hospital was obtained that revealed chronic ischemic white matter change. While the patient had failed to follow through on the neurosurgeon's other recommendations for further medical work-up of her cerebral vascular system, she was agreeable to a neuropsychological evaluation prior to initiation of counseling in order to better define her presenting complaints of memory impairment, word finding, difficulty switching from one subject to another, as well as her anxiety and depression. The patient's functioning level, as depicted in Table 9.11, was suggestive of significant decrease from her premorbid level of functioning as she remains the president of several companies, and had 14 years of education. A diagnostic conclusion of dementia with secondary depression was made, and later confirmed through improvement of cognitive abilities in response to improvement of depression through psychological counseling.

TABLE 9.11. Case #10—Age 69, Education 14, Sex F, Handedness R, Vocation Unknown

	Raw Score	Russell Ratings
Trailmaking Test		
Part A	47″	2
Part B	130″ (1 error)	3
Spatial Relations	2	1
Wechsler Memory Scale		
Semantic Immediate	13	4
Semantic Delayed	10	3
Figural Immediate	6	3
Figural Delayed	6	3
Associate Learning	[Easy/hard: 3/0, 6/1, 6/2]	
Digit Span	[Forward 6/Backward 5]	
Orientation	[Oriented × 3]	
Digit Symbol	[Scaled Score 6; Age Corrected 10]	
Immediate Recall	[Symbols 7; Pairs 7]	

	Raw Score	T-Score
Stroop Color Word Test		
Word	102	47
Color	73	45
Color–Word	41	46
Shipley Institute of Living Scale		
Vocabulary	38	67
Abstraction	22	58
Abs. Quot.		93

California Verbal Learning Test
List A (1–5): 5,7,7,6,7
List B: 3
Immed. Recall 6; Immed. Cued Recall 9
Delayed Recall 6; Delayed Cued recall 9
Delayed Recog. 15 (6 false positives)

MAE Controlled Oral Word Association Test
Raw Score 47 Percentile Rank 77–89

MAE Visual Naming Test
Raw Score 54 Percentile Rank 50

Category Test
85 errors

WAIS-R—Scaled Scores (Age Corrected)

Inf.	10 (10)	Pic. Com.	8 (11)
Dig. Sp.	10 (11)	Pic. Arr.	7 (11)
Voc.	10 (11)	B.D.	7 (10)
Arith.	10 (11)	O.A.	5 (8)
Comp.	12 (12)	Dig. Sym.	6 (10)
Sim.	9 (11)		

VIQ 107; PIQ 99; FSIQ 103

Beck Depression Inventory
Raw Score 13

POMS Depression Scale
Raw Score 6 T-Score 36

MAACL-R
Depression T-Score 87
Dysphoria T-Score 64
Positive Affect T-Score 30

Clinical Recommendations

As should be evident from the literature and cases presented in this chapter, there are no foolproof methods for detecting and quantifying the effects of depression on neuropsychological measures. With this caveat in mind, we offer the following suggestions for clinical practice:

1. Regularly include measures of depression among the tests administered to patients. However, as can be seen in cases #3, 4, and 5, self-report depression measures may be inconsistent with actual clinical presentation. Because of their face valid nature, low scores do not necessarily rule out depression.
2. Be aware of the behavioral characteristics often associated with pseudodementia.
3. Be particularly suspect of patients who are *too* impaired, or whose impairment is inconsistent with daily activities and responsibilities and/or with completely normal medical diagnostic tests (e.g., patient performs very severely on all measures administered, but successfully carries out normal adult daily life, including driving, banking, cooking, etc.). In addition to depression, these patients need to be evaluated with regard to possible secondary gain, and in some cases, even malingering.
4. Among patients who are depressed, use a more stringent "cutoff" before reaching a conclusion of brain dysfunction, especially on tests known to be strongly influenced by depression (e.g., Trails, Digit Symbol).
5. Among patients who are depressed, do not diagnose brain dysfunction only on the basis of such findings as decreased cognitive efficiency or mild attentional or memory problems. Instead, look for patterns *not* typically seen in depressed patients (e.g., clear aphasic sings, true "Stroop effect" as opposed to slowness on all three Stroop Color-Word pages, impaired recall *and* recognition, impaired incidental *and* intentional learning, impaired easy *and* hard paired associates).
6. When uncertain of the degree to which results may reflect poor effort, inattention, or other variables related to depression, readminister a portion of the measures on a different day. Look for significant changes from first to second administration.
7. If the diagnostic conclusion appears unclear despite all your best efforts, request a reevaluation of the depressed patient after at least some intervention (e.g., psychotherapy, antidepressant trial) has been carried out. Again look for emotional and cognitive changes across time.

SUMMARY

The neuropsychology of depression is a relatively new area of study and much work is still needed to understand the exact nature of the depression-related cognitive deficits described throughout this chapter. Future directions for research should be apparent, particularly with regard to studies further clarifying the influence of psychomotor retardation, motivational and attentional variables, and severity and subtype of depression. It is hoped that more will be learned about the clinical utility of administering some psychological measures (e.g., related to depression, motivation, or attention) in conjunction with neuropsychological measures to help clinicians tease out those deficits that are related to depression as opposed to brain damage. It would be of great clinical use to replicate and expand upon those studies offering specific neuropsychological measures that may effectively discriminate between depressed and brain-damaged groups (e.g., demented patients). Of particular interest is the further development of research methodologies directed at clarifying the influence of motivational factors upon neuropsychological test performance. In this regard, the research design of Richards and Ruff (1989), which allows evaluation of motivation as distinct from depression, holds particular promise.

With regard to our understanding of the neurobiology of depression, many recent developments in technology make this a very exciting time as advances are being made toward integrating findings from such areas as neuropsychology, neuropsychiatry, neurochemistry, and neuroendocrinology. For example, a recent study using MRI found that patchy white matter lesions (PWML) occur in unexpected abundance in the brains of individuals with affective disorder (e.g., Krishnan, Goli, Ellinwood, France, Blazer, & Nemeroff, 1988), suggesting that there may be specific brain changes that may account for some of the findings of depressive deficits outlined in this chapter. In the next few years, scientific advances and further clinical investigations will undoubtedly yield answers to many of the challenges faced by clinicians on a daily basis.

REFERENCES

Abrams, R., & Taylor, M. (1987). Cognitive dysfunction in melancholia. *Psychological Medicine, 17,* 359–362.

Adams, R., Craig, P., & Parsons, O. (1986). Neuropsychology of dementia. *Neurologic Clinics, 4*(2), 387–404.

Alves, W., Colohan, A., O'Leary, T., Rimel, R., & Jane, J. (1986). Understanding posttraumatic symptoms after minor head injury. *Journal of Head Trauma Rehabilitation, 1*(2), 1–12.

American Psychiatric Association. (1987). *Diagnostic and Statistical Manual of Mental Disorders* (3rd ed., rev.). Washington, D.C.:Author.

Atteberry-Bennett, J., Barth, J., Loyd, B., & Lawrence, E. (1986). *International Journal of Clinical Neuropsychology, 8,* 114–117.

Barber, J., Tomer, R., Sroka, H., & Myslobodsky, M. (1985). Does unilateral dopamine deficit contribute to depression? *Psychiatry Research, 15,* 17–24.

Baretz, R., & Stephenson, G. (1981). Emotional responses to multiple sclerosis. *Psychosomatics, 22,* 117–127.

Barnard, R., & Triggs, M. (1974). Corpus callosum in multiple sclerosis. *Journal of Neurology, Neurosurgery, and Psychiatry, 37,* 1259–1264.

Beatty, P., & Gange, J. (1977). Neuropsychological aspects of multiple sclerosis. *Journal of Nervous and Mental Disease, 164,* 42–50.

Benson, D., & Geschwind, N. (1975). Psychiatric conditions associated with focal lesions of the central nervous system. In M. Reiser (Ed.), *American Handbook of Psychiatry* (2nd ed., Vol. 4). (pp. 208–243). New York: Basic Books.

Bigler, E. (1988). *Diagnostic clinical neuropsychology* (2nd ed). Austin: University of Texas.

Blackburn, I. M. (1975). Mental and psychomotor speed in depression and mania. *British Journal of Psychiatry, 126*, 329–335.

Brown, G., & Wilson, W. (1972). Parkinsonism and depression. *Southern Medical Journal, 65*, 540–545.

Brownell, B., & Hughes, J. (1962). The distribution of plaques in the cerebrum in multiple sclerosis. *Journal of Neurology, Neurosurgery, and Psychiatry, 25*, 315–320.

Bryden, M., & Ley, R. (1983). Right-hemisphere involvement in the perception and expression of emotion in normal humans. In K. Heilman & P. Satz (Eds.), *Neuropsychology of human emotion.* (pp. 6–44). New York: Guilford Press.

Caine, E. (1981). Pseudodementia: Current concepts and future directions. *Archives of General Psychiatry, 38*, 1359–1364.

Calev, A., & Erwin, P. (1985). Recall and recognition in depressives: Use of matched tests. *British Journal of Clinical Psychology, 24*, 127–128.

Charcot, J. (1877). *Lectures on the diseases of the nervous system delivered at La Salpetriere.* London: New Sydenham Society.

Cohen, R., Weingartner, H., Smallberg, S., Pickar, D., & Murphy, D. (1982). Effort and cognition in depression. *Archives of General Psychiatry, 39*, 593–597.

Coughlan, A., & Hollows, S. (1984). Use of memory tests in differentiating organic disorder from depression. *British Journal of Psychiatry, 145*, 164–167.

Cronholm, B., & Ottoson, J. (1961). Memory functions in endogenous depression: Before and after electroconvulsive therapy. *Archives of General Psychiatry, 5*, 101–107.

Cummings, J. (1986). Subcortical dementia: Neuropsychology, neuropsychiatry, and pathophysiology. *British Journal of Psychiatry, 149*, 682–697.

Cummings, J., & Benson, D. (1984). Subcortical dementia: Review of an emerging concept. *Archives of Neurology, 41*, 874–879.

Feinberg, T., & Goodman, B. (1984). Affective illness, dementia, and pseudodementia. *Journal of Clinical Psychiatry, 45*, 99–103.

Finset, A. (1988). Depressed mood and reduced emotionality after right-hemisphere brain damage. In M. Kinsbourne (Ed.), *Cerebral hemisphere function in depression.* (pp. 51–64). Washington, D.C.: American Psychiatric Press.

Flor-Henry, P. (1979). On certain aspects of the localization of cerebral systems regulating and determining emotion. *Biological Psychiatry, 14*, 677–698.

Flor-Henry, P. (1983). *Cerebral basis of psychopathology.* Boston: Wright.

Flor-Henry, P. (1984). Hemispheric laterality and disorders of affect. In R. Post & J. Ballenger (Eds.), *Neurobiology of modo disorders.* (pp. 467–480). Baltimore: Williams & Wilkins.

Fogel, B., & Sparadeo, F. (1985). Focal cognitive deficits accentuated by depression. *Journal of Nervous and Mental Disease, 173*, 120–124.

Friedman, M., & Lipowski, Z. (1981). Pseudodementia in a young PhD. *American Journal of Psychiatry, 138*, 381–382.

Frith, C., Stevens, M., Johnstone, E., Deakin, J., Lawler, P., & Crow, T. (1983). Effect of ECT and depression on various aspects of memory. *British Journal of Psychiatry, 142*, 610–617.

Fromm, D., & Schopflocher, D. (1984). Neuropsychological test performance in depressed patients before and after drug therapy. *Biological Psychiatry, 19*(1), 55–72.

Fromm-Auch, D. (1983). Neuropsychological assessment of depressed patients before and after drug therapy: Clinical profile interpretation. In P. Flor-Henry & J. Gruzelier (Eds.), *Laterality and psychopathology.* (pp. 83–102). Amsterdam: Elsevier.

Gainotti, G. (1972). Emotional behavior and hemispheric side of the lesion. *Cortex, 8*, 41–55.

Gallagher, D., & Thompson, L. (1983). Depression. In P. Lewinson & L. Teri (Eds.), *Clinical geropsychology.* Elmsford, N.Y.: Pergamon Press.

Gass, C., & Russell, E. (1986). Differential impact of brain damage and depression on memory test performance. *Journal of Consulting and Clinical Psychology, 54*(2), 261–263.

Gennarelli, T. (1986). Mechanisms and pathophysiology of cerebral concussion. *Journal of Head Trauma Rehabilitation, 1*(2), 23–29.

Golden, C. (1981). *Diagnosis and rehabilitation in clinical neuropsychology.* Springfield, Ill.: Thomas.

Goldstein, K. (1942). *Aftereffects of brain injuries in war*. New York: Grune & Stratton.
Goodstein, R., & Ferrell, R. (1977). Multiple sclerosis presenting as depressive illness. *Diseases of the Nervous System, 38*, 127–131.
Goulet Fisher, D., Sweet, J., & Pfaelzer-Smith, E. (1986). Depression and neuropsychological impairment. *International Journal of Clinical Neuropsychology, VIII*(1), 14–18.
Gray, J., Dean, R., Rattan, G., & Cramer, K. (1987). Neuropsychological aspects of primary affective depression. *International Journal of Neuroscience, 32*, 911–918.
Gustafson, L. (1975). Psychiatric symptoms in dementia with onset in the presenile period. *Acta Psychiatrica Scandinavica [suppl.]*, (257):7–35.
Hale, W., & Strickland, B. (1976). Induction of mood states and their effect on cognitive and social behaviors. *Journal of Consulting and Clinical Psychology, 44*, 155.
Hart, R., Kwentus, J., Wade, J., & Hamer, R. (1987). Digit symbol performance in mild dementia and depression. *Journal of Consulting and Clinical Psychology, 55*(2), 236–238.
Hart, R., Kwentus, J., Taylor, J., & Hamer, R. (1988). Productive naming and memory in depression and Alzheimer's type dementia. *Archives of Clinical Neuropsychology, 3*, 313–322.
Haward, L. (1977). Cognition in dementia presinilis. In W. Smith & M. Kinsbourne (Eds.), *Aging and dementia*. (pp. 189–202). New York: Spectrum.
Heaton, R., & Crowley, T. (1981). Effects of psychiatric disorders and their somatic treatments on neuropsychological test results. In S. Filskov & T. Boll (Eds.), *Handbook of clinical neuropsychology*. (pp. 481–525). New York: Wiley.
Heaton, R., Baade, L., & Johnson, K. (1978). Neuropsychological test results associated with psychiatric disorders in adults. *Psychological Bulletin, 85*, 141–162.
Heaton, R., Nelson, D. L., Thompson, D., Burks, J., & Franklin, G. (1985). Neuropsychological findings in relapsing–remitting and chronic–progressive multiple sclerosis. *Journal of Consulting and Clinical Psychology, 53*, 103–110.
Heaton, S., & Heaton, R. (1981). Testing the impaired patient. In S. Filskov & T. Boll (Eds.), *Handbook of clinical neuropsychology*. (pp. 526–544). New York: Wiley.
Heilman, K., & Satz, P. (1983). *Neuropsychology of human emotion*. New York: Guilford Press.
Heilman, K., Watson, R., & Bowers, D. (1983). Affective disorders associated with hemispheric disease. In K. Heilman & P. Satz (Eds.). *Neuropsychology of human emotion*. (pp. 45–64). New York: Guilford Press.
Heinrichs, R. (1987). Does depression in patients with known or suspected cerebral disease contribute to impairment on the Luria–Nebraska Neuropsychological Battery? *International Journal of Neuroscience, 32*, 895–899.
Houlihan, J., Abrahams, J., La Rue, A., & Jarvik, L. (1985). Qualitative differences in vocabulary performance of Alzheimer versus depressed patients. *Developmental Neuropsychology, 1*(2), 139–144.
Hunt, J., & Cofer, C. (1944). Psychological deficit. In J. M. Hunt (Ed.), *Personality and the behavior disorders: A handbook based on experimental and clinical research*. (pp. 971–1032). New York: Ronald Press.
Johansen, A., Gustafson, L., & Risberg, J. (1985). Psychological evaluation in dementia and depression. *Danish Medical Bulletin, 32*(Suppl. 1), 60–62.
Kendell, R. (1974). The stability of psychiatric diagnoses. *British Journal of Psychiatry, 124*, 352–356.
Kennely, K., Hayslip, B., & Richardson, S. (1985). Depression and helplessness-induced cognitive deficits in the aged. *Experimental Aging Research, 11*(3), 169–173.
Kerry, R., McDermott, C., & Orme, J. (1983). Affective disorders and cognitive performance. *Journal of Affective Disorders, 5*, 349–352.
Kinsbourne, M. (1988). *Cerebral hemisphere function in depression*. Washington, D.C.: American Psychiatric Press.
Koenigsberg, H. (1984). Manic pseudodementia: Case report. *Journal of Clinical Psychiatry, 45*, 132–134.
Kopelman, M. (1986). Clinical tests of memory. *British Journal of Psychiatry, 148*, 517–525.
Krishnan, K., Goli, V., Ellinwood, E., France, R., Blazer, D., & Nemeroff, C. (1988). Leukoencephalopathy in patients diagnosed as major depressive. *Biological Psychiatry, 23*, 519–522.
Levin, H., Benton, A., & Grossman, R. (1982). *Neurobehavioral consequences of closed head injury*. New York: Oxford University Press.

Levin, H. Grafman, J., & Eisenberg, H. (1987). *Neurobehavioral recovery from head injury*. New York: Oxford University Press.

Lezak, M. (1983). *Neuropsychological assessment* (2nd ed.). New York: Oxford University Press.

Lipkin, M. (1985). Psychiatry and medicine. In H. Kaplan & B. Sadock (Eds.), *Comprehensive textbook of psychiatry (4th ed.)*. (pp. 1263–1277). Baltimore: Williams & Wilkins.

Lishman, W. (1968). Brain damage in relation to psychiatric disability after head injury. *British Journal of Psychiatry, 114*, 373–410.

Liston, E. (1977). Illness. *American Journal of Psychiatry, 138*, 1–13.

Livingston, M. (1987). Head injury: The relatives' response. *Brain Injury, 1*, 33–39.

Livingston, M., & Brooks, D. (1988). The burden on families of the brain injured: A review. *Journal of Head Trauma Rehabilitation, 3*, 6–15.

Lumsden, C. (1970). The neuropathology of multiple sclerosis. In P. Vinken & G. Bruyn (Eds.), *Handbook of clinical neurology* (Vol. 9, pp. 217–309). New York: American Elsevier.

Madden, J., Luhan, J., Kaplan, L., & Manfredi, H. (1952). Nondementing psychoses in older persons. *Journal of the American Medical Association, 150*, 1567–1570.

Malec, J. (1978). Neuropsychological assessment of schizophrenia versus brain damage: A review. *Journal of Nervous and Mental Disease, 166*, 507–516.

Marcopulos, B. (1987). Memory complaints in depressed and non-depressed elderly. Paper presented at the annual meeting of the American Psychological Association, New York.

Marsden, C., & Harrison, M. (1972). Outcome of investigation of patients with presenile dementia. *British Medical Journal, 2*, 249–252.

Marsh, G. (1980). Disability and intellectual function in multiple sclerosis patients. *Journal of Nervous and Mental Disease, 168*, 758–762.

Matthews, W. (1979). Multiple sclerosis presenting with acute remitting psychiatric symptoms. *Journal of Neurology, Neurosurgery, and Psychiatry, 42*, 859–863.

Mayeux, R. (1983). Emotional changes associated with basal ganglia disorders. In K. Heilman & P. Satz (Eds.), *Neuropsychology of human emotion*. (pp. 141–164). New York: Guilford Press.

McAllister, T. (1983). Overview: Pseudodementia. *American Journal of Psychiatry, 140*, 528–533.

McAllister, T. (1985). Recognition of pseudodementia. *American Family Physician, 32*, 175–181.

McCaffrey, R. Pollock, J., & Burns, P. (1987). An archival analysis of the needs of head injured survivors in New York State: Preliminary findings. *International Journal of Clinical Neuropsychology, 9*, 174–177.

McEvoy, J., & Wells, C. (1979). Conversion pseudodementia. *Journal of Clinical Psychiatry, 40*, 447–449.

McKinlay, W., Brooks, D., Martinage, D., & Marshall, M. (1981). The short-term outcome of severe blunt head injury as reported by relatives of the injured person. *Journal of Neurology, Neurosurgery, and Psychiatry, 44*, 527–533.

McLean, S. (1978). Assessing dementia. Part I: Difficulties, definitions, and differential diagnosis. *Australian and New Zealand Journal of Psychiatry, 21*, 142–174.

McMordie, W. (1988). Twenty-year follow-up of the prevailing opinion on the posttraumatic or postconcussional syndrome. *The Clinical Neuropsychologist, 2*, 198–212.

Miller, W. (1975). Psychological deficit in depression. *Psychological Bulletin, 82*, 238–260.

Mortimer, J., Christensen, K., & Webster, D. (1985). Parkinsonian dementia. In J. Fredericks (Ed.), *Handbook of clinical neurology: Neurobehavioral disorders (Vol. 2)*. (pp. 371–384). Amsterdam: Elsevier.

Mukherjee, S., Shukla, S., & Rosen, A. (1984). Neurological abnormalities in patients with bipolar disorder. *Biological Psychiatry, 19*(3), 337–345.

Nelson, J., & Charney, D. (1981). The symptoms of major depressive illness. *American Journal of Psychiatry, 138*, 1–13.

Newman, P., & Silverstein, M. (1987). Neuropsychological test performance among major clinical subtypes of depression. *Archives of Clinical Neuropsychology, 2*, 115–125.

Newman, P., & Sweet, J. (1986). The effects of clinical depression on the Luria–Nebraska Neuropsychological Battery. *International Journal of Clinical Neuropsychology, 7*(3), 109–114.

Nott, P., & Fleminger, J. (1975). Presenile dementia: The difficulties of early diagnosis. *Acta Psychiatrica Scandinavia, 51*, 210–217.

Peyser, J., & Poser, C. (1986). Neuropsychological correlates of multiple sclerosis. In S. Filskov & T. Boll (Eds.), *Handbook of clinical neuropsychology* (Vol. 2). (pp. 364–397). New York: Wiley.

Popkin, S., Gallagher, D., Thompson, L., & Moore, M. (1982). Memory complaint and performance in normal and depressed older adults. *Experimental Aging Research*, *8*(3), 141–145.

Prigatano, G. (1987). Psychiatric aspects of head injury: Problem areas and suggested guidelines for research. In H. Levin, J. Grafman, & H. Eisenberg (Eds.), *Neurobehavioral recovery from head injury* (pp. 215–231). New York: Oxford University Press.

Rabins, P., Brooks, B., O'Donnell, P., Pearlson, G., Moberg, P., Jubelt, B., Coyle, P., Dalos, N., & Folstein, M. (1986). Structural brain correlates to emotional disorder in multiple sclerosis. *Brain*, *109*, 585–597.

Rao, S. (1986). Neuropsychology of multiple sclerosis: A critical review. *Journal of Clinical and Experimental Neuropsychology*, *8*, 503–542.

Rees, R. (1988). How some families cope and why some do not. *Journal of Head Trauma Rehabilitation*, *3*, 72–77.

Reifler, B., Larson, E., & Hanley, R. (1982). Coexistence of cognitive impairment and depression in geriatric outpatients. *American Journal of Psychiatry*, *139*, 623–626.

Reitan, R., & Wolfson, D. (1985). *The Halstead–Reitan Neuropsychological Test Battery: Theory and clinical interpretation*. Tucson: Neuropsychology Press.

Richards, P., & Ruff, R. (1989). Motivational effects on neuropsychological functioning: A comparison of depressed versus non-depressed individuals. *Journal of Consulting and Clinical Psychology*, *57*, 396–402.

Robinson, R., & Price, T. (1982). Post-stroke depressive disorders: A follow-up study of 103 patients. *Stroke*, *13*, 635–641.

Robinson, R., Starr, L., Kubos, K., & Price, T. (1983). A two year longitudinal study of post-stroke mood disorders: Findings during the initial evaluation. *Stroke*, *14*, 736–741.

Robinson, R., Kubos, K., Starr, L., Rao, K., & Price, T. (1984). Mood disorders in stroke patients: Importance of location of lesion. *Brain*, *107*, 81–93.

Ron, M., Toone, B., Garralda, M., & Lishman, W. (1979). Diagnostic accuracy in presenile dementia. *British Journal of Psychiatry*, *134*, 161–168.

Ross, A., & Reitan, R. (1955). Intellectual and affective functions in multiple sclerosis. *Archives of Neurology and Psychiatry*, *73*, 663–677.

Ross, E. (1981). The aprosodias. *Archives of Neurology*, *38*, 561–569.

Ruckdeschel-Hibbard, M., Gordon, W., & Diller, L. (1986). Affective disturbances associated with brain damage. In S. Filskov & T. Boll (Eds.), *Handbook of clinical neuropsychology*. (pp. 305–337). New York: Wiley.

Rush, A., Weissenburger, J., Vinson, D., & Giles, D. (1983). Neuropsychological dysfunctions in unipolar nonpsychotic major depressions. *Journal of Affective Disorders*, *5*, 281–287.

Savard, R., Rey, A., & Post, R. (1980). Halstead–Reitan Category Test in bipolar and unipolar affective disorders: Relationship to age and phase of illness. *Journal of Nervous and Mental Disease*, *168*, 297–304.

Schaffer, C., Davidson, R., & Saron, C. (1983). Frontal and parietal electroencephalogram asymmetry in depressed and nondepressed subjects. *Biological Psychiatry*, *18*, 753–762.

Schiffer, R., & Babigian, H. (1984). Behavioral disorders in multiple sclerosis, temporal lobe epilepsy, and amyotrophic lateral sclerosis: An epidemiologic study. *Archives of Neurology*, *41*, 1067–1069.

Schiffer, R., Caine, E., Bamford, K., & Levy, S. (1983). Depressive episodes in patients with multiple sclerosis. *American Journal of Psychiatry*, *140*, 1498–1500.

Shipley, J., Kupfer, D. Spiker, D., Shaw, D., Coble, P., Neil, J., & Cofsky, J. (1981). Neuropsychological assessment and EEG sleep in affective disorders. *Biological Psychiatry*, *16*(10), 907–918.

Silberman, E., Weingartner, H., Targum, S., & Barnes, S. (1985). Cognitive functioning in the biological subtypes of depression. *Biological Psychiatry*, *20*, 654–661.

Singer, J., & Salovey, P. (1988). Mood and memory: Evaluating the network theory of affect. *Clinical Psychology Review*, *8*, 211–251.

Spicer, K., Roberts, R., & LeWitt, P. (1988). Neuropsychological performance in lateralized parkinsonism. *Archives of Neurology*, *45*, 429–432.

Spitzer, R., Endicott, J., & Robins, E. (1978). *Research diagnostic criteria (RDC) for a selected group of functional disorders* (3rd ed.). New York: New York State Psychiatric Institute, Biometrics Research.

Starkstein, S., & Robinson, R. (1988). Lateralized emotional response following stroke. In M. Kinsbourne (Ed.), *Cerebral hemisphere function in depression*. (pp. 25–47). Washington, D.C.: American Psychiatric Press.

Staton, R., Wilson, H., & Brumback, R. (1981). Cognitive improvement associated with tricyclic antidepressant treatment of childhood major depressive illness. *Perceptual and Motor Skills, 53*, 219–234.

Sternberg, D., & Jarvik, M. (1976). Memory functions in depression. *Archives of General Psychiatry, 33*, 219–224.

Stromgren, L. (1977). The influence of depression on memory. *Acta Psychiatrica Scandinavia, 56*, 109–128.

Strub, R., & Black, F. (1981). *Organic brain syndrome: An introduction to neurobehavioral disorders*. Philadelphia: Davis.

Sweet, J. (1983). Confounding effects of depression on neuropsychological testing: Five illustrative cases. *Clinical Neuropsychology, 5*, 103–109.

Tarter, R., Van Thiel, D., & Edwards, K. (1988). *Medical neuropsychology: The impact of disease on behavior*. New York: Plenum Press.

Teri, L., & Reifler, B. (1987). Depression and dementia. In L. Carstensen & B. Edelstein (Eds.), *Handbook of clinical gerontology*. (pp. 112–119). Elmsford, N.Y.: Pergamon Press.

Tucker, D. (1988). Neuropsychological mechanisms of affective self-regulation. In M. Kinsbourne (Ed.), *Cerebral hemisphere function in depression*. (pp. 101–131). Washington, D.C.: American Psychiatric Press.

Varney, N., Martzke, J., & Roberts, R. (1987). Major depression in patients with closed head injury. *Neuropsychology, 1*, 7–9.

Watts, F., Morris, L., & MacLeod, A. (1987). Recognition memory in depression. *Journal of Abnormal Psychology, 96*(3), 273–275.

Wechsler, D. (1987). *Wechsler Memory Scale—Revised (manual)*. New York: Psychological Corporation.

Weckowicz, T., Nutter, R., Cruise, D., Yonge, K., & Cairns, M. (1978). Speed in test performance in relation to depressive illness and age (An appendix). *Canadian Psychiatric Association Journal, 23*, 107–109.

Weingartner, H., & Silberman, E. (1982). Models of cognitive impairment: Cognitive changes in depression. *Psychopharmacology Bulletin, 18*(2), 27–42.

Weingartner, H., Cohen, R., Martello, J., & Gerdt, C. (1981). Cognitive processes in depression. *Archives of General Psychiatry, 38*, 42–47.

Weissman, M., & Boyd, J. (1985). Affective disorders: Epidemiology. In H. Kaplan & B. Sadock (Eds.), *Comprehensive textbook of psychiatry* (4th ed.). (pp. 764–769). Baltimore: Williams & Wilkins.

Wells, C. (1979). Pseudodementia. *American Journal of Psychiatry, 136*, 895–900.

West, R., Boatwright, L., & Schlester R. (1984). The link between memory performance, self-assessment, and affective status. *Experimental Aging Research, 10*(4), 197–200.

Whitehouse, P. (1986). The concept of subcortical and cortical dementia: Another look. *Annals of Neurology, 19*(1), 1–6.

Whitlock, F., & Siskind, M. (1980). Depression as a major symptom of multiple sclerosis. *Journal of Neurology, Neurosurgery, and Psychiatry, 43*, 861–865.

Williams, J., Little, M., Scates, S., & Blockman, N. (1987). Memory complaints and abilities among depressed older adults. *Journal of Consulting and Clinical Psychology, 55*, 595–598.

Wysocki, J., & Sweet, J. (1985). Identification of schizophrenic, brian-damaged, and normal medical patients using a brief neuropsychological screening battery. *International Journal of Clinical Neuropsychology, 7*, 40–44.

Zarit, S., & Zarit, J. (1983). Cognitive impairment. In P. Lewinsohn & L. Teri (Eds.), *Clinical Geropsychology*. (pp. 38–80). Elmsford, NY: Pergamon Press.

Zeigler, D. (1954). Cerebral atrophy in psychiatric patients. *American Journal of Psychiatry, 111*, 454–455.

Zung, W., & Krugman, A. (1968). Effect of electroconvulsive therapy on memory in depressive disorders. *Recent Advances in Biological Psychiatry, 10*, 160–178.

10

Schizophrenic Disorders

ELAINE WALKER, MARSHA LUCAS, and RICHARD LEWINE

INTRODUCTION

The conceptualization of schizophrenia as a brain disorder is long-standing. Kraepelin (1919/1971) emphasized the gradual cognitive deterioration in schizophrenia and argued that this "dementia" was organically based. Although Bleuler (1950) viewed "associative disturbance" as the core symptom in schizophrenia, like Kraepelin he presumed the symptoms of schizophrenia were a manifestation of underlying organic impairment. Since the times of Kraepelin and Bleuler, interest in organic determinants of schizophrenia has waxed and waned. Most recently, we have entered a new era of biological research on the disorder. The renewed concern with biological factors was, in part, spawned by the increasing sophistication of available techniques for assessing brain structure and function.

This chapter is concerned with the role of neuropsychology in the study, assessment, and treatment of schizophrenia. As the burgeoning field of neuropsychology broadened our understanding of brain–behavior relations, interest was stimulated in identifying the brain dysfunction subserving schizophrenia. The search began with the application of standardized clinical assessment batteries to groups of patients, often with the goal of differentiating psychiatric patients from those with neurological disorders or from normals. But, gradually, clinical neuropsychological assessment has been integrated into multimodal studies of schizophrenia that examine the relations between neuroanatomical and cognitive factors. In addition, experimental neuropsychological procedures have been used to investigate hemispheric asymmetry and interhemispheric transfer in schizophrenia. This work has generated several intriguing hypotheses regarding the nature of hemispheric functions in psychopathology.

ELAINE WALKER, MARSHA LUCAS, and RICHARD LEWINE • Departments of Psychiatry and Psychology, Emory University, Atlanta, Georgia 30322.

HANDBOOK OF NEUROPSYCHOLOGICAL ASSESSMENT: A Biopsychosocial Perspective, edited by Antonio E. Puente and Robert J. McCaffrey. Plenum Press, New York, 1992.

Our discussion of the research will address both the clinical and experimental neuropsychological literature on schizophrenia. The major competing hypotheses of brain dysfunction in schizophrenia will be highlighted; specifically, the hypotheses of (1) frontal lobe abnormality, (2) left hemisphere impairment, and (3) interhemispheric transfer deficit. Investigators have cited a number of other brain regions and processes as possible sources of schizophrenic pathology (e.g., the limbic system) and some of these will also be discussed, but the primary focus will be on the three hypotheses cited above. Finally, this chapter will address the role of neuropsychology in the assessment and treatment of schizophrenia.

A central point to be conveyed in this chapter is that neuropsychology holds great promise for contributing to our understanding of psychopathology. Contrary to the expectations of some psychopathologists, technologies such as computerized axial tomography, magnetic resonance imaging, and positron emission tomography have not provided conclusive evidence regarding the organic basis of schizophrenia. These techniques have, indeed, confirmed the existence of brain abnormalities in some psychiatric patients. However, the results of neuropsychological research had suggested this conclusion several decades before these brain-imaging technologies were available. It is now apparent that no single test or methodological approach holds the final answer to the riddle of schizophrenia. Instead, it appears that progress will depend upon multimodal approaches to research and clinical assessment.

HISTORY

Trends in Research on Cognitive Functions in Schizophrenia

In order to fully appreciate the evolving role of neuropsychology in our understanding of schizophrenia, we must begin with a brief overview of the literature on the cognitive deficits associated with the disorder. This research dates back to the 1930s when investigators first began to use standardized IQ tests to address the general question of whether schizophrenic patients are intellectually impaired. Laboratory-based procedures eventually began to play a role as researchers advanced more specific questions, such as whether attentional or memory dysfunction characterized schizophrenia.

Numerous studies have examined the performance of schizophrenic patients on standardized tests of intelligence. In an effort to synthesize the findings, we conducted a meta-analysis of the body of published data (Aylward, Walker, & Bettes, 1984). Combining the results across studies led to the following conclusions. First, compared to matched normal controls, schizophrenics manifest significant IQ deficits, although the mean scores for randomly selected groups of patients are well within the average range. Second, follow-back studies suggest that IQ deficits are characteristic of schizophrenic patients prior to the onset of symptoms. This is revealed when a patient's scores are compared to those of elementary-classroom peers, as well as when they are compared to those of siblings. There is little evidence of a decline in intellectual functioning following the onset of symptoms, nor does intellectual performance decline through the course of the disorder. In sum, intellectual performance deficits are associated with schizophrenia across the life span, suggesting that they may be linked with the organic vulnerability underlying the disorder.

The self-reports of patients frequently include references to problems with "concentration" or "attention" (Freedman, 1974). Such reports led investigators to hypothesize that attentional impairments may constitute the core deficit in schizophrenia. Many studies using laboratory-based tasks have demonstrated attentional problems in schizophrenic patients. Typically, these tasks are designed to assess a specific aspect of attention. For example, the continuous performance test is presumed to tap sustained visual attention, and investigations by several research groups have found that schizophrenics manifest significant performance deficits on this task (e.g., Walker & Shaye, 1982). There is also extensive evidence of selective attention deficits in schizophrenia, such that perception of relevant stimuli is impaired in the presence of distractors (Neale & Oltmanns, 1980). Given the attentional problems observed in schizophrenic patients, it is not surprising that they also manifest memory problems. This has been revealed in a variety of short-term recall tasks, such as the digit-span task, and it has been suggested that it is due to a failure in the organization of input (for a review, see Neale & Oltmanns, 1980).

The emergence of information processing theory in cognitive psychology alerted psychopathologists to the possibility of identifying a specific stage of processing deficiency in schizophrenia. This led to the application of new paradigms to the study of schizophrenic cognition. To date, the hope of identifying a stage-specific deficit has not been realized. Instead virtually all aspects of information processing that have been investigated in schizophrenic patients have been found to be deficient. This includes the very earliest stages of visual information processing, as measured with the backward masking procedure (Green & Walker, 1984) and sensory evoked potentials (Steinhauer & Zubin, 1982).

In sum, the vast literature on cognitive functions in schizophrenia has revealed a variety of performance deficits. The findings have led some to suggest that the disorder is characterized by generalized cognitive impairment, rather than any one specific deficit. In addressing this point, Chapman and Chapman (1978) have noted the difficulty of identifying differential deficits in performance. Specifically, in order to conclude that one has identified a deficit that is unique to a particular sample, it is necessary to administer multiple tasks that are equated on psychometric properties. Among the critical task parameters are mean item difficulty level and item variance. These factors determine the discriminative power of a task, i.e., the task's capacity to detect differences. When multiple tasks are administered in order to identify specific areas of impairment, which is typically the case in clinical neuropsychology, it is important that differences in task content not be confounded with differences in the discriminative power of the tasks. Unfortunately, this issue has received little attention from neuropsychologists. Undoubtedly, this is partially due to the fact that equating tasks on discriminative power when they are designed to tap disparate functions, such as psychomotor proficiency versus verbal memory, is both difficult and time-consuming.

THEORETICAL AND BASIC NEUROBIOLOGICAL ISSUES

Numerous researchers have used standardized neuropsychological batteries in studies of schizophrenia. Two general questions have dominated the literature: (1) Can schizophrenic patients be distinguished from brain-damaged patients on the basis of their performance? (2) Is it possible to differentiate among diagnostic subgroups of psychiatric patients? The first question originated in the debate regarding the neurological basis of schizophrenia. Schizophrenia was commonly referred to as a "functional" psychiatric disorder, implying the absence of an identifiable organic basis. Therefore, comparison of schizophrenic patients with neurological patients was viewed by some as a test of the validity of neuropsychological assessment. Of course, there is now strong evidence of brain abnormalities in a substantial subgroup of schizophrenic patients. As a result, the question is of limited theoretical relevance.

Comparison of Schizophrenic Patients with Other Diagnostic Groups

Several extensive reviews of the literature on clinical neuropsychological assessment of schizophrenia were published about a decade ago (Heaton, Baade, & Johnson, 1978; Lenzer, 1980; Malec, 1978). Most of the studies included in these reviews used the Halstead–Reitan (HRNB) or Luria–Nebraska Neuropsychological Battery (LNNB), and the focus was typically on overall level of performance rather than performance profiles. The general conclusion of the reviews was that schizophrenic patients could *not* be reliably distinguished from patients with organic diagnoses, although other psychiatric patients did perform significantly better than organic patients. It was therefore suggested that a substantial proportion of schizophrenic patients may, in fact, be suffering from brain impairment.

Since the time these reviews were published, several new studies comparing schizophrenic to brain-damaged patients have appeared in the literature. These investigations are characterized by methodological improvements, including more sophisticated statistical procedures and more careful documentation of the locus of brain damage in the comparison group. There have also been advances in psychiatric diagnosis; in contrast to earlier reports, most of the studies published after 1980 systematically rediagnose patients using some standard criteria. Although the specific criteria vary across studies, most recently published reports provide detailed information on the diagnostic procedures.

Some recent investigations show significant differences between schizophrenic and brain-damaged patients in overall performance, with schizophrenics performing better, but few yield evidence of differences in performance profiles. A study by Shelly and Goldstein (1983) replicated an earlier report (Purisch, Golden, & Hammeke, 1978) that the LNNB is capable of statistically discriminating schizophrenic from brain-damaged patients. However, although the combined scales were capable of discriminating the groups, no single scale achieved significant between-group differences. Moses, Cardellino, and Thompson (1983) administered the LNNB to samples of schizophrenic, schizoaffective, and brain-damaged patients and found that a few of the indices differentiated the groups, but discriminant analysis revealed no difference in profiles. They determined that group discriminability varied as a function of the inclusion criteria for the brain-damaged subjects, and suggest that differences in "hit rates" among studies are artifacts of sampling bias. Similar results are reported for the HRNB. Heaton (1979) and Chelune, Heaton, Lehman, and Robinson (1979) were able to differentiate schizophrenics from brain-damaged patients on the basis of overall impairment on the HRNB, but pattern analysis revealed no differences in profiles.

The results of an investigation by Taylor, Redfield, and Abrams (1981) constitute an exception to the general finding of no differences in performance profiles. These authors compared affective, schizophrenic, and brain-damaged patients using an abbreviated battery that included the WAIS, Peabody Picture Vocabulary, and Ravens Progressive Matrices. They found that schizophrenics performed below affective patients, but were comparable to brain-damaged patients, on the "dominant hemisphere tasks." On nondominant hemisphere tasks, schizophrenics fell midway between affective and brain-damaged patients, with only the affective and brain-damaged patients differing significantly.

Comparisons of schizophrenics with other psychiatric patients have generally revealed a continuum of neuropsychological impairment that corresponds to the severity of the disorder. This relation between severity and magnitude of performance deficits holds within the diagnostic category of schizophrenia (Benson & Stuss, 1982), as well as across categories. Schizophrenic patients perform more poorly than patients with affective disorders or other psychiatric disorders, and the latter groups perform below normals (e.g., Lawson, Waldman, & Weinberger, 1988; Maj, 1986; Taylor, Greenspan, & Abrams, 1979; Taylor *et al.*, 1981). There is, however, one diagnostic distinction that is not consistently associated with performance differences; namely, schizophrenia versus schizoaffective disorder (Maj, 1986; Moses, 1984). Controversy continues to surround the validity of this diagnostic distinction.

The notion that severity of disturbance is related to magnitude of neuropsychological impairment receives further support from the results of an investigation by Wooten (1983). The MMPI was administered along with a battery of neuropsychological tests to a group of 345 patients with known or suspected brain damage. Examination of the relation between MMPI scales and neuropsychological performance revealed a positive correlation between scores on the Schizophrenia scale of the MMPI and neuropsychological deficit.

Researchers have also approached the problem of identifying a unique performance profile among schizophrenic patients by contrasting them with other psychiatric patients. Taylor and colleagues (Taylor *et al.*, 1979, 1981; Taylor & Abrams, 1987) consistently report evidence of greater left temporal and temporo-parietal performance deficits among schizophrenics when compared to patients with affective disorders. Greater left hemisphere impairment in schizophrenics than in affective patients is also reported by Selin and Gottschalk (1983) and Dean, Gray, and Seretny (1987).

Consistent with the assumption that brain damage characterizes a substantial proportion of schizophrenic patients, numerous studies have shown that clinical neuropsychological assessment reliably differentiates groups of schizophrenics from normal controls (e.g., Kolb & Whishaw, 1983; Lewis, Golden, Purisch, & Hammeke, 1979; Strauss & Silverstein, 1986; Taylor *et al.*, 1979). There is also suggestive evidence of performance profile differences between the two groups. Taylor and colleagues (Taylor *et al.*, 1979; Taylor & Abrams, 1984) have used both the HRNB and LNNB and find evidence of greater deficits on tasks reliant on dominant frontotemporal regions. Performance profiles characteristic of left frontal deficits are also reported by authors using nonstandard batteries of neuropsychological tasks (Dean *et al.*, 1987; Levander, Bartfai, & Schalling, 1985). In contrast, Kolb and Whishaw (1983) reported that in comparison with normal controls, schizophrenic patients showed the greatest deficits on tasks tapping both left and right frontotemporal regions, but not parietal regions, and conclude that schizophrenia is associated with bilateral dysfunction.

The notion that frontal lobe pathology, particularly hypofrontality, is implicated in schizophrenia has been generated by both clinical observation and empirical data (Weinberger and Berman, 1988). The behavioral sequelae of frontal lobe lesions are well documented in the literature on brain damage. The frontal lobe patient is characterized by impaired social judgment and a lack of goal-directedness. A similar pattern of behavior has been observed in many schizophrenic patients. In fact, the notion of "negative" symptoms in schizophrenia is somewhat akin to the frontal syndrome. Negative symptoms are typically defined as behavioral deficits and include such signs as social withdrawal, blunted affect, poverty of speech, and anhedonia. Empirical support for the hypothesis of frontal lobe defects in schizophrenia comes, in part, from neuropsychological investigations.

There are several reports that schizophrenics perform below normals on the Wisconsin Card Sorting Test (Goldberg, Weinberger, & Berman, 1987; Kolb & Whishaw, 1983; Weinberger, Berman, & Zec, 1986), a measure that is presumed to be sensitive to lesions of the dorsolateral prefrontal cortex. In order to determine whether this performance deficit could be modified, Goldberg *et al.* (1987) provided schizophrenic patients with systematic instruction in the task. But repeated testing revealed no improvement in the performance of patients who showed initial deficits. These results were interpreted as providing support for the hypothesis of prefrontal abnormality in schizophrenia.

In summary, the findings from clinical neuropsychological studies of schizophrenic patients do not indicate a common or unique profile of performance. While schizophrenics show consistent deficits relative to normal and psychiatric controls, the nature of the functional impairment varies. When contrasted with affective patients, the most prevalent finding is dominant hemisphere dysfunction in schizophrenia. But when compared to normals, nonlateralized frontal and frontotemporal deficits are most apparent.

Distinguishing among Subgroups of Schizophrenic Patients

Although groups of schizophrenic patients manifest mean levels of performance on neuropsychological tasks that are consistently below those of normals, and most other psychiatric patients, there is clearly a subgroup of schizophrenics that shows no impairment. In a recent cluster-analytic study by Strauss and Silverstein (1986), 48% of schizophrenics scored in the impaired range on the LNNB, but the remaining 52% were indistinguishable from normal controls. A perusal of the cognitive literature on schizophrenia confirms that performance heterogeneity is a hallmark of randomly selected samples of patients. From a neuropsychological perspective, this lends support to the notion that patients diagnosed as schizophrenic by current criteria constitute a heterogeneous group with respect to the nature of organic involvement. As a result, randomly selected groups of patients fail to show a distinctive or "localizable" pattern of performance deficits. Instead, they manifest generalized deficits, although typically of a less severe nature than those shown by patients with known neurological conditions.

In order to shed light on the meaning of this heterogeneity, investigators have begun to examine the relation between clinical symptoms and the performance characteristics of patients. It has been shown that when schizophrenics are divided into paranoid and nonparanoid subgroups, the paranoid patients manifest better performance on clinical neuropsychological measures (Langell, Purisch, & Golden, 1987; Lewis, Nelson, & Eggertsen, 1979). Langell *et al.* (1987) concluded that paranoids show the greatest advantage over nonparanoids on tasks tapping processes subserved by the left frontal regions; specifically, motor functions, concentration, and processing of complex information. Along these same lines, Silverstein and Zerwic (1985) reported that schizophrenic patients who showed impairment on the LNNB had a *lower* incidence of delusions (i.e., were less paranoid) than patients who showed no neuropsychological impairment. In another study, Silverstein and Arzt (1985) examined the factors that differentiated neuropsychologically impaired and nonimpaired schizophrenic patients, and found that the impaired patients were characterized by significant reaction time deficits, but manifested no deficits on a word-association task. This finding converges with the results reported by Langell *et al.* (1987) that dominant frontal functions, particularly motor abilities, differentiate paranoid and nonparanoid patients.

The paranoid/nonparanoid distinction overlaps conceptually with the positive/negative symptom distinction. Positive symptoms are the florid signs of psychosis, such as hallucinations, delusions, and pressured speech. As indicated earlier, negative symptoms entail behavioral deficits, and include affective flattening, anhedonia, poverty of speech, and social withdrawal. By definition, then, paranoid patients tend to be characterized by greater positive symptoms, particularly delusions. Given this conceptual overlap, it is not surprising that the results of neuropsychological studies of positive and negative symptoms converge with the findings from studies of paranoid and nonparanoid subgroups.

Green and Walker (1985) administered symptom assessment scales and a diverse battery of neuropsychological tasks to a group of schizophrenic patients. The battery included the Purdue Pegboard, Block Design, Benton Visual Retention, Sentence Repetition, Graphesthesia, Bushke List Learning, and Token tests. The relations between ratings of positive and negative symptoms and performance on the individual tasks were examined. The results indicated that positive symptoms were predictive of deficits on measures of verbal function, especially short-term recall, whereas negative symptoms were predictive of deficits on perceptuo-motor and visual-analytic tasks. Consistent with these results, another group of investigators (Mayer, Alpert, Stastny, Perlick, & Empfield, 1985) found that affective flattening in schizophrenia was associated with performance deficits on neuropsychological measures of visual-spatial analysis and visual-motor skills. The relation between positive symptoms and performance deficits on measures of verbal recall has also been replicated (Liddle, 1987). These results lend support to the assumptions that (1) groups of schizophrenic patients are comprised of individuals who vary in the nature of their neuropsychological impairment and (2) variability in neuropsychological profiles may be linked with variability in symptom profiles.

As indicated earlier, our ability to distinguish among groups of subjects on the basis of task performance is determined by the psychometric properties of the tasks as well as the nature of the groups. Clinical neuropsychological batteries are comprised of diverse tasks that vary in their contribution to the discriminative power of the battery. A recent study by Donnelly (1984) illustrates this point with respect to the HRNB. This investigator administered the HRNB to a group of psychiatric patients, predominantly schizophrenics, and divided the sample into impaired and nonimpaired subgroups based on their performance. A subsequent discriminative function analysis using only two measures, Verbal IQ and Picture Arrangement Score, was able to predict subgroup membership with 100% accuracy. Thus, all of the variance in subgroup performance on the extensive HRNB was captured by performance indices from substantially briefer measures. We mention this study because the findings illustrate the importance of carefully examining the contribution of individual tasks to group differences.

The Effects of Medication on Performance

When comparing the performance of diagnostic groups, the problem of confounds is a salient one. Most of the studies discussed here controlled for the effects of demographic factors, such as sex and education. However, medication is, typically, not controlled. Because the majority of schizophrenic patients are medicated, and only rarely is medication withdrawn for research purposes, it is important to understand the impact of medication on cognitive performance. Studies that have examined the effects of neuroleptics on attentional processes find either no effect or a facilitatory effect (Neale & Oltmanns, 1980). Moses (1984) and Puente, Tune, Orrell, and Hendrickson (1984) compared the performance of medicated and nonmedicated schizophrenics on the LNNB and found no significant differences. However, there is evidence to suggest that patients who respond better to neuroleptics tend to perform better on neuropsychological tasks (Seeman, 1985).

Related to the issue of medication effects is the problem of tardive dyskinesia. The studies that have examined the relation between tardive dyskinesia and neuropsychological performance report conflicting results. An investigation by Wegner, Catalano, Gibralter, and Kane (1985) revealed significant performance differences between schizophrenic patients with and without tardive dyskinesia. Patients with tardive dyskinesia showed deficits on tasks measuring both dominant and nondominant hemisphere functions (e.g., WAIS Vocabulary, Trail-making, and Conceptual Analogies). However, the tardive dyskinesia patients also showed more neurological soft signs and poorer premorbid adjustment, so these factors may have contributed to their performance deficits. Consistent with the findings of Wegner *et al.* (1985), a study by Wade, Taylor, Kasprisin, and Rosenberg (1987*b*) revealed a significant, though modest, association between tardive dyskinesia and neuropsychological impairment. Myslobodsky (1985) found no performance differences between patients with and without tardive dyskinesia; however, the fact that the patients were prescreened to exclude those with extreme movement or cognitive disorder raises questions about the reliability of these findings. Clearly, additional research is needed to address the relationship between tardive dyskinesia and neuropsychological performance.

Structural Brain Abnormalities in Schizophrenia

The emergence of new technologies for imaging the human brain *in vivo* has marked a watershed in research on schizophrenia. It is no longer necessary to speculate on the existence of organic impairment in schizophrenia, as did Bleuler and Kraepelin, because we now have physical evidence. The questions that are currently confronting researchers are: (1) What structure(s) are impaired? (2) What are the clinical and neuropsychological correlates of these abnormalities? The latter is of critical relevance because the utility of neuropsychological assessment in psychiatry is partially dependent upon its ability to identify the subgroup of patients with detectable brain abnormalities. Before turning to a discussion of the relation between neuropsychological performance and brain abnormalities, we will first provide an overview of the results of computerized tomography (CT) and magnetic resonance imaging (MRI) studies of schizophrenia.

There is fairly consistent evidence from CT studies for an association between cerebellar abnormalities and severe psychosis in general (e.g., Yates, Jacoby, & Andreasen, 1987; Rieder, Mann, Weinberger, van Kammen, & Post, 1983; Weinberger, Torrey, & Wyatt, 1979*a*). The cerebellar vermis is a particularly relevant structure, due to evidence linking the superior vermis to a number of limbic structures, including the hippocampus, which has been suggested to play a role in positive schizophrenic symptoms (Weinberger, Wagner, & Wyatt, 1983).

In normal populations, it has been established that the two cerebral hemispheres of the human brain are morphologically asymmetrical, with larger right than left frontal areas, and larger left than right occipital areas (Galaburda, LeMay, Kemper, & Geschwind, 1978). There have been reports of a subgroup of schizophrenic patients with reversed cerebral asymmetry (Luchins, Weinberger, & Wyatt, 1979, 1982). A comparison between schizophrenic, medical, and neurologic patients showed that schizophrenics with reversed cerebral asymmetry had lower verbal than performance IQs compared to those with normal asymmetry (Luchins *et al.*, 1982). However, there has been a general failure to replicate these findings (Andreasen, Dennert, Olsen, & Damasio, 1982*a*; Jernigan, Zatz, Moses, & Cardellino, 1982*a*; Weinberger, DeLisi, Perman, Targum, & Wyatt, 1982).

Also highly inconclusive at this time are findings regarding brain density abnormalities in schizophrenia; reports indicate increased (Largen, Smith, Calderon, Baumgartner, Lu, Schoolar, & Ravichandran, 1984) as well as decreased (DeMeyer, Gilmor, Hendrie, DeMeyer, & Franco, 1984) brain tissue density in schizophrenic patients. There is some indication that cell loss and gliosis may lead to ventricular size abnormalities and increased tissue density (Dewan, Pandurangi, Lee, Ramachandran, Levy, Boucher, Yozawitz, & Major, 1986).

There is fairly consistent evidence of cortical atrophy in schizophrenia, and some patients with other psychiatric disorders also show this abnormality (for a review, see Shelton & Weinberger, 1986). In general, atrophy of the cerebral cortex is associated with a reduction in volume of the gyri, seen on brain scans as widening and deepening of the sulci, expansion of the fissures, and reduction of the gyri. It seems fairly clear that the atrophy observed in a subgroup of schizophrenic patients is not a manifestation of iatrogenic or treatment effects, since it is present in recently diagnosed, untreated patients, but is more likely due to brain impairment that predates the onset of symptoms (Williams, Reveley, Kolakowska, Ardern, & Mandelbrote, 1985).

There is some indication of structural abnormalities in the corpus callosum of schizophrenic patients (Nasrallah, Andreasen, Coffman, Olsen, Dunn,

Ehrhardt, & Chapman, 1986; Mathew, Partain, Prakash, Kulkarni, Logan, & Wilson, 1985). The primary fiber tract connecting the two hemispheres is easily visualized in MRI images, lending itself to measurement. However, there is considerable diversity in the nature of structural differences reported, including greater thickness (Nasrallah *et al.*, 1986), and abnormalities of length and shape (Mathew *et al.*, 1985).

Cortical ventricular enlargement (VE) is by far the most consistently replicated finding emerging from brain imaging studies of schizophrenic patients (e.g., Kelsoe, Cadet, Pickar, & Weinberger, 1988; Williams *et al.*, 1985; Pandurangi, Dewan, Lee, Ramachandran, Levy, Boucher, Yozawitz, & Major, 1984; Nasrallah, Kuperman, Hamra, & McCalley-Whitters, 1983; Andreasen, Smith, Jacoby, Dennert, & Olsen, 1982*b*; Johnstone, Crow, Frith, Husband, & Kreel, 1976), although there are some negative findings as well (Smith, Baumgartner, & Calderon, 1987; Jernigan, Zatz, Moses, & Berger, 1982*b*). VE has also been found in patients with psychiatric disorders other than schizophrenia (e.g., Luchins, Lewine, & Meltzer, 1984; Nasrallah, McCalley-Whitters, & Jacoby, 1982). Some (e.g., Waddington, 1985) have therefore suggested that VE may be a marker for nonspecific, psychiatric features.

The role of dopamine (DA) system abnormalities in schizophrenia has been of great interest to researchers. A particularly promising set of findings relates VE to DA activity abnormalities in schizophrenia (e.g., van Kammen, Mann, Sternberg, Scheinen, Ninan, Marder, van Kammen, Rieder, & Linnoila, 1983). It was originally thought that DA overactivation in subcortical structures was most relevant to schizophrenia, but now the DA pathways in the mesocortical–prefrontal area are proving to be an area of interest to investigators. This area has also been implicated as having poorer activation in schizophrenic patients in response to prefrontal cortex-specific tasks (e.g., Weinberger & Berman, 1988). Related to this, it has been suggested that differences in response to neuroleptics may indicate DA problems in two areas: insufficient DA activity in the frontal cortex, and DA hyperactivation in the limbic region (e.g., Davila, Manero, Zumarraga, Andia, Schweitzer, & Friedhoff, 1988; Weinberger & Berman, 1988).

There is a growing body of literature on neurophysiological correlates of schizophrenia that is based on technologies such as brain electrical activity mapping (BEAM), positron emission tomography (PET), and regional cerebral blood flow (RCBF) analysis. A review of this literature is beyond the scope of this chapter. Suffice it to say that at this point the findings are inconsistent, probably due in part to the nonstandardization of procedures. However, it should be noted that a reduction in frontal activity is one finding that has been demonstrated repeatedly (Weinberger *et al.*, 1986; Weinberger & Berman, 1988).

The relations between brain abnormalities and symptom type and severity have been examined by several research groups (for a review, see Walker & Lewine, 1988). The overall pattern of results suggests that VE, and other morphological abnormalities, are associated with greater negative symptoms in schizophrenic patients. This pattern of findings is consistent with the assumption that patients with greater negative symptoms represent a subtype with structural brain impairment (Crow, 1980).

In summary, just as the clinical neuropsychological literature reveals no localizable pattern of deficit in schizophrenia, brain-imaging studies indicate no specific structural impairment. The most consistent finding is VE; however, not all schizophrenic patients show VE, nor is it a phenomenon specific to schizophrenic disorders.

The Relation between Neuropsychological Performance and Brain Abnormalities

Several investigations have revealed a relation between global indices of neuropsychological deficit and "nonspecific" structural brain abnormalities in schizophrenia (Boucher, Dewan, Donnelly, Pandurangi, Bartell, Diamond, & Major, 1986; Donnelly, Weinberger, Waldman, & Wyatt, 1980; Freeland & Puente, 1984; Pandurangi, Dewan, Boucher, Levy, Ramachandran, Bartell, Bick, Phelps, & Major, 1986; Rieder, Donnelly, Herdt, & Waldman, 1979). There is also evidence of more specific relations between neuropsychological deficits and brain abnormalities. For example, Andreasen *et al.* (1986) reported that performance on tests of visual memory and frontal function (e.g., The Wisconsin Card Sort) correlated positively with cranial size and cerebral size in schizophrenic patients. Nyman, Nyback, Wiesel, Oxenstierna, and Schalling (1986) reported that test profiles indicative of left hemisphere dysfunction were associated with wider sylvian fissures and third ventricle enlargement, but not with the size of the lateral ventricles.

A commonly reported finding is a relation between global neuropsychological impairment and VE. Golden, Moses, Zelazowski, Graber, Zatz, Horvath, and Berger (1980; Golden, Graber, Coffman, Berg, Newlin & Bloch, 1981) and Kemali, Maj, Galderisi, and Salvati (1987) tested schizophrenic patients with and without VE, and found that those with VE scored more poorly on the LNNB. In addition, Kemali *et al.* found that those with VE had a longer duration of illness, and longer mean hospitalization. Lawson *et al.* (1988) found that schizophrenic patients with VE performed worse on both the HRNB and the WAIS than did other schizophrenic patients and controls. Berman, Weinberger, Shelton, and Zec (1987) found that schizophrenic subjects with VE exhibited lower prefrontal regional cerebral blood flow during the Wisconsin Card Sort Test. However, it is important to point out that not all studies find a relation between neuropsychological impairment and VE in schizophrenia (Bankier, 1985; Carr & Wedding, 1984; Kolakowska, Williams, Jambor, & Ardern, 1985; Obiols, Marcos, & Salamero, 1987).

In summary, then, there appears to be a relationship between structural abnormalities and neuropsychological deficits. Again, this is of critical importance for establishing the validity and potential clinical utility of neuropsychological assessment in psychiatry. However, as Adams, Jacisin, Brown, Boulos, and Silk (1984) have noted, while there is robust evidence for a link between neuropsychological dysfunctions and structural abnormalities in schizophrenia, the "biological dynamics, cause–effect relation, and clinical applicability . . . in the individual case . . . are far from clear" (p. 118). Clearly, further research is needed in order to elucidate the relations between specific neuropsychological functions and specific brain characteristics. We must also expand our understanding of the etiological and prognostic significance of neuropsychological factors.

Experimental Neuropsychological Studies of Schizophrenia

In contrast to the clinical neuropsychological research on schizophrenia, the experimental studies tend to be designed for the purposes of testing a specific hypothesis regarding the nature of brain dysfunction. Moreover, most of the experimental studies use tasks that assess only one sensory modality. For example, the dichotic listening paradigm has been used repeatedly to examine intra- and interhemispheric auditory processing, while the hemiretinal procedure has been used to study the same processes in the visual modality.

To understand this type of research, it is necessary to keep in mind the contralateral relationship between motor behavior and the subserving neural mechanism, namely that the left side of the brain dominates in the control of right-sided functions and the right side of the brain predominantly controls left-sided functions. Similarly, sensory input exhibits a predominantly contralateral relationship with cortical structures. Information input to the left ear, for example, is predominantly directed to the right hemisphere and input to the right ear is sent to the left hemisphere. The visual system has a pure contralateral organization; information from the right visual field (anything to the right of midline) is projected solely to the left hemisphere and information from the left visual field is projected solely to the right hemisphere. Furthermore, interhemispheric transfer studies capitalize on the tendency for verbal functions to be predominant in the left hemisphere and nonverbal functions to be predominant in the right hemisphere. Consider as one example that a visual stimulus presented in the left visual field would be projected to the right hemisphere; to be named correctly, information about this stimulus requires transfer from the right (nonverbal) hemisphere to be left (verbal) hemisphere.

Interest in the application of experimental neuropsychological procedures to the study of schizophrenia was stimulated, in part, by the success of such procedures in differentiating among patients with various types of brain damage. During the period between 1976 and 1981, a substantial number of these investigations were published. A critical review of this literature was published in 1982, focusing primarily on the dichotic listening, hemiretinal, and haptic studies (Walker & McGuire, 1982). The review was concluded by a reevaluation of the major hypotheses that generated the literature, namely defective interhemispheric transfer, left hemisphere overactivation, and left hemisphere dysfunction. We will briefly present these conclusions before turning to a discussion of the findings reported since the review was conducted.

Up to 1981, there was little support for the hypotheses of interhemispheric transfer deficits in schizophrenia. In fact, some findings in the literature were contradictory to this assumption. Several studies showed that schizophrenics manifested slower reaction times to both right ear and right visual field input, and this occurred whether the response was executed verbally or by either hand. Yet, studies of patients with lesions of the corpus callosum consistently show increased latencies only for responses executed by the hand ipsilateral to the sensory field receiving the stimulus (Bashore, 1981). Therefore, the absence of such a pattern of lateral asymmetry in response latency among schizophrenics would argue against an impairment in interhemispheric transfer.

Flor-Henry (1976) was among the first to propose that schizophrenia is related to left hemisphere impairment. His hypothesis was predicated on several lines of evidence, but particularly the reported association between left hemisphere lesions and schizophreniclike symptoms in epileptic patients.

The literature reviewed by Walker and McGuire (1982) showed moderate support for the notion of left hemisphere dysfunction in schizophrenia. There was little evidence of right ear or right visual field deficits in response accuracy; hemiretinal and dichotic listening studies of schizophrenic patients generally revealed the normative pattern of right sensory field advantage in the *accuracy* of processing of linguistic stimuli. However, as indicated above, when *reaction time* served as the dependent variable, there was evidence of increased latency in responding to visual, auditory, and haptic stimuli presented to the right sensory field. This could be interpreted as reflecting a slowdown in left hemisphere processing.

Finally, the literature on dichotic listening provided support for the notion of left hemisphere overactivation in schizophrenia. Specifically, several studies showed an exaggerated right ear advantage among schizophrenic patients, and an apparent inability to suppress attention to right ear input. A similar performance pattern has been demonstrated in normals under conditions of information overload (e.g., Wexler & Heninger, 1980), so the findings for schizophrenics are compatible with models postulating semantic information overload in the disorder (Shimkunas, 1978).

A cautionary note should be added to any attempts to interpret data on lateral performance asymmetries. Experimental neuropsychological investigations typically assume that both the direction and magnitude of asymmetries are reflective of hemispheric differences. Researchers often analyze laterality quotients that are based on differences between right and left side performance. The results of research on both normal and brain-damaged subjects indicate that it is valid to assume that the *direction* of performance asymmetries is reflective of differences in hemispheric dominance for certain functions (Walker & McGuire, 1982). However, recent research indicates that the *magnitude* of performance asymmetries may not be a valid index of "degree" of hemispheric dominance: there is little or no relation among measures of laterality derived from different tasks, including psychophysiological and perceptual measures (Schneider, 1983). Such findings challenge conventional assumptions regarding the meaning of lateral differences and point to the importance of further research on the determinants of performance asymmetries. Until we have a better understanding of the meaning of asymmetries, we must approach the interpretation of data with caution.

Recent Findings from Experimental Neuropsychological Research

Interhemispheric Transfer

The search for an interhemispheric transfer deficit in schizophrenia is commonly attributed to the conjunction of two lines of applied research. Numerous empirical investigations of "split-brain" patients, those whose corpus callosum has been sectioned to relieve otherwise intractable epileptic seizures, revealed both localization of function by hemisphere and transfer of information via the corpus callosum from one hemisphere to the other. For example, left hand anomia (the inability to name correctly an object held out of sight in the left hand, although being able to point correctly to a picture of that object) is a common characteristic of such patients and reflects the impairment of the left (verbal) hemisphere resulting from the loss of right (nonverbal) hemisphere information usually carried via the corpus callosum. The salience of cognitive disorder in schizophrenia led to the consideration of corpus callosum dysfunction as an underlying cause.

In 1972, Rosenthal and Bigelow reported the results of a postmortem study of schizophrenics which revealed a significant increase in the thickness of the corpus callosum. If structural changes in the corpus callosum could be replicated, it would be reasonable to expect a functional consequence. Until recently, however, with the introduction of MRI, which allows for midsagittal imaging, the simultaneous study of brain morphology and behavior has not been possible.

P. Green and colleagues have conducted one of the most extensive research efforts in this area (1978, 1983, 1987). In one of their early studies, they found that schizophrenic patients had more difficulty than normals in a tactual discrimination task requiring callosal transfer. Subsequent studies tended to confirm these findings. Moreover, Hatta, Yamamoto, and Kawabata (1984) ruled out the role of memory as a confounding factor by employing a manual matching, rather than learning, task. They found poorer performance when the matching was across hands; as before, the patients were also poorer on matching to the same hand.

Dichotic listening tasks, in which stimuli are presented separately to each ear, have also been used to assess interhemispheric transfer. In general, investigators have found that, for schizophrenics, binaural stimulus presentation resulted in either absolutely or relatively worse performance than monaural presentation (E. Green, 1985; P. Green, 1978, 1987; Green & Kotenko, 1980). For normals, binaural and monaural conditions yield similar performance levels. Hallett, Quinn, and Hewitt (1986) found a binaural deficit in children (mean age approximately 16) of schizophrenic parents, suggesting that this deficit may be indicative of vulnerability to schizophrenia. The results of these studies have led to the conceptualization of callosal "malconnection" rather than "disconnection."

The consistency in findings across studies is somewhat deceptive as there are several methodological problems that make inferences about callosal transfer problematic. The most serious methodological flaw is the failure to equate the various conditions for task complexity (Chapman & Chapman, 1978). That is, the conditions that test for interhemispheric transfer are also those that are arguably more inherently complex (Beaumont & Dimond, 1973). Thus, the schizophrenics' typically poorer performance on these tasks is more parsimoniously interpreted as increased performance impairment in the face of increased difficulty. Furthermore, many studies claiming to support interhemispheric transfer deficit also report that schizophrenics perform more poorly on intrahemispheric tasks. There may be, in other words, a general performance deficit, not a specific transfer deficit.

This assumption receives some support from the results of a doctoral dissertation by Tal (1988). She not only controlled for task difficulty, but also employed three different paradigms of interhemispheric transfer. It was found that schizophrenics, affective disordered patients, and normal controls (matched for educational and sociocultural background) did not differ on any of the interhemispheric tasks. In contrast, patients with major affective disorder showed a consistent right hemisphere impairment that was significantly different from both normal controls and schizophrenic patients.

The predominant model for the study of interhemispheric transfer deficit in schizophrenia has been that of the "split-brain" patient. However, as Craft, Willerman, and Bigler (1987) have argued, the split-brain model represents an acute disruption of callosal function in the mature brain, a condition unlikely to capture adequately the schizophrenic process, which probably has its roots in the early development of the individual. Corpus callosum agenesis is a congenital disorder marked by total or partial failure of corpus callosum development. A major difference between the commissurotomy and agenesis models is that the latter incorporates compensatory developmental processes so that the two conditions present with different clinical pictures. Craft *et al.* (1987) predicted that chronic schizophrenics would do more poorly than controls (normal and schizoaffective) on four tasks on which individuals with agenesis of the corpus callosum do poorly: associated movements test, cross-localization of touch, interocular transfer of visual spiral aftereffect, and transfer of blind formboard learning. Results indicated that schizophrenics and schizoaffectives did more poorly than normals on all but the formboard task; schizophrenics were significantly worse than schizoaffectives on the aftereffect task and showed a different pattern of deficits on the cross-localization task than did either of the other two groups. Unfortunately, Craft *et al.* did not include any tests specific to the commissurotomy model so that we cannot tell if the reported deficits are part of the generally poor performance profile found in schizophrenia.

In sum, the empirical evidence bearing on the corpus callosum transfer deficit model remains unconvincing, while tantalizing. The sharpening of the theoretical and conceptual models to be tested, as exemplified in the Craft *et al.* paper, should elucidate our search.

Left Hemisphere Dysfunction/Overactivation

There is little in the way of recent experimental support for the hypothesis of left hemisphere dysfunction in schizophrenia. Kugler and Caudrey (1983) found that schizophrenics performed below depressed patients and normals on a phonetic judgment task, and they interpreted their findings as indicating left hemisphere dysfunction. However, they did not include a "control" task for purposes of comparison, nor did they test for performance or processing asymmetries. The findings, therefore, provide only weak support for their conclusions.

The notion of left hemisphere overactivation in schizophrenia does receive support from the study by E. Green (1985). Binaural and monaural versions of a comprehension task were administered to chronic and acute schizophrenics and controls. Only the acute schizophrenics showed a right ear advantage in performance. This group also showed a performance decrement in the binaural relative to the monaural condition, leading the author to conclude that acute patients have greater difficulty focusing attention on input to the target ear in the presence of distraction. The presence of a right ear bias and susceptibility to distraction in acute patients is consistent with the findings of some earlier studies; specifically, reports of a right ear attentional bias in paranoid schizophrenics and greater susceptibility to distraction in patients with positive symptoms (Green & Walker, 1985; Walker & McGuire, 1982).

It has been suggested that the functional overactivation of the left hemisphere is reflective of dopaminergic overactivation (Gruzelier, 1984). However, there is no evidence of dopaminergic asymmetries in schizophrenia. In fact, the findings from a study of turning behavior in schizophrenics suggest right anterior dopaminergic overactivation rather than left side overactivation (Bracha, 1987). Bracha, noting that animals manifest a turning bias toward the hemisphere with lower striatal DA, concluded that schizophrenics' leftward rotational bias reflected a relative increase in right hemisphere DA activity.

In sum, while it is clear that schizophrenics manifest deficits on tasks that rely on left hemisphere processes, it is also apparent that performance on many right hemisphere tasks is deficient. Further, research on structural and physiological characteristics of the brain reveals no consistent evidence of left hemisphere dysfunction in schizophrenia. This does not negate the possibility that left hemisphere dysfunction subserves some cases of schizophrenia; however, it is unlikely that such dysfunction is generalizable to all patients.

The experimental neuropsychological literature has paid little attention to the issue of subgroups of schizophrenia patients. A notable exception is the work of Gruzelier (1984), which suggests that the positive/negative symptom distinction may be relevant to hemispheric function. Drawing on findings from psychophysiological as well as neuropsychological studies, Gruzelier concludes that there are two schizophrenic syndromes. A florid or positive-symptom syndrome is associated with left hemisphere overactivation, and a negative-symptom syndrome is subserved by right hemispheric overactivation. Although the evidence supporting this distinction is only suggestive, Gruzelier's approach is exemplary in its focus on the relation between symptom patterns and neuropsychological phenomena.

CLINICAL APPLICATIONS

The role of neuropsychological assessment in psychiatric diagnosis and treatment has been a topic of considerable controversy. Some have argued that the classification of psychiatric patients on the basis of neuropsychological profiles may have greater utility in treatment planning than does the application of traditional psychiatric labels (Townes, Martin, Nelson, Prosser, Pepping, Maxwell, Peel, & Preston, 1985). For example, these writers propose that such "competency-based" classifications would aid in decisions regarding the appropriateness of psychotherapies that rely on verbal skills and insight. In striking contrast, others have questioned the utility of neuropsychological assessment in psychiatry, particularly given the availability of new technologies for brain imaging. Between these two extreme positions, we are likely to find the future role of neuropsychology in psychiatry. The potential utility of neuropsychology is most apparent in the areas of rehabilitation and treatment planning.

Cognitive rehabilitation has its origins in the treatment of patients with brain damage. Over the past decade, rehabilitation programs have flourished in centers for the treatment of head injury patients. The notion of applying such programs to psychiatric patients has only recently been explored. Drawing on the literature on cognitive deficit in schizophrenia, Erickson and Binder (1986) have proposed an assessment battery for use in rehabilitative planning for schizophrenic patients. These authors emphasize the need to examine the patient's performance in terms of both successes and failures and to conceptualize rehabilitative interventions from the standpoint of the implications of cognitive deficits for problems faced in daily living.

A case study reported by Adams, Malatesta, Brantley, and Turkat (1981) illustrates a cognitive rehabilitation approach to schizophrenia. Although the authors used a behaviorally oriented interview, rather than neuropsychological assessment, to determine the patient's cognitive impairment, their intervention involved the use of some conventional neuropsychological tasks. These included attentional, digit span, verbal memory, and dichotic listening tasks. The "rehabilitation battery" was tailored to the patient's unique pattern of cognitive deficits. At the termination of a 6-month treatment program, the patient showed substantial improvement, with reduced distractibility and enhanced memory. Moreover, there appeared to be a generalization of effects, such that social functioning was also enhanced.

Clearly, the cognitive rehabilitation of psychiatric disorders is an undeveloped field. To date, there is little in the way of empirical support for its efficacy. Yet, the fact that cognitive deficits and abnormalities constitute a central feature of schizophrenia points to the importance of exploring strategies for modifying cognitive processes in this disorder. It may be that we will find that some deficits are not modifiable, while others are responsive to intervention. Such information would be important in its own right; cognitive deficits that are resistant to treatment may be more direct manifestations of underlying organic impairment.

There has been relatively little research on the use of neuropsychological assessment for planning treatment or predicting outcome in schizophrenia. However, the results of a recently completed study suggest that neuropsychological assessment may aid in patient management (Walker, 1988). In this investigation, a battery of neuropsychological and information-processing tasks was administered to a group of 40 inpatient schizophrenics. Cluster analysis of test scores revealed four patient clusters. Two of these clusters (1 and 3) were comprised of patients with relative deficits on perceptuo-motor tasks, but performance at or above the group mean on verbal memory tasks. Cluster 1 differed from cluster 3 in the degree of performance variability. The other two clusters (2 and 4) of patients showed the opposite pattern, namely deficits on auditory processing relative to their performance on perceptuo-motor tasks. Again, these two clusters differed in magnitude of performance variability, but not performance pattern.

The course of each patient's illness was examined approximately 1½ years after the assessment. Clusters 2 and 4 showed a lower incidence of medication noncompliance, a shorter duration of index hospitalization, and a lower rate of unemployment. The cluster 4 patients were also more likely to be described as showing good social functioning. In a final set of analyses, the predictive power of clinical symptom ratings and neuropsychological indices was examined. The results indicated that neuropsychological test scores were more powerful predictors of the outcome measures than were ratings of symptoms. Specifically, the presence of perceptuo-motor deficits was associated with poorer outcome, suggesting that patients with such deficits may be less responsive to traditional psychopharmacological intervention.

The results of this investigation highlight the need for further research on the predictive power of neuropsychological test results. The possibility that neuropsychological assessment may facilitate treatment planning, and thus play a greater role in psychiatric settings, deserves attention from researchers. Both clinical observation and empirical data demonstrate that schizophrenic patients do not respond in a uniform manner to neuroleptics. At this point, there is no basis for predicting treatment response, although many clinicians use information on symptoms as a basis for judging the likelihood of responsiveness to various psychopharmacological agents. The findings of Walker (1988) are encouraging in this regard because they suggest that variability in neuropsychological task performance has greater prognostic relevance than variability in symptoms.

SUMMARY

In summary, despite the proliferation of hypotheses linking schizophrenia to various localized brain abnormalities, there is little evidence that patients with this disorder share a common organic impairment. This does not, of course, mean that there is no "final common pathway" that produces schizophrenic symptomatology. Some patients may have acquired a vulnerability to schizophrenia through an insult to the CNS (e.g., viral infection, perinatal complications) that affected multiple structures. Consequently, some or all of the brain abnormalities noted in schizophrenic patients may bear no direct causal relation to their symptoms. But, at the same time, all patients may share an as yet undetected functional or structural impairment. On the other hand, it is possible that the differences we see among patients in the nature and course of their illness reflect important etiologic differences, and there may be no shared impairment.

Whatever the case, it is clear that neuropsychology has a great deal to contribute to the study of schizophrenia (Goldstein, 1986). It appears that neuropsychological performance profiles may be related to symptom profiles. This is an important issue to pursue in future investigations because it may provide insights into the cognitive deficits subserving specific symptoms. Research on the prognostic relevance of neuropsychological assessment should also be pursued. The cognitive rehabilitation of schizophrenic patients is another issue that has received little attention from researchers, yet it holds promises for making a significant contribution to treatment.

Finally, neuropsychological assessment may prove to be a valuable tool in pursuing the most important question in the field, namely the origins of schizophrenia. In our ongoing research (Walker & Lewine, 1990), we are conducting neuropsychological assessments and brain scans of schizophrenic patients, as well as collecting extensive data on the entire life-course. A critical component of the project is the use of childhood home-movies to examine the neuromotor development of patients. The films extend from infancy through adolescence, and they will allow us to determine whether neuromotor deficits in early childhood are associated with neuropsychological performance deficits and brain abnormalities in adulthood. If such an association were found, this would suggest that patients' neuropsychological deficits reflect a long-standing CNS impairment.

While there is little doubt that we are far from solving the riddle of schizophrenia, we must acknowledge that neuropsychology has already made a contribution to our understanding of the disorder. Long before brain-imaging technology revealed ventricular, frontal, and temporal abnormalities in schizophrenia, the results of clinical neuropsychological studies were telling us that schizophrenic and brain-damaged patients were not distinguishable. Thus, neuropsychology took the lead in verifying the theoretical assumptions of those who pioneered the study of schizophrenia, namely Kraepelin and Bleuler.

ACKNOWLEDGMENT. This work was supported in part by a grant from the Scottish Rite Foundation Schizophrenia Research Program.

REFERENCES

Adams, H., Malatesta, V., Brantley, P., & Turkat, I. (1981). Modification of cognitive processes: A case study of schizophrenia. *Journal of Consulting and Clinical Psychology, 49*, 460–464.

Adams, K. M., Jacisin, J. J., Brown, G. G., Boulos, R. S., & Silk, S. D. (1984). Neurobehavioral deficit and computed tomographic abnormalities in three samples of schizophrenic patients. *Perceptual and Motor Skills, 59*, 115–119.

Andreasen, N. C., Nasrallah, H. A., Dunn, S. C., Olson, S. C., Grove, W. M., Ehrhardt, J. C., Coffman, J. A., & Crossett, J. H. W. (1986). Structural abnormalities in the frontal system in schizophrenia. *Archives of General Psychiatry, 43*, 136–147.

Andreasen, N. C., Dennert, J. W., Olsen, S. A., & Damasio, A. R., (1982*a*). Hemispheric asymmetries and schizophrenia. *American Journal of Psychiatry, 139*, 427–430.

Andreasen, N. C., Smith, M. R., Jacoby, C. G., Dennert, J. W., & Olsen, S. A. (1982*b*). Ventricular enlargement in schizophrenia: Definition and prevalence. *American Journal of Psychiatry, 139*, 292–302.

Aylward, E., Walker, E., & Bettes, B. (1984). Intelligence in schizophrenia: A review and meta-analysis of the literature. *Schizophrenia Bulletin, 10*, 430–459.

Bankier, R. G. (1985). Third ventricle size and dementia in schizophrenia. *British Journal of Psychiatry, 147*, 241–245.

Bashore, T. (1981). Vocal and manual reaction time estimate of interhemispheric reaction time. *Psychological Bulletin, 89*, 352–368.

Beaumont, J. G., & Dimond, J. S. (1973). Brain disconnection and schizophrenia. *British Journal of Psychiatry, 123*, 661–662.

Benson, D. F., & Stuss, D. T. (1982). Motor abilities after frontal leukotomy. *Neurology, 32*, 1353–1357.

Berman, K. F., Weinberger, D. R., Shelton, R. C., & Zec, R. F. (1987). A relationship between anatomical and physiological brain pathology in schizophrenia: Lateral cerebral ventricular size predicts cortical blood flow. *American Journal of Psychiatry, 144*, 1277–1282.

Bleuler, E. (1950). *Dementia praecox or the group of schizophrenias*. New York: International Universities Press.

Boucher, M. L., Dewan, M. J., Donnelly, M. P., Pandurangi, A. K., Bartell, K., Diamond, T., & Major, L. F. (1986). Relative utility of three indices of neuropsychological impairment in a young, chronic schizophrenic population. *Journal of Nervous and Mental Disease, 174*, 44–46.

Bracha, S. (1987). Asymmetric rotational (circling) behavior. A dopamine-related asymmetry: Preliminary findings in unmedicated and never-medicated schizophrenic patients. *Biological Psychiatry, 22*, 105–114.

Carr, E. G., & Wedding, D. (1984). Neuropsychological assessment of cerebral ventricular size in chronic schizophrenics. *International Journal of Clinical Neuropsychology, 6*, 106–111.

Chapman, L. J., & Chapman, J. P. (1978). The measurement of differential deficit. *Journal of Psychiatric Research, 14*, 303–311.

Chelune, G. J., Heaton, R. K., Lehman, R. A. W., & Robinson, A. (1979). Level versus pattern of neuropsychological performance among schizophrenic and diffusely brain-damaged patients. *Journal of Consulting and Clinical Psychology, 47*, 155–163.

Craft, S., Willerman, L., & Bigler, E. D. (1987). Callosal dysfunction in schizophrenia and schizo-affective disorder. *Journal of Abnormal Psychology, 96*, 205–213.

Crow, T. J. (1980). Molecular pathology of schizophrenia: More than one disease process? *British Medical Journal, 280*, 66–68.

Davila, R., Manero, E., Zumarraga, M., Andia, I., Schweitzer, J. W., & Friedhoff, A. J. (1988). Plasma homovanillic acid as a predictor of response to neuroleptics. *Archives of General Psychiatry, 45*, 564–567.

Dean, R. S., Gray, J. W., & Seretny, M. L. (1987). Cognitive aspects of schizophrenia and primary affective depression. *The International Journal of Clinical Neuropsychology, 9*, 33–35.

DeMeyer, M. K., Gilmor, R., Hendrie, H., DeMeyer, W. E., and Franco, J. N. (1984). Brain densities in treatment-resistant schizophrenic and other psychiatric patients. *Journal of Operational Psychiatry, 15*, 9.

Dewan, M. J., Pandurangi, A. K., Lee, S. H., Ramachandran, T., Levy, B., Boucher, M., Yozawitz, A., & Major, L. (1986). A comprehensive study of chronic schizophrenic patients, I. Quantitative computed tomography: Cerebral density, ventricle and sulcal measures. *Acta Psychiatrica Scandinavica, 73*, 152–160.

Donnelly, E. F. (1984). Neuropsychological impairment and associated intellectual functions in schizophrenic and other psychiatric patients. *Biological Psychiatry, 19*, 815–824.

Donnelly, E. F., Weinberger, D. R., Waldman, I. N., & Wyatt, R. J. (1980). Cognitive impairment associated with morphological brain abnormalities on computed tomography in chronic schizophrenic patients. *Journal of Nervous and Mental Disease, 168*, 305–308.

Erickson, R. C., & Binder, L. M. (1986). Cognitive deficits among functionally psychotic patients: A rehabilitative perspective. *Journal of Clinical and Experimental Neuropsychology, 8*, 257–274.

Flor-Henry, P. (1976). Lateralized temporal limbic dysfunction and psychopathology. *Annals of the New York Academy of Science, 280*, 777–795.

Freedman, B. J. (1974). The subjective experience of perceptual and cognitive disturbances in schizophrenia. *Archives of General Psychiatry, 30*, 333–340.

Freeland, J., & Puente, A. E. (1984). Relative efficacy of the Luria–Nebraska Neuropsychological Battery and the Wechsler Adult Intelligence Scale in discriminating schizophrenics with and without brain damage. *International Journal of Neuropsychology, 6*, 261–263.

Galaburda, A. M., LeMay, M., Kemper, T. L., & Geschwind, N. (1978). Right–left asymmetries in the brain. *Science, 199*, 852–856.

Goldberg, T., Weinberger, D. R., & Berman, K. (1987). Further evidence for dementia of the prefrontal type in schizophrenia? A controlled study of teaching the Wisconsin Card Sorting Test. *Archives of General Psychiatry, 44*, 1008–1014.

Golden, C. J., Graber, B., Coffman, J., Berg, R. A., Newlin, D. B., & Bloch, S. (1981). Structural brain deficits in schizophrenia. *Archives of General Psychiatry, 38*, 1014–1017.

Golden, C. J., Moses, J. A., Zelazowski, R., Graber, B., Zatz, L. M., Horvath, J. B., & Berger, P. A. (1980). Cerebral ventricular size and neuropsychological impairment in young chronic schizophrenics. *Archives of General Psychiatry, 37*, 619–623.

Goldstein, G. (1986). The neuropsychology of schizophrenia. In I. Grant & K. Adams (Eds.), *Neuropsychological Assessment of Neuropsychiatric Disorders* (pp. 147–171). New York: Oxford University Press.

Green, E. J. (1985). Interhemispheric coordination and focused attention in chronic and acute schizophrenia. *British Journal of Clinical Psychology, 24*, 197–204.

Green, M., & Walker, E. (1984). Susceptibility to backward masking in schizophrenics with positive versus negative symptoms. *American Journal of Psychiatry, 141*, 1273–1275.

Green, M., & Walker, E. (1985). Neuropsychological performance and positive and negative symptoms in schizophrenia. *Journal of Abnormal Psychology, 94*, 460–470.

Green, P. (1978). Defective interhemispheric transfer in schizophrenia. *Journal of Abnormal Psychology, 87*, 472–480.

Green, P. (1987). Interference between the two ears in speech comprehension and the effect of an earplug in psychiatric and cerebral-lesioned patients. *Cerebral Dynamics, Laterality and Psychopathology*, 287–298.

Green, P., Hallett, S., & Hunter, M. (1983). Abnormal interhemispheric integration and hemispheric specialization in schizophrenia. In P. Flor-Henry & J. Gruzelier (Eds.), *Laterality and psychopathology* (pp. 131–150). Amsterdam: Elsevier.

Green, P., & Kotenko, V. (1980). Superior speech comprehension under monaural versus binaural listening conditions. *Journal of Abnormal Psychology, 89*, 399–408.

Gruzelier, J. (1984). Hemispheric imbalances in schizophrenia. *International Journal of Psychophysiology, 1*, 227–240.
Hallett, S., Quinn, D., & Hewitt, J. (1986). Defective interhemispheric integration and anomalous language lateralization in children at risk for schizophrenia. *The Journal of Nervous and Mental Disease, 174*, 418–427.
Hatta, T., Yamamoto, M., & Kawabata, Y. (1984). Functional hemispheric differences in schizophrenia: Interhemispheric transfer deficit of selective hemisphere dysfunction? *Biological Psychiatry, 19*, 1027–1036.
Heaton, R. K. (1979). Neuropsychological impairment with schizophrenia vs. acute and chronic cerebral lesions. *Journal of Clinical Psychology, 35*, 46–53.
Heaton, R. K., Baade, L. E., & Johnson, K. L. (1978). Neuropsychological test results associated with psychiatric disorders in adults. *Psychological Bulletin, 85*, 141–162.
Jernigan, T. L., Zatz, L. M., Moses, J. A., & Cardellino, J. P. (1982*a*). Computed tomography in schizophrenics and normal volunteers. II: Cranial asymmetry. *Archives of General Psychiatry, 39*, 771–773.
Jernigan, T. L., Zatz, L. M., Moses J. A., & Berger, P. A. (1982*b*). Computed tomography in schizophrenics and volunteers. I: Fluid volume. *Archives of General Psychiatry, 39*, 765–770.
Johnstone, E. C., Crow, T. J., Frith, C. D., Husband, J., & Kreel, L. (1976). Cerebral ventricular size and cognitive impairment in chronic schizophrenia. *Lancet, 2*, 924–926.
Kelsoe, J. R., Cadet, J. L., Pickar, D., & Weinberger, D. R. (1988). Quantitative neuroanatomy in schizophrenia. *Archives of General Psychiatry, 45*, 533–541.
Kemali, D., Maj, M., Galderisi, S., & Salvati, A. (1987). Clinical, biological, and neuropsychological features associated with lateral ventricular enlargement in DSM-III schizophrenic disorder. *Psychiatry Research, 21*, 137–149.
Kolakowska, T., Williams, A. O., Jambor, K., & Ardern, M. (1985). Schizophrenia with good and poor outcome: III. Neurological "soft" signs, cognitive impairment and their clinical significance. *British Journal of Psychiatry, 146*, 348–357.
Kolb, B., & Whishaw, I. Q. (1983). Performance of schizophrenic patients on tests sensitive to left or right frontal, temporal, or parietal function in neurological patients. *Journal of Nervous and Mental Disease, 171*, 435–443.
Kraepelin, E. (1971). *Dementia praecox and paraphrenia*. Huntington, N.Y.: Krieger.
Kugler, B. T., & Caudrey, D. J. (1983). Phoneme discrimination in schizophrenia. *British Journal of Psychiatry, 142*, 53–59.
Langell, M. E., Purisch, A. D., & Golden, C. J. (1987). Neuropsychological differences between paranoid and nonparanoid schizophrenics on the Luria–Nebraska Battery. *International Journal of Clinical Neuropsychology, 9*, 88–95.
Largen, J. W., Smith, R. C., Calderon, M., Baumgartner, R., Lu, R., Schoolar, J. C., & Ravichandran, G. K. (1984). Abnormalities of brain structure and density in schizophrenia. *Biological Psychiatry, 19*, 991–1013.
Lawson, W. B., Waldman, I. N., & Weinberger, D. R. (1988). Schizophrenic dementia: Clinical and computed axial tomography correlates. *Journal of Nervous and Mental Disease, 176*, 207–212.
Lenzer, I. I. (1980). Halstead–Reitan Test Battery: A problem of differential diagnosis. *Perceptual and Motor Skills, 50*, 611–630.
Levander, S. E., Bartfai, A., & Schalling, D. (1985). Regional cortical dysfunction in schizophrenic patients studied by computerized neuropsychological methods. *Perceptual and Motor Skills, 61*, 479–495.
Lewis, G., Golden, C. J., Purisch, A. D., & Hammeke, T. A. (1979). The effects of chronicity of disorder and length of hospitalization on the standardized version of Luria's Neuropsychological Battery in a schizophrenic population. *Clinical Neuropsychology, 1*, 13–18.
Lewis, R. F., Nelson, R. W., & Eggertsen, C. (1979). Neuropsychological test performances of paranoid schizophrenic and brain-damaged patients. *Journal of Clinical Psychology, 35*, 54–59.
Liddle, P. F. (1987). Schizophrenic syndromes, cognitive performance and neurological dysfunction. *Psychological Medicine, 17*, 49–57.

Luchins, D. J., Weinberger, D. R., & Wyatt, R. J. (1979). Schizophrenia: Evidence for a subgroup with reversed cerebral asymmetry. *Archives of General Psychiatry, 36*, 1309–1311.

Luchins, D. J., Weinberger, D. R., & Wyatt, R. J. (1982). Schizophrenia and cerebral asymmetry detected by computed tomography. *American Journal of Psychiatry, 139*, 753–757.

Luchins, D.J., Lewine, R., & Meltzer, H. (1984). Lateral ventricular size, psychopathology, and medication response in psychoses. *Biological Psychiatry, 19*, 29–44.

Maj, M. (1986). Neuropsychological functioning in schizoaffective disorder, depressed type. *Acta Psychiatrica Scandinavica, 74*, 524–528.

Malec, J. (1978). Neuropsychological assessment of schizophrenia versus brain damage: A review. *Journal of Nervous and Mental Disease, 166*, 507–516.

Mathew, R. J., Partain, C. L., Prakash, R., Kulkarni, M. V., Logan, T. P., & Wilson, W. H. (1985). A study of the septum pellicidum and corpus callosum in schizophrenia with MR imaging. *Acta Psychiatrica Scandinavica, 72*, 414–421.

Mayer, M., Alpert, M., Stastny, P., Perlick, D., & Empfield, M. (1985). Multiple contributions to clinical presentation of flat affect in schizophrenia. *Schizophrenia Bulletin, 11*, 420–426.

Moses, J. A. (1984). The effect of presence or absence of neuroleptic medication treatment on Luria–Nebraska Neuropsychological Battery performance in a schizophrenic population. *International Journal of Clinical Neuropsychology, 6*, 249–251.

Moses, J. A., Cardellino, J. P., & Thompson, L. L. (1983). Discrimination of brain damage from chronic psychosis by the Luria–Nebraska Neuropsychological Battery: A closer look. *Journal of Consulting and Clinical Psychology, 51*, 441–449.

Myslobodsky, M. S. (1985). Cognitive impairment in patients with tardive dyskinesia. *Journal of Nervous and Mental Disease, 173*, 156–160.

Nasrallah, H. A., McCalley-Whitters, M., & Jacoby, C. G. (1982). Cortical atrophy in schizophrenia and mania: A comparative CT study. *Journal of Clinical Psychiatry, 43*, 439–441.

Nasrallah, H. A., Kuperman, S., Hamra, B., & McCalley-Whitters, M. (1983). Clinical differences between schizophrenic patients with and without large cerebral ventricles. *Journal of Clinical Psychiatry, 44*, 407–409.

Nasrallah, H. A., Andreasen, N. C., Coffman, J. A., Olsen, S. C., Dunn, J. D., Ehrhardt, J. C., & Chapman, S. M. (1986). A controlled magnetic resonance imaging study of corpus callosum thickness in schizophrenia. *Biological Psychiatry, 21*, 274–282.

Neale, J., & Oltmanns, T. (1980). *Schizophrenia*. New York: Wiley.

Nyman, H., Nyback, H., Wiesel, F. A., Oxenstierna, G., & Schalling, D. (1986). Neuropsychological test performance, brain morphological measures and CSF monoamine metabolites in schizophrenic patients. *Acta Psychiatrica Scandinavica, 74*, 292–301.

Obiols, J. E., Marcos, T., & Salamero, M. (1987). Ventricular enlargement and neuropsychological testing in schizophrenia. *Acta Psychiatrica Scandinavica, 76*, 199–202.

Pandurangi, A. K., Dewan, M. J., Boucher, M., Levy, B., Ramachandran, T., Bartell, K., Bick, P. A., Phelps, B. H., & Major, L. (1986). A comprehensive study of schizophrenic patients. II: Biological, neuropsychological, and clinical correlates of CT abnormality. *Acta Psychiatrica Scandinavica, 73*, 161–171.

Pandurangi, A. K., Dewan, M. J., Lee, S. H., Ramachandran, T., Levy, B. F., Boucher, M., Yozawitz, A., & Major, L. (1984). The ventricular system in chronic schizophrenic patients: A controlled computed tomographic study. *British Journal of Psychiatry, 144*, 172–176.

Puente, A. E., Tune, L., Orrell, T., & Hendrickson, J. (1984). The relationship between the LNNB scale scores and neuroleptic dosage levels in schizophrenics. *International Journal of Clinical Neuropsychology, 7*, 69.

Purisch, A. D., Golden, C. J., & Hammeke, T. A. (1978). Discrimination of schizophrenic and brain-injured patients by a standard version of Luria's Neuropsychological Tests. *Journal of Consulting and Clinical Psychology, 46*, 1266–1273.

Rieder, R. O., Donnelly, E. F., Herdt, J. R., & Waldman, I. N. (1979). Sulcal prominence in young chronic schizophrenic patients: CT scan findings associated with impairment on neuropsychological tests. *Psychiatry Research, 1*, 1–8.

Rieder, R. O., Mann, L. S., Weinberger, D. R., van Kammen, D. P., & Post, R. M. (1983). Computed tomographic scans in patients with schizophrenia, schizoaffective, and bipolar affective disorder. *Archives of General Psychiatry, 40,* 735–739.

Rosenthal, R., & Bigelow, L. B. (1972). Quantitative brain measurements in chronic schizophrenics. *British Journal of Psychiatry, 121,* 259–264.

Schneider, S. J. (1983). Multiple measures of hemispheric dysfunction in schizophrenia and depression. *Psychological Medicine, 13,* 287–297.

Seeman, M. V. (1985). Clinical and demographic correlates of neuroleptic response. *Canadian Journal of Psychiatry, 30,* 243–245.

Selin, C. L., & Gottschalk, L. A. (1983). Schizophrenia, conduct disorder and depressive disorder: Neuropsychological, speech sample and EEG results. *Perceptual and Motor Skills, 57,* 427–444.

Shelly, C., & Goldstein, G. (1983). Discrimination of chronic schizophrenia and brain damage with the Luria–Nebraska Battery: A partially successful replication. *Clinical Neuropsychology, 5,* 82–85.

Shelton, R. C., & Weinberger, D. R. (1986). X-ray computerized tomography studies in schizophrenia: A review and synthesis. In H. A. Nasrallah & D. R. Weinberger (Eds.), *Handbook of schizophrenia* (Vol. I, pp. 207–250). Amsterdam: Elsevier.

Shimkunas, A. (1978). Hemispheric asymmetry and schizophrenic thought disorder. In S. Schwartz (Ed.), *Language and cognition in schizophrenia* (pp. 193–236). New York : Wiley.

Silverstein, M. L., & Arzt, A. T. (1985). Neuropsychological dysfunction in schizophrenia: Relation to associative thought disorder. *Journal of Nervous and Mental Disease, 173,* 341–346.

Silverstein, M. L., & Zerwic, M. J. (1985). Clinical psychopathologic symptoms in neuropsychologically impaired and intact schizophrenics. *Journal of Consulting and Clinical Psychology, 53,* 267–268.

Smith, R. C., Baumgartner, R., & Calderon, M. (1987). Magnetic resonance imaging studies of the brains of schizophrenic patients. *Psychiatry Research, 20,* 33–46.

Steinhauer, S., & Zubin, J. (1982). Vulnerability to schizophrenia information processing in the pupil and event-related potentials. In I. Hanin & E. Usdin (Eds.), *Biological markers in psychiatry and neurology* (pp. 239–253). Elmsford, N.Y.: Pergamon Press.

Strauss, B. S., & Silverstein, M. L. (1986). Luria–Nebraska measures in neuropsychologically nonimpaired schizophrenics: A comparison with normal subjects. *International Journal of Clinical Neuropsychology, 8,* 35–38.

Tal, C. (1988). *Intra- and inter-hemispheric dysfunction in schizophrenic and affective disorders.* Unpublished doctoral dissertation, Northwestern University.

Taylor, M. A., & Abrams, R. (1984). Cognitive impairment in schizophrenia. *American Journal of Psychiatry, 141,* 196–201.

Taylor, M. A., & Abrams, R. (1987). Cognitive impairment patterns in schizophrenia and affective disorders. *Journal of Neurology, Neurosurgery and Psychiatry, 50,* 895–899.

Taylor, M. A., Greenspan, B., & Abrams, R. (1979). Lateralized neuropsychological dysfunction in affective disorder and schizophrenia. *American Journal of Psychiatry, 136,* 1031–1034.

Taylor, M. A., Redfield, J., & Abrams, R. (1981). Neuropsychological dysfunction in schizophrenia and affective disease. *Biological Psychiatry, 16,* 467–478.

Townes, B. D., Martin, D. C., Nelson, D., Prosser, R., Pepping, M., Maxwell, J., Peel, J., & Preston, M. (1985). Neurobehavioral approach to classification of psychiatric patients using a competency model. *Journal of Consulting and Clinical Psychology, 53,* 33–42.

van Kammen, D. P., Mann, L. S., Sternberg, D. E., Scheinen, M., Ninan, P. T., Marder, S. R., van Kammen, W. B., Rieder, R. O., Linnoila, M. (1983). Dopamine-β-hydroxylase activity and homovanillic acid in spinal fluid of schizophrenics with brain atrophy. *Science, 220,* 974–977.

Waddington, J. L. (1985). Structural brain pathology and clinical features in schizophrenia: Further clues on the neurobiology of psychosis? *Trends in Neurosciences, 8,* 374–375.

Walker, E. (1988). Cognitive performance profiles and the course of schizophrenia. Unpublished manuscript.

Walker, E., & Lewine, R. J. (1988). The positive/negative symptom distinction in schizophrenia: Validity and etiologic relevance. *Schizophrenia Research, 1,* 315–328.

Walker, E., & Lewine, R. J. (1990). The prediction of adult-onset schizophrenia from childhood home-movies. *American Journal of Psychiatry, 147,* 1052–1056.

Walker, E., & McGuire, M. (1982). Intra- and interhemispheric information processing in schizophrenia. *Psychological Bulletin, 92,* 701–715.

Walker, E., & Shaye, J. (1982). Familial schizophrenia: A predictor of neuromotor and attentional dysfunction in schizophrenia. *Archives of General Psychiatry, 39,* 1153–1160.

Wegner, J. T., Catalano, F., Gibralter, J., & Kane, J. M. (1985). Schizophrenics with tardive dyskinesia–neuropsychological deficit and family psychopathology. *Archives of General Psychiatry, 42,* 860–865.

Weinberger, D. R., & Berman, K. F. (1988). Speculation on the meaning of cerebral metabolic hypofrontality in schizophrenia. *Schizophrenia Bulletin, 14,* 157–168.

Weinberger, D. R., Torrey, E. F., & Wyatt, R. J. (1979). Cerebellar atrophy in chronic schizophrenia. *Lancet, 1,* 718–719.

Weinberger, D. R., DeLisi, L. E., Perman, G. P., Targum, S., & Wyatt, R. J. (1982). Computed tomography in schizophreniform disorder and other acute psychiatric disorders. *Archives of General Psychiatry, 39,* 778–783.

Weinberger, D. R., Wagner, R. L., & Wyatt, R. J. (1983). Neuropathological studies of schizophrenia: A selective review. *Schizophrenia Bulletin, 9,* 193–212.

Weinberger, D. R., Berman, K. F., & Zec, R. F., (1986). Physiologic dysfunction of lateral prefrontal cortex in schizophrenia. *Archives of General Psychiatry, 43,* 114–125.

Wexler, B., & Heninger, G. R. (1980). Effects of concurrent administration of verbal and spatial visual tasks on a language related dichotic listening measure of perceptual asymmetry. *Neuropsychologia, 18,* 379–382.

Williams, A. O., Reveley, M. A., Kolakowska, T., Ardern, M., & Mandelbrote, B. M. (1985). Schizophrenia with good and poor outcome II: Cerebral ventricular size and its clinical significance. *British Journal of Psychiatry, 146,* 239–246.

Wooten, A. J. (1983). MMPI profiles among neuropsychology patients. *Journal of Clinical Psychology, 39,* 392–406.

Yates, W. R., Jacoby, C. G., & Andreasen, N. C. (1987). Cerebellar atrophy in schizophrenia and affective disorder. *American Journal of Psychiatry, 144,* 465–467.

11

Pseudoneurological and Psychosomatic Disorders

ARTHUR MACNEILL HORTON, JR.

INTRODUCTION

Professional neuropsychological consultation services are often provided on an acute neurology ward. There are at least two general categories of consultation requests. The first category concerns the further elucidation of the phenomena of brain impairment. For example, brain impairment could have been initially documented by computerized axial tomography (CT), magnetic resonance imaging (MRI), physical neurological evaluation, electroencephalogram (EEG), or some other neurodiagnostic technique and then the neurologist would seek to better understand the behavioral impairments associated with the documented brain damage. Often these consultation requests include questions about the ability to handle funds, operate complicated machinery, drive, or manage a household. This is a fairly traditional area well known to neuropsychologists (Horton & Wedding, 1984; see other chapters in this volume).

The second variety of consultation requests are particularly interesting and the focus of this chapter. In this category, the neurologist usually, after an exhaustive workup that would have included the physical neurological exam, extensive laboratory testing, CT scan, EEG, or other neurodiagnostic test, would still have difficulty correlating the objective test findings and the patient's complaints. Interestingly enough, the number of consultations for this category, at times, will rival that for the first category. Generally speaking, the neurologist wishes to determine whether psychological factors could be leading the patient

ARTHUR MACNEILL HORTON, JR. • Department of Psychiatry, University of Maryland Medical School, Baltimore, Maryland 21201. *Present Address*: Division of Clinical Research, National Institute of Drug Abuse, Rockville, Maryland 20857. Dr. Horton's contribution is in his private capacity and is neither supported nor endorsed by the federal government.

HANDBOOK OF NEUROPSYCHOLOGICAL ASSESSMENT: A Biopsychosocial Perspective, edited by Antonio E. Puente and Robert J. McCaffrey. Plenum Press, New York, 1992.

to present neurological symptoms without organic deficits. The problems could include either psychiatric difficulties or a simple desire to obtain secondary gain.

This pattern of late consultation for possible psychological factors masquerading as organic deficits is all too frequent. This is not appropriate, as it probably is effective to obtain neuropsychological consultation early in the course of a diagnostic workup in many of these cases. The purpose of this chapter is to outline some of the ways of discriminating individuals who may be presenting with organic deficits for psychological factors with the hope of educating colleagues, within neurology, psychiatry, and psychology, to this very important area. Generally speaking, relatively little attention has been paid to this area. A much greater degree of effort has been devoted to either the diagnosis of organic deficits by psychological means or the question of etiological factors or the further elucidation of various facets of brain injury upon behavioral competence. Improved neurodiagnostic technology such as MRI is now standard in neurological settings. It is entirely likely that given these new neurodiagnostic tools, the role of the neuropsychologist will evolve toward describing conditions and situations where the patient may have questionable motivations. A case can be made that the elucidation of emotional deficits, possibly secondary to brain injury, may be an important new area for consultation by neuropsychologists.

The plan of this chapter is as follows. First, some attention will be paid to the variety of pseudoneurological disorders that could lead a patient to present with neurological symptoms for psychological causes. In addition to psychological factors, situations where the expectation of secondary gain may cause a patient to present with neurological symptoms will be discussed as a possible second, but not totally exclusive, category. Then, discussion will focus on methods of discriminating between patients who actually have organic deficits and those who do not, even though both categories may be presenting with symptoms of organic deficits.

Two bodies of evidence will be considered. First, the results with respect to inspection of neuropsychological test batteries will be considered. This review will be brief as there has been relatively little work in this important area using comprehensive neuropsychological test batteries. The second section will be devoted to the use of personality measures to distinguish between patients who have symptoms of neurological disorder but who may or may not have objective signs. The Minnesota Multiphasic Personality Inventory (MMPI) will be the primary focus of this section for a number of reasons. First, the MMPI has a long history and has been the primary"workhorse" of neuropsychology in the area. Also, the objective nature of the test lends itself to research and there is a considerable body of literature on the MMPI dealing with pseudoneurological disorders. Moreover, some general conclusions regarding the adequacy of the current research base and possible suggestions for future research in this area will be considered. Finally, a general summary will be presented. The hope and expectation of this chapter is that it will provide some guidance in terms of improving neuropsychological methods in this very important area. It is perhaps worthy of note that clinical psychologists in general and clinical neuropsychologists in particular have a special expertise that would be of great value in this area.

HISTORY

The pseudoneurological disorders have a history as long as mental health itself. The Greeks of old times made the original conceptualization of hysteria as a "wandering uterus." In the Middle Ages, people thought the pseudoneurological disorders were caused by demonic possession. The first systematic study of neurotic disorders, however, began in the late 1800s in Jean Martin Charcot's clinic at the Salpêtrière in Paris, France (Nemiah, 1988). As is well known, the great psychoanalyst Sigmund Freud was first attracted to the study of mental process by a pseudoneurological disorder (Freud, 1894). Freud, whose initial emphasis in medicine was in the field of neurology, began his investigation of pseudoneurological disorders by examining a case of conversion hysteria (Nemiah, 1988). A young woman presented with conversion reaction symptoms and Freud was able to ameliorate her symptoms by hypnosis. From this therapy case, the modern study of pseudoneurological disorders began.

THEORETICAL PERSPECTIVES

Before discussing various sorts of psychological illnesses in patients who complain of organic symptoms, it would be most appropriate to point out the overall framework within which one works. For example, the question is sometimes inaccurately posed as to whether an individual might have a psychological illness or an organic illness. Almost the way the question is usually suggested presupposes a two-category solution. Actually, and by all logic, it would seem that a four-category solution would be most appropriate. For example, the various categories of patients could be (1) normal patients with neither psychological nor organic illness, (2) psychological illness, (3) organic illness, and (4) perhaps most important, some combination of psychological and organic illness. Very often, as in the question of dementia versus depression, there is a presupposition that only one condition can exist. Certainly, psychological illness is no barrier to organic illness and the opposite statement is no less true. Therefore, neuropsychologists, neurologists, psychiatrists, and other mental health and neuroscience professionals should consider all possible alternatives in answering this diagnostic question. While it is, for example, unlikely to have a normal person referred for evaluation, it is nonetheless possible.

Moreover, it is important to realize that an organic illness may not be immediately apparent. There is the possibility that underlying, unrecognized organic illness may not present itself in a characteristic way and would only become apparent after an extensive diagnostic workup. Studies of patients diagnosed as conversion reactions who have been followed over a considerable period of time have noted a 15 to 30% incidence of misdiagnosed organic disease (Ford & Folks, 1985). As mentioned, there is no reason to think, even in cases where a conversion disorder or some other psychological illness can be reliably determined, that the patient may not also have a concurrent neurological disorder. See Delay and Isaac (this volume) on peripheral neuropathies.

There are a number of physical conditions that on follow-up have been found to be present in patients who were earlier diagnosed as having hysterical symptoms. These often include conditions such as epilepsy, multiple sclerosis, and various CNS infections. In addition, the various musculoskeletal and connective tissue diseases, such as myasthenia gravis and syphilis, hyper- and hypothyroidism, and hypoglycemia, as well as pancrease disease are all conditions that are low base rate probabilities. When diagnosing a somatoform disorder, it is important to realize that usually such a disorder is a condition that presents uniformly throughout the life span. Clinicians should be particularly careful in terms of diagnosing somatoform disorders late in life when the likelihood of a number of age-related neurological conditions and various medical illnesses may increase significantly (Nolan, Swihart, & Pirozzolo, 1986).

At this point, consideration should be devoted toward various psychological conditions that mimic physical disease. In order to structure this discussion, the various disorders might be differentiated based on whether there is a presumed voluntary contribution by the patient. For example, the various somatoform disorders suggest that the patient is not aware in an active sense that he or she is simulating physical symptoms. On the other hand, there are various categories of disorder where the patient voluntarily, consciously, and actively mimics physical symptoms of organic conditions. The following discussion will first consider those categories where patients voluntarily and actively simulate organic conditions and then the category of disorder where patients, in a less active sense, complain for psychological reasons of organic deficits.

Voluntary Simulation of Organic Deficits

The two types of disorders in this group are malingering and factitious disorder with physical symptoms. Generally speaking, malingering is well known to mental health professionals.

DSM-III-R Criteria: V65.20

The essential feature of Malingering is intentional production of false or grossly exaggerated physical or psychological symptoms, motivated by external incentives such as avoiding military conscription or duty, avoiding work, obtaining financial compensation, evading criminal prosecution, obtaining drugs, or securing better living conditions.

Under some circumstances Malingering may represent adaptive behavior, for example, feigning illness while a captive of the enemy during wartime.

> Malingering should be strongly suspected if any combination of the following is noted:
>
> (1) medicolegal context of presentation, e.g., the person's being referred by his or her attorney to the physician for examination;
>
> (2) marked discrepancy between the person's claimed stress or disability and the objective findings;
>
> (3) lack of cooperation during the diagnostic evaluation and in complying with the prescribed treatment regimen;
>
> (4) the presence of Antisocial Personality Disorder.
>
> Malingering differs from Factitious Disorder in that the motivation for the symptom production in Malingering is external incentives, whereas in Factitious Disorder there is an absence of external incentives. Evidence of an intrapsychic need to maintain the sick role suggests Factitious Disorder. Thus, a diagnosis of Factitious Disorder excludes a diagnosis of Malingering.
>
> Malingering is differentiated from Conversion and other Somatoform Disorders by the intentional production of symptoms and by the obvious, external incentives. The person who is malingering is much less likely to present his or her symptoms in the context of emotional conflicts, and the presenting symptoms are less likely to be symbolically related to an underlying emotional conflict. Symptom relief in Malingering is not often obtained by suggestion, hypnosis, or an amobarbital interview, as it frequently is in Conversion Disorder. [DSM-III, 1987, pp. 205–206]

Very often, patients have specific reasons why they prefer some action (X) to occur and the easiest way to obtain X might be to fake an organic condition. This can range from something as simple as a homeless individual who, on a cold night, presents in a hospital emergency room complaining of generalized "chest pain." A more elaborate presentation would be a young woman with a minor head injury attempting to have a neuropsychologist write a letter explaining why she had not paid off her student loans even though the schedule of payments had been defaulted on prior to the head injury. Other common cases include patients who either wish to obtain drugs or avoid the legal consequences of their ill-considered actions. Often, borderline personality disorders, antisocial personality disorders, and alcohol and drug abuse are common diagnoses in patients presenting in this manner.

Factitious disorder with physical symptoms is often described as Munchhausen syndrome.

> **301.51 Factitious Disorder with Physical Symptoms**
>
> A. Intentional production or feigning of physical (but not psychological) symptoms.
>
> B. A psychological need to assume the sick role, as evidenced by the absence of external incentives for the behavior, such as economic gain, better care, or physical well-being.
>
> C. Occurrence not exclusively during the course of another Axis I disorder, such as Schizophrenia. [DSM-III-R, 1987, p. 177]

Basically, Baron Munchhausen would render "tall tales" regarding his exploits. The label has been generalized to patients who tell "tall tales" regarding their physical symptoms.

Generally speaking, these are patients who knowingly fake physical symptoms. On at least one level, they are less responsible for their actions than the malingerer but the end result is similar. Often they wish to assume a sick role to avoid difficulties or problems in their life and go from hospital to hospital (Henderson, Bell, & Miller, 1983). It is important to realize that patients with factitious disorder with physical symptoms often have personality difficulties and very real problems in terms of establishing interpersonal relationships. One particularly important issue is that patients with factitious disorder with physical symptoms may undergo multiple invasive medical procedures and are at risk for real tissue damage and possible iatrogenic drug addictions.

Common neurological complaints of patients with factitious disorders with physical symptoms include seizures and weakness.

Somatoform Disorders

Basically, in somatoform disorders there are a number of discrete, involuntary psychological conditions in which the patient involuntarily complains of symptoms of physical disease. The major conditions include conversion disorder, somatization disorder, somatoform pain disorder, and hypochondriasis.

Conversion disorder has also been known as hysterical neurosis, conversion type (Ford & Folks, 1985).

> **300.11 Conversion Disorder (or Hysterical Neurosis, Conversion Type)**
> A. A loss of, or alteration in, physical functioning suggesting a physical disorder.
> B. Psychological factors are judged to be etiologically related to the symptom because of a temporal relationship between a psychosocial stressor that is apparently related to a psychological conflict or need and initiation or exacerbation of the symptom.
> C. The person is not conscious of intentionally producing the symptoms.
> D. The symptom is not a culturally sanctioned response pattern and cannot, after appropriate investigation, be explained by a known physical disorder.
> E. The symptom is not limited to pain or to a disturbance in sexual functioning. [DSM-III-R, 1987, pp. 151–152]

A conversion disorder is an obvious loss of function in the nervous system without an identifiable neurological disorder. Frequently, conversion disorders can involve the motor or sensory systems. Conversion disorders may have various, poorly understood, psychological purposes. The usual notion is that there is a source of primary or secondary gain. Primary gain suggests that the patient is attempting to block out an unconscious wish or act or urge by the physical symptom. For example, if a patient wished to strike someone, the patient could lose the ability to use his/her arm.

Secondary gain operates in a similar way as for the malingerer. Essentially, the organic symptoms allow the patient to obtain some action or privilege that is, at least on the surface, positively reinforcing, e.g., receiving disability payments or being able to avoid some type of legal action. In a specific instance, a man who had embezzled over $200,000 subsequently developed a paralysis involving his right arm. It is often quite obvious to the clinician and others that there is a relationship between the symptoms and the person's circumstances. Apparently, the crucial point in making this diagnostic distinction is that the patient has no insight into the etiology of his/her condition.

A wide variety of neurological syndromes can be presented by the patient with a conversion reaction. These can include but are not limited to seizures, unconsciousness, paralysis, gait difficulties, sensory changes, and blindness. Associated features that often present with conversion reactions (Ford & Folks, 1985) include occurrence relatively early in the individual's life, a preexisting personality disorder, and often a history of similar conversion symptoms in the past, and symptoms may closely follow an acute stress episode.

At this point, attention can be shifted to the *somatization disorder*. This disorder has in the past been known as hysteria or Briquet's syndrome.

300.81 Somatization Disorder

A. A history of many physical complaints or a belief that one is sickly, beginning before the age of 30 and persisting for several years.

B. At least 13 symptoms from the list below. To count a symptom as significant, the following criteria must be met:

(1) no organic psychology or pathophysiologic mechanism (e.g., a physical disorder or the effects of injury, medication, drugs, or alcohol) to account for the symptom or, when there is related organic pathology, the complaint or resulting social or occupational impairment is grossly in excess of what would be expected from the physical findings

(2) has not occurred only during a panic attack

(3) has caused the person to take medicine (other than over-the-counter pain medication), see a doctor, or alter life-style

Symptoms list:

Gastrointestinal symptoms:

(1) vomiting (other than during pregnancy)
(2) abdominal pain (other than when menstruating)
(3) nausea (other than motion sickness)
(4) bloating (gassy)
(5) diarrhea
(6) intolerance of (gets sick from) several different foods

Pain symptoms:

(7) pain in extremities
(8) back pain
(9) joint pain
(10) pain during urination
(11) other pain (excluding headaches)

Cardiopulmonary symptoms:

(12) shortness of breath when not exerting oneself
(13) palpitations
(14) chest pain
(15) dizziness

Conversion or pseudoneurologic symptoms:

(16) amnesia
(17) difficulty swallowing
(18) loss of voice
(19) deafness
(20) double vision
(21) blurred vision
(22) blindness
(23) fainting or loss of consciousness
(24) seizure or convulsion

(25) trouble walking
(26) paralysis or muscle weakness
(27) urinary retention or difficulty urinating
Sexual symptoms for the major part of the person's life after opportunities for sexual activity:
(28) burning sensation in sexual organs or rectum (other than during intercourse)
(29) sexual indifference
(30) pain during intercourse
(31) impotence
Female reproductive symptoms judged by the person to occur more frequently or severely than in most women:
(32) painful menstruation
(33) irregular menstrual periods
(34) excessive menstrual bleeding
(35) vomiting throughout pregnancy
[DSM-III-R, 1987, pp. 153–154]

The syndrome has been reexamined in the recent versions of the *Diagnostic and Statistical Manual* of the American Psychiatric Association and some possible modifications of the traditional diagnosis of hysteria may be found. Generally speaking, patients with somatization disorder have numerous vague and very dramatic physical symptoms that involve a number of organic symptoms. Frequently, there are gastrointestinal and cardiopulmonary difficulties as well as various ill-defined pains. While symptoms may vary in their severity, the patient very forcefully presents them to his or her clinician. As noted by Tomb (1988), these patients often have a previous or current diagnosis of histrionic or antisocial personality disorder and this may be a chronic condition that often begins in adolescence and presents with frequent interpersonal and marital difficulties. Others (Cloninger, Martin, Guze, & Clayton, 1986) suggest that somatization disorder is more frequent in females than males. It is worth noting that follow-up studies find far fewer instances of later-diagnosed organic illness in cases of somatization disorder than in conversion disorder (Ford & Folks, 1985).

Somatoform pain disorder is defined as a pain that often presents following a stressor (DSM-III-R, 1987). There are some similarities with conversion disorder.

307.80 Somatoform Pain Disorder
A. Preoccupation with pain for at least six months
B. Either (1) or (2)
(1) appropriate evaluation uncovers no organic pathology or pathophysiologic mechanism (e.g., a physical disorder or the effects of injury) to account for the pain
(2) when there is related organic pathology, the complaint of pain or resulting social or occupational impairment is grossly in excess of what would be expected from the physical findings. [DSM-III-R, 1987, p. 155]

Hypochondriasis

Hypochondriacal neurosis had been an earlier term for hypochondriasis.

300.70 Hypochondriasis (or Hypochondriacal Neurosis)
A. Preoccupation with the fear of having, or the belief that one has, a serious disease,

based on the person's interpretation of physical signs or sensations as evidence of physical illness.
B. Appropriate physical evaluation does not support the diagnosis of any physical disorder that can account for the physical signs or sensations or the person's unwarranted interpretation of them, and the symptoms in A are not just symptoms of panic attacks.
C. The fear of having, or belief that one has, a disease persists despite medical reassurance.
D. Duration of the disturbance is at least six months.
E. The belief in A is not of delusional intensity, as in Delusional Disorder, Somatic Type (i.e., the person can acknowledge the possibility that his or her fear of having, or belief that he or she has, a serious disease is unfounded). [DSM-III-R, 1987, p. 259]

Essentially, these are individuals preoccupied with the idea that they are sick despite strong evidence to the contrary and they are often a source of great concern to the clinicians who treat them (Barsky, Wyshak, & Kellerman, 1986). These patients appear to wish to assume a role of being "sick" and will often "doctor shop" to find a physician who is willing to reassure them that they are ill. These patients are often extremely difficult for clinicians to deal with as their beliefs regarding their ill condition are quite fixed and difficult to change. This relatively common condition is chronic, may begin at adolescence or middle age, but it is common among the elderly and is for the most part relatively resistant to psychotherapy (Barsky *et al.*, 1986). Indeed, many physicians become quite angry and rejecting toward these patients.

CLINICAL APPLICATIONS

Generally speaking, there are two major strategies for differentiating psychological from organic illness in pseudoneurological syndromes. Always keeping in mind, of course, the four-category model previously mentioned, the possibilities for diagnosis are that the patient could be normal, organic, psychological, or both organic and psychological.

In summary, the diagnostic conditions of malingering, factitious disorder, somatoform disorder, conversion disorder, somatoform pain disorder, and hypochondriasis are all possible diagnostic categories within which to place the patients. Attention can now be directed toward the ways and means by which neuropsychologists make decisions as to which diagnostic category to place the patients. Put another way, the roadmap has been laid out; now the task is to obtain a means of transportation.

The following discussion will initially center on results of comprehensive neuropsychological test batteries that include cognitive, motor, and sensory/perceptual measures and then will consider the results of objective personality tests such as the MMPI. There has been relatively little research on the faking of brain damage on psychological tests. A small number of studies have utilized single tests, such as the Benton Visual Memory Test (Benton & Spreen, 1961) and the Bender-Gestalt (Bruhn & Reed, 1975). Those studies appeared to suggest that it is difficult to fake brain injury. It might be noted that Binder (Chapter 12) reviews the malingering literature from a different point of view. Binder (Chapter 12) examines malingering from the perspective of prank faking. This chapter examines the literature from the point of view of possible psychological processes presenting as organic conditions.

NEUROPSYCHOLOGICAL TEST RESULTS

Essentially two studies have used the Halstead–Reitan Neuropsychological Battery (HRNB) with regard to detecting malingering (Heaton, Smith, Lehman, & Vogt, 1978; Goebel, 1983).

In the first study (Heaton *et al.*, 1978), the results of 16 volunteer malingerers and 16 head trauma patients were compared. Both groups were administered the Wechsler Adult Intelligence Scale, the HRNB, and the MMPI. The malingerers did essentially as poorly as the head injury patients in terms of the overall level of neuropsychological test performance. For example, there were no significant differences among the groups on the Wechsler IQ values or the Halstead Impairment Index, or Average Impairment Rating. While the groups' levels of performance were relatively similar, there were some fairly clear differences in patterns of strengths and weaknesses. For example, the malingerers did worse on the Speech Sounds Perception Test, the Finger Tapping Test, Finger Agnosia, the Sensory Perception Exam, and the Strength of Grip Test than the other patients. In addition, with respect to personality testing, the malingerers showed a higher level on the F scale and six clinical scales of the MMPI suggesting greater emotional disturbance. By contrast, in the head injury group, the scores that were significantly worse than the malingerer group were on the Category Test, the error component of part B of the Trail Making Test, and on scores taken from the Tactual Performance Test (TPT).

In order to assess clinical judgment of neuropsychologists, a group of ten neuropsychologists were instructed to make blind judgments based on test protocol data as to whether each subject's data were those of a malingerer or a head injury patient. The ten neuropsychologist judges differed widely in terms of clinical experience. The levels of clinical experience ranged from less than 1 year to almost two decades. It should be noted that this research procedure differs significantly from the usual clinical situation where the patient is usually present and his or her behavior directly observed.

The neuropsychologists making blind judgments ranged in terms of their diagnostic accuracy from chance level prediction to about 20% better than chance. While one would consider the possibility that the amount of experience in neuropsychology was an important factor in the judges' diagnostic accuracy, the data do not strongly support this notion. For example, the relationship between the diagnostic accuracy of the judges and their experience in neuropsychology had a correlation of 0.27, which was not meaningful. There was, however, a slight tendency for those judges with greater experience to more accurately assess the subjects. Another method of classifying the subjects was also used by the investigators. They attempted to see whether discriminate function analysis (a multivariable statistical technique) could be used with greater accuracy. The discriminate function analysis proved valuable in that it was better able to correctly classify the subjects. The HRNB was able to correctly classify 100% of the subjects in both groups. Moreover, using the MMPI alone, 94% of the subjects in both groups were correctly classified. It should be noted, however, that these discriminate functions were based on a small number of subjects in each group and were not completely cross-validated. To use them clinically without complete cross-validation would be inconsistent with good scientific methodology.

It is noteworthy that Heaton *et al.* (1978) did conduct a partial cross-validation of the discriminate functions. A group of head injury patients who were either involved or not involved in court actions and/or had given clinical evidence of faking were assessed on the statistical measures and demonstrated discriminate functions that were used in the partial cross-validation. However, there was a significant decrease in terms of accuracy of the discriminate functions as less than seven of ten subjects were correctly identified. The authors noted that the discriminate functions should *only* be employed with respect to the "head injury/malingerer distinction." As a test of the generalizability of their results, the authors used a group of patients who had suffered strokes as well as head injuries to assess the power of the discriminate functions. Applying the discriminate functions, the group of stroke patients was classified as malingerers by the neuropsychological tests. It would appear that the discriminate functions may be effective only for discriminating head trauma patients from malingerers, and not stroke patients.

The second study, which examined the diagnosis of faking on the HRNB, was done by Goebel (1983). Goebel attempted to build on the work of Heaton *et al.* (1978) by using a larger sample size, a control group, and a heterogeneous group of brain-damaged patients. In addition, he also examined whether malingering patients could fake lateralized or diffuse patterns of neuropsychologically impaired abilities.

This study utilized two relatively large groups: 52 brain-impaired patients and 202 nonimpaired volunteers. The volunteers were assigned to five groups: a control group where the volunteers were requested to do their best on the neuropsychological test battery, and four groups differing in terms of the types of brain damage that the volunteers were requested to fake. Two groups were requested to fake unilateral brain damage to either the right or left hemisphere and a third group was asked to fake damage to both hemispheres and a fourth group was simply requested to fake brain damage. The analysis of data used both "blind" clinical judgment and statistical methodology.

A possible weakness of the study is that only one clinical judge was used (i.e., the study's author) and that he had previously seen the brain-impaired profiles. In terms of diagnosing whether a brain-impaired profile was either faked or not, the author was correct in approximately 94% of the profiles. This is significantly different from the earlier results in the Heaton *et al.* (1978) study.

Of the three specific groups, patients, controls, and fakers, the following results were typical. In the patient group, 79.1% were correctly classified as brain impaired and 20.9% as nonimpaired. Similarly, in the control group, excellent results were obtained with 100% of the group found to be nonimpaired. In addition, in the faking group, 98% were found to be nonimpaired and a mere 2% of the fakers were assessed as brain-injured. While these results are certainly positive evidence in favor of clinical judgment in neuropsychology, it would have been much better if the level of diagnostic accuracy had been achieved with a number of judges. The fact that the single rater had not been entirely blind to the neuropsychological test profiles is an extremely serious methodological flaw.

In terms of the statistical analysis, discriminate functions were calculated at five different base rates of malingering. These range from 1 out of 3 to 1 out of 50. The accuracy changed rather drastically depending on the base rate assumed. At a base rate of 1 out of 3, the discriminate functions achieved a reasonably good correct rate of 78%. By contrast, at a base rate of 1 out of 50, the overall rate fell to 48.8% correct or about what one would expect in terms of chance. Interestingly, the ability to discriminate between patients and nonpatients remained high regardless of the malinger base rate. The overall correct rate was, in all cases, approximately 95% when the control versus faking distinction was ignored by pooling the nonpatient data.

The author (Goebel, 1983) very appropriately cautioned his readers about generalization of these results to the clinical setting. He pointed out the possible differences in the motivation to fake between the volunteers in his studies and "true malingerers." He did, however, make the point that the ability to fake deficits on neuropsychological test results is not solely a matter of motivation. Rather, the successful faking of neuropsychological deficits probably requires a certain amount of knowledge and awareness of what the particular tests require as many of these tests are quite complex.

There is one particularly interesting point of similarity between the Heaton *et al.* (1978) and Goebel (1983) studies. For instance, both found the TPT particularly difficult to fake. Indeed, all of the various measures associated with the TPT (i.e., time, memory, and localization) were relatively insensitive to the effects of faking. Moreover, in the Goebel study, the TPT nondominant hand time was a particularly important variable in distinguishing between brain-impaired and nonimpaired individuals. Future efforts in clinical neuropsychological practice might involve careful assessment of TPT performance when malingering is suspected. Goebel (1983) also points out the possible potency of "test time" as a discriminating variable in distinguishing between malingerers and brain-impaired subjects. Brain-damaged subjects in his study required, on the average, more than one-half hour longer to complete the HRNB than neurologically unimpaired volunteers. Moreover, in his study, the faking volunteers either were unable to, or just did not, consider the possibility of lengthening the test time. Thus, future research in this area might carefully look at both the amount of time it takes a possible malingerer to complete the nondominant hand trial of the TPT of the HRNB and also the amount of time taken to complete the entire HRNB.

With regard to studies of faking of neuropsychological deficits, only one utilizing the Luria–Nebraska Neuropsychological Test Battery (LNNB) could be found. Mensch and Woods (1986) used a number of clinical judges and had subjects (of at least normal intelligence) take the Luria–Nebraska on two separate occasions. On each occasion, different instructions were given. One time, the subjects were requested to fake brain damage, and at the other time, they were asked not to fake brain damage. Generally speaking, the results demonstrated that the sensory/motor items of the motor, rhythm, and tactile scales were most often faked.

While not a typical neuropsychological test, the symptom validity testing of Binder and Pankratz (1987) is certainly useful. In their study, they used 100 trials of visual or auditory stimuli with distraction to assess the faking of memory problems. They appear to have been relatively successful in detecting the faking of memory problems.

Efforts to examine malingering in children and adolescents have been almost nonexistent. The studies that have been done had difficulty in identifying malingering in children (Faust, Hart, & Guilmette, 1988*a*) and adolescents (Faust, Hart, Guilmette, & Arkes, 1988*b*).

Personality Test Results

In this section, results based on the MMPI will be considered. Generally speaking, the MMPI is the most widely used and carefully researched objective instrument in the personality assessment literature. It is a test with a long history in clinical neuropsychology and a vast number of studies (Hathaway & McKinley, 1951; Dahlstrom, Welsh, & Dahlstrom, 1975).

With respect to the use of the MMPI, different strategies have been employed. The two major strategies are (1) using both the validity and clinical scales that are most commonly scored or (2) looking at special scales for elucidating more subtle relationships. In this section, the results, with respect to the special scales, will be considered after examination of the value of the validity and clinical scales.

The most careful work in terms of detecting faking on the MMPI has used the F and K scales (Gynther, 1961). Generally speaking, it has been suggested that the F minus K dissimilation index would be more sensitive than either the F or K alone. The F scale is a measure of "faking bad." Usually, high F scores are obtained by patients who wish to look worse than they are. It is one of the classic validity scales and is particularly valuable in discriminating invalid profiles. By contrast, the K scale was initially developed as a "correction factor" for more carefully identifying schizophrenic patients who were missed by the MMPI (McKinley, Hathaway, & Meehl, 1948). One way of understanding the K scale is to think of it as a "subtle lie" scale. The more classically developed L scale, which was supposed to identify patients who were attempting to appear in better mental health than they actually were, has proven to be relatively insensitive to "subtle lies." In other words, it missed, in many cases, the patients it was supposed to identify. Therefore, the K scale was developed to correct this deficiency.

In a normal population, Grow, McVaugh, and Enco (1980) found that an F minus K index ≥ 7 was useful in detecting test subjects who wished to look worse than they were while an F minus K ≤ -11 suggested individuals who were attempting to fake good. Using organic subjects, the previously discussed Heaton *et al.* (1978) study suggested that an F minus K index < 5 would be useful in detecting patients who wish to fake. Along these same lines, Greene (1978) developed a special scale that he termed the "Carelessness scale." Its purpose was to detect the effects of lack of interest or poor attention on the MMPI.

At this point, some attention should be devoted to the attempts to develop special scales on the MMPI to distinguish various sorts of emotional disturbance. Perhaps the most valuable work has been that of Watson (1971). Initially, he developed the Schizophrenia versus Organic or "Sc–O" scale, which has proved generally useful in distinguishing organic from schizophrenic patients. Watson was, however, also interested in looking at more general varieties of psychiatric illness and discriminating those patients from organic patients. Therefore, he attempted to develop a more broad-ranging MMPI special scale. Watson and Plemel (1978) developed the Psychiatric–Organic or "P–O" special scale of the MMPI to distinguish general psychiatric patients from organically impaired patients. They demonstrated a success rate of roughly 65% with this scale in a relatively young psychiatric population. The results were cross-validated by Horton and Wilson (1981) in an elderly Department of Veterans Affairs domiciliary population with a correct rate of 78%. Watson and other colleagues (Watson, Gasser, Schaefer, Burnen, & Woll, 1981) again cross-validated the P–O scale and found comparable results of approximately 69% in a slightly younger population than that studied by Horton and Wilson. [See Watson (1984) for an excellent comprehensive review of the Sc–O and P–O MMPI scales.]

In terms of the specific question of pseudoneurotic disorders, there is a scale that specifically looks at brain-damaged versus non-brain-damaged persons with neurological symptoms (Shaw & Matthews, 1965). One study found correct classification of 67% of the non-brain-damaged subjects and 78% of the brain-damaged subjects. These results would suggest some value of the Ps–N scale, but there is a need for cross-evaluation of this instrument in the future. Review of the available literature failed to identify a replacement except for Puente, Rodenbough, and Horton (1989), which will be discussed later in this chapter.

It should be noted by way of caution that very often certain neurological disorders will demonstrate impaired profiles on the MMPI (Mack, 1979). There is, of course, the question of whether or not these emotional disturbances are a result of having a neurological disease or simply brain-related emotional disturbances. For example, multiple sclerosis patients in exacerbation very often demonstrate a classic conversion reaction 1–3 MMPI profile (Dodge & Kolstoe, 1971). In addition, ALS patients frequently present a 1–2–3 MMPI profile and myasthenia gravis patients often present a 3–2–1 profile.

In a recent quasi-experimental multiple-group study, Puente *et al.* (1989) demonstrated the particular value of the P–O scale in distinguishing various sorts of neurological and somatoform illnesses.

In this research study, Puente *et al.* (1989) assembled four groups of outpatients. The groups included brain-damaged patients (N = 35), brain-damaged schizophrenic patients (N = 10), non-brain-damaged schizophrenics (N = 15), and patients with somatoform disorders (N = 45). All patients were administered the MMPI and four carefully selected MMPI scales were scored. These were the Schizophrenic–Organic (Sc–O), Psychiatric–Organic (P–O), Pseudo–Neurological (P–N) special scales and the Schizophrenic (Sc) clinical scale. The two most exciting methodological features of this study were the inclusion of a brain-damaged schizophrenic group to control for the combination of these conditions and the inclusion of the somatoform disorder group to control for psychological causation of organic complaints.

In order to control for demographic variables, the data were analyzed in two ways. First, statistics were computed on the clinical groups as they were composed, and second, the patients with various diagnostic categories were matched in groups (N = 10) on the basis of age, gender, race, and education. In the unmatched group, analysis of the data suggested that the Sc clinical scale was able to differentiate brain-damaged schizophrenic patients from patients with brain damage or somatoform disorders. By contrast, with the matched group data the Sc clinical scale was able to discriminate brain-damaged schizophrenics from other clinical groups and the P–O scale was able to discriminate the non-brain-damaged schizophrenics from patient groups with brain damage or somatoform disorders. Unfortunately, the P–N scale was not able to differentiate somatoform disorders from brain-damaged patients. Also, the Sc–O scale could not discriminate the clinical groups when matched group data were used.

While the study of Puente *et al.* (1989) will certainly require independent cross-validation with a larger sample size, its data are clearly supportive of the value of the P–O special scale. Just as clearly, it called into question the relative efficacy of the P–N special scale of the MMPI. However, further research is needed to better elucidate the relative strengths and weaknesses of these and other MMPI special scales.

It would be appropriate at this point to mention the Keane MMPI scale for the assessment of combat-related posttraumatic stress disorder (PTSD). Using an empirical procedure, Keane with Malloy and Fairbank (1982) developed an MMPI scale that has been rather effective in distinguishing patients with combat-related PTSD from those without the disorder. While there might be a question of whether PTSD could be considered as a neurological or pseudoneurological syndrome (Everly & Horton, 1989), nonetheless, one point of view would be that this is certainly an area in which faking is likely to be done. Moreover, there is a developing school of thought suggesting that PTSD represents an extensive interaction between biological substances and social events (see Everly, 1990, for a review).

The MMPI on which this research was generated has been recently revised. Major changes have been made to remove sex bias in the items and to delete out-of-date terms. Also, a new normative sample of 2600 persons (1462 females and 1138 males) was selected to reflect the national population (Butcher, Dahlstrom, Graham, Tellegen, & Kaemmer, 1989). The MMPI-2 (Hathaway & McKinley, 1989) has only been available for general clinical use in the last year. Therefore, it is too early to draw any conclusions with regard to the clinical utility of the MMPI-2 in identifying pseudoneurological disorders (Graham, 1990). It will be necessary to replicate many of the studies previously reviewed with the MMPI-2 prior to rely on the latter to make these judgments in clinical situations. Also, the available research suggests the MMPI-2 generates different profiles from the MMPI. The worth of these new profiles remains to be demonstrated. It is worth noting, however, that new scales for PTSD and Type A behavior will be routinely scored in the MMPI-2.

Comment

In addition to neuropsychological test batteries and personality test results, an essential element in the detection of malingering and pseudoneurological disorders from organically impaired patients is extensive history-taking. It is essential for the neuropsychologist to take a careful history from each and every patient covering social, emotional, biological, vocational, educational, and avocational aspects. In addition, evidence from significant others and individuals who have extensively interacted with the patient is particularly helpful. The use of the history is that of a picture frame, in which to look at the test results presented by the patient. For example, the individual who had been a varsity letter-winning first baseman in college and then presents with severe motor deficits but an unimpaired Category test score after a questionable head injury without loss of consciousness will need to do a great deal of explaining.

SUMMARY

Generally speaking, the available neuropsychological and personality test research, with respect to assessment of pseudoneurological disorders, is still at a relatively embryonic level. The few helpful suggestions that can be gleaned from the scant research literature include close analysis of the TPT scores of the HRNB and the F scale of the MMPI. At this point, there is considerable room for careful research on the detection of psychoneurological disorders.

For example, it would appear quite clear that the entire neuropsychological literature on psychoneurological disorders consists of a small number of studies. Indeed, the methodological quality of the studies would serve to render almost any conclusion suspect, except for the need for additional research. Such research in this area might profit from careful review of methodological flaws of previous studies. While certainly not an exhaustive list of suggestions, future researchers in this area might consider the following points. First, use multiple control group designs and include combinations of psychological and organic factors. Second, control both for other common psychiatric conditions and for expert faking knowledge as per Keane and his colleagues. Moreover, in clinical judgment studies it will be crucial for researchers to use multiple, *blind* raters with varied training and experience in clinical neuropsychology and large numbers of subject profiles.

Finally, researchers should cross-validate their results over different types of brain damage, psychiatric conditions, settings, and judges. Indeed, so little is known that perhaps the best approach is to echo Paul Meehl's words in a paper on "Psychotherapy" in the *Annual Review of Psychology* in 1955, when he stated that "the only proper attitude is one of maximum experimentation" (p. 375).

REFERENCES

American Psychiatric Association. (1987). *Diagnostic and statistical manual* (3rd ed., rev.). Washington, D.C.: Author.

Barsky, A. J., Wyshak, G., & Kellerman, G. L. (1986). Hypochondriasis. *Archives of General Psychiatry, 43*, 483–500.

Benton, A. L., & Spreen, O. (1961). Visual memory test; the simulation of mental incompetence. *Archives of General Psychiatry, 18*, 79–83.

Binder, L. M., & Pankratz, L. (1987). Neuropsychological evidence of a factitious memory complaint. *Journal of Clinical and Experimental Neuropsychology, 8*, 323–346.

Bruhn, A. R., & Reed, M. R. (1975). Simulation of brain damage on the Bender Gestalt by college students. *Journal of Personality Assessment, 39*, 244–255.

Butcher, J. N., Dahlstrom, W. G., Graham, J. R., Tellegen, A., & Kaemmer, B. (1989). *Manual for the restandardized Minnesota Multiphasic Personality Inventory: MMPI-2. An administrative and interpretative guide.* Minneapolis: University of Minnesota Press.

Cloninger, C. R., Martin, R. L., Guze, S. B., & Clayton, P. J. (1986). A prospective follow-up in family study of somatization in men and women. *American Journal of Psychiatry, 143*, 873–876.

Dahlstrom, W. G., Welsh, G. S., & Dahlstrom, L. E. (1975). *An MMPI handbook* (Vol. II, rev. ed.). Minneapolis: University of Minnesota Press.

Dodge, G. R., & Kolstoe, R. H. (1971). The MMPI in differentiating early multiple sclerosis and conversion hysteria. *Psychological Reports, 29*, 155–159.

Everly, G. S. (1990). Post-traumatic stress disorder as a disorder of arousal. *Psychology and Health, 4*, 135–145.

Everly, G. S., & Horton, A. M. (1989). Neuropsychology of post traumatic stress disorders: A pilot study. *Perceptual and Motor Skills, 68*, 807–810.

Faust, D., Hart, K., & Guilmette, T. J. (1988*a*). Pediatric malingering: the capacity of children to fake believable deficits of neuropsychological testing. *Journal of Consulting and Clinical Psychology, 56*, 578–582.

Faust, D., Hart, K., Guilmette, T. J., & Arkes, H. T. (1988*b*). Psychologist's capacity to detect adolescent malingerers. *Professional Psychology: Research and Practice, 14*, 508–545.

Ford, C. V., & Folks, T. G. (1985). Conversion disorders: An overview. *Psychosomatics, 26*, 371–383.

Freud, S. (1894). The neuro-psychiatric defenses. In J. Strachey (Ed.), *The Works of Sigmund Freud, standard edition* (Vol. 3). London: Hogarth Press, 1962.

Goebel, R. A. (1983). Detection of faking on the Halstead–Reitan Neuropsychological Test Battery. *Journal of Clinical Psychology, 39,* 331–342.

Graham, J. R. (1990). *Assessing personality and psychopathology.* New York: Oxford University Press.

Greene, R. C. (1978). An empirically derived MMPI carelessness scale. *Journal of Clinical Psychology, 34,* 408–410.

Grow, R., McVaugh, W., & Enco, T. P. (1980). Faking and the MMPI. *Journal of Clinical Psychology, 36,* 910–917.

Gynther, M. (1961). The clinical utility of invalid MMPI F-scores. *Journal of Consulting Psychology, 25,* 540–542.

Hathaway, S. R., & McKinley, J. C. (1951). *MMPI manual.* New York: Psychological Corporation.

Hathaway, S. R., & McKinley, J. C. (1989). *MMPI-2 manual.* Minneapolis: National Computer Services.

Heaton, R. K., Smith, H. H., Jr., Lehman, R. A. W., & Vogt, A. T. (1978). Prospects for faking believable deficits on neuropsychological testing. *Journal of Consulting and Clinical Psychology, 46,* 892–900.

Henderson, L. M., Bell, B. A., & Miller, J. D. (1983). A neurosurgical Munchausen tale. *Journal of Neurology, Neurosurgery, and Psychiatry, 46,* 437.

Horton, A. M., Jr., & Wedding, D. (1984). *Clinical and behavioral neuropsychology.* New York: Praeger.

Horton, A. M., Jr., & Wilson, F. M. (1981). Cross validation of the Psychiatric–Organic (P–O) special scale of the MMPI in a V. A. domiciliary setting. *Clinical Neuropsychology, 3,* 1–3.

Keane, T. M., Malloy, P. F., & Fairbank, J. A. (1982). The empirical development of an MMPI-subscale for the assessment of combat related post traumatic stress disorder. *Journal of Consulting and Clinical Psychology, 52,* 888–891.

Mack, J. L. (1979). The MMPI and neurological dysfunction. In C. S. Newmark (Ed.), *MMPI: Clinical and Research Trends* (pp. 53–79). New York: Praeger.

McKinley, J. C., Hathaway, S. R., & Meehl, P. E. (1948). The MMPI: VI. The K Scale. *Journal of Consulting Psychology, 12,* 20–31.

Mensch, A. J., & Woods, D. J. (1986). Patterns of faking brain damage on the Luria–Nebraska Neuropsychological Battery. *International Journal of Clinical Neuropsychology, 8,* 59–63.

Nemiah, J. C. (1988). Psychoneurotic disorders. In A. M. Nicholi (Ed.), *The new Harvard guide to psychiatry.* Cambridge, Mass.: Harvard University Press.

Nolan, B. H., Swihart, A. A., & Pirozzolo, F. J. (1986). The neuropsychology of normal aging and dementia: An introduction. In D. Wedding, A. M. Horton, Jr., & J. S. Webster (Eds.), *The neuropsychology handbook* (pp 410–440). New York: Springer.

Puente, A. E., Rodenbough, J., & Horton, A. M., Jr. (1989). Relative efficacy of the Sc-O, P-O, P-N, and Sc MMPI scales in differentiating brain damage, brain damage schizophrenic, schizophrenic, and somatoform disorders in an outpatient setting. *Journal of Clinical Psychology, 45,* 99–105.

Shaw, D. J., & Matthews, C. G. (1965). Differential MMPI performance of brain damaged versus pseudoneurological groups. *Journal of Clinical Psychology, 21,* 405–408.

Tomb, D. (1988). *The House Officers guide to psychiatry* (2nd ed.). Baltimore: Williams & Wilkins.

Watson, C. G. (1971). An MMPI scale to separate brain damage from schizophrenic men. *Journal of Consulting and Clinical Psychology, 46,* 1127–1132.

Watson, C. G. (1984). The schizophrenic–organic (Sc–O) and psychiatric–organic (P–O) MMPI scale: A review. *Journal of Clinical Psychology, 40,* 1010–1021.

Watson, C. G., & Plemel, D. (1978). MMPI scale to separate brain-damaged from functional psychiatric patients in neuropsychiatric settings. *Journal of Consulting and Clinical Psychology, 46,* 1127–1132.

Watson, C. G., Gasser, D., Schaefer, A., Burnen, C., & Woll, T. (1981). Separation of brain-damaged from psychiatric patients with ability, and personality measures. *Journal of Clinical Psychology, 37,* 347–353.

12

Deception and Malingering

LAURENCE M. BINDER

INTRODUCTION

This chapter describes the evaluation of the possibility of malingering in neuropsychological assessment. Cases with financial incentives will be emphasized—e.g. workers compensation, personal injury litigation, and Social Security disability. Although malingering in criminal forensic and military settings will not be discussed, this material is relevant to those settings. Assessment of the patient who is attempting to feign mental health will not be examined.

Malingering is defined as the intentional production of symptoms for the purpose of obtaining an external incentive such as financial compensation, dodging of military duty, or avoidance of punishment for criminal behavior (American Psychiatric Association, 1987). Malingering is not considered a mental disorder although it frequently coexists with mental disorders. Unlike malingering, in Munchhausen syndrome and other factitious disorders the incentive is to play the patient role rather than to obtain an external incentive (Pankratz, 1981).

Historically, observations of malingering were first recorded in biblical times. The development of the legal concepts of the tort and negligence in medieval times, followed by development of workers compensation systems in Europe and the United States in the 19th century, brought monetary gain into prominence as incentive for malingering. The advent of the railroads led to numerous high-velocity accidents and the industrialization of the workplace led to both more dangerous workplaces and less self-employment. Contemporary debates about malingering are parallel to those of the 19th century (Trimble, 1981). According to Trimble (1981), the work of Erichsen (1882) was enormously

LAURENCE M. BINDER • Psychology Service, Veterans Administration Medical Center, Portland, Oregon 97207.

HANDBOOK OF NEUROPSYCHOLOGICAL ASSESSMENT: A Biopsychosocial Perspective, edited by Antonio E. Puente and Robert J. McCaffrey. Plenum Press, New York, 1992.

influential in providing credence to the notion that an injury did not have to be visible to be compensable. Erichsen (1882) introduced the concept of "spinal concussion," which he viewed as pathology at the molecular level. Shortly afterward, Page (1885) argued that the origin of much of the disability associated with the entity of "spinal concussion" was psychological and criticized Erichsen for the lack of evidence of neuropathological damage.

Clearly, in the past many clinicians felt poorly equipped to make the diagnosis and to distinguish between hysterical reactions and malingering (McMahon & Satz, 1981). Research reviewed in this chapter showed that the average clinician generated unacceptable error rates when attempting to diagnose malingering, at least in the past. More recently, our understanding of both clinical manifestations of poor motivation and diagnostic accuracy have improved substantially.

The actual incidence of malingering is unknown because past research has been hampered by difficulty in ascertaining that all cases have been identified. Opinions in the literature state that it is rare after head injury (Bigler, 1986; Cartlidge & Shaw, 1981), common and virtually synonymous with accident neurosis (Miller, 1961), and probably common in neuropsychological examinations of compensable head trauma (Heaton, Smith, Lehman, & Vogt, 1978). In a sample of 2500 industrial accident cases of all types of injuries (Braverman, 1978), 38% were judged by unspecified criteria to be malingerers. The incidence differs across settings and populations. A literature review of malingering cited incidence estimates ranging from 1 to 50% (Resnick, 1988). It may be less common in severe traumatic brain injury patients who have no trouble proving disability than in minor head trauma patients. A review of 33 cases of financially compensable mild head injuries evaluated in the author's independent practice revealed that 5 patients generated results on forced choice memory testing (described later) that were diagnostic of malingering while an additional patient confessed to malingering. By these conservative diagnostic criteria the incidence rate was 18%. By less conservative criteria the incidence of poor motivation was 26% in an extension of the same series (Binder & Willis, 1991).

Clinician Attitudes and the Need for Differential Diagnosis

Psychologists and psychiatrists sometimes seem reluctant to make the diagnosis that implies that symptoms are exaggerated or totally factitious and induced by a desire to obtain money or other incentive. Yet, a recent survey revealed that most psychologists and neurosurgeons felt that financial incentives played some role in the postconcussive syndrome (McMordie, 1988). Many clinicians fail to appreciate the reinforcing value of money and all too quickly dismiss the possibility of malingering. Society pays people to perform honest tasks that, in some ways, are more disagreeable than simulating illness. Although mental health professionals tend to regard work highly, not all people share these values. Some people do things for money that are more unpleasant than malingering. Why shouldn't some patients malinger?

There have been multiple reasons for the clinically observed infrequency of diagnosis of malingering in some settings. Perhaps mental health professionals found it difficult to be skeptical and therapeutic at the same time. Or, skepticism may have translated into functional diagnoses such as depression or conversion reaction rather than malingering.

Anger is the frequent reaction of a treating clinician whose patient is labeled as a malingerer by another diagnostician. Clinicians who diagnose malingering sometimes are considered callous, mercenary, and countertherapeutic. In reality, the reaction of the clinician labeling the behavior as malingering may be sorrow over the patient's pathetic adaptation to life. With many of these patients, it is not the existence of distress that is in dispute, but the nature and cause of the distress. Mislabeling psychopathology as brain damage may also be countertherapeutic. Nonetheless, perhaps some clinicians avoid the diagnosis out of concern for a negative reaction from a colleague or referral source.

One would expect that anger is a common reaction of patients who receive the diagnosis of malingering. Although no systematic research exists on the subject, one Australian patient murdered two orthopedic surgeons and wounded a third after receiving a malingering diagnosis in connection with complaints of back pain. The patient committed suicide and the autopsy did not demonstrate organic back pathology, providing some data in support of the diagnosis by the physician-victims (Parker, 1979). Some clinicians may fear the possibility of a professional negligence lawsuit if they anger the patient by diagnosing malingering, providing an additional disincentive for making the diagnosis.

The best method of avoiding the outrage of colleagues, if not patients, is to minimize diagnostic errors. Neuropsychologists are vulnerable to diagnostic errors if they fail to make a systematic differential diagnosis. Merely forming an impression regarding the presence or absence of brain damage, an all too common clinical practice, inevitably leads to ignoring psychological factors that provide alternative explanations for cognitive deficits. Neuropsychology developed means of detecting brain damage that are superior, in some ways, to those available to medicine. However, use of neuropsychological tests without ruling out various psychiatric diagnoses will lead to false-positive diagnoses of brain damage. For example, differential diagnosis after mild head injury includes depression, somatoform disorders, anxiety disorders, substance abuse, vestibular dysfunction, malingering and brain injury (Binder & Rattok, 1989). (See Part II for further information.)

The only sensible procedure for the clinician is to consider the possibility of malingering in every patient who has any monetary or other external incentive for faking bad on a neuropsychological examination. Any other tactic is indefensible (American Psychiatric Association, 1987; Binder, 1990; Ziskin & Faust, 1988). Malingerers often are cunning and experienced deceivers who have much to lose if they are detected. Consequently, they take pains to avoid discovery. The clinician must employ systematic procedures to enhance the probability of detection of possible patient deception. Before diagnosing malingering, alternative diagnoses must be considered such as depression, conversion reaction, and somatoform disorders. Diagnostic issues are discussed in detail in the remainder of the chapter.

Unfortunately, although the presence of malingering can be proved, the nonexistence of malingering is demonstrably highly unlikely in some cases, but cannot be disproved. The notion that a single test could rule out brain damage was dispelled long ago and the same is true for simulation of mental deficits. Motivation must be evaluated throughout the neuropsychological examination, and not just in a single task.

RESEARCH ON SIMULATION IN NEUROPSYCHOLOGICAL TESTING

Experimental studies consistently have demonstrated the ability of normal subjects to perform on a variety of neuropsychological tests at the level of brain-damaged patients after receiving brief instructions to simulate. Yet, in an otherwise excellent discussion of forensic neuropsychology, the ability of patients to successfully fake neurological disorders was questioned (Bigler, 1986). In an early study of the Benton Visual Retention Test, simulators fell below the brain-damaged group (Benton & Spreen, 1961). Impaired performance by simulators also was found on the Halstead–Reitan (Heaton *et al.*, 1978) and the Luria–Nebraska battery (Mensch & Woods, 1986). One study seemed to show that simulators performed more like the normal controls than the brain-damaged patients, but the brain-damaged group clearly was severely impaired, suggesting that the simulators failed to go far enough (Goebel, 1983). Not only can deficits on effortful tasks be simulated, but supposedly involuntary neurological responses such as the patellar reflex can be brought under voluntary control to fool trained observers (Stam, Speelman, & van Crevel, 1989).

Some quantitative and qualitative differences between brain-damaged and simulating subjects exist. Compared with head trauma patients, simulators had more deficits on sensorimotor measures including Speech-Sounds Perception, finger tapping, finger localization, grip strength, and sensory extinctions and less deficits on the Category Test and Tactual Performance Test measures of total time, memory, and location (Heaton *et al.*, 1978). The mean WAIS FSIQ of simulators was in the average range, but the mean was 17 points lower than the estimate of their mean actual IQ based on Shipley–Hartford data obtained prior to asking them to fake (Heaton *et al.*, 1978). Simulators had more distortion errors and fewer omission, perseverative, and size errors on the Benton Visual Retention Test than brain-damaged patients (Benton & Spreen, 1961). On the Bender-Gestalt unspecified qualitative indicators were more helpful than scores for an expert attempting to distinguish between simulators and brain-damaged patients (Bruhn & Reed, 1975). Bizarre, inconsistent, and approximate answers are given by simulators on intelligence tests (Schretlen, 1988).

The studies of simulation of brain damage have provided some interesting hypotheses about malingering that require validation with clinical samples.

Simulators will fake selectively, rather than mimicking global, severe mental impairment. Although IQ scores may be lowered by faking, the IQ scores may remain quite average. The measures that simulators choose to demonstrate deficits may not always be those that are most sensitive to organic impairment. Instead, they tend to fake on sensorimotor measures (Heaton *et al.*, 1978).

Studies of the ability of clinicians to diagnose malingering on traditional neuropsychological measures have shown poor rates of detection. Clinicians with varying levels of experience received test protocols including the WAIS, Halstead–Reitan Battery, and the MMPI (Heaton *et al.*, 1978). Despite knowledge that the base rate for malingering in the series was 50%, the hit rates ranged from the chance level to just 20% above chance. A discriminant function analysis was able to separate the two groups accurately, but methodological problems probably created a spuriously high classification rate (Adams, 1979). In the only study of this question on pediatric cases, none of the 42 clinicians correctly diagnosed simulation (Faust, Hart, & Guilmette, 1988). Previous research on detection of malingering with neuropsychological tests has been reviewed elsewhere in more detail (Franzen, Iverson, & McCracken, 1990; Schretlen, 1988).

Forced Choice Testing

The work of Loren Pankratz was seminal in demonstrating that forced choice testing is the most powerful technique for the detection of malingering. In forced choice testing of memory the patient is presented with a recognition memory task. The number of foils (incorrect choices) determines the probability of guessing correctly on each item. Performance significantly worse than chance results from the deliberate production of wrong answers; the probability of an explanation other than malingering is nil (Rogers, 1988). Forced choice testing has been applied to hearing loss (Pankratz, Fausti, & Peed, 1975), blindness (Grosz & Zimmerman, 1965; Pankratz, 1979), tactile sensation loss (Miller, 1986; Pankratz, Binder, & Wilcox, 1987), and memory complaints (Binder, 1990; Binder & Pankratz, 1987; Binder & Willis, 1991; Brandt, 1988; Hiscock and Hiscock, 1989; Pankratz, 1983, 1988).

The most useful treatment of data from forced choice testing is the application of the binomial theorem (Siegel, 1956). The formula is

$$z = \frac{(x - 0.5) - NP}{\text{square root of } (NPQ)}$$

where N equals the number of test items, P and Q are the expected proportions of right and wrong answers, and x is the number of errors. The inclusion of the correction for continuity of 0.5 in the formula is controversial, unless x is close in value to N (G. Sexton, personal communication, 1990). Elimination of the correction makes the formula slightly more powerful. When using the z tables available in most textbooks of statistics, the more powerful, one-tailed test is justified by the prediction that the patient will perform worse than chance. A large number of test items will provide a test of performance when the error rate approximates 60%. If 36 items are administered, then 23 errors is significant at the 0.07 level, for example. Fifty-nine errors out of one hundred is significant at the 0.05 level. Extreme performances become significant quickly. For example, 11 errors in 14 items is significant at the 0.03 level. All of these examples were computed using the 0.5 correction.

Case studies of malingering documented by statistically significant results on forced choice testing of memory have been described. The first published case (Binder & Pankratz, 1987) of a compensation claimant who malingered on such a procedure involved repeated presentations of either a pen or a pencil followed by interpolated mental activity and recognition testing. Unfortunately, this method of forced choice testing is not very sensitive. Most malingerers are wary of being caught and may view this procedure as too easy to risk a performance below the level of chance. An improved method was first suggested by Hiscock and Hiscock (1989). Their forced choice task contained increasing levels of difficulty which provide a more compelling invitation to fake bad than the earlier procedure. Their patient did not perform below chance level until the more difficult level of the test was reached.

The Portland Digit Recognition Test (PDRT) was developed (Binder, 1990; Binder & Willis, 1991) in order to improve the sensitivity of forced choice testing and was based upon the work of Hiscock and Hiscock (1989). Each item requires recognition of a five-digit number from among two possibilities; the probability of guessing correctly is 0.5. The test has three levels of difficulty. The patient is told before the second and third levels that the task will become more difficult. The patient counts backwards for 5 sec in the first block of 18 items, for 15 sec in the second block of 18 items, and for 30 sec in the third and fourth blocks which each have 18 items. Statistical significance is assessed in the 36 most difficult group of items or in the test total of 72 items. This test is recommended whenever compensation is a potential issue including all personal injury, workers compensation, and disability examinations.

A large number of claimants perform within the range of chance on forced choice procedures such as the PDRT. From a rational viewpoint, chance level performance on a recognition task is comparable to zero correct on a recall task, and calls motivation into question. Observations in this laboratory on the early version of forced choice testing and on the PDRT indicated that normal subjects instructed to simulate usually performed at the chance level and rarely significantly below the chance level (Binder & Willis, 1991). One patient tested several months after a mild concussion performed at the chance level on the newer procedure, scored below the lowest normative levels on most Wechsler Memory Scale–Revised index scores, and confessed to faking. Brandt (1988) has also observed that normal-fakers often perform at the chance level on a forced choice task. Clearly, chance level performance does not rule out faking bad.

Standardization data (Binder & Willis, 1991) show that some brain dysfunction patients with no motivation for compensation performed as poorly as 54% correct overall and within the range of chance, but only if they have severe cognitive deficits, abnormalities on neurological examination, and documented structural brain damage. The mean brain dysfunction group performance was significantly better than the mean performances by minor head trauma patients seeking compensation for their injury, brain-damaged patients seeking compensation, and normals instructed to simulate. Patients with affective disorders had a deficit similar to the brain dysfunction patients not seeking compensation, and performed better than minor head trauma patients. On the most difficult items the worst brain-damaged patient performance in the group not seeking compensation was 50% correct.

The standardization data for the PDRT now include 67 brain-damaged subjects who were not applying for compensation and the cutoff scores (Binder, unpublished data) of 50% correct on the 36 30-sec items and 54% correct on the total of 72 items have not changed. These cutoff scores can be used to judge the effort on this test of a patient. Of course, objective indices of neurological injury that are independent of patient effort and cooperation such as CT and MRI scans should not be ignored. For example, a patient falling just below the cutoff scores on the PDRT is unlikely to have fully recovered from a massive traumatic brain injury with severely impaired coma level scores, coma of long duration, and massive hemorrhages shown on CT scanning, regardless of his or her motivation during the PDRT. In contrast, a patient suffering a minor head trauma with no loss of consciousness or period of posttraumatic amnesia and normal brain scan who falls below the PDRT cutoff scores many months after the injury probably is poorly motivated, at least on the PDRT.

It may be difficult in some cases to evaluate the diagnostic significance of chance level performance in the presence of well-documented structural brain damage or definite neurological abnormalities. In the absence of clear evidence of cerebral dysfunction from neurodiagnostic studies, however, the clinician should be suspicious of performance below the cutoffs of 39 of 72 total correct or 18 of 36 correct on the 30-sec items.

Another method of analyzing chance level performance has been described (Miller, 1986). In forced choice testing of tactile sensory loss, 120 trials were divided into 24 blocks of five items. An expected chance level distribution of errors, based upon the binomial theorem, would have included some blocks with zero, one, four, and five errors. Miller's patient produced 22 blocks with either two or three errors. Comparison of the expected and the observed values with the chi-square statistic was significant, indicating that the performance did deviate from chance.

Simulation on the MMPI

The MMPI probably has been the most widely used test of emotional functioning by neuropsychologists and simulation on the MMPI has been exhaustively studied. Some of the information in this brief review may generalize to the MMPI-2.

Caveats for use of the MMPI in neurological settings include the tendency of brain-damaged patients to have elevations on Scales One, Two, Three, and, to a lesser extent, Seven and Eight (Mack, 1979). Mack (1979) called for more research on the behavioral correlates of profiles that have traditionally been interpreted in nonneurological settings, but also judged the test to be useful for brain-damaged patients.

Normal simulators obtained higher scores on Scales F, One, Three, Six, Seven, Eight, and Zero than head-injured patients who were not in litigation (Heaton *et al.*, 1978). The mean F scale *t*-score for the simulators was 80 (S.D. 19) compared with the head-injured mean of 64 (S.D. 12). These data from a small sample suggest that F scores above 90 on the MMPI are rare in the head-injured population who are not pursuing compensation claims. The MMPI-2 scales now have a uniform T-score distribution and a recommended cutoff score of 65 rather than 70. One would assume that F scores above 90 will be no more common on the MMPI-2 than the MMPI, and research on this issue is under way.

The MMPI yields three measures of exaggeration and faking. The best known is the Gough Dissimulation (F minus K) index. The recommended cutting score for invalidating a profile using this index is 16 for Lachar (1974), 10–11 for Caldwell (1975), and 9 for Gough (1950). However, with a cutting score of 10, only 72% of simulated profiles will be detected while a cutting score of one correctly classifies 88% of both the genuine and simulated profiles (Gough, 1950). More recently, a cutting score of zero resulted in correct classification of 88% of patients and 70% of simulators (Anthony, 1971), but in a psychiatric setting 38% of the patients had F minus K scores above zero and 16% had scores greater than 10 (Greene, 1988). In short, the index may often reflect both real distress and exaggeration and simply measures the response set or the way the patient wishes to be perceived, or could reflect random responding or lack of comprehension of the items. In combination with other data it might show evidence of malingering. The F scale measures symptoms that generally are in the psychotic realm and would not be expected to assess the malingering of nonpsychotic states. An F score of greater than 90, without reference to K, casts doubt on the validity of a profile (Butcher, Dahlstrom, Graham, Tellegen, & Kaemmer, 1989).

The Wiener and Harmon subtle and obvious items may also provide some evidence of exaggeration (Greene, 1988; Wiener & Harmon, 1946). T scores above 70 on all five obvious scales and scores near 50 on all five subtle scales suggest exaggeration (Greene, 1988). If the only exception to this rule of thumb is on Scale Four, the patient may be trying to maximize reports of current symptoms while minimizing reports of preinjury family and behavioral problems. The subtle–obvious distinction needs more research to determine its validity in compensation cases when only Scales Two and Three show higher obvious than subtle scores. The subtle–obvious scales have been retained on the MMPI-2, but concerns about their validity have been expressed (Weed, 1989).

The Gough Dissimulation Scale–Revised consists of 40 items that distinguished neurotics from simulators (Greene, 1988). It was more accurate than the F minus K index in detecting simulation (Anthony, 1971), but could lead to many false-positive diagnoses of malingering in an inpatient psychiatric setting (Greene, 1988). On the MMPI-2, 34 of the 40 original items have been retained.

SUBTYPES OF MALINGERING

Not all malingerers are alike, and a clinician will err by retaining an overly specific notion of malingering. The disorder is colored by the adaptive and maladaptive personality traits of the individual. Some subtypes of malingering are akin to the personality disorders. The existence of organic injury and the relationship of the injury to the compensable accident provide two additional dimensions for subtyping the disorder.

Braverman (1978) identified five subtypes. Among the subtypes was decoy malingering with the deception serving to draw the attention of the patient away from a very real and threatening injury. In hysterical malingering the patient suffers an initially unconscious regression toward hopelessness about recovery and dependence upon others for assistance, but elements of conscious deception are also present. Psychotic malingerers use malingered symptoms to defend against a fantasied danger. Organic malingerers have actual brain injuries that affect their abilities to understand their own feelings and invent symptoms in order to convince themselves that they are real, feeling persons. Only in the fraudulent subtype is the deception totally conscious. In the other subtypes there is extensive psychopathology with the symptoms often serving to defend against awareness of some damage or inadequacy. About 80% of the malingerers were categorized as hysterical, but explicit diagnostic criteria were not provided.

Inaccurate statements and outright lying can be explained by the phenomena of specific personality disorders (Ford, King, & Hollender, 1988). In histrionic personality disorder, inattention to detail and disdain for facts are characteristic. Among other features, narcissistic persons have feelings of entitlement, exploit others, and often feel that they do not have to play by the rules governing others. Pathological lying, termed pseudologia fantastica, in persons with borderline personality may result from poor tolerance of the anxiety caused by telling the truth, poor self-esteem, and poor impulse control (Snyder, 1986). The anger and tendency to project of the borderline personality lead to blaming others for actions for which the patient is responsible. It is difficult to determine if these lies result from delusional thinking or a desire to deceive. These patients may falsely claim that clinicians seen previously have diagnosed disorders that suit their primitive needs. One woman claimed that she had received a diagnosis of epilepsy and that diazepam was the anticonvulsant of choice (Snyder, 1986). In reality, she was dependent on diazepam.

The diagnosis of a personality disorder is problematic if a patient is inclined to minimize preinjury problems. In a medicolegal examination, sufficient data to make a personality disorder diagnosis may only come from the records, if they are available at all. The cases described below generally had insufficient information regarding preinjury functioning to justify a DSM III-R Axis II diagnosis of personality disorder, but clearly had maladaptive personality traits.

Case One: Mixed Personality Disorder

A man was seen 3 years after an on-the-job low back injury. Chronic pain was the major disabling feature, but a neuropsychological examination was requested to determine if cognitive abilities limited his potential for retraining. He reported a series of head injuries and complained of memory problems. Physicians had noted vagueness and poor memory in routine history taking. Testing revealed problems with concept formation and shifting, memory, and reading comprehension and malingering was not suspected.

He was seen again at the request of the insurer 4 years after the initial examination. Investigation had revealed considerable deception about his medical history. Records showed a 20-year history of treatment for opiate abuse and a 6-year history of treatment for narcolepsy. The diagnosis of narcolepsy was in doubt because it was based upon his report; he probably had lied about narcolepsy symptoms in order to obtain amphetamines. No single set of his three sets of doctors (back, drug abuse, narcolepsy) were aware of the existence of the other disorders or doctors until the investigation. The chief psychiatrist at the drug abuse facility, who had known him for the 20 years he had been treated, commented upon his deterioration in mental abilities and diagnosed an organic brain syndrome secondary to his polydrug abuse. The second neuropsychological examination showed cognitive deterioration and confused, chaotic thinking on the Rorschach. His claim for psychological damage secondary to the back injury was finally denied with the denial upheld after 7 years of disability payments.

After reviewing the records 3 years after the second examination, this writer is not certain that he did not malinger on testing given the primitive methods of detection available at the time of the examination. Sociopathic and borderline features were obvious by the time of the second examination. A fascinating feature of both examinations was his antisocial responses to questions on the WAIS-R. When asked to identify Martin Luther King he responded with a racial slur. He responded that he would look at the contents if he found an envelope that was sealed, addressed, and stamped.

A clinician can request that a patient provide, without advance warning, a urine sample to a medical laboratory. In this writer's experience no patient has refused, and some analyses have been positive, indicating recent drug use that had been denied in the interview.

Case Two: Histrionic Traits

A woman reported sustaining a concussion at work in an accident that occurred just 3 months after she had returned from a lengthy convalescence from back surgery. Her return to her skilled manual trade from the back injury had been difficult because she felt unable to perform all of her normal duties. After the concussion she complained of severe pain in her cervical region and was returned to temporary disability. Almost a year after her injury she was seen by a psychologist for memory complaints and was found to have both a psychogenic memory problem and signs of a frontal lobe syndrome and psychotherapy sessions for depression and anxiety were initiated. More than a year after the reported concussion she began to report intermittent episodes of vision loss. At various times she described these as consisting of loss of peripheral vision, feeling like being in a fog, and inability to recognize a toothbrush held in her hand. Multiple EEGs, an MRI scan, and a CT scan were all normal and her neurologist concluded that her spells were functional.

When seen for examination she acknowledged driving the approximately 8-mile distance to the office from her home. She claimed that her visual fog had suddenly disappeared recently and specified the precise date and time of her abrupt cure. However, an investigative report stated that she had been driving prior to her cure more extensively than she acknowledged. She continued to complain of loss of peripheral vision. A forced choice technique was devised to test her visual complaint and she announced after a few items that she could only be wrong half the time and performed accordingly. On the PDRT she also performed at the chance level. In addition, this procedure led to her complaining that she was losing her vision and going into a fog, but her vision reportedly returned after a 2-min rest. In marked contrast to her chance level performance on the PDRT was her entirely normal performance on the Rey Auditory Verbal Learning Test where she was able to recall 14 of 15 unrelated words after five presentations. Other test data were also average including intelligence and memory scores. No problems on visual tasks were observed. The only other deficit was on immediate recall of geometric designs on the Visual Reproductions I subtest of the Wechsler Memory Scale–Revised, but she performed significantly better on delayed recall, recalling material that she had not recalled earlier on immediate recall.

The histrionic features included her visual complaints and response to the forced choice technique of temporary blindness. In addition, records noted that she had reported responding to tiny doses of psychotropic medications with marked side effects. Just 10 mg of doxepine, an antidepressant that is therapeutic in doses of 150–300 mg, caused her to sleep for 3 days, she claimed.

The diagnosis of malingering was based upon her bizarre response to the forced choice technique, which was interpreted as an attempt to avoid a task that placed her in a dilemma, her chance level performance on the same task (when she could see the response cards), which was worse than the performance of patients with documented brain damage and similar to normal simulators, her inconsistent performance on visual recall with immediate memory inferior to delayed recall, and her continued driving of her motor vehicle despite her visual complaints. The visual deficits she reported were incompatible with her claim of a blow to the head with brief loss of consciousness and no confusion or amnesia coupled with the negative neurodiagnostic studies. The late onset of her visual deficits was also suspicious. After the examination it was learned that an investigator had observed her traveling regularly to an office and staying inside for several hours on a regular basis. It was alleged by the insurer that she was employed while she was fraudulently receiving total disability payments. The case was settled before the evidence of fraud was presented in hearing.

Case Three: Pathological Lying

An industrial painter was diagnosed as suffering from occupational asthma after reporting that he had been overcome by fumes at work. He was referred for neuropsychological examination because of complaints of memory and concentration problems. He reported receiving bachelor's and master's degrees in literature.

The examination process took several weeks because he missed several appointments due to reported pulmonary and other physical symptoms. Testing revealed a number of subtle discrepancies between above-average abilities on tasks usually resistant to the effects of cerebral dysfunction and mild impairment on many tasks more sensitive to cerebral dysfunction, with some of the more sensitive tasks showing normal scores. For example, his Verbal IQ was 110 with age-corrected scale scores one standard deviation above average on Digit Span and Arithmetic. He was average on the Purdue Pegboard, a measure of manual dexterity, and faster than average on the Seguin–Goddard Formboard, a forerunner of the Tactual Performance Test. No visual constructional impairment existed and he was average on other measures including the Wisconsin Card Sort Test. Trail Making, and Babcock Story Recall. He was more than a standard deviation below the mean on both the written and oral administrations of the Symbol Digit Modalities Test and on the Serial Digit Learning Test. The latter was in contrast to his better-than-average performance on Digit Span where he could retain as many as eight forward and seven backwards. He was also mildly impaired on the Rey Auditory Verbal Learning Test.

I diagnosed a toxic encephalopathy and recommended supportive psychotherapy because he appeared in the interviews and on an objective inventory to be in great distress and reported feeling suicidal. He never returned for psychotherapy after he was informed of the diagnosis. During the interviews he had denied, and later admitted, serving in the military in Vietnam.

Two years later he was seen at the request of the insurer by an allergist and another neuropsychologist (Dr. Ruth Matarazzo performed the second examination) who noted a large number of inconsistent reports and apparent fabrications in his communications to various examiners. He had claimed that he had obtained a doctorate and then worked as a surgical assistant and taught at the college level. School transcripts revealed that he had failed to graduate from college and the college where he claimed to have taught had no record of his employment. The hospital where he said he had worked as a surgical assistant only had records of him working as an orderly. Furthermore, he had concealed a history of cigarette smoking from several medical examiners and had claimed, and then later denied, that his father had died of emphysema. His ex-wife reported to an investigator that he regularly smoked marijuana and took mescaline when they first married. Some of this history undoubtedly would have influenced the physician who had diagnosed the occupational asthma 2 years earlier.

In the second neuropsychological examination he claimed he could not remember where he had obtained a bachelor's degree and that he was unable to fill out a simple history questionnaire. On testing his performance was consistent in many respects with the first examination. His Verbal IQ was 110 and his Performance IQ was 93. His Wechsler Memory Scale Memory Quotient was 114 with no intelligence or memory subtests showing abnormalities except for mild impairments on Digit Symbol and Object Assembly. His total time on the Tactual Performance Test of 8.45 min, 23 Category Test errors, and zero Rhythm Test errors were better-than-average scores, but he expressed confusion on some of the other tests. On the Rey Auditory Verbal Learning Test he recalled 5, 7, 10, 7, and 6 words out of 15 over the five learning trials. The examiner correctly noted that it was difficult to explain this recall deficit on anything but a motivational basis and was also skeptical of his zero recall on the Tactual Performance Test, failure to recall simple autobiographical information, and nonanatomical errors on perception of tactile double simultaneous stimulation. He complained of intermittent confusion during testing, but this complaint was inconsistent with the mostly normal performances noted above. The allergist felt that he had airway disease attributable to tobacco and marijuana usage, and both the neuropsychologist and the allergist felt that the probability of malingering was high.

When the attorney for the claimant asked for a review of the reports of the allergist and neuropsychologist, this writer agreed that the patient was malingering. By this time he reportedly had been granted Social Security and was pursuing a claim for damages against the manufacturer of the allegedly toxic material to which he had been exposed. Clearly, this man could not buttress his claim of industrial injury by lying about his educational or occupational background, but fatally damaged his credibility through his deception.

The many normal test scores obtained in both examinations did nothing to disprove this clear-cut case of deception. In reviewing the initial test data there is no evidence of poor motivation. In retrospect, however, his inconsistent report about military service in Vietnam, failure to return to multiple appointments because of his claimed symptomatology, and lack of follow-through with psychotherapy despite reporting suicidal ideation might have raised some questions about his motivation. This case illustrates the fact that the absence (or near absence) of evidence of malingering is not evidence for absence of malingering.

This case also demonstrates the value of repeat examinations in the detection of malingering. Only on the second examination was malingering apparent. The case underscores the need to request permission to obtain educational transcripts from many patients in compensation cases. This patient probably would have refused permission to obtain a transcript, but this refusal would have provided valuable information. Not long after seeing this patient this writer began to routinely obtain educational transcripts of patients. Failure to obtain educational records is exhaustively criticized in a book designed to assist attorneys in destroying the credibility of expert testimony of psychologists and psychiatrists (Ziskin & Faust, 1988).

CONVERSION DISORDER IN RELATION TO MALINGERING AND COMPENSATION ISSUES

Exaggeration is common to both conversion reactions (formerly termed hysteria) and malingering. As Henry Miller (1961) stated, "differentiation between conscious and unconscious purpose is quite insusceptible to any form of scientific inquiry. . . . To compensate a man financially because he is stated to be deceiving himself as well as trying to deceive others is strange equity and stranger logic" (p. 993). Miller viewed the postconcussive syndrome as one form of accident neurosis and believed that the symptoms were inversely related to the severity of the head injury. Although he recognized that these patients presented in a spectrum ranging from conversion reactions to malingering, he vigorously disputed the notion that all motivation in conversion reactions was unconscious, noting that these patients were well aware of financial considerations. For Miller, "these disproportionate results of trivial injury are not seen except where financial compensation is in question" (p. 995). He ridiculed those who maintained that clinicians could distinguish between conscious and unconscious motivation in such cases, and argued that the distinction mattered little, because the symptoms of 50 patients whom he followed almost invariably cleared up after legal settlement.

In response to Miller it was shown that postconcussive symptoms could continue long after settlement of a claim (Merskey & Woodforde, 1972). More recently, data confirm that the distinction between patients in litigation and those who are not is based upon subjective complaints rather than objective measures of organic damage (Cartlidge & Shaw, 1981; Fee & Rutherford, 1988), but also replicate the finding that settlement does not lead to symptom relief after concussion (Fee & Rutherford, 1988).

The distinction between a conversion reaction and malingering becomes easy if the patient is observed functioning in a manner that he/she claims he/she cannot. Examples of claimed loss of function in a hand being disbelieved because of nicotine stains on fingers have been cited (McMahon & Satz, 1981; Miller, 1961). Performance significantly worse than chance on forced choice testing and other gross inconsistencies in testing are also examples of the patient performing much better than he/she says he/she is able.

In many cases of prolonged symptoms of conversion reaction after a traumatic injury there is little doubt that elements of malingering are present (Walsh, 1985). Some patients may convince themselves that they are suffering from their symptoms (McMahon & Satz, 1981), a bit of self-deception that surely cuts two ways because it increases both their suffering and the worth of their claim.

A diagnosis of conversion reaction does not rule out the presence of organic disease. A review by Pankratz (1988) demonstrates that, in a neurological setting, neurological disease can be demonstrated in a large number of patients with hysterical findings. Presumably, patients in a psychiatric setting with hysterical findings are less likely to have neurological disease than those in a neurological setting. Two features commonly thought to indicate psychogenic sensory loss were common in organic patients complaining of hemifacial numbness (Rolak, 1988). Diminished vibratory sensation in the forehead was found in 86% of the organic patients and facial midline splitting of sensory loss was found in 7.5% of the organic patients compared with 20% of the purely psychogenic patients.

Case Four: Conversion Reaction

Occasionally, careful study leads to a conclusion that a disorder might be motivated by unconscious factors. A man was treated at a VA Medical Center for intractable seizures and was admitted for video-telemetry monitoring of his seizures. Neuropsychological testing found a conversion V on the MMPI, convincing evidence of cerebral dysfunction, and negative findings on the PDRT and forced choice testing of his stocking distribution tactile sensation loss on both lower extremities. The latter was attributed to a peripheral neuropathy probably caused by his Dilantin. The brain damage was reportedly attributable to an unconfirmed cerebral hemorrhage, but the patient was known in the past to have had an alcohol abuse problem. He was receiving Social Security disability payments and was not claiming that his seizures were military service connected. Video-telemetry EEG monitoring revealed that he had two types of seizures, both epileptic and pseudoepileptic (nonorganic).

CASE EXAMPLES OF MALINGERING OF SPECIFIC DISORDERS

Case Five: Malingering after Low Back Injury

Cognitive abilities are of relevance in back injury cases if the patient is expected to be physically unable to return to his/her previous occupation and must receive vocational retraining. This patient was judged unemployable by a vocational consultant because of his illiteracy and his back condition. However, the attorney for the workers compensation suspected malingering from information in the medical record and requested a neuropsychological evaluation.

The medical record contained a number of observations by orthopedic surgeons of functional overlay, pain behavior, pain responses to mild palpitation, positive Waddell signs (Waddell, McCulloch, Kummel, & Venner, 1980), and giveway weakness. A CT scan showed impingement on the right-side L3 nerve root, lumbar spinal stenosis, and marked osteoarthritis. Electromyography (EMG) demonstrated mild right L5 denervation. He had a history of two low back surgeries 18 and 20 years before.

A physical capacities examination found that he did not exceed 10 consecutive minutes of sitting or standing. His maximum lift from waist to chest was 2.5 pounds with pain complaints and he carried 4 pounds just 50 feet with pain complaints. His grip strength was 7 pounds in the right hand and 20 pounds in the left. Surely, a man with no demonstrable pathology above the lumbar level should have demonstrated greater arm and hand strength. His maximum walking distance was 0.2 mile and his maximum walking speed on a treadmill was less than 1 mile per hour. His claim that he did not have the strength to attempt to balance on one leg was not consistent with his demonstrated ability to walk, no matter how slowly or briefly he could endure. On a vocational interest blank he left 41 items blank and the other 121 items were marked as disliked. In short, he reported that there was no work that he could perform. At a pain treatment center, alcohol abuse was suspected because he was observed to be intoxicated by a fellow patient and he was judged to be generally uncooperative with the program.

A previous psychological examiner observed that pain behavior coincided only with verbal cognitive tasks and that visual tasks led to a temporary cessation of pain behavior. Because of inconsistent test performance and other observations, this previous examiner felt that the patient was malingering. A more recent exam at the request of the patient's attorney led to a diagnosis of major depressive episode secondary to his work injury and disability.

Neuropsychological testing provided strong evidence of malingering. He missed 42 of 72 items on the PDRT ($p < 0.10$), and at one point missed 9 consecutive items. Compared with the testing by the first examiner a year before, he declined two standard deviations on both Picture Completion and Block Design. On the Rey Auditory Verbal Learning Test he recalled 5, 4, 8, 5 and 5 words out of 15 on five consecutive learning trials. He recalled 3 after a brief interference task and 3 twenty minutes later, and recognized 7 correctly with 10 false-positive recognition errors. His poor level of recall, decline in recall from the third to the fourth trials, and his poor recognition memory performance suggested poor motivation. His Wechsler Memory Scale–Revised index scores were all two to three standard deviations below the mean. On Arithmetic he was asked how much is $4 plus $5 and, after 24 sec, he asked if the question was how much is $4 from $5. When the question was repeated he answered "20." Failure on this item is unusual except for some aphasics and delirious patients and he was well oriented and had no language deficit. His apparent multiplication instead of addition is not typical of brain-injured patients. On subsequent arithmetic items, his pattern was to wait an extreme amount of time and then ask for a repetition of the question, and then say that he did not know or give a wrong answer. In the first exam his finger tapping speed was reported to be normal, but in the second exam he averaged 22 with his dominant hand and 20 with his nondominant hand. He was abnormal on all measures of tactile sensation.

The diagnosis of major depression did not seem appropriate because he denied appetite disturbance and anhedonia. However, if one simply accepted his self-report, he did meet the diagnostic criteria for major depression.

Case Six: Malingering in a Patient with a Diagnosis of Vestibular Dysfunction

Literature reviewed elsewhere (Binder, 1986) shows that injury to the vestibular system is a common sequel of head injury. This man was referred by his workers compensation insurer for evaluation 2 years after a head injury that did not result acutely in a clear-cut loss of consciousness, confusion, or loss of memory. A neuro-otologist made a diagnosis of vestibular dysfunction, benign paroxysmal positional nystagmus, and bilateral perilymph fistulas (leaking in the oval window of the ear). Some of these findings were disputed by vestibular specialists who reviewed the records for the insurer. The patient was complaining chiefly of cervical pain rather than vestibular problems, but also reported memory loss.

The examination was remarkable for his pain behavior and extreme hostility. He appeared to perform less than his best on Block Design, for example, rotating item number four after he was told that rotations were not permitted on the second item. Otherwise, his test performance on measures including the Wechsler Memory Scale–Revised, WAIS-R, and other tests did not show clear evidence of poor motivation.

On the PDRT, he was incorrect on 54 of 90 items ($p < 0.05$) and 36 of the 54 most difficult items ($p < 0.02$). This case has been reported elsewhere (Binder, 1990).

THE DIAGNOSTIC PROCEDURE

Review of the Medical Record and the Interview

A question of malingering will often be raised by a review of the medical record or by interview data. Late onset of neuropsychological symptoms may make no neurological sense, but could be explained by malingering or a conversion reaction. Resistance to evaluations and treatment may indicate lack of cooperation, guardedness, or desire to remain ill. Reports of neurological and orthopedic examinations should be scrutinized for mention of functional findings such as giveway weakness, marked pain behavior, and nondermatomal sensory loss. The presence of three or more Waddell signs (Waddell *et al.*, 1980) including nonanatomic and superficial tenderness, simulation of movement that reportedly causes pain, distraction tests to check for the consistency of pain complaints, regional weakness or sensory loss on a nonanatomic basis, and overreaction suggest a nonorganic basis for the complaints. The diagnosis of pseudoepileptic seizures confirms the presence of nonorganic factors.

Lying strongly suggests the possibility of malingering. The patient who is untruthful about autobiographical details also may be untruthful about symptomatology or not give his/her best effort during testing. The medical record or interview sometimes will contain evidence of untruthfulness or statements that can be checked against employment, school, or military records. Exaggerated or totally fabricated combat experience (Sparr & Pankratz, 1983), military intelligence work, athletic exploits, police employment, or other "macho" experiences may be described. The loss of a loved one may be feigned in an apparent attempt to elicit sympathy or attention (Snowdon, Solomons, & Druce, 1978) and may be associated with a history of factitious physical symptoms (Phillips, Ward, & Ries, 1983). Two disorders that are strongly associated with deception—antisocial personality disorder (American Psychiatric Association, 1987) and substance abuse (Sierles, 1984)—greatly increase the likelihood of malingering.

Some malingerers report symptoms that originally began on an organic basis. The early existence of these symptoms trains the patient to convincingly describe them to clinicians after they have disappeared.

Signs of Deception on Neuropsychological Testing

Walsh (1985) noted that the demand characteristics of some situations are more likely than others to elicit exaggerated performance deficits. Forced choice testing probably is the single most useful tool for eliciting evidence of malingered performance deficits (Rogers, 1988). Research on this strategy has been summarized above.

Gross discrepancies between what is expected after an injury and what is reported or observed on testing require explanation. Within broad parameters the severity of neuropsychological deficits can be predicted from knowledge of the acute brain injury. Mild head injury, one of the most common forms of compensable injury seen by neuropsychologists, provides an example of prediction of deficit. Within several weeks of mild head injury the subjective complaints normally outweigh the objective cognitive deficits (Dikmen, McLean, & Temkin, 1986; Levin, Mattis, Ruff, Eisenberg, Marshall, Tabaddor, High, & Frankowski, 1987) and controlled studies show no evidence of any statistically significant cognitive deficits. Yet, brain damage in the form of contusions and diffuse axonal injury clearly can occur. From these studies it can be concluded that mild or even moderate neuropsychological deficits might be observed within a few weeks of seemingly mild head injury. Substantial improvement will occur in the first 3 months. Some cases of head injury, classified as mild because the acute Glasgow Coma Scale score is normal or close to normal or because the loss of consciousness and confusional state (amnesia) is less than an hour (Binder, 1986), actually are more serious because of contusions that go undetected in the absence of an acute MRI scan. Nonetheless, if the clinician has experience with the deficits of severe head injury and knows the usual strong improvement these patients make over the first year (Dikmen, Temkin, McLean, Wyler, & Machamer, 1987), then one knows that the deficits of the plateaued mildly injured patient, at worst, will be comparable to the best of the plateaued severely injured patient. Cases of malingering after mild head injury were described here and elsewhere (Binder, 1990).

Knowing the general parameters of expected deficit after an injury and the general patterns of performance provides the basis for knowing what is unexpected and requires explanation. Missing easy items from measures of previously acquired verbal or visual skills would be unexpected for most forms of brain damage and this sign has received some empirical support (Schretlen, 1988). Similarly, failure to correctly answer simple autobiographical questions can be found among normal fakers (Brandt, 1988). The Information and Orientation subtest of the Wechsler Memory Scale–Revised (Wechsler, 1987) provides a well-standardized measure of easy general and autobiographical information. Bizarre responses are deserving of special note. For example, rotational errors on WAIS-R Digit Symbol or the arithmetic errors of Case Five are unusual after many forms of brain injury.

Marked inconsistencies in testing are usually explained on a psychological, and often on a motivational, basis. Examples of these inconsistencies are numerous. Apparently intact recall for symptoms and the history of the illness on interview probably is compatible with a mild memory deficit, but certainly not a severe one. Severe slowing on finger tapping with scores about 20 (less than 50% of the mean for most age groups) is probably inconsistent with normal performance on Digit Symbol, a measure requiring graphomotor speed. Digit span performance usually is not severely impaired in an alert patient with a severe organic amnesia (Brandt, 1988) and should only be mildly impaired in most patients typically seen for forensic assessment. The Dot Counting test (Lezak, 1983) is a motivational test that assumes that it is easier to count dots in a geometric pattern than dots randomly arrayed. Unfortunately this writer is not aware of any evidence that it identifies fakers, but the strategy of comparing performance on two tasks of different difficulty levels is sensible. The same strategy can be applied to Trail Making, single and double simultaneous sensory stimulation, and other procedures. Inconsistencies across repeated medicolegal examinations in conditions that should be stable, such as head trauma more than a year after the injury, usually are explained psychologically. For this reason, the examiner should make an effort to replicate much of a previous examiner's efforts.

SUMMARY

Failure to correctly diagnose malingering often will be avoided simply by constantly attending to the issue of financial motivation and ruling out deception and character pathology. In every case with possible financial or other external incentives it is critical to assess all data for evidence of poor motivation and faking of any kind. Clinicians can sometimes detect untruthfulness and exaggeration merely from the interview, but judgments from the interview will yield many false-negative diagnostic errors. Specific test procedures, careful review of the medical record, and observation of interview and test behavior may provide evidence of deception. Extensive knowledge of neuropsychological syndromes enables the clinician to make predictions about deficits from information about the acute injury. Performance below expectations requires explanation. All cases require differential diagnosis rather than simply attributing deficits to brain damage. The presence of an organic disorder does not rule out malingering.

It may be impossible to assess the extent of real neuropsychological deficits in a patient who is malingering. Just as the clinical scales of an invalid MMPI should not be interpreted (Greene, 1988), the interpretation of neuropsychological test data should stop with a diagnosis of malingering. An estimate of the patient's functional status can be attempted from knowledge of the severity of the brain injury as measured by neurological and neuroradiological findings.

REFERENCES

Adams, K. M. (1979). Linear discriminant analysis in clinical neuropsychology research. *Journal of Clinical Neuropsychology, 1,* 259–272.

American Psychiatric Association. (1987). Diagnostic and statistical manual III–revised. Washington., D.C.: Author.

Anthony, N. (1971). Comparison of client standard exaggerated and matching MMPI profiles. *Journal of Consulting and Clinical Psychology, 36,* 100–103.

Benton, A. L., & Spreen, O. (1961). Visual memory test: The simulation of mental incompetence. *Archives of General Psychiatry, 4,* 79–83.

Bigler, E. D. (1986). Forensic issues in neuropsychology. In D. Wedding, A. M. Horton, Jr., & J. Webster (Eds.), *The neuropsychology handbook* (pp. 526–547). Berlin: Springer.

Binder, L. M. (1986). Persisting symptoms after mild head injury: A review of the postconcussive syndrome. *Journal of Clinical and Experimental Neuropsychology, 8,* 323–346.

Binder, L. M. (1990). Malingering following minor head trauma. *The Clinical Neuropsychologist, 4,* 25–36.

Binder, L. M., & Pankratz, L. (1987). Neuropsychological evidence of factitious memory complaint. *Journal of Clinical and Experimental Neuropsychology, 9,* 167–171.

Binder, L. M., & Rattok, J. (1989). Assessment of the postconcussive syndrome after mild head injury. In M. D. Lezak (Ed.), *Assessment of the behavioral consequences of head injury* (pp. 37–48). New York: Lisse.

Binder, L. M., & Willis, S. C. (1991), Assessment of motivation after compensable minor head trauma. *Psychological Assessment: A Journal of Consulting and Clinical Psychology, 3,* 175–181.

Brandt, J. (1988). Malingered amnesia. In R. Rogers (Ed.), *Clinical assessment of malingering and deception* (pp. 65–83). New York: Guilford Press.

Braverman, M. (1978), Post-injury malingering is seldom a calculated ploy. *Occupational Health and Safety, 47,* 36–48.

Bruhn, A. R., & Reed, M. R. (1975). Simulation of brain damage on the Bender-Gestalt test by college students. *Journal of Personality Assessment, 39,* 244–255.

Butcher, J. N., Dahlstrom, W. G., Graham, J. R., Tellegen, A., & Kaemmer, B. (1989). *MMPI-2 manual for administration and scoring.* Minneapolis: University of Minnesota.

Caldwell, A. B. (1975). *A handbook of MMPI personality types*. Santa Monica: Clinical Psychological Services.

Cartlidge, N. E. F., & Shaw, D. A. (1981). Head injury. Philadelphia: Saunders.

Dikmen, S., McLean, A., & Temkin, N. (1986). Neuropsychological and psychosocial consequences of minor head injury. *Journal of Neurology, Neurosurgery, and Psychiatry, 49*, 1227–1232.

Dikmen, S., Temkin, N., McLean, A., Wyler, A., & Machamer, J. (1987), Memory and head injury. *Journal of Neurology, Neurosurgery, and Psychiatry, 50*, 1613–1618.

Erichsen, J. E. (1882). *On concussion of the spine: Nervous shock and other obscure injuries of the nervous system in their clinical and medico-legal aspects*. London: Longmans, Green.

Faust, D., Hart., K., & Guilmette, T. J. (1988). Pediatric malingering: The capacity of children to fake believable deficits on neuropsychological testing. *Journal of Consulting and Clinical Psychology, 56*, 578–582.

Fee, C. R., & Rutherford, W. H. (1988). A study of the effect of legal settlement on post-concussion symptoms. *Archives of Emergency Medicine, 5*, 12–17.

Ford, C. V., King, B. H., & Hollender, M. H. (1988). Lies and liars: Psychiatric aspects of prevarication. *American Journal of Psychiatry, 145*, 554–562.

Franzen, M. D., Iverson, G. L., & McCracken, L. M. (1990). The detection of malingering in neuropsychological assessment. *Neuropsychology Review, 1*, 247–279.

Goebel, R. A. (1983). Detection of faking on the Halstead–Reitan neuropsychological test battery. *Journal of Clinical Psychology, 39*, 731–742.

Gough, H. (1950). The F minus K dissimulation index for the Minnesota Multiphasic Personality Inventory. *Journal of Consulting Psychology, 14*, 408–441.

Greene, R. L. (1988). Assessment of malingering and defensiveness by objective personality inventories. In R. Rogers (Ed.), *Clinical assessment of malingering and deception* (pp. 123–158). New York: Guilford Press.

Grosz, H. J., & Zimmerman, J. (1965). Experimental analysis of hysterical blindness. *Archives of General Psychiatry, 13*, 256–260.

Heaton, R. K., Smith, H. H., Jr., Lehman, R. A. W., & Vogt, A. J. (1978). Prospects for faking believable deficits on neuropsychological testing. *Journal of Consulting and Clinical Psychology, 46*, 892–900.

Hiscock, M., & Hiscock, C. K. (1989). Refining the forced-choice method for the detection of malingering. *Journal of Clinical and Experimental Neuropsychology, 11*, 967–974.

Lachar, D. (1974). *The MMPI: Clinical assessment and automated interpretation*. Los Angeles: Western Psychological Services.

Levin, H. S., Mattis, S., Ruff, R. M., Eisenberg, H. M., Marshall, L. F., Tabaddor, K., High, W. M., & Frankowski, R. F. (1987). Neurobehavioral outcome of minor head injury: A three center study. *Journal of Neurosurgery, 66*, 234–243.

Lezak, M. D. (1983). *Neuropsychological assessment*. New York: Oxford University Press.

Mack, J. L. (1979). The MMPI and neurological dysfunction. In C. S. Newmark (Ed.), *MMPI: Current clinical and research trends* (pp. 53–79). New York: Praeger.

McMahon, E. A., & Satz, P. (1981). Clinical neuropsychology: Some forensic applications. In S. J. Filskov & T. J. Boll (Eds.). *Handbook of clinical neuropsychology* (pp. 686–701). New York: Wiley.

McMordie, W. R. (1988). Twenty-year follow-up of the prevailing opinion on the posttraumatic or postconcussional syndrome. *The Clinical Neuropsychologist, 2*, 198–212.

Mensch, A. J., & Woods, D. J. (1986). Patterns of feigning brain damage on the LNNB. *The International Journal of Clinical Neuropsychology, 8*, 59–63.

Merskey, H., & Woodforde, J. M. (1972). Psychiatric sequelae of minor head injury. *Brain, 95*, 521–528.

Miller, E. (1986). Detecting hysterical sensory symptoms: An elaboration of the forced choice technique. *British Journal of Clinical Psychology, 25*, 231–232.

Miller, H. (1961). Accident neurosis. *British Medical Journal, 1*, 919–925, 992–998.

Page, H. (1885). *Injuries of the spine and spinal cord without apparent mechanical lesion*. London: Churchill.

Pankratz, L. (1979). Symptom validity testing and symptom retraining: Procedures for the assessment and treatment of functional sensory deficits. *Journal of Consulting and Clinical Psychology, 47*, 409–410.

Pankratz, L. (1981). A review of the Munchausen syndrome. *Clinical Psychology Review, 1*, 65–78.

Pankratz, L. (1983). A new technique for the assessment and modification of feigned memory deficit. *Perceptual and Motor Skills, 57*, 367–372.

Pankratz, L. (1988). Malingering on intellectual and neuropsychological measures. In R. Rogers (Ed.), *Clinical assessment of malingering and deception* (pp. 169–192). New York: Guilford Press.

Pankratz, L., Fausti, S. A., & Peed, S. (1975). A forced choice technique to evaluate deafness in a hysterical or malingering patient. *Journal of Consulting and Clinical Psychology, 43*, 421–422.

Pankratz, L., Binder, L. M., & Wilcox, L. M. (1987). Evaluation of an exaggerated somatosensory deficit with symptom validity testing. *Archives of Neurology, 44*, 787.

Parker, N. (1979). Malingering: A dangerous diagnosis. *Medical Journal of Australia, 1*, 568–569.

Phillips, M. R., Ward, N. G., & Ries, R. K. (1983). Factitious mourning: Painless patienthood. *American Journal of Psychiatry, 141*, 420–425.

Resnick, P. J. (1988). Malingering of post-traumatic disorders. In R. Rogers (Ed.), *Clinical assessment of malingering and deception* (pp. 84–103). New York: Guilford Press.

Rogers, R. (1988). Current status of clinical methods. In R. Rogers (Ed.), *Clinical assessment of malingering and deception* (pp. 293–308). New York: Guilford Press.

Rolak, L. A. (1988). Psychogenic sensory loss. *The Journal of Nervous and Mental Disease, 176*, 686–687.

Schretlen, D. J. (1988). The use of psychological tests to identify malingered symptoms of mental disorder. *Clinical Psychology Review, 8*, 451–476.

Siegel, S. (1956). *Nonparametric statistics*. New York: McGraw–Hill.

Sierles, F. S. (1984). Correlates of malingering. *Behavioral Sciences and the Law, 2*, 113–118.

Snowdon, J., Solomons, R., & Druce, H. (1978). Feigned bereavement: Twelve cases. *British Journal of Psychiatry, 133*, 15–19.

Snyder, S. (1986). Pseudologia fantastica in the borderline patient. *American Journal of Psychiatry, 143*, 1287–1289.

Sparr, L., & Pankratz, L. D. (1983). Factitious posttraumatic stress disorder. *American Journal of Psychiatry, 140*, 1016–1019.

Stam, J., Speelman, H. D., & van Crevel, H. (1989). Tendon reflex asymmetry by voluntary mental effort in healthy subjects. *Archives of Neurology, 46*, 70–73.

Trimble, M. R. (1981). *Post-traumatic neurosis*. New York: Wiley.

Waddell, G., McCulloch, J. A., Kummel, E., & Venner, R. M. (1980). Non-organic physical signs in low-back pain. *Spine, 5*, 117–125.

Walsh, K. W. (1985). *Understanding brain damage*. Edinburgh: Churchill Livingstone.

Wechsler, D. (1987). *Wechsler Memory Scale–Revised manual*. New York: Psychological Corporation.

Weed, N. (1989). Why "subtle scales" should not be used in clinical assessment. In J. N. Butcher & J. R. Graham (Eds.) *Topics in MMPI-2 interpretation* (pp. 54–56). Minneapolis: MMPI-2 Workshops and Symposia.

Wiener, D. N., & Harmon, L. R. (1946). Subtle and obvious keys for the MMPI: Their development. *Advisement Bulletin, 16*. Minneapolis: Regional Veterans Administration Office.

Ziskin, J., & Faust, D. (1988). *Coping with psychiatric and psychological testimony*. Marina del Rey: Law and Psychology Press.

III

Biological and Environmental Factors

Introduction

In Part III, selected biological and environmental factors are discussed. The chapter by Delay and Isaac reviews the pathology associated with the peripheral nervous system. This chapter is important since many symptoms associated with dysfunction in the peripheral nervous system may be confused with dysfunction secondary to central nervous system damage. The chapter by Lorig reviews the literature on the role of cardiovascular and somatic disorders as they affect neuropsychological functioning. Neurosurgical interventions and the differentiation of premorbid from postsurgical factors are presented in an in-depth and scholarly chapter by Uzzell.

The neuropsychological sequelae associated with the use of psychoactive drugs in the treatment of psychotic and affective disorders are presented by Medalia and Gold. This chapter highlights a number of important variables with a history of psychotic and/or affective disorders. Finally, the psychobiological foundations of neuropsychological toxicology are presented by Hartman. In this chapter, the major toxins and their effects on brain functioning are discussed.

13

Pathology of the Peripheral Nervous System

EUGENE R. DELAY and WALTER ISAAC†

INTRODUCTION

While pathology of the peripheral nervous system (PNS) is not usually considered to be within the province of the neuropsychologist, such pathology may complicate, or confuse, an attempt to evaluate a dysfunction of the central nervous system (CNS). Many PNS disorders, or *neuropathies*, often go unrecognized since they produce symptoms similar to other functional and organic disorders that the neuropsychologist frequently encounters. In addition, the types of processes that result in CNS dysfunction also are capable of affecting the PNS, including trauma (e.g., compression or entrapment injuries), toxins, infectious diseases, malnutrition, alcoholism, and genetic disorders. Not being aware of some of the more common disorders involving the PNS can lead to misdiagnosis and inappropriate treatment for the patient thought to have a CNS disorder. As with any medical disorder, precise evaluation and treatment of neuropathies should be done by a practitioner competent to do so. However, a familiarity with the general features of peripheral neuropathies is essential for the neuropsychologist to identify the presence of these disorders, distinguish between peripheral and central symptoms and signs, and at the same time, recognize potential limitations imposed by a peripheral disorder on procedures used to assess CNS functions. The intent of this chapter is to provide information that can help neuropsychologists address these issues.

†Deceased.

EUGENE R. DELAY • Department of Psychology, Regis University, Denver, Colorado 80221.
WALTER ISAAC • Department of Psychology, University of Georgia, Athens, Georgia 30602.

HANDBOOK OF NEUROPSYCHOLOGICAL ASSESSMENT: A Biopsychosocial Perspective, edited by Antonio E. Puente and Robert J. McCaffrey. Plenum Press, New York, 1992.

HISTORY

In 1787 Lettson gave the first description of a peripheral neuropathy associated with alcohol consumption (cited in Delwaide, 1987). By the middle of the 19th century, disorders of the PNS were receiving considerable attention from neuroscientists and clinicians alike. One important disorder, characterized by inflammation of portions of the PNS was initially identified by Landry in 1859 and was elaborated further by Guillain, Barré, and Strohl in 1916 (cited in Schonberger, Hurwitz, Katona, Holman, & Bregman, 1981). This disease became known as Guillain–Barré–Strohl syndrome and more recently as Guillain–Barré syndrome. Largely due to the identification of histopathological and clinical effects of Guillain–Barré syndrome and other neuropathies known in the 19th century, disorders of the PNS were generally classified as "neuritis." However, it soon became apparent that many peripheral nerve disorders were the result of noninflammatory processes such as degeneration due to toxic reactions. By the 1930s, Wechsler (1933, 1938) and others were suggesting that a new term, *peripheral neuropathy*, was nomenclature more appropriate for classification of peripheral nerve disorders, of which neuritis was but one form. Still, as recently as 1958 Wartenberg argued that the term *neuropathy* was too general and that the term *neuritis* was more descriptive of the processes associated with a damaged or diseased peripheral nerve. Nevertheless, today a disorder of the PNS is known as a peripheral neuropathy.

Throughout the 1800s, the medical profession became increasingly aware of the susceptibility of the PNS to disruption. By the end of the 19th century, the number of clinically documented PNS disorders led Church (1890) to write that "The causes of multiple neuritis are legion" (p. 639). Extensive lists of agents that could damage peripheral nerves were published. These lists included etiologies such as medicines and home remedies, bacteriotoxins, deficiency states, honeybee stings, viruses, and chemical substances such as industrial compounds along with other well-established etiologies such as alcohol, diabetes, and compressed nerves (Wartenberg, 1958). Today, if a complete list of etiological agents of peripheral neuropathies could be compiled, it would probably reach into the thousands.

Advances in experimental and clinical technology have led to more rapid identification and characterization of peripheral neuropathies and to vastly improved methods for clinical diagnosis of neuropathies. For instance, early clinical work revealed that the ability to detect vibrating stimuli often was reduced or abolished, particularly in the distal portion of the limbs, by many of the peripheral neuropathies (Williamson, 1922). Initially, clinicians used tuning forks to assess vibration thresholds. However, the need for better quantification of vibration thresholds led to the evolution of standardized methods for measuring these thresholds that can lead to early diagnosis of subclinical neuropathies (Goldberg & Lindblom, 1979). Along different lines, after Dawson and Scott (1949) described the first procedure for measuring nerve conduction in intact humans, advances in electrophysiological techniques dramatically improved the accuracy of diagnosis of peripheral neuropathies (Hodes, Larrabee, & German, 1948; McDonald, 1963). Today, a combination of clinical, electrophysiological, and peripheral nerve biopsy techniques are employed to diagnose and study peripheral neuropathies. Nowhere is this more evident than in the vast array of technology focused in recent years on the peripheral neuropathies associated with the acquired immunodeficiency syndromes (AIDS). Moreover, as our understanding of the nature of peripheral neuropathies increases, it is becoming more apparent that these disorders can alter behavior in ways that can pose diagnostic headaches for the clinical neuropsychologist. An awareness of the major features of prominent peripheral neuropathies is essential for the clinician who needs to accurately differentiate between PNS and CNS signs and symptoms.

THEORETICAL AND BASIC NEUROBIOLOGICAL ISSUES

Peripheral neuropathies may be *mononeuropathic*, involving a single peripheral nerve, *mononeuropathic multiplex* (multifocal neuropathy), in which several individual nerves are damaged, or *polyneuropathic*, in which there is systemic involvement of peripheral nerves. Thus, it should not be surprising to find that, as with any aspect of neuropsychology, a background in neuroanatomy, neurophysiology, and a working knowledge of systemic physiology and gross anatomy are elementary to the understanding of peripheral neuropathies as well as to the identification of patients exhibiting symptoms of a peripheral neuropathy. Since the characteristics of each component of the PNS often hold the key to the disorders to which each is susceptible and to the pattern of symptoms most likely to emerge, a brief overview of the PNS will be presented before the discussion of specific neuropathic disorders. Although there are many interesting and even exotic peripheral neuropathies, only those common neuropathies that might be of interest to, or are likely to be confronted by, the practicing neuropsychologist will be discussed. More complete descriptions of these and other disorders can be found elsewhere (e.g., Matthews, 1987; Schaumburg, Spencer, & Thomas, 1983; Stewart, 1987).

General Anatomical Considerations

The term *peripheral nervous system* includes all neural structures outside of the brain and spinal cord. This portion of the nervous system consists of the cranial nerves, the dorsal and ventral roots of the spinal nerves, the spinal nerves and their dorsal and ventral rami, the plexuses, and the peripheral nerves, as well as the peripheral portions of the autonomic nervous system. Because of the anatomical relationships among these structures, pathology affecting any one of these structures produces a pattern of symptoms that is distinguishable from a pattern seen with pathology involving any other structure. Unfortunately for the neuropsychologist, many of these patterns of symptoms may resemble syndromes of a functional nature or may be confused with the consequences of CNS dysfunction.

Even though cranial nerves have a variety of unique physiological, anatomical, and functional characteristics, many of these nerves also share some common functions (see Table 13.1). Some of the cranial nerves (CN I, II, and VIII) are totally sensory, some (CN III, IV, VI, XI and XII) are purely motor. The others are mixed motor and sensory, although the relative magnitude of the two components may vary. Some of the cranial nerves (CN III, VII, IX, X, and XI) include motor components that are part of the parasympathetic division of the autonomic nervous system. Cranial nerves with sensory functions have sensory ganglion and the rest do not. Further, the distribution of the cranial nerves varies from those that supply specific structures, such as the optic nerve (CN II), to those that have a wide distribution, such as the vagus nerve (CN X).

In comparison to the cranial nerves, the portion of the PNS that leaves the CNS at the level of the spinal cord has several common characteristics. At each level of exit there is a ventral root (mainly motor) and a dorsal root (mainly sensory). The ventral root contains the large-diameter, myelinated neurons of the spinal motor neurons and the small-diameter, myelinated fibers of the

TABLE 13.1 Overview of the Cranial Nerves and Their Functions

Cranial nerve	Functions
I. Olfactory	Sensory: Smell
II. Optic	Sensory: Vision
III. Oculomotor[a]	Motor: All intrinsic (lens, pupils) and most extrinsic muscles that rotate the eye
IV. Trochlear	Motor: Superior oblique muscle, rotates eye
V. Trigeminal	Sensory: Somatosensory receptors to the face, forehead, eye, upper and lower jaws Motor: Muscles of mastication, external meatus, tympanic membrane, parotid and lacrimal glands
VI. Abducens	Motor: Lateral rectus muscle, rotates eye
VII. Facial[a]	Sensory: Taste from anterior ⅔ of tongue and soft palate; somatosensory from external meatus; proprioception from facial muscles Motor: Muscles of expression (bilateral cortical control of upper facial muscles, contralateral control of lower facial muscles), salivary and lacrimal glands
VIII. Vestibulocochlear	Sensory: Vestibular and auditory
IX. Glossopharyngeal[a]	Sensory: Taste posterior ⅓ of tongue; somatosensory from pharynx, tonsils, pharyngeal part of tongue, tympanic cavity, auditory canal Motor: Stylopharyngeus and pharyngeal musculature, parotid glands
X. Vagus[a]	Sensory: Heart, GI tract, larynx, pharynx, trachea, lungs, bronchi, external ear, tympanic membrane, some meninges Motor: Heart, GI tract, pharynx, lungs, bronchi
XI. Accessory[a]	Motor: Sternocleidomastoid, trapezius
XII. Hypoglossal	Motor: Ipsilateral tongue muscles

[a]Parasympathetic.

sympathetic nervous system. The dorsal root includes the cell bodies of unipolar afferent neurons that form the dorsal root ganglion. Some of these neurons are large-diameter, myelinated fibers responsible for cutaneous and proprioceptive input while others have small-diameter fibers that can be either myelinated (e.g., temperature afferents) or nonmyelinated (e.g., pain afferents). These roots unite to form a spinal nerve as they leave the spinal column through the intervertebral foramen, the openings between the vertebrae. The spinal nerve then divides and forms a dorsal and a ventral ramus. The dorsal rami supply the back and the ventral rami supply the limbs and ventrolateral parts of the neck and body wall. Fibers of the rami of the cervical and lumbar–sacral levels intermingle to form plexuses, from which major peripheral nerves arise. Most prominent of these include the brachial, lumbar, and sacral plexuses. The brachial plexus is formed from spinal nerves exiting the spinal cord at the cervical (C5–8) and upper thoracic (T1) levels. The median, ulnar, and radial nerves arise from the brachial plexus to innervate the hands, arms, and shoulder region. The lumbar and sacral plexuses, formed by fibers from L1–S4, give rise to the femoral, the sciatic, and other nerves serving the lower limbs. In contrast, the ventral rami of the thoracic nerves (T2–T12) do not form plexuses. Instead, they innervate the body trunk in a circular or radial manner at the approximate level that the spinal nerves exit the spinal column.

The parasympathetic and sympathetic divisions of the autonomic nervous system differ not only in terms of function but also in terms of anatomical and physiological makeup. Axons of the cell bodies of the parasympathetic division that leave the CNS at the cranial and sacral levels, end in ganglia located in, or near, the structure they innervate. Thus, the postganglionic fibers are relatively short and their distribution is restricted. Acetylcholine functions as the neurotransmitter for both the pre- and postganglionic axons. The sympathetic division of the autonomic nervous system follows a different pattern, however. Axons of the cell bodies of this division lie within the lateral horn of the spinal cord at the thoracolumbar levels of the spinal cord (T1–L2). These small-diameter myelinated axons exit at those levels by way of the ventral roots and end in a series of interconnected ganglia, known as the sympathetic chain, located outside of the vertebral column. The sympathetic chain extends from the base of the skull to the coccyx, or from the upper limits of the spinal column to the lower limits. The chain is joined to the ventral rami by pairs of rami communicantes, bundles of axons that travel to the ganglia and from the ganglia back to the ventral rami. Like the plexuses discussed above, the fibers traveling to the ganglia intermingle a great deal. Other sympathetic ganglia also occur in the plexuses and have the same structure and function as the ganglia of the sympathetic truck. As a result of the intermingling of the fibers within the ganglia, the response of the sympathetic nervous system is more widespread than the parasympathetic division. Since the ganglia are located closer to the spinal cord, the sympathetic postganglionic fibers are longer than those of the parasympathetic division. Acetylcholine serves as the neurotransmitter for the preganglionic fibers while epinephrine and norepinephrine serve as the neurotransmitters for the postganglionic synapses at most target tissues. One exception to this is the sweat gland where acetylcholine is the neurotransmitter. Acetylcholine is also the neurotransmitter of the sympathetic fibers innervating the adrenal medulla. When the adrenal medulla is activated, it releases epinephrine and norepinephrine into the cardiovascular system. Once released, these hormones produce generalized "postganglionic" adrenergic effects that intensify and prolong the sympathetic response wherever these hormones function as neurotransmitters.

Cranial Nerve Neuropathies

In view of the broad range of functions in which cranial nerves are involved (see Table 13.1), it is not surprising that neuropathies of these nerves can have quite diverse effects. However, only the most frequently encountered symptoms and signs of cranial nerve neuropathies will be discussed.

Three cranial nerves control the muscular functions of the eyes. The oculomotor nerve (CN III) innervates the intraocular muscles (pupillary and ciliary), most of the extraocular muscles controlling the rotation of the eye in its socket, and the levator muscle of the upper lid of each eye. Palsies associated with CN III damage often result in a lack of pupillary response with the pupils dilated (mydriasis), an inability to focus on near objects, and an inability to rotate the eye upward or medially. Ptosis, a drooping of the upper eyelid as the result of muscular paralysis, also is seen. If the lesion is unilateral, all of these effects will be seen on the ipsilateral side of the lesion. In addition, conjugate motion of the eyes will be disrupted and the person may experience diplopia, the perception of two images of a single object. The trochlear nerve (CN IV) innervates the contralateral superior oblique muscle which assists in turning the eye downward and outward while the abducens nerve (CN VI) innervates the ipsilateral lateral rectus muscle, which rotates the eye outward. Palsies associated with damage to each of these nerves reduce or prevent the normal rotation of the eye from occurring and can result in diplopia. Frequently, all three nerves are damaged during head trauma injuries (Trautmann & Barnett, 1984), either directly or through increased intracranial pressure following the injury. For example, sudden shifts in the location of the brain during impact may stretch or avulse (tear away) the nerves. Total or partial ophthalmoplegia (paralysis of the eye muscles), ipsilateral paresis (muscular weakness), and diplopia are among the symptoms that frequently occur with trauma injuries. It should be noted that infections, neoplasms, vascular accidents, and other sources of injury also can cause these symptoms.

Neuropathies of the trigeminal nerve (CN V) can produce diminished somatosensory sensitivity or paresthesias (abnormal sensations) of the facial areas, the cornea, and the tongue. Since this nerve has three major branches serving different areas of the face and head, not all of these symptoms may appear together. In addition to the sensory symptoms, paralysis of the muscles of mastication also is common if the mandibular branch of CN V is damaged.

Trigeminal sensory neuropathies may or may not be accompanied by pain, but if present it is usually a constant, dull ache or burning sensation. Occasionally, this pain may mimic the paroxysm of the trigeminal neuralgia (tic douloureux) disorder of CN V. The pain paroxysms of trigeminal neuralgia are brief, lasting from a few seconds to a few minutes, and may recur after a brief interval. Episodes of this disorder may last days or even months followed by pain-free periods. The neuralgia is typically unilateral and can be triggered by specific sensory or motor stimuli.

Bell's palsy is the most common neuropathy associated with disorders of the facial nerve (CN VII). The palsy is a widespread, rapidly developing unilateral facial paralysis that results in a distortion of facial expression. Facial movements are often accompanied by unintentional movement (synkinetic movements). For example, when the patient is smiling, the eyelids may close on the side of the face affected by the palsy. Hyperacusis (acute hearing), abnormal taste sensations, and reduced lacrimal secretions also may be present. The more proximal the nerve damage is to the brain stem, the more likely it is that the latter three symptoms will occur (Schaumburg *et al.*, 1983). In a recent study, 20 of 28 patients diagnosed as having Bell's palsy also showed evidence of reduced functioning of the trigeminal nerve during the acute phase of the palsy (Hanner, Andersen, Frisén, Rosenhall, & Edström, 1987). Further testing revealed that over half of the 28 patients had symptoms indicating an etiology involving other cranial nerves (usually CN V), brain-stem structures, or both, in addition to the facial nerve. These data suggest that before a facial paralysis can be considered a symptom of CNS deficits, one needs to examine the functional integrity of the facial nerve and other cranial nerves.

Motor dysfunctions are characteristic of disorders of cranial nerves IX–XII. For instance, the accessory nerve (CN XI) innervates muscles of the neck and shoulder. Damage to this nerve results in weakness of head rotation to the side opposite the damage and in paresis of shoulder muscles. Of far more interest to the neuropsychologist, however, are the neuropathies involving cranial nerves IX, X, and XII since each nerve innervates some aspect of the peripheral speech apparatus (Newsom-Davis, Thomas, & Spalding, 1984). For example, the glossopharyngeal nerve (CN IX) serves the stylopharyngeus muscle and occasionally other parts of the pharynx. The vagus nerve (CN X) also has motor efferents serving pharyngeal as well as palate musculature and unilateral lesions of this nerve may lead to defective elevation of the palate and uvula during phonation. Lesions in both nerves will result in dysphagia (difficulty in swallowing) and flaccid dysarthria. Flaccid dysarthria is indicated by speech production that is low intensity or weak-sounding, is nasal or hoarse, and tires easily. Other signs include reduced variation in pitch, slow and imprecise consonant production, and distorted vowel production such as a "fluttering," prolonged /a/ (see Darley, Aronson, & Brown, 1969; Hartman, 1984, for further details). These dysarthric symptoms appear to be more severe in adults than in children (van Dongen, Arts, & Yousef-Bak, 1987). Dysphagia and a variety of autonomic disturbances (see the section on Diabetic Neuropathies) also are symptomatic of CN X damage. The hypoglossal nerve (CN XII) serves the ipsilateral tongue muscles. Unilateral damage to CN XII will cause the tongue to deviate to the ipsilateral side when protruded and over time one may see atrophy of the ipsilateral tongue musculature if nerve regeneration does not occur. Bilateral damage can produce severe dysarthria and dysphagia. Moreover, the patient will probably have difficulty protruding the tongue.

The optic nerve (CN II) is embryologically part of the CNS, but as the cranial nerve responsible for afferent visual stimulation, it is appropriate to consider some of the peripheral neuropathies associated with the optic nerve, particularly since they can be problematic in the diagnosis of central visual functioning. With penetrating head injuries, obvious visual neuropathies can result from trauma to the eye or the optic nerve. However, neuropathies resulting from indirect optic nerve trauma from nonpenetrating injury to the head are less obvious but still well documented (Kline, Morawetz, & Swaid, 1984; Lessell, 1989). For example, even though the skull may not be fractured, the nerve may be stretched during a bicycle fall or automobile accident or edema may develop after the injury. These injuries can produce loss of visual acuity, visual field cuts, pupillary dysfunctions, and dyschromatopsia (color vision dysfunction), either unilaterally or bilaterally. Metabolic disturbances can lead to retinopathy as well. An example of this is the loss of vision associated with uremia. Deterioration of visual function may be abrupt and bilateral and may or may not be reversed by correction of the uremic condition (Hamed, Winward, Glaser, & Schatz, 1989). Optic neuropathy also can develop from ischemia following an infarction of the vessels within the retina. The onset of visual dysfunction is usually sudden and painless, although deterioration may continue for several days or weeks after the initial visual loss. Depending upon the location of the infarction, visual deficits for the afflicted eye range from minor loss of visual acuity in a specific area of the visual field to a full field loss. Inferior nasal losses are most frequent but central scotomas also are common. People over 50 years of age appear to be more susceptible to optic ischemia (Boghen & Glaser, 1975). Occasionally, an involved eye will have recurrent episodes of ischemia which will lead to progressive field loss over time (Kao, Huang, & Chen, 1989). Another neuropathy, optic neuritis, is an inflammatory condition that may be seen either unilaterally or bilaterally, and either in isolation or in association with infectious diseases such as herpes zoster, or demyelinating pathological processes such as multiple sclerosis (Sandberg-Wollheim, Bynke, Cronqvist, Holtas, Platz, & Ryder, 1990). It can affect the optic nerve inside the eyeball (neuropapillitis) or the segment of the nerve just behind the eyeball (retrobulbar). Patients with optic neuritis may complain of reduced visual acuity. Moreover, high-contrast stimuli will appear dimmer to the patient and the apparent contrast between stimuli will be diminished. In fact, threshold and suprathreshold visual contrast testing is becoming a standard procedure for detecting optic neuritis (Lorance, Kaufman, Wray, & Mao, 1987). Optic neuritis can lower suprathreshold apparent contrast sensitivity and elevate contrast thresholds, especially for stimuli of intermediate and high spatial frequencies

(Sjöstrand & Abrahamsson, 1982). At low spatial frequencies the magnitude of the threshold deficit appears to be attenuated when the temporal frequency of the stimulus is increased (Hess & Plant, 1983). Besides these neuropathies of the optic nerve, there are many other causes of dysfunction within the peripheral portion of the visual system. Generally, cognitive functions will not be disturbed in these patients unless the optic neuropathy is associated with a disorder affecting the CNS such as multiple sclerosis (Lyon-Caen, Jouvent, Hauser, Chaunu, Benoit, Widlöcher, & Lhermitte, 1989). However, care should be taken to assure that assessment of central visual functioning is not hampered by field cuts, reduced acuity, lower contrast sensitivity, or other visual processes affected by optic neuropathies.

The eighth cranial nerve is a sensory nerve involved in auditory and vestibular modalities. Even though these modalities are quite different experientially, the sensory apparatus and transduction processes for each system are remarkably similar. Loss of auditory sensitivity, reduced frequency discrimination, and tinnitus are characteristic of damage to the cochlear apparatus and the eighth nerve. Speech perception is often reduced, although the degree of this deficit is variable (Luxon, 1986) and depends upon how much of the peripheral auditory system is damaged and whether the damage is unilateral or bilateral. Damage to the cochlea (but not nerve damage) will produce a symptom called loudness recruitment. Loudness recruitment is an abnormally rapid increase in apparent loudness when a sound stimulus is increased in intensity; that is, the sound appears to increase in intensity faster than it really does. On the other hand, adaptation to a sound occurs much more rapidly than normal if the nerve is damaged, but not when the cochlea is damaged. Patients with nerve damage will hear a constant tone (e.g., vibrating tuning fork) for only a few seconds compared to people with normal hearing or with cochlear damage. Involvement of the vestibular branch of the eighth nerve will result in dysequilibrium, vertigo, and asymmetrical nystagmus. While the two branches of the eighth nerve may be affected simultaneously, bilateral vestibulopathy without associated hearing loss has been described (Baloh, Jacobson, & Honrubia, 1989). Since the path of the eighth nerve is close to the facial nerve, penetrating or closed head trauma injuries to the eighth nerve also may be accompanied by facial paralysis (Bell's palsy). In addition to trauma, the eighth nerve also is susceptible to invasion by bacterial (e.g., meningitis) and viral (e.g., mumps, herpes zoster) agents. It should be noted that although vestibular dysfunction is often symptomatic of multiple sclerosis, studies have suggested that these symptoms are due to central rather than peripheral involvement (Luxon, 1986; Ward, Cannon, & Lindsay, 1965).

The cranial nerves function as primary afferents or efferents for many of our most complex behavioral functions such as vision and speech. Numerous neuropsychological tests used for CNS assessment, as well as the people administering the tests, implicitly depend upon intact cranial nerve function. When these nerves are dysfunctional, performance on most of these tests will be affected. It then becomes necessary to discriminate between the behavioral deficits due to central disorders and those due to peripheral disorders before an accurate diagnosis is possible.

Compression and Entrapment Neuropathies

While compression or entrapment neuropathies can occur at many locations throughout the PNS, the most frequently occurring compression mononeuropathies involve the nerves innervating the limbs. In the course of traveling long distances to serve each limb, the nerves are often protected only by the overlying skin and subcutaneous tissues where they are vulnerable to external pressure, stretching, or other forms of physical trauma. At other locations a nerve may travel through a narrow anatomical passage where physical abnormalities may "entrap" the nerve, resulting in a compression that inhibits the normal functioning of the nerve. Impairment of each major nerve will produce a characteristic localized pattern of sensory and motor symptoms (e.g., pain, numbness, paresthesia, weakness) that is related to the area each nerve serves and that can help the psychologist distinguish this pattern of symptoms from other disorders.

One such nerve is the median nerve, which travels down the forearm to innervate a portion of the skin surface and some of the muscles of the hand (see Fig. 13.1). Because of the anatomical arrangement of the wrist, it is often the site of compression or entrapment neuropathies. Perhaps the most common of the neuropathies associated with the wrist is the carpal tunnel syndrome resulting from compression of the median nerve as it travels through the carpal tunnel. This "tunnel" is located just proximal to the base of the palm and is formed by the small carpal bones of the wrist and a thick, broad fibrous band (flexor retinaculum). Tendons, blood vessels, and nerves fill the tunnel. When the volume of the contents of the tunnel is greater than the size of the tunnel, the pressure increases within the tunnel and compresses the nerve fibers of the median nerve. The median nerve innervates the medial region of the hand; that is, a portion of the thumb as well as the palmar region and the dorsal surface of tips of the index, the middle, and the radial half of the ring fingers (see Fig. 13.1). Since the median nerve is composed of about 94% sensory fibers, it is not surprising that patients may first complain of numbness and tingling in this region, then of pain. The pain initially is experienced at night, and can be relieved by hanging, rubbing, shaking, or exercising the hands. Elevations in vibration and pressure thresholds have been noted at early stages of the syndrome while changes in two-point thresholds are generally not seen until more advanced stages. Also, as the thenar muscles atrophy and weaken, motor symptoms appear as the coordination between the thumb and index finger deteriorates. Even simple tasks such as buttoning clothes, sewing, or grasping small objects are affected, especially during the morning, although some improvement generally occurs during the day. Symptoms can occur in one, or often both hands, and can generally be aggravated by repetitive or strenuous use of the hands (Szabo, 1989).

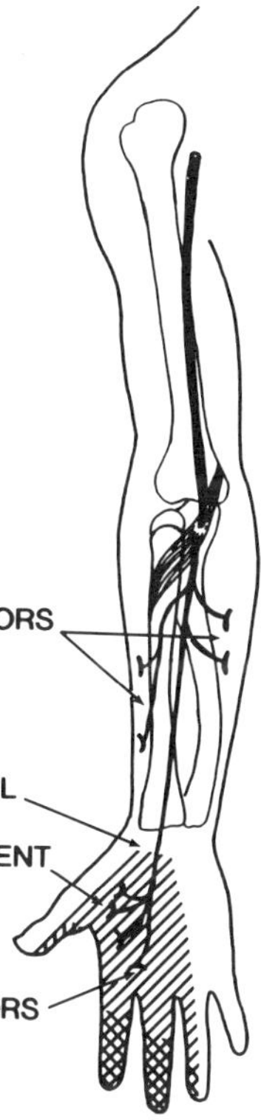

FIGURE 13.1. Schematic view of the median nerve and its primary motor supply as it travels down the arm to the hand. Also, the sensory innervation of the palmar or volar (///) and the dorsal (\\\) surfaces of the hand are shown.

A wide variety of etiologies have been described for the carpal tunnel syndrome. Factors that can increase the pressure within the carpal tunnel, such as fluid retention during pregnancy, arthritis, diabetes (Entin, 1968), or long-term hemodialysis (Schwarz, Keller, Seyfert, Pool, Molzahn, & Distler, 1984), have been implicated. In addition, there is an increased risk of the syndrome for people whose occupations require repetitive or strain-producing movements of the wrists or fingers, or the use of vibrating hand tools or musical instruments (Bleecker, Bohlman, Moreland, & Tipton, 1985; Cannon, Bernacki, & Walter, 1981; Falck & Aarnio, 1983; Feldman, Goldman, & Keyserling, 1983; Lederman, 1989; Spaans, 1970). A careful examination of the presenting symptoms combined with attention to the person's occupation or other physical activities can aid in the detection of this syndrome.

Compression of the ulnar and radial nerves in the arms can result in neuropathies somewhat similar to the carpal tunnel syndrome, but at different locations. The ulnar nerve is most vulnerable to damage at the elbow and at the wrist. As the ulnar nerve courses the length of the arm (see Fig. 13.2), it passes the cubital tunnel at the elbow. At the wrist the nerve travels a narrow path (Guyon's canal) between the hook of the hamate bone and the pisiform bone and through a canal formed by several ligaments. A dorsal cutaneous branch arises

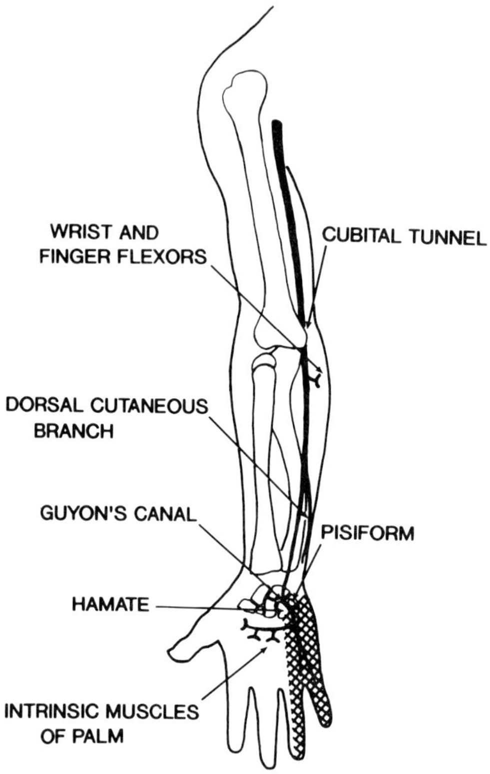

FIGURE 13.2. Schematic view of the course of the ulnar nerve in the forearm. The primary motor innervation of the nerve as well as the palmar (///) and dorsal (\\\) sensory distribution of the nerve are shown.

below the elbow and above the wrist which bypasses the canal. The motor components of the nerve at the wrist innervate most of the intrinsic muscles in the hand while the sensory components innervate the lateral half of the fourth finger and all of the fifth finger. Compression syndromes of the ulnar nerve generally result in sensory disturbances of the fourth and fifth fingers and lateral sides of the hand. Pain also may be present and, depending upon the location of the compression, the pain may extend up to the elbow. Other signs of compression at the elbow include a weakening of the intrinsic muscles of the hand which may be indicated by impaired ability to open (abduction) or close (adduction) the fingers when the palm is flat and fingers are extended and by an impaired ability to pick up small objects between the thumb and the index fingers. In more severe cases, the fourth and fifth digits may become deformed ("claw-hand") as muscles within the hand weaken further. Ulnar damage located at the wrist can affect different branches of the nerve and may result in sensory loss without motor deficits, motor deficits without sensory loss, or both sensory and motor losses. Compression injuries of the ulnar nerve have been associated with activities that require repetitive flexion and extension movements of the arms (e.g., hammering, shoveling), with external pressure from prolonged resting of the elbow on a hard surface (e.g., bedridden patients), chronically leaning or pressing on the elbows (e.g., office clerks) or the base of the hands (e.g., bicycle riders), and with occupations that require workers (e.g., plumbers, musical instrumentalists) to maintain their arms in flexed and restricted positions (Eckman, Perlstein, & Altrocchi, 1975; Feldman *et al.*, 1983; Lederman, 1989; Spaans, 1970). Many other factors have been associated with ulnar neuropathies including fractures, dislocation of the elbow, soft tissue injury, masses such as tumors, and physical deformities (Stewart, 1987).

The radial nerve winds around the posterior humerus bone of the upper arm to the lateral side (see Fig. 13.3). Upon reaching the elbow region the nerve divides into a deep motor branch serving the extensor muscles of the hand and wrist, and a superficial sensory branch that bypasses the wrist compartments en route to the dorsolateral surface of the thumb and the dorsal aspects of the first two fingers of the hand. The nerve innervates muscles of both the upper and lower forearm and has a cutaneous sensory distribution running from the dorsal upper arm to the wrist. As a result of its course in the arm, neuropathies of the radial nerve occur less often than either the median or ulnar nerves and are generally due to external pressure rather than entrapment in an anatomical

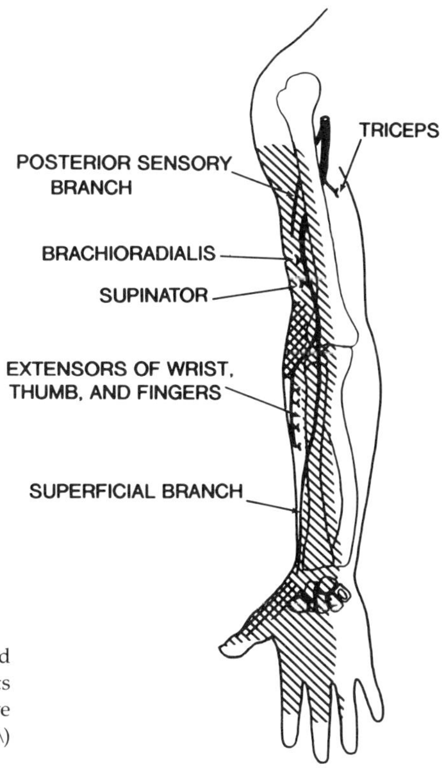

FIGURE 13.3. Schematic view of the motor and sensory distribution of the radial nerve along its path down the forearm. The nerve has extensive cutaneous innervation to much of the dorsal (\\\) area of the forearm and to small volar (///) areas.

compartment. Compression injuries of the radial nerve are sometimes associated with disorders such as "resistant tennis elbow" (Stewart, 1987). This is usually accompanied by pain in the extensor portion of the forearm which is worse at night. Manual workers can suffer from this syndrome when the occupation requires repetitive or forceful extension of the forearm. Even prolonged use of a walker has been reported to produce upper arm paralysis due to radial nerve compression (Ball, Stempien, Pasupuleti, & Wertsch, 1989). "Wrist-drop" syndrome occurs when compression of the radial nerve impairs wrist extension by weakening the extensor muscles in the arm and wrist. Sensory response along the dorsal surface of the hand may or may not be affected, depending upon the location of the compression. This syndrome can be distinguished from stroke-related symptoms since the strength in the muscles of the arm, wrist, and hand innervated by the median and ulnar nerves remains intact in this syndrome. A lesion restricted to the sensory branch of the radial nerve produces paresthesias within the area served by the nerve and may include causalgia, or a "burning pain" symptom.

While the syndromes described above have fairly discrete patterns of symptoms that are dictated by the distribution of each nerve, the picture becomes more complicated when injuries involve several peripheral nerves or the brachial plexus. This is especially apparent when the cause of the lesion is a traction injury occurring when the head and neck are forced in directions opposite that of the shoulder and arm, such as during a fall or a motorcycle accident. For example, on impact a motorcyclist's body momentarily moves or rotates off the cycle while the arms remain on the handlebars, severely stretching the plexus or even avulsing the spinal roots from the cord. This damage can be further aggravated by subsequent impact with the ground or with the oncoming vehicle in a head-on accident (Wynn Parry, 1987). In avulsion cases, paralysis is seen in the portion of the arm innervated by the severed roots and is accompanied by extreme burning pain with shooting pains in an area otherwise lacking cutaneous sensitivity (Wynn Parry, 1980). Milder injuries may result in only partial damage of the plexus or its associated roots and nerves. Clinical pictures tend to be mixed. For example, damage limited to the upper portion of the plexus often results in more paralysis or paresis in the upper arm than in the hand, and cutaneous sensitivities may be fully intact or segmentally absent. In contrast, damage to the lower portion of the plexus typically produces paralysis or paresis of the hand and fingers which is almost always accompanied by a loss of cutaneous sensitivity and by Horner's syndrome (Schaafsma, 1970).

There are a number of neuropathies of the lower limbs that are of interest to the neuropsychologist. Probably the most common and best known of these mononeuropathies involve compression or traction of points along the branches of the sciatic nerve and the femoral nerves. The sciatic nerve originates from the ventral rami of spinal roots L4–S3 and at about midthigh divides into two major nerve trunks, the tibial nerve and the common peroneal nerve, and several other lesser branches. The tibial nerve and its branches innervate the muscles and skin surfaces of the back and lateral sides of the lower leg, the lateral sides of the ankle and foot, most of the sole of the foot as well as the ventral surface and the nail bed of the big toe, the second and third toes, and the medial portion of the fourth toe (see Figs. 13.4 and 13.5). Branches of the common peroneal nerve innervate the lateral anterior muscles and skin of the lower leg, the dorsal surfaces of the foot, the big toe, toes 2–4, and the dorsomedial surface of the

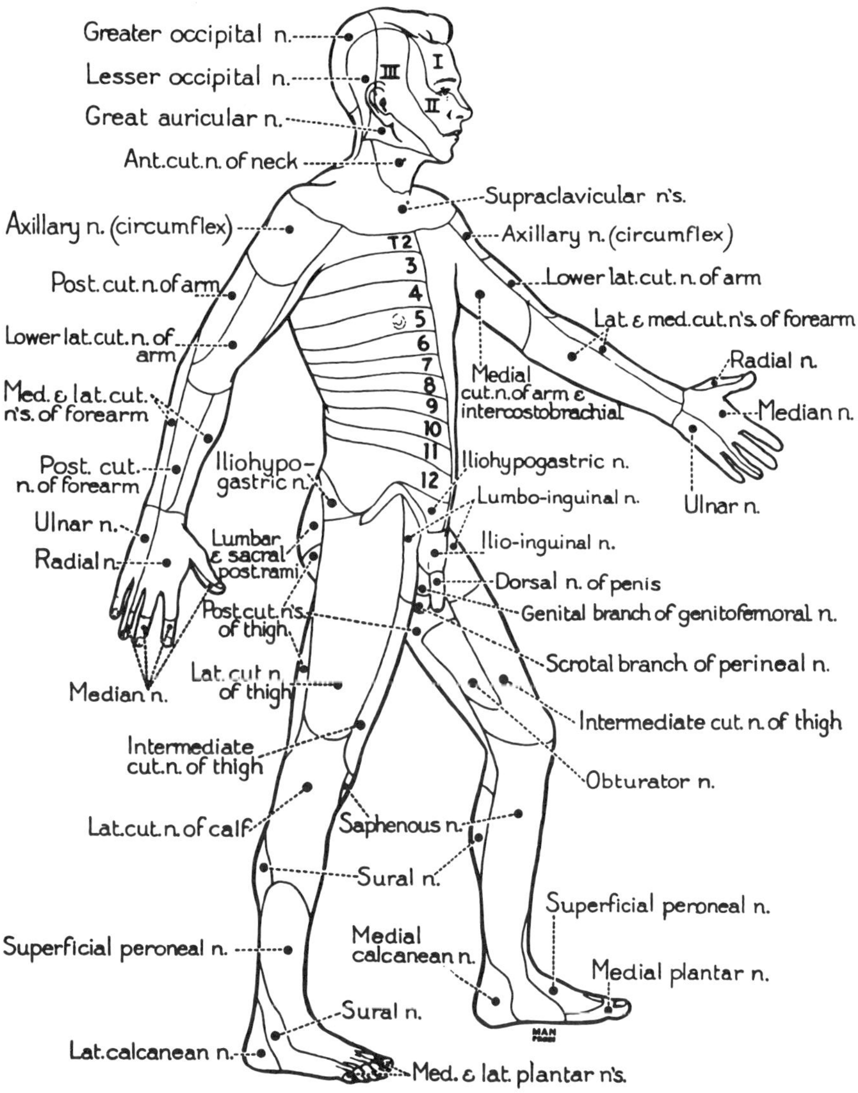

FIGURE 13.4. A side view of the body surface showing the distribution of cutaneous innervation by each of the major peripheral nerves. From *Peripheral nerve injuries* (p. 40) by W. Haymaker and B. Woodhall, 1953. Philadelphia: Saunders. Reprinted by permission.

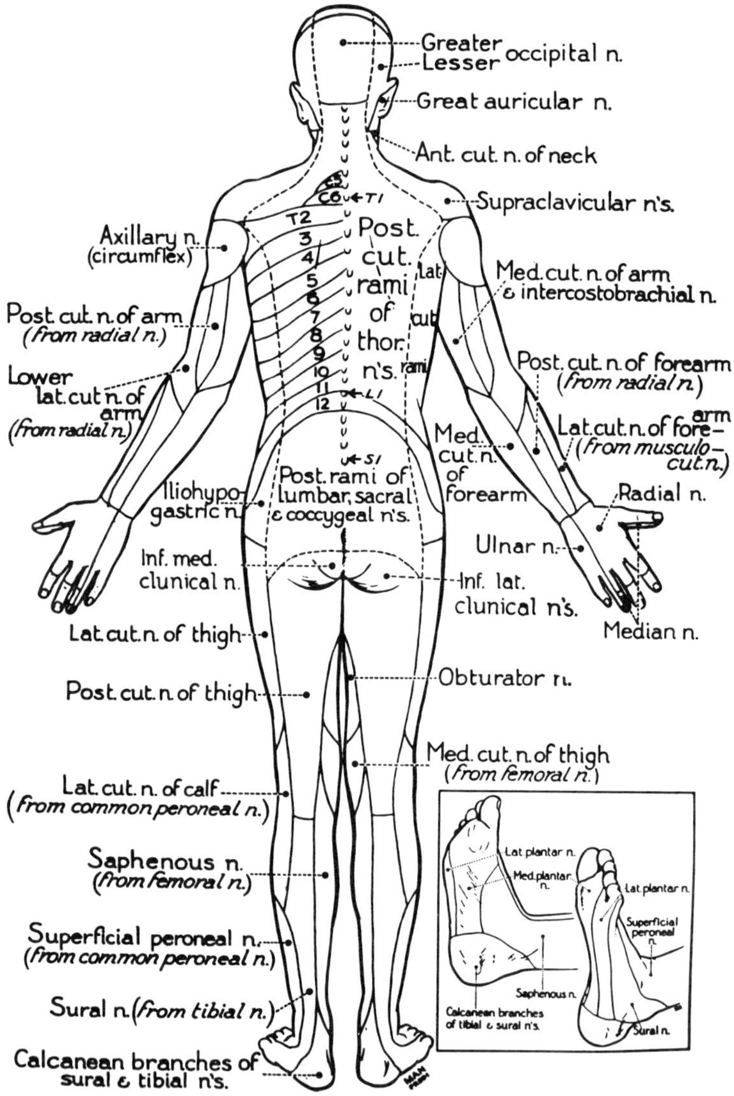

FIGURE 13.5. A posterior view of the body surface showing the distribution of cutaneous innervation by each of the major peripheral nerves. The contemporary names for inferior lateral and inferior medial clinical nerves are perineal branches of the posterior cutaneous nerve of the thigh. From *Peripheral nerve injuries* (p. 43) by W. Haymaker and B. Woodhall, 1953. Philadelphia: Saunders. Reprinted by permission.

small toe. Trauma is the most common cause of sciatic nerve damage and is generally accompanied by loss of motor and sensory function in the areas innervated by the nerve distal to the site of injury. External compression also can cause injury to the sciatic nerve and result in muscle weakness, footdrop (dropping of the foot due to paralysis of the anterior muscles of the legs), pain, and paresthesias. Compression is generally due to a tissue mass or hematoma, unusual and prolonged work posture such as kneeling or sitting on a hard surface, excessive exercise, or from lying in a position that compresses the nerve, e.g., when a person is bedridden or comatose (Spaans, 1970, 1987). Entrapment also can occur at several locations and can cause severe pain. One example of this is the "painful heel syndrome," which involves one or more of the branches of the tibial nerve. This pain worsens when the person is carrying weight on the heel. Like other entrapment syndromes, the pain is most intense at night and in the morning. It may gradually improve before worsening again as the day progresses (Mann & Plattner, 1989).

The lateral femoral cutaneous nerve and the femoral nerve are the major sources of innervation of the thigh region (see Figs. 13.4 and 13.5). The lateral femoral nerve is entirely sensory and serves the lateral thigh region. Nerve compression may produce symptoms of burning paresthesia and hyperpathia (exaggerated subjective response to painful stimuli) on the outer thigh which can be aggravated by prolonged standing or walking (Staal, 1970). Elevation of touch, pain, and temperature thresholds but not pressure thresholds frequently is reported (Ecker & Woltman, 1938). The femoral nerve innervates the musculature and skin surfaces of the anterior thigh area and knee, and the anteriomedial portion of the lower leg and ankle. Given its location, external compression injuries of this nerve and its branches are rare, but pressure from other factors such as a hematoma and trauma can cause a disruption of motor and sensory function within the area of distribution. The femoral nerve is also a primary site of diabetic neuropathy but a diabetic etiology results in a more widespread disruption of limb functioning than does a focal injury which confines its effects to the area supplied by the nerve (see the section on Diabetic Neuropathies).

Thus, peripheral nerve neuropathies with sensory and/or motor dysfunctions can result from compression, entrapment, or other forms of acute trauma. More importantly, traumatic injury to the brain is often accompanied by injury to peripheral nerves which can complicate neuropsychological diagnostic and therapeutic processes (Cosgrove, Vargo, & Reidy, 1989; Wilmot, Cope, Hall, & Acker, 1985). Detecting and distinguishing mononeuropathies from disorders affecting the CNS can be done by a careful examination of the pattern of sensory and motor symptoms, combined with a study of the patient's occupational, sport, and other physical activities. The more distal the focal point of the injury is from the spinal cord, the more specific the pattern of disturbance is to the local pattern of innervation. Moreover, cognitive capacity is unaffected unless the neuropathy is the early clinical manifestation of an infectious disease, alcoholism, or some other systemic disorder. However, it should be noted that if a peripheral nerve is severed and does not regenerate, cortical somatosensory fields appear to reorganize, changing significantly the topographical representation of the body surface on the cortex. Somatosensory cortex deprived of sensory input from the severed peripheral nerve may begin to respond to stimulation of new areas of the body surface and there is a change in the shape and size of surface representation in the cortical tissues adjacent to the deprived cortex (Merzenich & Kaas, 1982).

Infectious Neuropathies

A variety of infections of the PNS are known to result in neuropathies, but only a few of the more frequently occurring disorders will be described. Globally, leprosy is the most common treatable neuropathy (Schaumburg *et al.*, 1983) but since it is relatively rare in Western countries, it will not be discussed.

One of the best known and most frequently diagnosed of the infectious neuropathies is Guillain–Barré syndrome. Guillain–Barré syndrome is a worldwide disease, with an annual occurrence of 0.95 case per 100,000 population in the United States (Schonberger *et al.*, 1981). While people of all ages can be affected, the age distribution is bimodal and somewhat skewed toward younger people. Young adults 16–25 years of age are most susceptible to the disease, followed to a lesser extent by people between 45 and 60. Although the exact etiology of the syndrome is unknown, epidemiological findings have discovered a rather remarkable relationship between antecedent events and the occurrence of the disease. In one study, over two-thirds of the patients reported having a viral-like infection, typically either a respiratory or a gastrointestinal illness or both, within the 8-week period prior to the onset of Guillain–Barré (Hurwitz, Holman, Nelson, & Schonberger, 1983). Another 4.5% of the patients had received vaccinations and 5% had undergone a surgical procedure within the same period. The list of antecedent events that may trigger Guillain–Barré syndrome includes some bacterial diseases, a wide variety of childhood viral diseases such as measles, chicken pox, and mumps, and possibly vaccination for viral diseases such as poliomyelitis (Dowling, Blumberg, & Cook, 1987; Kinnunen, Färkkilä, Hovi, Juntunen, & Weckström, 1989). To date, however, the exact nature of the link between these and Guillain–Barré syndrome has not been established with any degree of certainty.

Guillain–Barré syndrome is referred to as an inflammatory *myelinopathy* since it results in the destruction of the Schwann cell myelin sheath of the peripheral nerves (Schaumburg *et al.*, 1983). These cells are thought to be the target of an immune-mediated attack. Segments of the myelin sheath along an axon are attacked and destroyed, usually leaving the axon intact but unable to function properly. While the inflammatory process tends to be irregularly scattered throughout the PNS, and generally does not affect the myelin of the CNS, it is usually more pronounced in the proximal roots close to the dorsal root ganglia, the autonomic ganglia, and the distal portion of the peripheral nerves. The remaining Schwann cells can divide and remyelinate the axon but it may take several weeks to several months for the inflammation to subside and the remyelination process to take place. Recent research has suggested a potential genetic involvement in the regulation of the immune response to Guillain–Barré and other inflammatory demyelinating neuropathies (Feeney, Pollard, McLeod, Stewart, & De Lange, 1989).

The symptoms of Guillain–Barré develop rapidly, reaching maximum disruption within 3 weeks of the onset of the disease in about 80% of the cases. Typically the symptoms are predominantly motor, but in most cases these are accompanied by some autonomic and mild sensory symptoms. Usually (but not always) they begin with a weakening of the distal lower limbs which leads to complaints of difficulty in walking. The gait may become unsteady with a wide-based waddling motion. As the disease progresses, the muscular weakening and areflexia (loss of reflexes) spread upward to cover the entire body. The degree of paralysis can vary from minimal paresis to total paralysis in which the individual will require aid in respiration. Bilateral weakening of the facial muscles (facial diplegia), which can affect speech production and indicates cranial nerve involvement, is present in over half of the cases. Up to 10% of the patients will show signs of extraocular muscle paralysis. Sensory symptoms may take longer to appear than the motor symptoms and commonly occur in the form of "stocking–glove" paresthesias in the feet or hands and an elevation of vibratory and pin–prick thresholds. Often the patient will have difficulty sensing and reproducing joint positions. Pain similar to that experienced with overexercise is often reported in the lower back, thighs, and buttocks. Autonomic nervous system symptoms probably stem from involvement of myelinated preganglionic fibers and the ganglia. Imbalances between the sympathetic and parasympathetic division may result in abnormalities in cardiac functioning, blood pressure, bladder and bowel control, and sweating. Generally, autonomic nervous system symptoms are minor, but in a few patients, sudden, unexpected fluctuations in blood pressure or cardiac dysrhythmias occur that are life-threatening (Albers & Kelly, 1989; Dowling *et al.*, 1987). The fatality rate for the disease is 3–5% as a result of the autonomic and respiratory problems. Patients contracting Guillain–Barré syndrome can fully recover in time, usually within a year. However, as many as 50% of the patients continue to exhibit signs of PNS damage, including paresis, facial asymmetry, or dysesthesia (Schaumburg *et al.*, 1983), and these abnormalities need to be considered in any subsequent neuropsychological evaluation.

Although several variants of Guillain–Barré syndrome have been noted, probably the most important is the chronic inflammatory demyelinating polyneuropathy. This disorder is characterized by chronic inflammation of the peripheral nerves and, except for the temporal development of the symptoms, the diagnostic criteria for this syndrome are essentially the same as those for Guillain–Barré syndrome (Albers & Kelly, 1989; Dyck & Arnason, 1984). The disease tends to follow either a chronic, monophasic, slowly progressive course or a cycle of relapses and remissions of the illness. To date, no antecedent events have been clearly linked to this disorder. Another interesting clinical variant of Guillain–Barré syndrome is a pure sensory neuropathy. Patients will experience severe and progressive proprioceptive and vibratory sensory loss and paresthesias, usually beginning in the distal portion of the limbs. Light touch and temperature thresholds may be mild to moderately depressed. These patients may lose any perception of position, graphesthesia, and stereognosia. In addition, they will exhibit gait and limb ataxia even though motor functions remain normal. Histological and nerve conduction evidence suggests that these deficits are due to neuronal loss in the dorsal root ganglia rather than to demyelination (Dawson, Samuels, & Morris, 1988; Sterman, Schaumburg, & Asbury, 1980). This syndrome is essentially indistinguishable from the sensory neuronopathy sometimes reported as a remote effect of various forms of carcinoma (Donofrio, Alessi, Albers, Knapp, & Blaivas, 1989; Kaufman, Hopkins, & Hurwitz, 1981; Vallat, 1989).

Another example of an infectious neuropathy is herpes zoster or varicella zoster neuritis, a disease with the same viral agent as chicken pox. After recovery from chicken pox (primary varicella infection), the virus is believed to remain dormant in the dorsal root ganglia and maybe in other peripheral locations. If it becomes active again, it can cause a sensory neuritis which is restricted to a single dermatome or the sensory field of a cranial nerve. In varicella zoster sensory radiculitis, paresthesias and dermatomal pain followed by edema generally precede the development of a rash within the infected dermatome. The rash becomes encrusted within 5 to 10 days before it disappears. Pain, however, may persist after the disappearance of the rash. The thoracic dermatomes and the cranial nerves are the most common sites of the infection. Zoster motor radiculitis may appear within 2 weeks after a rash. Essentially this is a rapidly developing segmental paresis or paralysis of the muscles served by the infected spinal roots. Of the cranial nerves, the trigeminal (CN V) and facial (CN VII) nerves are common sites of infection. Typically the infection involves the sensory portions of these nerves first and then spreads to the motor portions. When this happens within the facial nerve, a Bell's palsy will be evident. In addition, the vestibulocochlear nerve (CN VIII) often is infected and the patient may suffer partial deafness and dysequilibrium (Schaumburg *et al.*, 1983; Swift & Rivner, 1987). As a result of the multisegmental nature of the zoster neuritis, it is often described as a *polyradiculoneuropathy*.

Each of the inflammatory diseases discussed above can have widespread and profound effects on the functioning of the PNS. In most cases, however, these disorders do not affect cognitive capacity. Recently, interest in these diseases has increased since several of them have been identified among the more frequent opportunistic infections that can accompany AIDS (Dix & Bredesen, 1988; see the section on AIDS and ARC Neuropathies).

Alcohol Neuropathy

Alcohol neuropathy is a polyneuropathy associated with chronic abuse of alcohol. The exact incidence of alcohol neuropathy has not been established. However, it has been estimated that about 10% of people suffering from chronic alcoholism show peripheral neuropathic signs (Delwaide, 1987), making it one of the leading causes of peripheral neuropathies.

The pathological effect of chronic alcohol intake on the peripheral nerves is often described as a "dying back" of the peripheral nerve. While both myelin and axons undergo degeneration in the nerves, at least some evidence suggests that the axon degenerates (axonopathy) first followed by the myelin sheath (Behse & Buchthal, 1977). The distal portion of the nerve is affected initially, but in severe cases, more proximal portions of the nerve will be involved. In many instances, the axonopathy appears to be the result of nutritional deficiencies but it is unclear whether it is a vitamin deficiency (vitamin B group), disrupted pancreatic functioning, or some other factor or combination of factors. In addition, alcohol probably has neurotoxic effects on the axon since some patients develop neuropathic symptoms even though malnutrition does not appear to be at issue (Behse & Buchthal, 1977), a conclusion also supported by nonhuman animal research (Walker, Hunter, & Abraham, 1981).

The first symptoms of alcohol polyneuropathy typically appear between the ages of 40 and 60 (Kemppainen, Juntunen, & Hillbom, 1982) since a long period of excessive alcohol consumption is usually required before the polyneuropathy develops. The symptoms of this polyneuropathy are diverse but generally they are symmetrical sensory or mixed sensorimotor. Initially they involve the distal portions of the legs, later spreading to the arms. Although these symptoms may worsen suddenly after bouts of heavy drinking, they are progressive and appear to follow a somewhat systematic pattern of development as long as the consumption of alcohol is continued (Hawley, Kurtzke, Armbrustmacher, Saini, & Manz, 1982). Early signs are primarily sensory and may be subclinical. When questioned carefully, a patient may describe mild symptoms of numbness or paresthesias in the lower legs and feet, most notably at night. As the polyneuropathy progresses, the existing sensory symptoms become more intense and may include some pain. When the polyneuropathy is fully developed, sensory deficits can be seen across all modalities and may follow a "stocking–glove" pattern in which the distribution of sensory loss is symmetrical with blurred and indistinct borders. Once the sensory loss has reached the knees, signs of sensory disturbance or loss may begin to appear in the tips of the fingers (Hawley *et al.*, 1982). In patients without pain, this may produce reduced discriminability in the fingers which may be the first deficit that they notice. For many patients, pain will develop in the feet and legs, intensifying over time, and can result in "painful anesthesia" (Delwaide, 1987). In some cases the pain may be accompanied by the "burning feet" syndrome. In this syndrome the pain in the soles of the feet may be described as prickly or stabbing, and develop into an intense burning sensation. The soles are extremely sensitive to touch, making the pressure of footgear intolerable. The symptoms usually spread first to the dorsal surface of the foot and then to the rest of the leg.

In addition to the early sensory disturbances, many patients may exhibit signs of distal muscular impairment that become prominent in the more advanced stages of the polyneuropathy. Fatigue and muscle weakness of the legs are often early complaints. Other motor signs, such as loss of reflexes, footdrop or wristdrop, and muscular atrophy, may occur and eventually can interfere with walking or use of the hands. With advancement of the polyneuropathy, motor symptoms will progress proximally from the lower legs to the thighs, and, if the hands are symptomatic, to the forearms. Involvement of the lower cranial nerves (e.g., CN X) may produce dysphagia and flaccid dysarthria. Clinical and subclinical autonomic symptoms also may be present. For example, the patient may show signs of hyper- or hypohidrosis (abnormal amounts of perspiration), suggesting sympathetic involvement (Delwaide, 1987), while neuropathy of the parasympathetic portion of the vagus nerve appears to be associated with higher than normal mortality rates (Johnson & Robinson, 1988). Finally, the neuropsychologist should be aware of the potential for compression injuries of peripheral nerves in chronic alcoholic patients. Kemppainen *et al.* (1982) found that generally these injuries have an acute onset and develop during sleep following a heavy drinking bout. Compression of the radial nerve was the most frequent injury reported. This was followed by injury to the brachial plexus and to the peroneal nerve of the leg and foot. These injuries may be the first detectable symptoms of an alcohol neuropathy or may be superimposed on those of a more generalized alcohol polyneuropathy already in evidence.

The presence of alcohol peripheral polyneuropathy can complicate the issues confronting the neuropsychologist concerned with the analysis of CNS functioning, particularly when other neurological disorders exist simultaneously. For instance, gait and lower limb ataxia may be the result of cerebellar degeneration associated with chronic alcohol consumption or the deterioration of peripheral polyneuropathy or both. Also, Wernicke's encephalopathy may coexist with alcoholic polyneuropathy. While cerebral atrophy appears to be correlated with the level of peripheral neurophysiological dysfunction in chronic alcoholic patients (Meldgaard, Andersen, Ahlgren, Danielsen, & Sørensen, 1984), attempts to correlate deficits on a wide variety of cognitive tests with peripheral nerve damage have been unsuccessful (e.g., Franceschi, Truci, Comi, Lozza, Marchettini, Galardi, & Smirne, 1984). Generally, however, if the patient refrains from further alcohol consumption, the prognosis for complete or nearly complete recovery from the polyneuropathy appears to be good and is independent of the age of the patient (Hawley *et al.*, 1982; Hillbom & Wennberg, 1984).

Diabetic Neuropathies

Neuropathies are associated with several disorders of the endocrine glands, such as disorders of the thyroid and pituitary glands, but by far the most common are those associated with diabetes mellitus. Even though estimates of the incidence of peripheral neuropathies vary widely, most studies suggest that it is probably high for both insulin-dependent, Type I (juvenile) and non-insulin-dependent, Type II (mature) diabetes (Hogenhuis, 1987), as well as for malnutrition-related diabetes mellitus (Sutjahjo, Taniguchi, Hendromartono, Tjokroprawiro & Baba, 1988). A number of factors contribute to the risk of diabetic peripheral neuropathies. One critical factor is the duration of the disease. Several studies have found a linear increase in the likelihood of neuropathic symptoms with duration of the disease. In a carefully conducted, large-scale longitudinal study, Pirart (1978*a*,*b*) reported that 7.5% of his patients showed clinical signs of neuropathy at the time of initial diagnosis, over 10% of the patients exhibited clinical signs within 5 years of the initial diagnosis, and by 25 years after the diagnosis, the number of patients exhibiting such signs had increased to 50%. In a more recent study, diabetic retinopathy increased from 15% of the patients with diabetes for less than 5 years to 100% in patients with the disease for over 30 years (Karma, Gummerus, Kujansuu, & Pitkäjärvi, 1987). Several other risk factors have been identified, including exposure to toxic substances (e.g., alcohol), age of the patient, hypertension, the degree of metabolic control over the disease, and even the height of the individual. Although the pathogenic basis for the axonopathy seen with diabetes has not yet been firmly established, evidence suggests that a chronic hyperglycemic state produces abnormalities in vascular functioning, particularly at the capillary level, and in metabolic processes occurring within the nerve cell that probably result in irreversible structural and functional changes in the nerve (Bays & Pfeifer, 1988). In spite of considerable research efforts, the pathological effects of diabetes remain unclear. Axonal degeneration and regeneration, demyelination and remyelination as well as a variety of other pathological signs have been reported. At the more advanced stages of the disease, loss of myelinated and unmyelinated fibers within the peripheral nerves is well established and there is some evidence that there may be a selectivity for certain axonal types (Hogenhuis, 1987).

Diabetic neuropathies are often divided into three basic clusters of syndromes: symmetrical polyneuropathies, asymmetrical mononeuropathies or mononeuropathy multiplexes, and autonomic neuropathies (see Table 13.2). Each of these can be further divided into clinically relevant syndromes depending upon the population of nerve fibers affected by the disease and the corresponding clinical symptoms and signs detected. For example, the symmetrical polyneuropathies can be subdivided into distal sensory, motor, and mixed sensorimotor syndromes as well as a proximal motor syndrome. The distal symmetrical polyneuropathies are the most common forms of diabetic neuropathies. In general, the symptoms and signs of these polyneuropathies first appear bilaterally in the most distal distributions of the peripheral nerves ("stocking–glove" pattern), generally beginning in the feet or toes. Once the disturbances have reached the knees in these polyneuropathies, the nerves serving the hands (median, ulnar, and radial) also become involved. Eventually, symptoms are noted on the trunk of the body. Sensory fibers tend to be the most susceptible to diabetic pathological effects. Progression of the distal neuropathies typically follows a fiber-length-dependent proximal course along the lower

TABLE 13.2. Peripheral Neuropathies Associated with Diabetes Mellitus

Symmetrical polyneuropathies
Distal sensory
Distal motor
Distal sensorimotor (mixed)
Proximal motor (amyotrophy)
Asymmetrical mononeuropathies or mononeuropathy multiplexes
Individual peripheral nerves
Truncal
Cranial nerves
Autonomic neuropathies
Cardiovascular
Gastrointestinal
Genitourinary
Sudomotor

and the upper limbs. Curiously, the taller the patient, the more likely the patient is to exhibit the distal sensory neuropathy, presumably because the longer peripheral nerves in tall people are more susceptible to diabetic ischemic or metabolic effects (Sosenko, Gadia, Fournier, O'Connell, Aguiar, & Skyler, 1986).

Symptoms of the distal sensory neuropathies are determined by the diameter of the sensory fibers involved. When large-diameter, myelinated sensory fibers are affected, typical symptoms include elevated vibration thresholds (Sosenko, Gadia, Natori, Ayyar, Ramos, & Skyler, 1987), impaired balance, decreased perception of limb position, and loss of tendon reflexes. Usually pain and paresthesias are not present unless they are the result of a neurological complication such as neuropathic ulceration (Greene & Brown, 1987). Involvement of small-diameter, myelinated or nonmyelinated fibers can produce a somewhat different set of symptoms. Early complaints often include numbness (e.g., "dead feet"), tingling, and other forms of paresthesias in the feet. Elevated pain and temperature thresholds can lead to repeated injury of the feet and fingers (e.g., burnt fingers from cigarettes, cooking utensils, or hot water). Other patients may complain of hyperesthesia to touch, intense superficial pain, or a deep aching pain, all of which are more noticeable at night. The pain can become so severe that it may become disabling.

Clinical motor symptoms in diabetes usually do not appear early in the course of the disease although nerve conduction studies may detect a slowing of velocity and a reduction of amplitude (Hogenhuis, 1987). Pure *distal motor polyneuropathy* is extremely rare in diabetic patients (Brown & Greene, 1984; Hogenhuis, 1987). However, a mixed *symmetrical distal sensorimotor polyneuropathy* is very common. Sensory symptoms dominate and cross modalities, suggesting both large- and small-fiber involvement. Typically, sensory symptoms include paresthesias and threshold elevations for light touch, pain, and temperature, as well as poor sensing of limb position. Muscular weakness occurs later in the course of the disease and is first detected in the most distal intrinsic muscles of the feet and hands. This syndrome is often accompanied by autonomic neuropathies which are discussed below. A recent multivariate analysis of clinical and neurofunctional data suggested that the sensory, motor, and autonomic components of the mixed syndrome may be separate entities that develop in parallel during the course of the disease (Sasaki, Nanjo, Yamada, Naka, Bessho, Kikuoka, Satogami, Matsumoto, Emoto, & Miyamura, 1988).

A *symmetrical proximal motor polyneuropathy* (also known as diabetic amyotrophy or Bruns–Garland syndrome) may be seen in older, mildly diabetic patients. Patients with this syndrome will develop an intense, incapacitating pain in the upper leg and pelvic region. The syndrome will progress slowly over a period of 6–12 months generally after the patient has undergone weight loss or a period of hyperglycemia. The greatest loss of power and atrophy will be seen in muscles innervated by the femoral nerve and to a lesser extent in muscles innervated by the sciatic and other nerves in the upper leg.

Diabetic *asymmetrical mononeuropathies* or *mononeuropathy multiplexes* have many features that can occur alone or with the symmetrical neuropathies. For instance, unilateral femoral neuropathy may have most of the characteristics of symmetrical proximal motor neuropathy. This will appear as a unilateral thigh pain with sudden onset, followed by muscular weakness and patchy sensory loss within the distribution area of the nerve. Like the unilateral femoral neuropathy, cranial neuropathies also are common in older diabetic patients. CN III, IV, and VI are the cranial nerves most frequently affected and result in ophthalmoplegia without necessarily altering pupillary responding. This condition is accompanied by pain in about half of the cases (Thomas & Eliasson, 1984). Occasional involvement of other cranial nerves with their associated nerve palsies also may be seen. Nearly all of the spinal nerves are susceptible to the effects of diabetes, singly as well as in combination. Entrapment neuropathies of the type described earlier are found in as many as 40% of diabetic patients (Brown & Greene, 1984). In addition, episodes of truncal neuropathy, primarily sensory, may be seen with other diabetic neuropathies. With truncal neuropathy the patient may complain of severe pain and dysesthesia (e.g., "scald" or "bad sunburn") of the chest, rib cage, upper back, or abdomen which tend to worsen at night and may be accompanied by a weakening of the abdominal muscles (Ellenberg, 1978; Kikta, Breuer, & Wilbourn, 1982; Sun & Streib, 1981). While patients generally experience some relief from this neuropathy in time, some patients may have recurrent episodes in which the afflicted area may blend with that of previous episodes or may be quite different. The topography of the neuropathy tends to follow the distribution of the rami of the spinal nerves rather than a dermatomal distribution (Stewart, 1989).

Although *autonomic neuropathies* can occur alone (see Appenzeller, 1987; Low, 1987), they are frequently associated with diabetic polyneuropathies (Bays & Pfeifer, 1988). When this happens, most of the autonomic nervous system can be affected and can be influential in the final prognosis of the disease. The most important symptoms would, of course, reflect the involvement of the cardiovascular system. A few of the major cardiovascular symptoms include exercise intolerance resulting from reduced cardiac output due to impaired parasympathetic or sympathetic control or both, resting tachycardia resulting from denervation of vagal control over cardiac function, and orthostatic (postural) hypotension resulting from a decrease in diastolic or in systolic blood pressure when the patient shifts from a lying to an upright position. These symptoms are associated with increased risk of "silent" ischemic heart disease and other major cardiovascular disorders. Hypertension also appears to increase the probability of proliferative retinopathy in patients having diabetes for a long period of time (Matzen, Larsen, & Frøland, 1986). Other autonomic neuropathic dysfunctions that produce complaints among diabetic patients include gastrointestinal symptoms such as diarrhea, constipation, vomiting, postprandial nausea, and early satiation. Genitourinary complaints also are common. These include impotence and retrograde ejaculation in males and decreased vaginal lubrication in females during sexual activities which may result in dyspareunia and orgasmic dysfunction. As the bladder's sensory mechanisms are affected, a reduction in urinary frequency may be noted. Later, as the efferent system becomes involved, complaints of incomplete or difficult bladder emptying are made. Disruption of sympathetic control over sudomotor (sweating) function is frequently observed among diabetic patients. Although hyperhidrosis (excessive sweating) has been reported, partial or complete anhidrosis (lack of sweating) is probably the most common impairment (Scott, Bennett, & MacDonald, 1987). Several discrete patterns of anhidrosis have been described which correlate well with the area and the severity of autonomic dysfunction and painful truncal neuropathy, and to a lesser extent with the distribution of distal neuropathic dysfunction (Fealey, Low, & Thomas, 1989). In addition, if the adrenal gland is affected, its normal response of releasing epinephrine to help maintain glucose levels during acute hypoglycemic states is impaired. This can lead to coma and other widespread autonomic dysfunction.

Again, as with other systemic polyneuropathies, the existence of diabetic neuropathies can make neuropsychological issues more complex. Diabetic polyneuropathies can present a wide variety of peripheral neuropathic syndromes which usually become more complex with increased duration of the illness, even for patients in which the disease is well-controlled. To complicate issues even more and paralleling the direct neuronal effects of the disease, diabetic patients can develop premature and severe atherosclerosis and other vascular abnormalities, are subject to an increased tendency toward stroke, and generally have a poorer prognosis for recovery of function following cerebral injury. Depending upon the diagnostic questions, neuropsychological assessments may require the clinical investigator to determine the behavioral effects of diabetic peripheral polyneuropathies before an accurate assessment of CNS functioning can be made.

AIDS and ARC Neuropathies

There is little doubt that the nervous system is highly susceptible to AIDS and AIDS-related complex (ARC), both of which are thought to be due to infection with the human immunodeficiency viruses (HIV), and to a variety of opportunistic infections and neoplasms that may contribute to the AIDS clinical picture. Identification of the AIDS dementia complex in a large number of AIDS patients has stimulated considerable interest in the neurological effects of HIV-related CNS disease among neuropsychologists. Recent reports have begun to clarify the nature of the neuropsychological deficits associated with AIDS (Gabuzda & Hirsch, 1987; Janssen, Saykin, Cannon, Campbell, Pinsky, Hessol, O'Malley, Lifson, Doll, Rutherford, & Kaplan, 1989; Miller, Selnes, McArthur, Satz, Becker, Cohen, Sheridan, Machado, Van Gorp, & Visscher, 1990; Navia, Jordan, & Price, 1986; Sidtis & Price, 1990; Van Gorp, Miller, Satz, & Visscher, 1989). After the AIDS dementia complex, peripheral neuropathies are the most frequently occurring neurological disorders with as many as 50% of AIDS patients exhibiting some clinical symptoms. In addition, people identified as seropositive for the HIV antibody but who are still asymptomatic for AIDS may already be experiencing early peripheral neuropathy (Jakobsen, Smith, Gaub, Helweg-Larsen, & Trojaborg, 1989; Simpson & Bender, 1988). The pathogenesis of most of these disorders is still unknown but the peripheral neuropathies are so varied that it is unlikely that there is a single pathogenic agent responsible for all of them. While most of these neuropathies are probably related to immune-mediated syndromes, patients may suffer from neuropathies caused by secondary opportunistic pathogens such as cytomegalovirus (CMV) and the varicella zoster viruses (Miller, Kiprov, Parry, & Bredesen, 1988*a*) or by the neurotoxic effects of drugs used during therapy (Dubinsky, Yarchoan, Dalakas, & Broder, 1989). Compared to other forms of peripheral neuropathies, discovery of HIV neuropathies is relatively new and their clinical descriptions are sometimes incomplete or details appear to be conflicting. However, several rather distinct neuropathies related to AIDS and ARC have emerged (see Table 13.3). Others are likely to be identified as HIV is better understood and the clinical pictures of AIDS and ARC are clarified.

Of all the neuropathies associated with AIDS and ARC, the *symmetrical distal polyneuropathies* have been described most often and of these, the *symmetrical distal sensory polyneuropathy* is the most prevalent. Cornblath and McArthur

TABLE 13.3. Peripheral Neuropathies Associated with AIDS and ARC

Symmetrical distal polyneuropathies
Sensory
Pain
Sensorimotor
Motor
Symmetrical proximal motor neuropathy (myopathy)
Inflammatory demyelinating polyneuropathies
Acute
Chronic
Progressive polyradiculoneuropathies
Mononeuropathy multiplexes
Autonomic neuropathies

(1988) characterized this polyneuropathy from the cases of 40 patients diagnosed as simultaneously having the HIV and distal sensory polyneuropathy. Pain dysesthesias, particularly in the soles of the feet, were reported by 62% of the patients and often took the form of "burning feet." This caused the patients to walk on their heels or to wear loose-fitting slippers to avoid pressure on their soles. Light touch or other types of contact made the pain more intense. Other forms of paresthesias were reported, generally for the dorsal surface of the feet as well as the soles. Cornblath and McArthur also found pain and vibration thresholds elevated in 85% of the patients and the knee jerk reflex was absent or reduced in 96% of the patients. The symptoms were symmetrical except at the onset when they might appear in one foot before the other. Through serial examinations, they found that the symptoms were progressive but seldom extended above the ankles and no symptoms appeared in the hands. In addition, intrinsic weakness of foot musculature was found in only 31% of the patients. More recently, Fuller, Jacobs, and Guiloff (1989) noted that a few of the patients in the Cornblath and McArthur study may have had another distal sensory polyneuropathy which they identified as *painful peripheral neuropathy*. In the symmetrical distal sensory neuropathy, pain can be just one of several sensory abnormalities. However, in painful peripheral neuropathy, it is the primary sensory symptom and starts in the toes as a stiffness before it progresses to a painful tingling or burning sensation. Vibratory and position senses as well as muscular strength may show little or no impairment (Fuller *et al.*, 1989; Lange, Britton, Younger, & Hays, 1988). Fuller *et al.* (1989) found that in 75% of their patients the onset of pain occurred within a month or less of the first symptoms of CMV infection. This temporal relationship along with pathological and electrophysiological evidence suggest that painful peripheral neuropathy may be due to CMV infection of the dorsal root ganglia (Fuller *et al.*, 1989; Rance, McArthur, Cornblath, Landstrom, Griffin, & Price, 1988). To date, it is not known whether CMV also might be the pathogenic agent for other distal sensory polyneuropathies.

While Cornblath and McArthur (1988) found some signs of neuromuscular involvement in about a third of their patients, other reports have cited higher incidences of paresis among patients diagnosed with symmetrical distal sensory polyneuropathy. Miller *et al.* (1988*a*) found that the sensory loss and paresis beginning in the toes gradually spread proximally. Once these effects reached the knees, the hands became affected. It seems likely that the Miller group may have been reporting data that are more in agreement with a *symmetrical distal sensorimotor polyneuropathy* than with a distal sensory neuropathy. The features of symmetrical distal sensorimotor neuropathy include motor weakness, distal sensory loss, and paresthesias of the lower extremities (Bailey, Baltch, Venkatesh, Singh, & Bishop, 1988). These patients have elevated thresholds for tactile discrimination and vibration, hyporeflexia, and weakness of intrinsic foot muscles. Weakness and atrophy of the leg muscles have been seen in some of the patients. The hands also may show weakness of intrinsic muscles and sensory involvement but not to the same extent as the lower limbs. Evidence of progressive demyelination and degeneration of the peripheral nerves and dorsal root ganglia has been found in patients with these syndromes (Chaunu, Ratinahirana, Raphael, Hénin, Leport, Brun-Vezinet, Léger, Brunet, & Hauw, 1989; Cornblath & McArthur, 1988; de la Monte, Gabuzda, Ho, Brown, Hedley-Whyte, Schooley, Hirsch, & Bhan, 1988; Mah, Vartavarian, Akers, & Vinters, 1988; Miller, Parry, Pfaeffl, Lang, Lippert, & Kiprov, 1988*b*; Rance *et al.*, 1988). In contrast to the distal symmetrical polyneuropathies, some patients develop a *symmetrical proximal motor neuropathy*. This is characterized by moderate to severe weakening predominantly of the proximal limb muscles, but facial and neck muscles also may be affected. Some distal sensory symptoms may accompany this neuropathy (Simpson & Bender, 1988).

Acute and chronic forms of *inflammatory demyelinating polyneuropathies* also have been reported in AIDS and ARC patients. The acute or subacute form may be identical, or at least similar, to Guillain–Barré syndrome in that this neuropathy appears to have the basic temporal relationship with the HIV infection that Guillain–Barré syndrome has with its antecedent viral infection. Although some researchers have suggested that these two syndromes may have the same pathogenesis since both appear to involve pathology of an autoimmune nature (Cook & Dowling, 1981), it should be noted that they do not necessarily have the same effects on protein levels in the cerebral spinal fluid (Cornblath, McArthur, Kennedy, Witte, & Griffin, 1987). Moreover, the acute HIV inflammatory syndrome generally is not accompanied by autonomic disturbances. A chronic form of inflammatory demyelinating polyneuropathy appears to be associated more with asymptomatic HIV infection or ARC. Patients with the chronic polyneuropathy often do not progress to AIDS in contrast to people having distal symmetrical polyneuropathies who almost invariably already have AIDS (de la Monte *et al.*, 1988). Moreover, like the non-HIV chronic inflammatory polyneuropathy, the course of the HIV chronic polyneuropathy is progressive, although for some patients periods of improvement and relapses occur spontaneously. The clinical symptoms and signs of AIDS and ARC inflammatory demyelinating polyneuropathies are similar to those described earlier for non-HIV inflammatory polyneuropathies (see the section on Infectious Neuropathies). Cornblath *et al.* (1987) found that most of the symptoms exhibited by their AIDS patients were moderate to severe motor disturbances accompanied by mild sensory loss. These include generally symmetrical, moderate to severe weakness in both proximal and distal muscle groups in the arms and/or legs. Motor problems are experienced while walking, climbing stairs, or standing from a seated position. If the arms and hands are affected, then reaching, grasping and manipulating objects are impaired as are other fine motor movements. Sensory symptoms are usually mild and include areflexia and a generalized loss of cutaneous and proprioceptive sensations. These lead to poor object identification as well as poor limb and digit position sensing. Pain symptoms are relatively infrequent compared to some other HIV-related neuropathies but when they are reported, patients may complain of "burning," aching, or some form of sharp pain. Involvement of several of the cranial nerves with their associated symptom patterns has been observed as well (Miller *et al.*, 1988*a*; Lipkin, Parry, Kiprov, & Abrams, 1985).

Other forms of HIV-related neuropathies appear to be distinctive clinical phenomena but have been reported with less frequency than the previously described syndromes. Patients with a *progressive polyradiculoneuropathy* exhibit progressive sensory and motor symptoms that begin in the areas innervated by the lumbar and sacral nerves and spread to the thoracic and cervical areas. Other early symptoms are impaired sphincter and bladder control (Miller *et al.*, 1988*a*). Symptoms often progress rapidly and the prognosis for these patients is poor (Miller *et al.*, 1988a; Parry, 1988). This neuropathy may be caused by CMV infection after the responsiveness of the immune system is suppressed (Wiley, 1989). A few cases of *mononeuropathy multiplex* involving a variety of spinal and cranial nerves, particularly CN V and VII, have been described (Chaunu *et al.*, 1989; Cornblath *et al.*, 1987; Lipkin *et al.*, 1985; Miller *et al.*, 1988*b*). Generally, symptoms of paresthesia or paresis develop rapidly and the size of the involved areas increases periodically as new mononeuropathies with different distributions appear. For example, a patient may experience sudden onset of facial muscle weakness, footdrop, and numbness and burning sensations on areas of the trunk. Later, other symptoms may suddenly appear (Miller *et al.*, 1988*a*). Eye movement abnormalities and other ophthalmic diseases such as retinal vascular disease or retinitis are particularly prevalent in HIV patients and may be an initial indication of the onset of AIDS (Currie, Benson, Ramsden, Perdices, & Cooper, 1988; Freeman, Henderly, Lipson, Rao, & Levine, 1989; Winward, Hamed, & Glaser, 1989). CMV retinitis, found in up to 46% of AIDS patients, is the only common opportunistic retinal infection (Hennis, Scott, & Apple, 1989; Holland & Kreiger, 1988). There appear to be two types of CMV retinitis and both have devastating effects on the retina. Type I CMV retinitis progresses steadily from the periphery to the optic disc cutting the visual field as it advances and producing permanent loss of vision within 6 months if not treated. Type II CMV retinitis is an infection of the head of the optic nerve and can cause rapid and complete loss of visual acuity and optic atrophy within days (Gross, Sadun, Wiley, & Freeman, 1989). *Autonomic neuropathies* have been reported infrequently, but a recent study found cardiovascular symptoms indicating autonomic neuropathy in several patients (Craddock, Pasvol, Bull, Protheroe, & Hopkin, 1987). Further research may reveal more autonomic neuropathies since AIDS is often accompanied by diarrhea, abnormal sweating, and impotence that cannot be explained by other means.

AIDS-related peripheral neuropathies have received little attention until recently since the early research and clinical emphases were placed on more pressing medical problems associated with AIDS. As the number of AIDS and ARC cases increases, however, and as the survival rate and the survival period of AIDS patients increase, clinical psychologists and neuropsychologists will become more involved in the diagnosis and management of these patients. An awareness of the features of CNS and PNS symptoms associated with AIDS and ARC will be essential for that involvement.

Other Peripheral Neuropathies

Like the CNS, the PNS is susceptible to the adverse effects of many factors beyond those etiologies described above. Some of the more commonplace etiologies have hereditary bases while others can be any number of substances found in our environment. Hereditary peripheral neuropathies form a heterogeneous group of diseases. In some, peripheral neuropathy may be a predominant feature while in others it may be relatively rare. Charcot–Marie–Tooth disease, Dejerine–Sottas disease, Morvan's disease, Riley–Day syndrome, or familial dysautonomia are just a few of the older labels given hereditary sensory and motor neuropathies. Currently, the general label of hereditary motor and sensory neuropathies (HMSN), with types subdivided and identified with numbers I, II, III, and so on, are used. For instance, HMSN I (Charcot–Marie–Tooth disease) is a fairly common, predominantly motor, peripheral neuropathy with some sensory and autonomic symptoms. It is a slowly progressing, chronic polyneuropathy featuring weakness and atrophy of distal limb muscles and foot deformity. Years after the disease has advanced in the lower limbs, the hands may begin to show signs of involvement. This and other hereditary neuropathies have been reviewed by several authors (see Dyck, 1984; Schaumburg *et al.*, 1983).

Many of the neurotoxic chemicals found in the workplace and the general environment have been implicated in peripheral neuropathies. For example, *n*-hexane and methyl-*n*-butyl-ketone, both neurotoxic hexacarbons, are widely used solvents and can be found in glues, glue thinners, and lacquers. Peripheral distal symmetrical polyneuropathies have been reported after deliberate inhalation (glue sniffing) or after occupational exposure. Glue sniffing can produce a subacute, primarily motor neuropathy while prolonged occupational exposure may produce both sensory and motor peripheral symptoms that develop more slowly. Autonomic symptoms have been reported after glue sniffing but not in occupational cases (Schaumburg *et al.*, 1983). Many other neurotoxic substances, including heavy metals such as gold, mercury, and lead, as well as certain pharmacological agents such as ethambutol (used in the treatment of tuberculosis), streptomycin, neomycin, and other antimicrobial agents, have been linked to peripheral neuropathies (see Critchley, 1987; Windebank, 1987). A complete listing of environmental and pharmacological neuropathic agents is probably impossible to prepare considering the rapidly expanding number of new products being developed, and the lack of systematic investigation of these products. Moreover, any such list would be unable to take into account the potential environmental impact of different industries seen within geographic regions. For example, a neuropsychologist practicing in a region heavily involved in chemical manufacturing may see neuropathies associated with those industries whereas one practicing in a mining region may encounter different job-related neuropathies. Therefore, it is probably wisest to be vigilant for potential neurotoxic effects of environmental and drug agents that might be the basis for difficult-to-explain symptoms indicating PNS dysfunction (see Chapter 17 for further information on neurotoxins).

CLINICAL APPLICATIONS

In the previous section, descriptions were made of many of the major symptoms and signs observed when individual cranial and spinal nerves of the autonomic nervous system are dysfunctional. Symptom patterns also were presented for some of the more common polyneuropathies that involve the PNS on a larger or systemic scale. In addition, some of the major clinical implications of each of these disorders were discussed above. Consequently, the remarks here will deal with more general concerns.

It should be clear that an understanding of the PNS and its disorders is vitally important to the neuropsychologist. The CNS receives most of its sensory input through the afferent portions of the PNS and exerts control over behavior through the efferent portions of the PNS. Dysfunctions within the PNS can alter the information received by the CNS and/or can prevent or distort CNS control over behavioral expression. Even if the CNS is capable of normal function, a wide range of behavioral functions can be disrupted by peripheral dysfunction, including (but certainly not limited to) functions such as receptive and expressive aspects of language, somatosensory discrimination, gait, and fine motor skills involving the hands. Thus, during an assessment of CNS functions, a neuropsychologist unfamiliar with the effects of peripheral neuropathies may unknowingly mistake a behavioral deficit produced by a peripheral neuropathy for a deficit produced by the CNS. These errors can be avoided, however, if several basic issues are addressed during an assessment. Initially, sensory and motor signs and symptoms must be carefully identified and characterized. Then these symptoms and signs, along with the medical and case histories of the patient, should be examined for patterns that differentiate peripheral disorders from central or functional disorders. If a peripheral neuropathy is suspected and a physical examination has not been conducted, it is important to enlist medical support to identify the specific neuropathy, to characterize the state of the neuropathy, and to render appropriate treatment, especially if the neuropathy is a rapidly progressive or potentially fatal disease. If it is determined that a peripheral neuropathy exists, then one must ask whether the neuropathy will place any restrictions on the testing of the CNS or limitations on the interpretation of the test results. Should there be restrictions or limitations, then alternative means of assessment should be considered.

There are many documented peripheral neuropathies and, while one cannot be familiar with all of these neuropathies, a familiarity with the PNS and with some of the more common neuropathies can be of immense benefit to the practicing neuropsychologist. Symptoms of peripheral neuropathies can assume a variety of patterns, each depending upon the etiology and the portion of the PNS affected. Mononeuropathies of the cranial nerves or the individual peripheral nerves result in important but fairly discrete symptom patterns that are related to the specific functions and the distribution fields of the affected nerve; patterns that are unlikely to develop with the dysfunctions of the sensory or motor areas of the cortex. Moreover, mononeuropathies do not directly disrupt cognitive processes. Also, there is often an identifiable occupational or physical activity that might result in compression, entrapment, or some other form of trauma to a nerve that may be responsible for the symptoms. All of these characteristics can help the neuropsychologist distinguish symptoms of peripheral mononeuropathies from symptoms of cortical dysfunction.

Broad motor, sensory, or autonomic impairment often is indicative of a disorder affecting the CNS. However, when these symptoms coincide with infections, alcoholism, diabetes mellitus, or other systemic disorders, one must consider the possibility that a peripheral mononeuropathy multiplex or a polyneuropathy is contributing to, or is the basis for, these observed impairments. Since many systemic disorders are illnesses associated with abnormalities or deterioration of CNS functioning and often require neuropsychological assessment, the clinician must be able to recognize and distinguish the symptoms of peripheral dysfunction from those of a central origin. Many of the peripheral neuropathies seen with systemic peripheral disorders tend to appear as distal symmetrical and predominantly sensory polyneuropathies, but other patterns of symptoms and signs for these disorders also are well documented. Peripheral involvement can further complicate the assessment process by restricting the number of sensory or motor response modes available for testing CNS functions in patients with these disorders. For example, if a disorder has affected the functioning of cranial nerves (e.g., CN VII, VIII, X), basic receptive and expressive features of language may be affected and could hinder examination of central language functions as well as limit tests of other cognitive skills. However, by themselves, peripheral neuropathies do no affect cognitive capacity, and assessment tools that avoid utilizing dysfunctional aspects of the PNS should provide accurate assessment of cognitive functioning in a systemic disease. As with mononeuropathies, a familiarity with typical patterns of neuropathies associated with a specific medical illness can be immensely helpful to the clinician confronted with these problems.

SUMMARY

In view of the wide range of disorders of the PNS it is highly probable that a clinical neuropsychologist will encounter a number of peripheral neuropathies in an active clinical environment. These disorders can occur as simple mononeuropathies involving single peripheral nerves or in more complex or systemic forms as mononeuropathy complexes or as polyneuropathies. A few of the more common neuropathies have been described in this chapter to assist in the understanding of the nature of these disorders. It should be evident from these descriptions that while peripheral neuropathies do not alter cognitive functions directly (although they may be associated with a CNS disorder that does), neuropathies disrupt the sensory input and the motor output of the CNS. Consequently, peripheral neuropathies can hamper assessment of CNS functioning, or, if undetected, can result in an erroneous clinical evaluation. By combining a working knowledge of the PNS and some of the more common neuropathies with careful attention to symptom patterns, and the occupation, physical activities, and medical history of the patient, the neuropsychologist can distinguish between the deficits produced by PNS and CNS injury. Discriminating between these two types of deficits has important implications for accurate diagnosis and for subsequent treatment and long-term management of patients with neuropsychological impairments.

ACKNOWLEDGMENTS. The authors thank Rona J. Delay and Dr. Martha H. Ashmore for their critical reading of earlier manuscripts. Their helpful comments and thoughtful suggestions were crucial to the presentation of the material and were greatly appreciated. The authors also thank Keith Easterling for his assistance to Walter Isaac in the early stages of the manuscript. Unfortunately, Dr. Isaac died before this chapter could be completed. He constantly stimulated the curiosity of those around him; but more importantly, he insisted that logic and scientific rigor be practiced in the laboratory and in the clinic by his students and his colleagues. He was a friend who is sorely missed. And so is his storytelling.

REFERENCES

Albers, J. W., & Kelly, J. J., Jr. (1989). Acquired inflammatory demyelinating polyneuropathies: Clinical and electrodiagnostic features. *Muscle & Nerve, 12*, 435–451.

Appenzeller, O. (1987). Autonomic neuropathies. In W. B. Matthews (Ed.), *Handbook of clinical neurology, Vol. 7 (51): Neuropathies* (pp. 475–490). Amsterdam: Elsevier.

Bailey, R. O., Baltch, A. L., Venkatesh, R., Singh, J. K., & Bishop, M. B. (1988). Sensory motor neuropathy associated with AIDS. *Neurology, 38*, 886–891.

Ball, N. A., Stempien, L. M., Pasupuleti, D. V., & Wertsch, J. J. (1989). Radial nerve palsy: A complication of walker usage. *Archives of Physical Medicine and Rehabilitation, 70*, 236–238.

Baloh, R. W., Jacobson, K., & Honrubia, V. (1989). Idiopathic bilateral vestibulopathy. *Neurology, 39*, 272–275.

Bays, H. E., & Pfiefer, M. A. (1988). Peripheral diabetic neuropathy. *Medical Clinics of North America, 72*, 1439–1464.

Behse, F., & Buchthal, F. (1977). Alcoholic neuropathy: Clinical, electrophysiological, and biopsy findings. *Annals of Neurology, 2*, 95–110.

Bleecker, M. L., Bohlman, M., Moreland, R., & Tipton, A. (1985). Carpal tunnel syndrome: Role of carpal canal size. *Neurology, 35*, 1599–1604.

Boghen, D. R., & Glaser, J. S. (1975). Ischaemic optic neuropathy. The clinical profile and natural history. *Brain, 98*, 689–708.

Brown, M. J., & Greene, D. A. (1984). Diabetic neuropathy: Pathophysiology and management. In A. K. Asbury & R. W. Gilliatt (Eds.), *Neurology 4. Peripheral nerve disorders: A practical approach* (pp. 126–153). London: Butterworths International Medical Reviews.

Cannon, L. J., Bernacki, E. J., & Walter, S. D. (1981). Personal and occupational factors associated with carpal tunnel syndrome. *Journal of Occupational Medicine, 23*, 255–258.

Chaunu, M.-P., Ratinahirana, H., Raphael, M., Hénin, D., Leport, C., Brun-Vezinet, F., Léger, J.-M., Brunet, P., & Hauw, J.-J. (1989). The spectrum of changes on 20 nerve biopsies in patients with HIV infection. *Muscle & Nerve, 12*, 452–459.

Church, A. (1890). Multiple neuritis. *Journal of the American Medical Association, 15*, 636–640.

Cook, S. D., & Dowling, P. C. (1981). The role of autoantibody and immune complexes in the pathogenesis of Guillain–Barré syndrome. *Annals of Neurology, 9 (Suppl.),* 70–79.

Cornblath, D. R., & McArthur, J. C. (1988). Predominantly sensory neuropathy in patients with AIDS, and AIDS-related complex. *Neurology, 38,* 794–796.

Cornblath, D. R., McArthur, J. C., Kennedy, P. G. E., Witte, A. S., & Griffin, J. W. (1987). Inflammatory demyelinating peripheral neuropathies associated with human T-cell lymphotropic virus type III infection. *Annals of Neurology, 21,* 32–40.

Cosgrove, J. L., Vargo, M., & Reidy, M. E. (1989). A prospective study of peripheral nerve lesions occurring in traumatic brain-injured patients. *American Journal of Physical Medicine and Rehabilitation, 68,* 15–17.

Craddock, C., Pasvol, G., Bull, R., Protheroe, A., & Hopkin, J. (1987, July 4). Cardiorespiratory arrest and autonomic neuropathy in AIDS. *The Lancet, 2* (8549), 16–18.

Critchley, E. M. R. (1987). Neuropathies due to drugs. In W. B. Matthews (Ed.), *Handbook of clinical neurology, Vol. 7 (51): Neuropathies* (pp. 293–314). Amsterdam: Elsevier.

Currie, J., Benson, E., Ramsden, B., Perdices, M., & Cooper, D. (1988). Eye movement abnormalities as a predictor of the acquired immunodeficiency syndrome dementia complex. *Archives of Neurology, 45,* 949–953.

Darley, F. L., Aronson, A. E., & Brown, J. R. (1969). Differential diagnostic patterns of dysarthria. *Journal of Speech and Hearing Research, 12,* 246–269.

Dawson, D. M., Samuels, M. A., & Morris, J. (1988). Sensory form of acute polyneuritis. *Neurology, 38,* 1728–1731.

Dawson, G. D., & Scott, J. W. (1949). The recording of nerve action potentials through skin in man. *Journal of Neurology, Neurosurgery, and Psychiatry, 12,* 259–267.

de la Monte, S. M., Gabuzda, D. H., Ho, D. D., Brown, R. H., Jr., Hedley-Whyte, E. T., Schooley, R. T., Hirsch, M. S., & Bhan, A. K. (1988). Peripheral neuropathy in the acquired immunodeficiency syndrome. *Annals of Neurology, 23,* 485–492.

Delwaide, P. J. (1987). Alcoholic neuropathy. In W. B. Matthews (Ed.), *Handbook of clinical neurology, Vol. 7 (51): Neuropathies* (pp. 315–320). Amsterdam: Elsevier.

Dix, R. D., & Bredesen, D. E. (1988). Opportunistic viral infections in acquired immunodeficiency syndrome. In M. L. Rosenblum, R. M. Levy, & D. E. Bredesen (Eds.), *AIDS and the nervous system* (pp. 221–261). New York: Raven Press.

Donofrio, P. D., Alessi, A. G., Albers, J. W., Knapp, R. H., & Blaivas, M. (1989). Electrodiagnostic evolution of carcinomatous sensory neuronopathy. *Muscle & Nerve, 12,* 508–513.

Dowling, P. C., Blumberg, B. M., & Cook, S. D. (1987). Guillain–Barré syndrome. In W. B. Matthews (Ed.), *Handbook of clinical neurology, Vol. 7 (51): Neuropathies* (pp. 239–262). Amsterdam: Elsevier.

Dubinsky, R. M., Yarchoan, R., Dalakas, M., & Broder, S. (1989). Reversible axonal neuropathy from the treatment of AIDS and related disorders with 2′,3′-dideoxycytidine (ddC). *Muscle & Nerve, 12,* 856–860.

Dyck, P. J. (1984). Inherited neuronal degeneration and atrophy affecting peripheral motor, sensory, and autonomic neurons. In P. J. Dyck, P. K. Thomas, E. H. Lambert, & R. Bunge (Eds.), *Peripheral neuropathy, Vol. II* (pp. 1600–1642). Philadelphia: Saunders.

Dyck, P. J., & Arnason, B. G. W. (1984). Chronic inflammatory demyelinating polyradiculoneuropathy. In P. J. Dyck, P. K. Thomas, E. H. Lambert, & R. Bunge (Eds.), *Peripheral neuropathy, Vol. II* (pp. 2101–2114). Philadelphia: Saunders.

Ecker, A. D., & Woltman, H. W. (1938). Meralgia paraesthetica: A report of one hundred and fifty cases. *Journal of the American Medical Association, 110,* 1650–1652.

Eckman, P. B., Perlstein, G., & Altrocchi, P. H. (1975). Ulnar neuropathy in bicycle riders. *Archives of Neurology, 32,* 130–131.

Ellenberg, M. (1978). Diabetic truncal mononeuropathy—A new clinical syndrome. *Diabetes Care, 1,* 10–13.

Entin, M. A. (1968). Carpal tunnel syndrome and its variants. *Surgical Clinics of North America, 48,* 1097–1112.

Falck, B., & Aarnio, P. (1983). Left-sided carpal tunnel syndrome in butchers. *Scandinavian Journal of Work, Environment and Health, 9,* 291–297.

Fealey, R. D., Low, P. A., & Thomas, J. E. (1989). Thermoregulatory sweating abnormalities in diabetes mellitus. *Mayo Clinic Proceedings, 64*, 617–628.

Feeney, D. J., Pollard, J. D., McLeod, J. G., Stewart, G. J., & De Lange, G. G. (1989). Gm haplotypes in inflammatory demyelinating polyneuropathies. *Annals of Neurology, 26*, 790–792.

Feldman, R. G., Goldman, R., & Keyserling, W. M. (1983). Peripheral nerve entrapment syndromes and ergonomic factors. *American Journal of Industrial Medicine, 4*, 661–681.

Franceschi, M., Truci, G., Comi, G., Lozza, L., Marchettini, P., Galardi, G., & Smirne, S. (1984). Cognitive deficits and their relationship to other neurological complications in chronic alcoholic patients. *Journal of Neurology, Neurosurgery, and Psychiatry, 47*, 1134–1137.

Freeman, W. R., Henderly, D. E., Lipson, B. K., Rao, N. A., & Levine, A. M. (1989). Retinopathy before the diagnosis of AIDS. *Annals of Ophthalmology, 21*, 468–474.

Fuller, G. N., Jacobs, J. M., & Guiloff, R. J. (1989, October 21). Association of painful peripheral neuropathy in AIDS with cytomegalovirus infection. *The Lancet*, 2(8669), 937–941.

Gabuzda, D. H., & Hirsch, M. S. (1987). Neurologic manifestations of infection with human immunodeficiency virus. *Annals of Internal Medicine, 107*, 383–391.

Goldberg, J. M., & Lindblom, U. (1979). Standardized method of determining vibratory perception thresholds for diagnosis and screening in neurological investigation. *Journal of Neurology, Neurosurgery, and Psychiatry, 42*, 793–803.

Greene, D. A., & Brown, M. J. (1987). Diabetic polyneuropathy. *Seminars in Neurology, 7*, 18–29.

Gross, J. G., Sadun, A. A., Wiley, C. A., & Freeman, W. R. (1989). Severe visual loss related to isolated peripapillary retinal and optic nerve head cytomegalovirus infection. *American Journal of Ophthalmology, 108*, 691–698.

Hamed, L. M., Winward, K. E., Glaser, J. S., & Schatz, N. J. (1989). Optic neuropathy in uremia. *American Journal of Ophthalmology, 108*, 30–35.

Hanner, P., Andersen, O., Frisén, L., Rosenhall, U., & Edström, S. (1987). Clinical observations of effects on central nervous system in patients with acute facial palsy. *Archives of Otolaryngology, Head and Neck Surgery, 113*, 516–520.

Hartman, D. E. (1984). Neurogenic dysphonia. *Annals of Otology, Rhinology, and Laryngology, 93*, 57–64.

Hawley, R. J., Kurtzke, J. F., Armbrustmacher, V. W., Saini, N., & Manz, H. (1982). The course of alcoholic-nutritional peripheral neuropathy. *Acta Neurologica Scandinavica, 66*, 582–589.

Hennis, H. L., Scott, A. A., & Apple, D. J. (1989). Cytomegalovirus retinitis. *Survey of Ophthalmology, 34*, 193–203.

Hess, R. F., & Plant, G. T. (1983). The effect of temporal frequency variation on threshold contrast sensitivity deficits in optic neuritis. *Journal of Neurology, Neurosurgery, and Psychiatry, 46*, 322–330.

Hillbom, M., & Wennberg, A. (1984). Prognosis of alcoholic peripheral neuropathy. *Journal of Neurology, Neurosurgery, and Psychiatry, 47*, 699–703.

Hodes, R., Larrabee, M. G., & German, W. (1948). The human electromyogram in response to nerve stimulation and the conduction velocity of motor axons. *Archives of Neurology and Psychiatry, 60*, 340–365.

Hogenhuis, L. A. H. (1987). Endocrine polyneuropathies. In W. B. Matthews (Ed.), *Handbook of clinical neurology, Vol. 7 (51): Neuropathies* (pp. 497–528). Amsterdam: Elsevier.

Holland, G. E., & Kreiger, A. E. (1988). Neuroophthalmology of acquired immunodeficiency syndrome. In M. L. Rosenblum, R. M. Levy, & D. E. Bredesen (Eds.), *AIDS and the nervous system* (pp. 103–120). New York: Raven Press.

Hurwitz, E. S., Holman, R. C., Nelson, D. B., & Schonberger, L. B. (1983). National surveillance for Guillain–Barré syndrome: January 1978–March 1979. *Neurology, 33*, 150–157.

Jakobsen J., Smith, T., Gaub, J., Helweg-Larsen, S., & Trojaborg, W. (1989). Progressive neurological dysfunction during latent HIV infection. *British Medical Journal, 299*, 225–228.

Janssen, R. S., Saykin, A. J., Cannon, L., Campbell, J., Pinsky, P. F., Hessol, N. A., O'Malley, P. M., Lifson, A. R., Doll, L. S., Rutherford, G. W., & Kaplan, J. E. (1989). Neurological and neuropsychological manifestations of HIV-1 infection: Association with AIDS-related complex but not asymptomatic HIV-1 infection. *Annals of Neurology, 26*, 592–600.

Johnson, R. H., & Robinson, B. J. (1988). Mortality in alcoholics with autonomic neuropathy. *Journal of Neurology, Neurosurgery, and Psychiatry, 51*, 476–480.

Kao, L. Y., Huang, L., & Chen, T. T. (1989). Anterior ischemic optic neuropathy—Recurrent attacks in one eye in a bilateral case. *Annals of Ophthalmology, 21*, 71–74.

Karma, A., Gummerus, S., Kujansuu, E., & Pitkäjärvi, T. (1987). Predicting diabetic retinopathy. *Acta Opthalmologica, 182* (Suppl.), 136–139.

Kaufman, M. D., Hopkins, L. C., & Hurwitz, B. J. (1981). Progressive sensory neuropathy in patients without carcinoma: A disorder with distinctive clinical and electrophysiological findings. *Annals of Neurology, 9*, 237–242.

Kemppainen, R., Juntunen, J., & Hillbom, M. (1982). Drinking habits and peripheral alcoholic neuropathy. *Acta Neurologica Scandinavica, 65*, 11–18.

Kikta, D. G., Breuer, A. C., & Wilbourn, A. J. (1982). Thoracic root pain in diabetes: The spectrum of clinical and electromyographic findings. *Annals of Neurology, 11*, 80–85.

Kinnunen, E., Färkkilä, M., Hovi, T., Juntunen, J., & Weckström, P. (1989). Incidence of Guillain–Barré syndrome during a nationwide oral poliovirus vaccine campaign. *Neurology, 39*, 1034–1036.

Kline, L. B., Morawetz, R. B., & Swaid, N. S. (1984). Indirect injury of the optic nerve. *Neurosurgery, 14*, 756–764.

Lange, D. J., Britton, C. B., Younger, D. S., & Hays, A. P. (1988). The neuromuscular manifestations of human immunodeficiency virus infections. *Archives of Neurology, 45*, 1084–1088.

Lederman, R. J. (1989). Peripheral nerve disorders in instrumentalists. *Annals of Neurology, 26*, 640–646.

Lessell, S. (1989). Indirect optic nerve trauma. *Archives of Ophthalmology, 107*, 382–386.

Lipkin, W. I., Parry, G., Kiprov, D., & Abrams, D. (1985). Inflammatory neuropathy in homosexual men with lymphadenopathy. *Neurology, 35*, 1479–1483.

Lorance, R. W., Kaufman, D., Wray, S. H., & Mao, C. (1987). Contrast visual testing in neurovisual diagnosis. *Neurology, 37*, 923–929.

Low, P. A. (1987). Autonomic neuropathy. *Seminars in Neurology, 7*, 49–57.

Luxon, L. M. (1986). Disorders of hearing. In A. K. Asbury, G. M. McKhann, & W. I. McDonald (Eds.), *Diseases of the nervous system: Clinical neurobiology* (pp. 544–560). Philadelphia: Saunders.

Lyon-Caen, O., Jouvent, R., Hauser, S., Chaunu, M.-P., Benoit, N., Widlöcher, D., & Lhermitte, F. (1986). Cognitive function in recent-onset demyelinating diseases. *Archives of Neurology, 43*, 1138–1141.

Mah, V., Vartavarian, L. M., Akers, M.-A., & Vinters, H. V. (1988). Abnormalities of peripheral nerve in patients with human immunodeficiency virus infection. *Annals of Neurology, 24*, 713–717.

Mann, R. A., & Plattner, P. F. (1989). Nerve entrapment syndromes of the foot and ankle: Part I. In R. M. Szabo (Ed.), *Nerve compression syndromes: Diagnosis and treatment* (pp. 273–291). Thorofare, N.J.: Slack.

Matthews, W. B. (Ed.). (1987). *Handbook of clinical neurology, Vol. 7 (51): Neuropathies*. Amsterdam: Elsevier.

Matzen, L. E., Larsen, J. B., & Frøland, A. (1986). Hypertension—A risk factor for proliferative retinopathy. *Transplantation Proceedings, 18*, 1571.

McDonald, W. I. (1963). The effects of experimental demyelination on conduction in peripheral nerve: A histological and electrophysiological study. *Brain, 86*, 501–524.

Meldgaard, B., Andersen, K., Ahlgren, P., Danielsen, U. T., & Sørensen, H. (1984). Peripheral neuropathy, cerebral atrophy, and intellectual impairment in chronic alcoholics. *Acta Neurologica Scandinavica, 70*, 336–344.

Merzenich, M. M., & Kaas, J. H. (1982). Reorganization of mammalian somatosensory cortex following peripheral nerve injury. *Trends in Neuroscience, 5*, 434–436.

Miller, E. N., Selnes, O. A., McArthur, J. C., Satz, P., Becker, J. T., Cohen, B. A., Sheridan, K., Machado, A. M., Van Gorp, W. G., & Visscher, B. (1990). Neuropsychological performance in HIV-1-infected homosexual men: The multicenter AIDS cohort study (MACS). *Neurology, 40*, 197–203.

Miller, R. G., Kiprov, D. D., Parry, G., & Bredesen, D. E. (1988*a*). Peripheral nervous system dysfunction in acquired immunodeficiency syndrome. In M. L. Rosenblum, R. M. Levy, & D. E. Bredesen (Eds.), *AIDS and the nervous system* (pp. 65–78). New York: Raven Press.

Miller, R. G., Parry, G. J., Pfaeffl, W., Lang, W., Lippert, R., & Kiprov, D. (1988*b*). The spectrum of peripheral neuropathy associated with ARC and AIDS. *Muscle & Nerve, 11*, 857–863.

Navia, B. A., Jordan, B. D., & Price, R. W. (1986). The AIDS dementia complex: I. Clinical features. *Annals of Neurology, 19*, 517–524.

Newsom-Davis, J., Thomas, P. K., & Spalding, J. M. K. (1984). Diseases of the ninth, tenth, eleventh, and twelfth cranial nerves. In P. J. Dyck, P. K. Thomas, E. H. Lambert, & R. Bunge (Eds.), *Peripheral neuropathy, Vol. II* (pp. 1337–1350). Philadelphia: Saunders.

Parry, G. J. (1988). Peripheral neuropathies associated with human immunodeficiency virus infection. *Annals of Neurology, 23* (Suppl.), S49–S53.

Pirart, J. (1978*a*). Diabetes mellitus and its degenerative complications: A prospective study of 4400 patients observed between 1947 and 1973. (Part 1). *Diabetes Care, 1*, 168–188.

Pirart, J. (1978*b*). Diabetes mellitus and its degenerative complications: A prospective study of 4400 patients observed between 1947 and 1973. (Part 2). *Diabetes Care, 1*, 252–263.

Rance, N. E., McArthur, J. C., Cornblath, D. R., Landstrom, D. L., Griffin, J. W., & Price, D. L. (1988). Gracile tract degeneration in patients with sensory neuropathy and AIDS. *Neurology, 38*, 265–271.

Sandberg-Wollheim, M., Bynke, H., Cronqvist, S., Holtås, S., Platz, P., & Ryder, L. P. (1990). A long-term prospective study of optic neuritis: Evaluation of risk factors. *Annals of Neurology, 27*, 386–393.

Sasaki, H., Nanjo, K., Yamada, M., Naka, K., Bessho, H., Kikuoka, H., Satogami, E., Matsumoto, G., Emoto, M., & Miyamura, K. (1988). Diabetic neuropathy as a heterogeneous syndrome: Multivariate analysis of clinical and neurological findings. *Diabetes Research and Clinical Practice, 4*, 215–222.

Schaafsma, S. J. (1970). Plexus injuries. In P. J. Vinken & G. W. Bruyn (Eds.), *Handbook of clinical neurology, Vol. 7: Diseases of nerves, Part I* (pp. 402–429). Amsterdam: North-Holland.

Schaumburg, H. H., Spencer, P. S., & Thomas, P. K. (1983). *Disorders of peripheral nerves*. Philadelphia: Davis.

Schonberger, L. B., Hurwitz, E. S., Katona, P., Holman, R. C., & Bregman, D. J. (1981). Guillain–Barré syndrome: Its epidemiology and associations with influenza vaccination. *Annals of Neurology, 9* (Suppl.), 31–38.

Schwarz, A., Keller, F., Seyfert, S., Pool, W., Molzahn, M., & Distler, A. (1984). Carpal tunnel syndrome: A major complication in long-term hemodialysis patients. *Clinical Nephrology, 22*, 133–137.

Scott, A. R., Bennett, T., & MacDonald, I. A. (1987). Diabetes mellitus and thermoregulation. *Canadian Journal of Physiology and Pharmacology, 65*, 1365–1376.

Sidtis, J. J., & Price, R. W. (1990). Early HIV-1 infection and the AIDS dementia complex. *Neurology, 40*, 323–326.

Simpson, D. M., & Bender, A. N. (1988). Human immunodeficiency virus-associated myopathy: Analysis of 11 patients. *Annals of Neurology, 24*, 79–84.

Sjöstrand, J., & Abrahamsson, M. (1982). Suprathreshold vision in acute optic neuritis. *Journal of Neurology, Neurosurgery, and Psychiatry, 45*, 227–234.

Sosenko, J. M., Gadia, M. T., Fournier, A. M., O'Connell, M. T., Aguiar, M. C., & Skyler, J. S. (1986). Body stature as a risk factor for diabetic sensory neuropathy. *American Journal of Medicine, 80*, 1031–1034.

Sosenko, J. M., Gadia, M. T., Natori, N., Ayyar, D. R., Ramos, L. B., & Skyler, J. S. (1987). Neurofunctional testing for the detection of diabetic peripheral neuropathy. *Archives of Internal Medicine, 147*, 1741–1744.

Spaans, F. (1970). Occupational nerve lesions. In P. J. Vinken & G. W. Bruyn (Eds.), *Handbook of clinical neurology, Vol. 7: Diseases of nerves, Part I* (pp. 326–343). Amsterdam: North-Holland.

Spaans, F. (1987). Compression and entrapment neuropathies. In W. B. Matthews (Ed.), *Handbook of clinical neurology, Vol. 7 (51): Neuropathies* (pp. 85–118). Amsterdam: Elsevier.

Staal, A. (1970). The entrapment neuropathies. In P. J. Vinken & G. W. Bruyn (Eds.), *Handbook of clinical neurology, Vol. 7: Diseases of nerves, Part I* (pp. 285–325). Amsterdam: North-Holland.

Sterman, A. B., Schaumburg, H. H., & Asbury, A. K. (1980). The acute sensory neuronopathy syndrome: A distinct clinical entity. *Annals of Neurology, 7*, 354–358.

Stewart, J. D. (1987). *Focal peripheral neuropathies*. Amsterdam: Elsevier.

Stewart, J. D. (1989). Diabetic truncal neuropathy: Topography of the sensory deficit. *Annals of Neurology, 25*, 233–238.

Sun, S. F., & Streib, E. W. (1981). Diabetic thoracoabdominal neuropathy: Clinical and electrodiagnostic features. *Annals of Neurology, 9*, 75–79.

Sutjahjo, A., Taniguchi, H., Hendromartono, Tjokroprawiro, A., & Baba, S. (1988). High frequency of autonomic as well as peripheral neuropathy in patients with malnutrition-related diabetes mellitus. *Diabetes Research and Clinical Practice, 5*, 197–200.

Swift, T. R., & Rivner, M. H. (1987). Infectious diseases of nerve. In W. B. Matthews (Ed.), *Handbook of clinical neurology, Vol. 7 (51): Neuropathies* (pp. 179–194). Amsterdam: Elsevier.

Szabo, R. M. (1989). Carpal tunnel syndrome. In R. M. Szabo (Ed.), *Nerve compression syndromes: Diagnosis and treatment* (pp. 101–120). Thorofare, N.J.: Slack.

Thomas, P. K., & Eliasson, S. G. (1984). Diabetic neuropathy. In P. J. Dyck, P. K. Thomas, E. H. Lambert, & R. Bunge (Eds.), *Peripheral neuropathy, Vol. II* (pp. 1773–1810). Philadelphia: Saunders.

Trautmann, J. C., & Barnett, C. R. (1984). Diseases of the third, fourth, and sixth cranial nerves. In P. J. Dyck, P. K. Thomas, E. H. Lambert, & R. Bunge (Eds.), *Peripheral neuropathy, Vol. II* (pp. 1203–1223). Philadelphia: Saunders.

Vallat, J. M. (1989). Sensory Guillain–Barré syndrome. *Neurology, 39*, 879.

van Dongen, H. R., Arts, W. F. M., & Yousef-Bak, E. (1987). Acquired dysarthria in childhood: An analysis of dysarthric features in relation to neurologic deficits. *Neurology, 37*, 296–299.

Van Gorp, W. G., Miller, E. N., Satz, P., & Visscher, B. (1989). Neuropsychological performance in HIV-1 immunocompromised patients: A preliminary report. *Journal of Clinical and Experimental Neuropsychology, 11*, 763–773.

Walker, D. W., Hunter, B. E., & Abraham, W. C. (1981). Neuroanatomical and functional deficits subsequent to chronic ethanol administration in animals. *Alcoholism: Clinical and Experimental Research, 5*, 267–282.

Ward, P. H., Cannon, D., & Lindsay, J. R. (1965). The vestibular system in multiple sclerosis. *The Laryngoscope, 75*, 1031–1047.

Wartenberg, R. (1958). *Neuritis, sensory neuritis, neuralgia*. New York: Oxford University Press.

Wechsler, I. S. (1933). Etiology of polyneuritis. *A.M.A. Archives of Neurology and Psychiatry, 29*, 813–827.

Wechsler, I. S. (1938). Multiple peripheral neuropathy versus multiple neuritis. *Journal of the American Medical Association, 110*, 1910–1913.

Wiley, C. A. (1989). Neuromuscular diseases of AIDS. *The FASEB Journal, 3*, 2503–2511.

Williamson, R. T. (1922). The vibrating sensation in diseases of the nervous system. *American Journal of Medical Science, 164*, 715–727.

Wilmot, C. B., Cope, D. N., Hall, K. M., & Acker, M. (1985). Occult head injury: Its incidence in spinal cord injury. *Archives of Physical Medicine and Rehabilitation, 66*, 227–231.

Windebank, A. J. (1987). Peripheral neuropathy due to chemical and industrial exposure. In W. B. Matthews (Ed.), *Handbook of clinical neurology, Vol. 7 (51): Neuropathies* (pp. 263–292). Amsterdam: Elsevier.

Winward, K. E., Hamed, L. M., & Glaser, J. S. (1989). The spectrum of optic nerve disease in human immunodeficiency virus infection. *American Journal of Ophthalmology, 107*, 373–380.

Wynn Parry, C. B. (1980). Pain in avulsion lesions of the brachial plexus. *Pain, 9*, 41–53.

Wynn Parry, C. B. (1987). Brachial plexus injuries. In W. B. Matthews (Ed.), *Handbook of clinical neurology, Vol. 7 (51): Neuropathies* (pp. 143–155). Amsterdam: Elsevier.

14

Cardiovascular and Somatic Disorders

TYLER S. LORIG

INTRODUCTION

Neuropsychological testing has experienced enormous growth in recent years. It is a standard procedure for pre- and postassessment of neurosurgical patients in most medical centers and many smaller hospitals. Referrals for neuropsychological testing from neurologists and neurosurgeons are growing and are a testament to the usefulness of these assessment batteries. While the use of these tests presently enjoys some success, the continued growth and potential of neuropsychological testing is limited by injudicious interpretation. One factor contributing to problems with these tests is the false-positive, the case where a neuropsychological problem is found when none actually exists. A variant of this problem is the case where a neuropsychological deficit is found and attributed to closed, or other, head trauma when the actual deficit is due to other pathology affecting the nervous system. Such is the case with many somatic illnesses. Hall, Popkin, Devaul, Faillace, and Stickney (1978), for instance, report that 9.1% of psychiatric referrals are actually somatic diseases producing psychiatric symptoms. And, as Tarter, Edwards, and van Thiel (1989*a*) point out, even though the number of acute illnesses have declined, chronic illnesses have increased thus exacerbating the risk of neurological complications from somatic disease.

Consider the hypothetical, but common, case of a patient complaining of memory loss. This patient is a 54-year-old male with a history of treated

---

TYLER S. LORIG • Department of Psychology, Washington and Lee University, Lexington, Virginia 24450.

HANDBOOK OF NEUROPSYCHOLOGICAL ASSESSMENT: A Biopsychosocial Perspective, edited by Antonio E. Puente and Robert J. McCaffrey. Plenum Press, New York, 1992.

hypertension and cardiac arrest. The patient is moderately overweight, has recently stopped smoking, and has a long history of alcohol use and occasional abuse. After approaching his family physician about recent memory problems, the patient is referred to a neurologist for evaluation. The neurological battery and EEG are inconclusive as is the computed tomography (CT) and magnetic resonance imaging (MRI), which shows asymmetrical evolution of the occipital lobe. As a precaution and because of carotid restriction suspected by the family physician, the neurologist refers the patient to a local neuropsychologist who administers several subtests of the Halstead–Reitan and Luria–Nebraska batteries. The findings of the neuropsychological evaluation indicate that the patient is suffering from moderate loss of recent memory, slight constructional apraxia, and flattened affect. There are now several questions that the neuropsychologist must face: What was found, what does it mean, and what should be said about it? In the case of this hypothetical patient with a series of inconclusive tests and history of medical problems, the primary goal of the neuropsychologist is to determine whether or not any neuropathological conditions exist. It is not a goal of the assessment, however, to tell the physician that any neuropsychological deficit is due to some specific etiology but rather to suggest a subset of possibilities.

In the present case, the report should mention that most of the observed deficits are not typical of focal lesions. This simple and obvious statement (to the neuropsychologist) would help substantiate the assertion that the asymmetry observed in the CT and MRI was insignificant. Any other information that can be added by the neuropsychologist can also be very helpful to the physician who, ultimately, must prescribe a treatment course for the individual. For example, in the assessment of this hypothetical patient, one might say that "the observed deficits suggest limited and diffuse cerebral involvement and might be the result of transient cerebral ischemia (TCI)." This would suggest to the neurologist that the observations of the family physician concerning carotid insufficiency could have been correct. This, however, could also be misleading. Diffuse deficits such as those observed in our patient could be the result of many problems including the onset of multi-infarct dementia, Alzheimer's disease, or poisoning. To point out that cerebral ischemia could be the cause of the problem is to give undue weight to one of the many etiologies suggested by this subject's history. Careful examination of the medical record indicates at least three somatic problems of this patient other than TCI that could account for the observed neuropsychological deficits. This subject has a long history of self-reported alcohol use and occasional abuse. It is likely that the occasions of abuse are underreported because of societal concerns and stigma. Thus, it is possible that this subject is suffering from early symptoms of Korsakoff's dementia. Another possibility is that the subject's hypertension, even though being treated, accounts for the deficits since treated and untreated hypertensives show some memory loss and constructional apraxia (King & Miller, 1990). Finally, the casual mention that this individual has had a history of cardiac arrest should immediately alert the neuropsychologist to the possibility of post-cardiac arrest hypoxia, a condition that contributes to significant diffuse cortical damage among cardiac arrest victims who have been resuscitated (Cowan, 1986).

The purpose of this example has been to suggest the necessity of the neuropsychologists' familiarity with somatic illnesses and their neuropsychological sequelae. Neuropsychologists approaching this hypothetical case who are unaware of the effects of hypertension or cardiac arrest could have misattributed the causes of the patient's problem. While it is not appropriate for the neuropsychologist to make medical diagnoses, it is appropriate for the neuropsychologist to act as a consultant and provide a list of reasonable possibilities for observed deficits. To do this job of consulting well requires knowledge of problems that arise from illness since it is rare to receive a referral for evaluation who is in perfect health. This knowledge will be even more important as the sensitivity of neuropsychological batteries increases.

HISTORY

In a recent review of the progress of neuropsychology, Boll (1985) points out the rapidity with which tests have become more sophisticated. He cites studies such as those by Vaernes and Eidsvik (1982) in which deep-sea divers with normal IQs were found to have neuropsychological deficits. Other studies such as those by Casson and colleagues (Casson, Siegel, Sham, Campbell, Tarlau, & DiDomenico, 1984) have, not surprisingly, found deficits in boxers. What is surprising is the degree of pathology uncovered by this neuropsychological testing. For instance, no individual in their sample scored in the normal range for the Wechsler Memory Scale. These findings indicate great sensitivity of neuropsychological tests. This sensitivity is bound to increase in coming years. As the sophistication of neuropsychological batteries has increased so have the findings of impairment. For instance, the Benton timing task was once widely used but has fallen into some disfavor since it is relatively insensitive to all but the most devastating cortical damage (Benton, van Allen, & Fogel, 1964). As more factor analytic studies of existing tests are accomplished, the neuropsychologist's arsenal will become more specific and less time-consuming. Additional tests and new ways of testing such as coupling EEG mapping with cognitive/behavioral measures should tremendously increase the sensitivity of our tests. As this occurs, more deficits will be found. It is vitally important to make proper causal attributions concerning this increasing number of observed deficits for the sake of the patient and, consequently, the sake of the field. Consider a neuropsychological battery capable of detecting any damage to the brain. The testing of a single normal subject would indicate a variety of deficits associated with many areas of the cortex. Such findings would appear to be false-positives unless plausible explanations for observed neuropsychological deficits were available.

THEORETICAL AND BASIC NEUROBIOLOGICAL ISSUES

Cardiovascular Pathology

Cardiovascular pathology is one of the most common health concerns among Western cultures. Neuropsychological sequelae of cardiovascular disorders take several forms and although little is known about the exact pathophysiology that results in the behavioral deficits, cardiovascular problems should immediately suggest to the neuropsychologist, the possibility of cerebral damage.

Hypertension

The history of the effects of hypertension on neuropsychological function is long and complex. In an early study, Apter, Halstead, and Heimburger (1951) reported that "impairment of cerebral function equivalent to that seen in patients with surgical resection of the frontal lobes may occur early in the course of essential hypertension without neurological signs." More recent hypertension research has focused on several topics that are of interest for present purposes. The first point addressed in current research is whether the neuropsychological deficits observed in hypertension are a primary or a secondary effect of the disease. For instance, neuropsychological problems might arise from increased pressure in cerebral arteries which would alter capillary action in neural tissue. This would be an example of a primary effect of hypertension. Secondary effects might be due to the increased pressure on capillary walls which leads to infarcts. Another secondary cause of neuropsychological difficulties could be due to atherosclerosis, which increases blood pressure and may result in cerebral artery thrombosis. Research by Goldman and colleagues (Goldman, Kleinman, Snow, Bidus, & Korol, 1974) has suggested that hypertension alone is the primary cause of neuropsychological deficits. In this study, hypertensive subjects were assessed before and after biofeedback reduction of blood pressure. Findings indicated significant improvement on a variety of neuropsychological tasks for those subjects who were able to reduce diastolic pressure. Similar results were obtained by Shapiro, Miller, King, Ginchereau, and Fitzgibbon (1982) and Mazzucchi, Mutti, Poletti, Ravanetti, Novarini, and Parma (1986) using drug intervention. At first inspection, the improvement in neuropsychological function with pressure reduction would indicate that hypertension was the primary cause of deficits. This may not be the case. Drug effects are difficult to interpret and conflicts arise in the findings of the studies mentioned above. While Mazzucchi *et al.* (1986) report general improvement in subjects on antihypertensive medications and subjects on low-sodium diets, their data indicate that the drugs improve performance on some tasks while decreasing performance on others such as finger tapping and street name completion. And, while Shapiro *et al.* (1982) found improvement in subjects under treatment, these subjects still exhibited differences in neuropsychological task performance when compared to matched controls. There may also be problems in nondrug approaches, such as biofeedback, to the problem of direct affects of hypertension. Since only those subjects responding to treatment may be used in comparisons, an important subject variable may select out those subjects who remain impaired. Results of these studies and many others (see King & Miller, 1990, for review) suggest that the etiololgy of neuropsychological effects of hypertension is complex and probably due to both primary and secondary causes. King and Miller (1990) also both point out the relevance of personality and other individual differences in neuropsychological response to hypertension therapies. A second question addressed in the hypertension literature concerns the nature of deficits observed in these patients. Some investigators (Wilkie & Eisdorfer, 1971; Apter *et al.*, 1951) have suggested severe alterations in task performance for hypertensive individuals. Others have noted less marked deficits. Of all neuropsychological measures associated with hypertension, the most consistent and pronounced finding is that of response slowing (see Light, 1980, for review). This variable affects a variety of neuropsychological tasks such as finger tapping, pegboard completion, reaction time, and many other tests of dexterity. Cognitive impairments such as lowered IQ have also been noted (Wilkie & Eisdorfer, 1971) as have deficits on Wechsler Memory Scales, Categories test, Trail Making test, and many others used in neuropsychological assessment (King & Miller, 1990; Elias, Robbins, Schultz, & Streeten, 1986; Light, 1980). Personality changes of note to the neuropsychologist have not been studied extensively, but have been suggested in the literature (Harris & Singer, 1968; Kalis, Harris, Bennett, & Sokolow, 1968). These include increased hostility coupled with some flattening of affect.

Of primary interest to this discussion of hypertension is its relevance to causal attributions made in the neuropsychological assessment of the single case. For this reason, the extent of the decline in performance noted in hypertension is important as is the treatment method employed in its control. Several studies have indicated that even mild hypertension (diastolic blood pressure of 90–95 mm Hg) can affect neuropsychological performance (Miller, Shapiro, King, Ginchereau, & Hosutt, 1984; Shapiro *et al.*, 1982) as can the drugs used to treat this disorder (Mazzucchi *et al.*, 1986; Miller *et al.*, 1984). Drug treatment for this problem falls into two major categories: beta-blocking agents and diuretics. King and Miller (1990), surveying this literature, report that beta-blockers do not produce the response-slowing characteristic of diuretics and other drug treatments. King and Miller (1990) and Light (1980) have warned, however, that some studies exploring the effects of hypertensive medication have used normotensive subjects as controls and may produce misleading conclusions about these medications if patient constitutional factors interact with drug actions.

The clinical neuropsychologist faced with the assessment of an individual with treated or untreated hypertension should consider that observed deficits in almost any area of test performance could be due to the hypertensive conditions. It is also true, however, that statistically significant differences in hypertensives and controls may be misleading when it comes to the individual case.

King and Miller (1990, p. 55) describe a reasonable approach to the assessment of an individual patient. "The primary practical consideration for the clinical neuropsychologist which derive from the experimental investigations of hypertension as an abnormal brain state, would not at the present seem to lie in diagnosis, differential diagnosis, or prediction, as the deficiencies observed appear to be much too slight and too much like those of other chronic diseases. . . . Nevertheless, it would be prudent to explore the drug history of any hypertensive patient displaying neuropsychological deficiency."

Cardiac Disease

Another problem producing neuropsychological abnormalities is associated with cardiac dysfunction. Neuropsychological deficits may arise from a variety of problems relating to the heart and blood. Atherosclerosis may increase blood pressure and lead to multi-infarct dementia or may result in a major focal thromboembolism. Restriction of these vessels may also produce hypoxic or ischemic episodes. Because of the greater numbers of patients surviving cardiopulmonary resuscitation, the incidence of damage due to prolonged cerebral hypoxia has risen. Cowan (1986) studied subjects surviving resuscitation without recognized brain injury and found decreased performance IQs. Barclay, Weiss, Mattis, Bond, and Blass (1988) report that cardiovascular disease may account for 20 to 35% of all dementias reported in the elderly, and Garcia, Tweedy, and Blass (1984) found that 17% of patients admitted for cardiac ischemia without diagnosed strokes had significant cognitive impairments. These statistics suggest the high likelihood of CNS impairment in cardiac rehabilitation patients referred for neuropsychological evaluation.

The nature of deficits observed in these patients is varied and, as might be expected, appears diffuse rather than focal. In the study by Barclay *et al.* (1988), 20 patients admitted for cardiac rehabilitation without known stroke or dementia were examined. Sixty percent of these subjects showed fine motor deterioration, and 40% showed memory and perservative problems.

Sickle-Cell Anemia

This genetic disorder is characterized by sickle-shaped red blood cells which can carry less oxygen and therefore produce anemia. The disease is more common in males than females and much more common in blacks than other racial groups. Incidence rate for African-Americans is approximately 8% (Serjeant, 1985). Neuropathology arises from hypoxia and Gilroy and Meyer (1979) report that neurologic abnormalities arise in about 25% of these patients. These abnormalities include peripheral and central neuropathologies such as sudden deafness or blindness, seizures, and cranial nerve palsies. Multi-infarct dementia may also appear in this disease due to the abnormal shape of the cells and their difficulty in passing through small capillaries (Gilroy & Meyer, 1979). While the neuropsychological literature in this area is limited, studies with young children suffering from this disease have indicated reading and spelling deficits as well as attentional and visuomotor problems in older children (Fowler, Whitt, Lallinger, Nash, Atkinson, Wells, & McMillian, 1988).

Cancer

Cancer has been a major health concern for many years but the neuropsychological sequelae of this broad class of diseases remain relatively unstudied. This is in part due to the diffuse nature of the disease and its many different forms. Neoplasms outside the nervous system may affect any organ system and thus may be highly idiosyncratic in their involvement of CNS activities. One way in which tumors may act on the CNS suggests that autoimmune antibodies that attack the tumor may pass the blood–brain barrier and compromise CNS integrity. Other effects may include alteration of endocrine systems by tumors that secrete endocrinelike substances that mimic naturally occurring endocrines and thus throw the system into disregulation. Both autoimmune and endocrine-related problems may produce symptoms of cortical dementia in some patients (Davis, Fernandez, Adams, Holmes, Levy, Lewis, & Neidhart, 1987). These authors report that 71% of their sample of treated cancer victims referred for neuropsychiatric evaluations met criteria for organic mental disease. Others have reported smaller proportions in otherwise normal cancer populations (Derogatis, Morrow, & Fetting, 1983).

Several problems should immediately suggest themselves to the neuropsychologist upon learning that a patient has cancer. These include iatrogenic treatment effects and metastasies. Metastatic tumors arising from tumors in the lungs, breasts, and gastrointestinal tract may invade the nervous system and produce focal, space-occupying lesions. Metastatic tumors of the lung seem to have a special affinity for nervous tissue. den Hollander, Van Hulst, Meerwaldt, and Haasjes (1989) report two patients with metastatic tumors of the limbic system arising from small-cell tumors of the lung. While this particular form of tumor is relatively rare, the authors suggest using the presence of neuropsychiatric symptoms as a warning sign for the possibility of metastatic tumors.

Presently, three main approaches are used to treat cancer. These include resection, chemotherapy, and radiation. Of these, resection is the most discrete and produces the most limited CNS involvement, assuming the original tumor was outside the nervous system.

Chemotherapy has only recently been studied regarding its neuropsychological effects. A variety of commonly used antineoplastic agents have been found to produce memory, motor, and other CNS deficits (Weiss, Walker, & Wienik, 1974). Hwang and colleagues (Hwang, Yung, Estey, & Fields, 1985) found similar affects for the drug Ara-C, often used in cancer treatment. Davis *et al.* (1987) report that the long-held belief that "chemotherapeutic agents do not cross the blood–brain barrier" is in need of reevaluation.

The neuropsychological effects of radiation have been studied for many years owing to questions concerning effects of radioactive fallout and whole body irradiation. The use of modern radiotherapy in cancer treatment is somewhat different. In these cases, X or gamma rays are focused on particular body areas and little incidental radiation results. This incidental radiation may have minor affects on neuropsychological function. In recent experiments with children (Bordeaux, Dowell, Copeland, Fletcher, Francis, & van Eys, 1988), no direct effects of radiotherapy were found. Even limited cranial radiotherapy may have few measurable neuropsychological consequences. In a subsequent investigation (Copeland, Dowell, Fletcher, Bordeaux, Sullivan, Jaffe, Frankel, Reid, & Cangir, 1988), cranial radiotherapy interacted with chemotherapy to produce deficits in neuropsychological performance which they attributed to peripheral neuropathy induced by the chemotherapy.

A difficulty in accurate diagnosis may also arise in the flattened affect seen in many cancer victims. Cavanaugh and Wettstein (1989) report that cancer victims often experience profound depression as do individuals with gastrointestinal and orthopedic problems.

Metabolic and Endocrine Pathology

There are many metabolic and endocrine disorders that may cause neuropsychological deficits. Because of the pervasiveness of these disorders, it would be prudent of the neuropsychologist to assume that the metabolic or endocrine problem of the patient affects the nervous system activity in some way. If a patient presents with some problem with which the neuropsychologist is unfamiliar, the neurological concomitant of the disease can often be found in a medical neurology text such as Gilroy and Meyer (1979) or the recent neuropsychology text edited by Tartar, van Thiel, and Edwards (1989). While medical texts typically do little to elaborate on neuropsychological problems beyond dementia, they do indicate pathological conditions that could cause focal lesions or diffuse problems.

Diabetes Mellitus

Diabetes is often an insidious disease that can affect patients for several years without their knowledge. Strider (1982) reports that 50% of chronic diabetics develop significant neurologic complications. Often, these complications involve the peripheral nervous system and there is some evidence that peripheral neuropathies develop in all diabetics. These neuropathies first develop at the lower extremities, then the upper extremities, and spread proximally (Ellenburger, 1976). Often they consist of motor loss from pathology occurring in individual motor units, but they can, and often do produce paresthesias, distal burning, and pain. The effects of diabetes mellitus on the CNS are somewhat more complicated. One investigator (Locke, 1971) has even stated that diabetes has no effect on the CNS. This statement seems unlikely given that the result of insulin shock is stupor and coma. There is a confluence of evidence that significant CNS effects are due directly and indirectly to diabetes.

Indirect effects result from chronic blood pressure alteration, atherosclerosis, acute myocardial infarction, microangiopathy, and retinopathy (Strider, 1982). Other indirect effects result from toxemia due to kidney failure. Direct effects from atherosclerosis and microangiopathy may also be found and result in diffuse damage to the CNS such as multi-infarct dementia. Another direct CNS effect due to lowered insulin levels is the production of ketone bodies. These bodies are toxic to neural tissue and may produce both peripheral and central effects (Strider, 1982). Ketoacidosis resulting from disregulated insulin production may also produce cerebral dysfunction because of brain edema. This may be the precipitating factor in diabetic stupor and coma.

Studies by Grunnett (1963) and others (Alex, Baron, Goldberg, & Blumenthal, 1962) found an increased incidence of cerebrovascular accidents in diabetics. These accidents are also more likely to appear earlier in life for diabetics. The findings suggest that in addition to generalized deficits, diabetics may have specific and focal losses due to stroke. Diffuse cerebral degeneration, meningeal thickening, and basal ganglia calcification have also been reported (Reske-Nielsen, Lindback, & Rafaelsen, 1966).

Neuropsychological testing of diabetics has indicated several distinct deficits. The degree of a patient's hypoglycemia has been related to performance on the Walton–Black New Word learning test (Bale, 1973) with increasing severity of the disorder associated with greater difficulty in learning new words. Strider (1982) found that 32% of diabetics tested showed mild to moderate impairment on the Luria–Nebraska neuropsychological battery. The deficits observed in that study indicated temporal and parieto-occipital involvement, areas served by the middle cerebral artery. Impairment was also related to length of illness, with complications increasing rapidly after 12–15 years of illness. These findings are in agreement with those of Ireland, Thompson and Williamson (1980). As might be expected, those patients with a history of poor insulin regulation or noncompliance with therapy tended to show increased deficits (Strider, 1982).

In summary, diabetics do show CNS effects. These effects may be focal and are often related to cerebrovascular insufficiency due to infarction or atherosclerosis. The severity of the neuropsychological effects is related to the severity of the disease and the compliance of the patient. The approach to be taken when testing diabetic patients is best summarized by Strider (1982): "Because the brain damage is subtle in most persons in the diabetic group . . ., the clinician or others dealing with these patients may not suspect their impairment."

Hypoglycemia

Hypoglycemia is a common disorder and may result from a variety of problems such as malnutrition, malabsorption, drug use, and liver dysfunction. It is a serious problem and can result in permanent cerebral damage. Because the brain requires large amounts of glucose for proper cerebral metabolism, systemic reductions in glucose result in symptoms similar to cerebral hypoxia. While there is little information available regarding neuropsychological test performance of nondiabetic hypoglycemic patients, Lester and Fishbein (1989) report a variety of symptoms associated with a hypoglycemic attack. These include emotional disturbances, hysteria, depression, and hypochondriasis. Holmes, Koepke, and Thompson (1986) also found that while simple perceptual and motor responses are not measurably affected by high hypoglycemia, more complex tasks require longer latencies for completion. Repeated hypoglycemic episodes produce chronic damage which is similar to repeated hypoxic episodes, and thus one might expect a pattern of diffuse impairment such as recent memory loss, and inattention similar to that observed in professional deep-sea divers (Vaernes & Eidsvik, 1982) or patients with chronic pulmonary disease (Prigatano, Parsons, Wright, Levin, & Hawryluk, 1983).

Renal Failure

Temporary kidney failure is a relatively common condition that may result from a variety of viral and other illnesses that directly or indirectly affect the kidneys. As yet, there are no data that implicate temporary renal failure in cerebral dysfunction. Chronic kidney failure, however, does produce neuropsychological deficits and, in some cases, very severe dysfunction. This disorder, known as uremic encephalopathy, is probably the result of the chronic acidosis accompanying the disease. A variety of neuropsychological symptoms such as fatigue, decreased alertness, and an inability to concentrate are associated with the disease. In later stages patients may suffer apathy, memory problems, perceptual and hallucinatory problems. Hart, Pederson, Czerwinski, and Adams (1983) report that untreated victims of renal failure were impaired on a variety of neuropsychological measures including the Wechsler Memory Scale and digit-symbol tasks.

A related problem in patients with renal failure arises from dialysis treatment. Some patients may present severe reactions to dialysis which begin 14 months to 7 years after treatment (Gilroy & Meyer, 1979). This encephalopathy is probably the result of cerebral edema and produces early symptoms of apraxia and aphasia coupled with a progressive dementia. Prognosis for these patients is poor since the condition is insidious. Death may occur 3 to 15 months after onset.

Liver Failure

Hepatic encephalopathies may be exceptionally severe and abrupt or may linger depending upon their specific etiology. Acute hepatic coma occurs as the result of viral or toxic hepatitis and is often fatal. Other hepatic encephalopathies can result from cirrhosis or as the result of long-standing liver disease. In these cases, failure of the liver to remove toxic metabolic and environmental agents results in cerebral dysfunction. Materials such as ammonia, methionine, and some biogenic amines which are not degraded by a diseased liver affect the CNS and produce clinical signs including stupor, waxing and waning of consciousness and may also produce constructional apraxia in less symptomatic patients (Gilroy & Meyer, 1979). Rehnstrom and Simart (1977) have also found intellectual impairment in subjects with chronic liver disease. An excellent review of the neuropsychological literature concerning liver dysfunction is provided by Tarter, Edwards, and van Thiel (1989*b*).

Oral Contraceptives

Oral contraceptive use is widespread and remains a highly controversial topic among health care professionals. Early contraceptives employed large doses of estrogen and/or progesterone and have been associated with many health problems. The most notable of these problems for the purposes of this chapter are the effects on the cardiovascular system. Early studies found increased blood pressure and subarachnoid hemorrhage in females using these drugs (Royal College, 1977). These effects were greatest for those females using the drugs the longest and those who smoked. Others (Seigel & Corfman, 1968) found increased evidence of stroke in oral contraceptive users. These results have, however, been disputed (Drill, 1972). Neuropsychological findings on oral contraceptive users have indicated mild alterations in verbal reaction times (Garrett & Elder, 1984). These investigators suggest that cognitive, rather than motor deficits occur in these women. While controversy on this topic continues, long-term use of oral contraceptives especially if coupled with smoking should suggest to the neuropsychologist the possibility of behavioral deficits associated with cerebrovascular problems.

Pulmonary Disease

Chronic Airflow Obstruction (CAO)

Chronic pulmonary disease may arise from a variety of problems such as smoking, viral and bacterial infections (e.g., pneumonia). The resulting conditions of emphysema and chronic bronchitis are often known as chronic airflow obstruction (formerly chronic obstructive pulmonary disease) and produce varying levels of hypoxia. Patients with this type of disease often experience psychological problems such as depression because of altered life-style and reduced coping. These psychological symptoms can be quite consistent. Kinsman and co-workers (Kinsman, Fernandez, Schocket, Dirks, & Covino, 1983) found that cluster analyses of 11 descriptors such as fatigue, poor memory, irritability, and anxiety were highly predictive and reliable for individuals suffering from CAO. Neuropsychological problems arising from CAO are probably the result of decreased oxygenation of the blood leading to diffuse cerebral damage. Prigatano *et al.* (1983), in a study of 100 COPD patients, found mild neuropsychological deficits on the Halstead–Reitan battery for patients compared with normal controls. These deficits were highly correlated with observed oxygen partial pressure. Recently, Grant and colleagues (Grant, Prigatano, Heaton, McSweeny, Wright, & Adams, 1987) found that 10% of mildly hypoxic patients showed some form of neurologic impairment while moderate and severely hypoxic individuals had rates of 25 and 40%, respectively.

Acquired Immune Deficiency Syndrome (AIDS)

While still affecting a proportionally small number of the patients who may be referred for neuropsychological evaluation, the number of patients testing positive for human immunodeficiency virus (HIV) is growing rapidly. Sato, Chin, and Mann (1989) report that while less than 1% of the population may be HIV positive, rates in high-risk populations may grow to 50% by the year 2000 in North America, western Europe, and Australia. Because of the severe nature of this medical problem and the public concern over its consequences, federal funding and research in this area has been accelerated dramatically. As a result, many new findings have emerged concerning neuropsychological sequelae of this disorder. The first report of neuropsychological deficits observed in AIDS victims was that of Snider and colleagues (Snider, Simpson, & Nielsen, 1983). While a preliminary report, this study described an AIDS dementia consisting primarily of motor symptoms and some behavioral deficits. Because of the nature of these deficits, the investigators suggested that AIDS dementia was similar to Parkinson's and Huntington's diseases and might be a subcortical dementia. Subsequent investigations found similar results.

At first the motoric and behavioral deficits were attributed to secondary opportunistic infection of the CNS but studies by Levy, Shimabukuro, Hollander, Mills, and Kaminsky (1985) assayed cerebrospinal fluid and brain tissue and found AIDS-related viruses, thus suggesting a direct mechanism for the observed deficits. In a large autopsy study of AIDS patients, Navia, Jordan, and Price (1986) found that 66% of their sample showed degenerative subcortical changes even after patients with focal or secondary CNS diseases were eliminated from the study. Neuropsychological studies of AIDS victims have been relatively consistent in indicating mild motor deficits (Saykin, Janssen, Sprehn, Kaplan, Spira, & Weller, 1988; Ayers, Abrams, Newell, & Friedrich, 1987). Additionally, Saykin *et al.* (1988) found naming and word fluency deficits in these subjects. An excellent review of the neuropsychological sequelae of AIDS may be found in a recent paper by Kaemingk and Kaszniak (1989).

Not all investigators have agreed as to the nature of AIDS dementia. Bruhn (1987), for instance, has argued that most studies have not used matched control subjects and that observed deficits are due to fatigue and reaction to the disease. His findings indicated no differences in AIDS victims and matched controls on a limited neuropsychological battery. This battery was, however, deficient on motor and simple language tasks. The neuropsychologist should consider the possibility that AIDS patients, even in the early stages of the disease, may exhibit mild motoric and language deficits.

Possibly more important as a source of confusion in making causal attributions concerning neuropsychological deficits related to AIDS were the findings of Silberstein and colleagues (Silberstein, McKegney, O'Dowd, Selwyn, Schoenbaum, Drucker, Feiner, Cox, & Friedland, 1987). They found that even subjects who were asymptomatic for AIDS showed neuropsychological deficits on a brief screening battery. Another important consideration concerns the patient group. Haitian-born AIDS patients are 3.7 times more likely to develop neurologic impairment than other AIDS victims (Kaemingk & Kaszniak, 1989). Blacks and intravenous drug users with AIDS are also more likely to show deficits than other victims (Levy, Janssen, Bush, & Rosenblum, 1988). Such findings are difficult to interpret but may suggest that neuropsychological deficits found in these AIDS patients may be additive to previously existing neuropathology due to nutritional or other factors present in individuals of low socioeconomic status (Tarter, Edwards, & van Thiel, 1989*a*).

CONCLUSIONS

The foregoing discussion has not been intended to be a complete description or literature review of the neuropsychological affects of these diseases. Rather, it is intended to alert the neuropsychologist to the variety of factors that may adversely affect performance on neuropsychological tests. Awareness of the effects of these disease processes should increase the accuracy and especially the utility of neuropsychological testing for the health services community.

REFERENCES

Alex, M., Baron, E. K., Goldberg, S., & Blumenthal, H. T. (1962). An autopsy study of cerebrovascular accident in diabetes mellitus. *Circulation, 25,* 663–673.

Apter, N., Halstead, W., & Heimburger, R. (1951). Impaired cerebral function in essential hypertension. *American Journal of Psychiatry, 107,* 808–813.

Ayers, M. R., Abrams, D. I., Newell, T. G., & Friedrich, F. (1987). Performance of individuals with AIDS on the Luria–Nebraska Battery. *International Journal of Clinical Neuropsychology, 9,* 101 105.

Bale, R. N. (1973). Brain damage in diabetes mellitus. *British Journal of Psychiatry, 122,* 337–341.

Barclay, L. L., Weiss, E. M., Mattis, S., Bond, O., & Blass, J. P. (1988). Unrecognized cognitive impairment in cardiac rehabilitation patients. *American Geriatrics Society, 36,* 22–28.

Benton, A. L., van Allen, M. W., & Fogel, M. L. (1964). Temporal orientation in cerebral disease. *Journal of Nervous and Mental Disease, 139,* 110–119.

Boll, T. J. (1985). Developing issues in clinical neuropsychology. *Journal of Clinical and Experimental Neuropsychology, 7,* 473–485.

Bordeaux, J. D., Dowell, R. E., Jr., Copeland, D. R., Fletcher, J. M., Francis, D. J., & van Eys, J. (1988). A prospective study of neuropsychological sequelae in children with brain tumors. *Journal of Child Neurology, 3,* 63–68.

Bruhn, P. (1987). AIDS and dementia: A quantitative neuropsychological study of unselected Danish patients. *Acta Neurologica Scandinavica, 76,* 443 447.

Casson, T. R., Seigel, O., Sham, R., Campbell, E. A., Tarlau, M., & DiDomenico, A. (1984). Brain damage in modern boxers. *Journal of the American Medical Association, 251,* 2263–2667.

Cavanaugh, S. V., & Wettstein, R. M. (1989). Emotional and cognitive dysfunction associated with medical disorders. *Journal of Psychosomatic Research, 33,* 505–514.

Copeland, D. R., Dowell, R. E., Jr., Fletcher, J. M., Bordeaux, J. D., Sullivan, M. P., Jaffe, N., Frankel, L. S., Reid, H. L., & Cangir, A. (1988). Neuropsychological effects of childhood cancer treatment. *Journal of Child Neurology, 3,* 53–62.

Cowan, D. M. (1986). Neuropsychological sequelae of post-cardiac arrest hypoxia. Unpublished dissertation, University of Detroit.

Davis, B. D., Fernandez, F., Adams, F., Holmes, V., Levy, J. K., Lewis, D., & Neidhart, J. (1987). Diagnosis of dementia in cancer patients. *Psychosomatics, 28,* 175–179.

den Hollander, A., Van Hulst, A., Meerwaldt, J., & Haasjes, J. (1989). Limbic encephalitis: A rare presentation of the small-cell lung carcinoma. *General Hospital Psychiatry, 11,* 388–392.

Derogatis, L. R., Morrow, S. R., & Fetting, H. (1983). The prevalence of psychiatric disorders among cancer patients. *Journal of the American Medical Association, 249,* 751–757.

Drill, V. A. (1972). Oral contraceptives and thromboembolitic disease I: Prospective and retrospective studies. *Journal of the American Medical Association, 219,* 583–596.

Elias, M. F., Robbins, M. A., Schultz, N. R., Jr., & Streeten, D. (1986). A longitudinal study of neuropsychological test performance for hypertensive and normotensive adults: Initial findings. *Journal of Gerontology, 41,* 503–505.

Ellenburger, M. (1976). Diabetic neuropathies: Clinical aspects. *Metabolism,* 25, 1627–1655.

Fowler, M. G., Whitt, J. K., Lallinger, R. R., Nash, K. B., Atkinson, S. S., Wells, R. J., & McMillian, C. (1988). Neuropsychologic and academic functioning of children with sickle cell anemia. *Developmental and Behavioral Pediatrics, 9,* 213–220.

Garcia, C. A., Tweedy, J. R., & Blass, J. P. (1984). Underdiagnosis of cognitive impairments in a rehabilitation setting. *Journal of the American Geriatric Society, 32,* 339–342.

Garrett, K. F., & Elder, S. T. (1984). The menstrual cycle from a bio-behavioral approach: A comparison of oral contraceptive and non-contraceptive users. *International Journal of Psychophysiology, 1,* 209–214.

Gilroy, J., & Meyer, J. S. (1979). *Medical neurology* (3rd ed.). New York: Macmillan Co.

Goldman, H., Kleinman, K., Snow, M., Bidus, D., & Korol, B. (1974). Correlation of diastolic blood pressure and signs of cognitive dysfunction in essential hypertension. *Disorders of the Nervous System, 35,* 571–572.

Grant, I., Prigatano, G. P., Heaton, R. K., McSweeny, A. J., Wright, E. C., & Adams, K. M. (1987). Progressive neuropsychological impairment and hypoxia. *Archives of General Psychiatry, 44,* 999–1006.

Grunnett, M. L. (1963). Cerebrovascular disease: Diabetes and cerebral atherosclerosis. *Neurology, 13,* 486–491.

Hall, R. C. W., Popkin, M. K., Devaul, R. A., Faillace, L. A., & Stickney, S. K. (1978). Physical illness presenting as psychiatric disease. *Archives of General Psychiatry, 35,* 1315–1320.

Harris, R., & Singer, M. (1968). Interaction of personality and stress in the pathogenesis of essential hypertension. *Hypertension: Neural Control of Arterial Blood Pressure, 16,* 104–115.

Hart, R. P., Pederson, J. A., Czerwinski, A. W., & Adams, R. L. (1983). Chronic renal failure, dialysis and neuropsychological function. *Journal of Clinical Neuropsychology, 5,* 301–312.

Holmes, C. S., Koepke, K. M., & Thompson, R. G. (1986). Simple versus complex performance at three glucose blood levels. *Psychoneuroendocrinology, 11,* 353–357.

Hwang, T., Yung, A. W. K., Estey, E. H., & Fields, W. S. (1985). Central nervous system toxicity with high-dose Ara-C. *Neurology, 35,* 1475–1479.

Ireland, J. T., Thompson, W. S., & Williamson, J. (1980). *Diabetes today: A handbook for the clinical team.* Berlin: Springer.

Kaemingk, K. L., & Kaszniak, A. W. (1989). Neuropsychological aspects of human immunodeficiency virus infection. *The Clinical Neuropsychologist, 3,* 309–326.

Kalis, B., Harris, R., Bennett, C., & Sokolow, M. (1968). Personality and life history in persons who are potentially hypertensive. *Journal of Nervous and Mental Disease, 132,* 457–468.

King, H. E., & Miller, R. E. (1990). Hypertension and behavior. *Neuropsychological Review, 1,* 31–73.

Kinsman, R. A., Fernandez, E., Schocket, M., Dirks, J. F., & Covino, N. A. (1983). Multidimensional analysis of the symptoms of chronic bronchitis and emphysema. *Journal of Behavioral Medicine, 6,* 339–357.

Lester, M. L., & Fishbein, D. H. (1989). Nutrition and childhood neuropsychological disorders. In R. E. Tarter, D. H., van Thiel, & K. L. Edwards (Eds.), *Medical neuropsychology: The impact of disease on behavior* (pp. 291–336). New York: Plenum Press.

Levy, J. A., Shimabukuro, J., Hollander, H., Mills, J., & Kaminsky, L. (1985). Isolation of AIDS associated retro-virus from cerebrospinal fluid and brains of patients with neurological symptoms. *Lancet, 2*, 586–588.

Levy, J. A., Janssen, R. S., Bush, T. J., & Rosenblum, M. L. (1988). Neuroepidemiology of acquired immunodeficiency syndrome. *Journal of Acquired Immunodeficiency Syndrome, 1*, 31–40.

Light, K. (1980). Hypertension and response slowing. In M. Elias & D. Streeten (Eds.), *Hypertension and cognitive processes* (pp. 17–32). Mount Desert, Maine: Beech Hill Press.

Locke, S. (1971). The nervous system and diabetes. In A. Marble, P. White, R. F. Bradly & L. P. Krall (Eds.), *Joslin's diabetes mellitus*. Philadelphia: Lea & Febiger.

Mazzucchi, A., Mutti, A. Poletti, A., Ravanetti, C., Novarini, A., & Parma, M. (1986). Neuropsychological deficits in arterial hypertension. *Acta Neurologica Scandinavica, 73*, 619–627.

Miller, R. E., Shapiro, A. P., King, H. E., Ginchereau, E. H., & Hosutt, J. A. (1984). Effect of antihypertensive treatment on the behavioral consequences of elevated blood pressure. *Hypertension, 6*, 202–208.

Navia, B. A., Jordan, B. D., & Price, R. W. (1986). The AIDS dementia complex I: Clinical features. *Annals of Neurology, 19*, 517–524.

Prigatano, G. P., Parsons, O., Wright, E., Levin, D. C., & Hawryluk, G. (1983). Neuropsychological test performance in mildly hypoemic patients with chronic obstructive pulmonary disease. *Journal of Clinical and Consulting Psychology, 54*, 108–116.

Rehnstrom, S., & Simart, G. (1977). Chronic hepatic encephalopathy: A psychometric study. *Scandinavian Journal of Gastroenterology, 12*, 305–311.

Reske-Nielsen, E,. Lindback, K., & Rafaelsen, O. J. (1966). Pathological changes in the central and peripheral nervous systems of young long-term diabetics I: Diabetic encephalopathies. *Diabetologia, 1*, 233–241.

Royal College (1977). Recommendation from the findings by the RCGP oral contraceptive study on the mortality risks of oral contraceptive users. *British Medical Journal, 12*, 947.

Sato, P. A., Chin, J., & Mann, J. M. (1989). Review of AIDS and HIV infection: Global epidemiology and statistics. *AIDS 1989, 3* (Suppl.), S301–307.

Saykin, A. J., Janssen, R. S., Sprehn, G. C., Kaplan, J. E., Spira, T. J., & Weller, P. (1988). Neuropsychological dysfunction in HIV-infection: Characterization in a lymphadenopathy cohort. *International Journal of Clinical Neuropsychology, 10*, 81–95.

Seigel, D., & Corfman, P. (1968). Epidemiological problems associated with studies with the safety of oral contraceptives. *Journal of the American Medical Association, 203*, 950–954.

Serjeant, G. R. (1985). *Sickle cell disease*. Oxford: Oxford University Press.

Shapiro, A. P., Miller, R. E., King, H. E., Ginchereau, E. H., & Fitzgibbon, K. (1982). Behavioral consequences of mild hypertension. *Hypertension, 4*, 355–360.

Silberstein, C. H., McKegney, F. P., O'Dowd, M. A., Selwyn, P. A., Schoenbaum, E., Drucker, E., Feiner, C., Cox, C. P. & Friedland, G. (1987). A prospective longitudinal study of neuropsychology and psychological factors in a symptomatic individual at risk for HTLV-III/LAV infection in a methadone program: Preliminary findings. *International Journal of Neuroscience, 32*, 669–676.

Snider, W. D., Simpson, D. M., & Nielsen, S. (1983). Neurological complications of acquired immune deficiency syndrome: Analysis of 50 patients. *Annals of Neurology*, 14, 403–418.

Strider, M. A. (1982). Neuropsychological concomitants of diabetes mellitus. Unpublished dissertation, University of Nebraska, Lincoln.

Tarater, R. E., Edwards, K. L., & van Thiel, D. H. (1989*a*). Perspective and rationale for neuropsychological assessment of medical disease. In R. E. Tarter, D. H. van Thiel, & K. L. Edwards (Eds.), *Medical neuropsychology: The impact of disease on behavior* (pp. 1–10). New York: Plenum Press.

Tarter, R. E., Edwards, K. L., & van Thiel (1989*b*). Neuropsychological dysfunction due to liver disease. In R. E. Tarter, D. H. van Thiel, & K. L. Edwards (Eds.), *Medical neuropsychology: The impact of disease on behavior* (pp. 75–98). New York: Plenum Press.

Vaernes, R. J., & Edisvik, S. (1982). Central nervous dysfunction after near miss accident in diving. *Aviation, Space and Environmental Medicine, 1982*, 803–807.

Weiss, H. D., Walker, M. D., & Wienik, P. H. (1974). Neurotoxicity of commonly used antineoplastic agents. *New England Journal of Medicine, 291*, 75–127.

Wilkie, F., & Eisdorfer, C. (1971). Intelligence and blood pressure in the aged. *Science, 172*, 959–962.

15

Neurosurgical Interventions and Neuropsychology

B. P. UZZELL

INTRODUCTION

The purpose of this chapter is to focus on neurosurgical interventions and their associated neuropsychological sequelae. Traditionally, knowledge accumulated in this area has converged upon correspondences between brain and behavior, although alternate interpretations are possible.

Since neurosurgical treatments are frequently associated with rapidly occurring life-threatening events, particularly trauma, neuropsychological implications often are not addressed prior to treatment inception. However, this does not diminish the importance of neuropsychological outcomes in relationship to surgery. Through the years, neuropsychological observations made prior, during, or following neurosurgical treatments have fostered an understanding of brain–behavior relationships. Generally, accumulated neuropsychological feedback has been appreciated by neurosurgeons who have modified surgical procedures in ways to minimize adverse clinical outcomes.

Similarly, over the years neurosurgical techniques have changed as well. The introduction of surgical microscopes in human neurosurgical operative rooms in the 1960s and neuroimaging developments in the 1970s, and their widespread usages thereafter, have led to modern-day changes of neurosurgical and neuroradiological procedures, and subsequently clinical findings. No longer have clinical findings been interpreted on the basis of limited visualization of brain morphology from neurosurgical notes, as had been done prior to the inception of surgical microscopes in the operating rooms; or poor resolution, technetium-99*m* brain scans, as had been done prior to the introduction of

B. P. UZZELL • Del Oro Institute, Houston, Texas 77054.

HANDBOOK OF NEUROPSYCHOLOGICAL ASSESSMENT: A Biopsychosocial Perspective, edited by Antonio E. Puente and Robert J. McCaffrey. Plenum Press, New York, 1992.

computed tomography (CT). By providing direct visualization, the surgical microscope has led to the development of microvascular neurosurgery techniques for conditions such as extracranial–intracranial anastomosis; the ease of obliteration of aneurysms and arteriovenous malformations; and the improvement of surgical approaches, for instance, to the posterior fossa and transsphenoid areas.

Appearing in the mid-1970s, CT technology provided a clearer definition of anatomical structures and the presence of pathology in *in vivo* brain structures than had ever been seen prior to that time. Arrival of magnetic resonance imaging (MRI) during the 1980s has refined tomographic resolution of anatomical structures by the counting of atomic nucleus rotations and alignment, rather than capturing photon decay of an ionizing X-ray beam, as had been done with CT measurements. Simultaneously with CT and MRI developments, attempts have been made to apply the tomography methodology to examine *in vivo* brain functioning with positron emission tomography (PET) and single-photon emission computed tomography (SPECT) techniques. However, none of these new imaging techniques have become a panacea for improving correlations between brain and behavior. Instead, many new findings have raised additional questions, such as whether all existing lesions have been visualized, whether the boundaries of observed lesions are truly representative, and why some lesions in certain brain areas do not correlate with clinical findings, while lesions in other areas produce unexpected correlations.

After a brief historical review, this chapter will focus on theoretical issues and clinical applications. The purpose is to examine the strengths and vulnerability of neurosurgical–neurobehavioral interrelationships in identifying brain lesions.

HISTORICAL FOUNDATIONS

Since neuropsychology and neurosurgery have been linked inquisitively over the years with functional brain localizations, the following review is selective, not exhaustive. The long history of correlating behavioral observations with specific brain locations in man is beyond the scope of this chapter.

Neurosurgery and neuropsychology have enjoyed a scientific association spanning thousands of years. Neurosurgery origins can be traced back in time through archeological discoveries of human skulls with craniectomy defects as early as the Neolithic Period, 7000 to 3000 B.C. An Egyptian, Imhotep, living in approximately 1600–1700 B.C., described behavioral observations obtained from some records as early as 3500 B.C. that related to anatomical locations following head injuries (Sondhaus & Finger, 1988).

From these early times to the present day, both neurosurgeons and neuropsychologists have had mutual interests in the correspondences between two functions, namely, language and memory, and their respective cerebral cortex locations. Since these two functions have been vital to the everyday lives of human beings, it has been critical that brain tissues responsible for these functions be respected, not resected, if at all possible during neurosurgical intervention. Since language, as well as the transfer of stored information from one generation to the next, have been a part of human behavior, it is understandable that through the years neuropsychologists have been curious about the locations of brain regions underlying these two functions. From these beginnings of mutually shared interests in localizing vital human functioning, it is understandable that neurosurgeons and neuropsychologists have maintained and strengthened their scientific associations.

The outset of modern neurological surgery has been attributed to Victor Horsley, known as the "father of neurosurgery," who at the turn of the 20th century developed in London a method to localize certain nervous structures mechanically with reference to a three-dimensional coordinate system without direct visual control. This pioneering work of stereotaxic surgery (Horsley & Clarke, 1908) was later adapted for ablative treatment of subcortical structures pertaining to movement disorders, intractable pain, epilepsy, and psychiatric illness (Wilkins & Rengachary, 1985). While stereotaxic usage with its lack of direct visualization has been objectionable to some, its minimization of surgical trauma has been appealing to others. Stereotaxic surgery has survived, and combined with CT, MRI, PET, and/or laser beam guidance to increase visual accuracy, has had a recent resurgency of usage for biopsies, implantation of focal radioactive seeds into tumor sites and thromboses of aneurysms to prevent bleeding. While Horsley's work laid the foundations for surgical epilepsy therapy, Harvey Cushing's work which began in the United States during the 1900s, provided operative standards, some of which are still used today, for modern neurosurgery.

Not neglected, however, have been the concerns of neurosurgeons about relationships between cerebral locations and language and memory functioning. Nowhere is this more apparent than in the neurosurgical literature of intractable epilepsy. Penfield's book (Penfield & Jasper, 1954) and Scoville and Milner's (1957) article were the most frequently cited neurosurgical publications during a 15-year period (1965 to 1979), when counts of scientific citations were recorded (Davis, 1987).

Temporal Lobe Surgery

While tendencies toward epileptogenicity have varied within human cortical regions, neural structures within the medial temporal lobe have shown a high degree of susceptibility (Wieser, 1986). The first report of neuropsychological findings following bilateral hippocampal resections raised considerable concern (Scoville & Milner, 1957). Observations of global amnesia (Milner, 1972) in the now-famous case of H.M., and other cases, following radical bilateral medial temporal lobe resections that included the uncus, amygdala, and anterior two-thirds of the hippocampus and parahippocampal gyrus, changed the course of future neurosurgical treatment of intractable epilepsy.

Curiously, these cases showed no lowering of IQ, as measured by standardized tests, no perceptual difficulties, normal recall of early life events, no motor learning problems, and an intact immediate memory, as measured by digit span. At the same time, performances on neuropsychological tasks of one-trial recognition, delayed comparisons and matching, and 28-choice point stylus maze demonstrated short-term memory losses (Milner, 1971).

Thereafter, unilateral anterior temporal lobectomies, not bilateral medial temporal lobe resections, were surgically performed for treatment of intractable epilepsy. Resections were also confined to the anterior two-thirds of the temporal lobe. The essential temporal lobe structure held responsible for short-term memory was the hippocampus, perhaps Sommer's sector of the hippocampus, and neurosurgeons felt it should remain intact unilaterally to prevent a major cognitive deficit (Milner, 1972; Penfield & Mathieson, 1974).

These unilateral neurosurgical procedures afforded neuropsychologists opportunities to investigate material-specific memory deficits (Smith & Milner, 1984). Verbal learning and recall were found to be impaired after left anterior temporal lobectomies that spared the speech area in patients who had left hemisphere speech localization. Correspondingly, removal of the temporal lobe from the right hemisphere impaired the recognition and recall of complex visual and auditory patterns of nonsense figures, unfamiliar faces and melodies. The import of these investigations was that patients with left temporal lobectomies were impaired on verbal recall tasks, but not visual recall tasks. Reverse findings were obtained in patients with right temporal lobectomies (Milner, 1971, 1972).

Follow-up studies began investigating the size of the lateral hippocampal excisions in relationship to cognitive functioning. Findings with Peterson and Peterson's (1959) task of recalling consonants after varied intervals filled with activity showed the expected relationship: namely, the larger the hippocampal excision, the greater the reduction in recall (Milner, 1972). In keeping with material-specific tasks, patients with large right hippocampal excisions showed deficits in learning and recalling abstract designs (Jones-Gotman, 1986). Recall only of the last few items from a word list by left temporal lobectomized patients (Milner, 1978) and the last few abstract designs from a list by right temporal lobectomized patients (Jones-Gotman, 1986) confirmed the presence of recency, but not primacy, of serial positions and the material-specific hypothesis. The import of these studies weakens support for a unitary concept of memory.

The Surgically Avoided Language Areas

The bulk of the early descriptions of language dysfunctioning was based on clinical observations; some of which followed surgical therapy, others did not. In about 30 A.D., alexia was recognized by a Roman author, Valerius Maximus, following a traumatic head injury. However, credit for the first description of alexia without agraphia goes to Gerolamo Mercuriale who during the 16 and 17th centuries observed such dysfunctioning after an epileptic seizure. It remained for Jean-Baptiste Bouillaud (1796–1881) to derive a classification of aphasia into two basic types: articulatory and amnesic, which are now conceived as nonfluent and fluent (Benton & Joynt, 1960).

On the other hand, while disruption of language functioning was noted during ancient times following head injury, relationships between left hemisphere injuries and aphasia were not recognized until sometime later (Sondhaus & Finger, 1988). Articulate speech was one of the first functions to be localized (Broca, 1863), and this localization was initially to the frontal lobes (Berker, Berker, & Smith, 1986). Subsequently, the left hemisphere was declared dominant for speech following Broca's (1865) assertion that the seat for language was in the left hemisphere. This declaration of speech localization was confirmed 119 years later with a CT scan of the brain of Tan, Broca's famous patient (Signoret, Castaigne, Lhermitte, Abelanet, & Lavorel, 1984). Wernicke's description of fluent aphasia, which bears his name, appeared in 1874, and was localized to the left hemisphere in the posterior part of the first temporal gyrus (Benton, 1981). Pure word deafness, which has never been found to be "pure" with formal testing, was first described by Lichtheim (1885).

Following Broca's description of language localization, the expression, "left hemisphere dominance," appeared. By implication, functioning of the right nondominant hemisphere was considered less important. Subsequently, neuropsychological studies of patients following cerebral commissurotomies provided knowledge about specialized functions of each cerebral hemisphere (Sperry, 1961; Milner & Taylor, 1968, 1972; Cronin-Golomb, 1986; Wale & Geffen, 1986). Fortunately, significances of nonlanguage functioning have been recognized, and the misnomers *dominant* and *nondominant* have gradually begun to dissipate. Nowadays, use of the term *dominance* in relationship to functioning requires specification, i.e., dominance for what?

Almost at the same time as Broca's discovery, a qualifier was added that the left hemisphere was dominant for speech only for right-handed individuals (Benton, 1981). More recently, it has been estimated that 95% of right-handers and 60% of left-handers have language localized in the left hemisphere. The remaining 5% of right-handers have language localized in the right hemisphere or bilaterally (Albert, Goodglass, Helm, Rubens, & Alexander, 1981). For the remaining 40% of left-handers, the split is about even for right hemisphere or bilateral speech dominance (Friberg, 1989). (See Chapter 5 for further details.)

Because of the vital communicational aspects of language to the lives of human beings and anatomical variations of speech locations among individuals, a functional method for localizing language in a potential candidate for neurosurgical treatment was needed. Such a localization method was found following unilateral intracarotid injection of sodium amytal (Wada, 1949), which produces contralateral hemiparesis, speech arrest, and memory deficits (Ojemann & Dodrill, 1985). The method was used with intractable epilepsy patients to determine their suitability prior to neurosurgical intervention (Wada & Rasmussen, 1960). Although language functioning includes many acts besides object naming, when temporal lobe resections avoid areas essential to naming, there have been less overall verbal performance decrements postoperatively (Ojemann, 1986).

Relationships between neuropsychologists and neurosurgeons have been intense in the area of intractable epilepsy, where precise localization of language and memory functioning has been a hallmark of these relationships, as well as excision size (Miller & Milner, 1985). The early reports of the 1950s and 1960s correlating neuropsychological and neurosurgical findings were exemplary at the time of completion. As is the case with much pioneering work, these studies produced previously unheard-of data which raised new questions.

THEORETICAL AND BASIC NEUROBIOLOGICAL ISSUES

Imaging and Localization

A basic neurobiological issue is the agreement between lesion locations and functioning. Correlations are better with focal lesions, such as tumors (Hom & Reitan, 1984), than with diffuse lesions. But the correspondence is not always precise even with tumors, as the surgery itself may produce direct damage, or the damage may arise from secondary effects, such as brain swelling and intracranial hypertension. It is well known by neurosurgeons that the brain swells following evacuations. On the other hand, certain surgical techniques, such as a transcallosal parafornicial approach for removing third ventricle tumors, produce no neuropsychological disruption (Petrucci, Buchheit, Woodruff, Karian, & DeFilipp, 1987). Localization issues are compounded by remote effects, where tissue damage in one area produces dysfunctioning in another remote brain region because of CNS interconnections.

While pioneering studies called attention to cognitive and psychosocial devastations following surgical removal of certain cortical areas, localization of postsurgical tissue losses in these studies was not precise. Drawings of lesions made from surgical notes are not as accurate as viewing lesions firsthand with CT and MRI technology, which were not available at the time of the pioneering studies. Since the 1980s, imaging techniques have been commonplace, and are now preferred for greater accuracy of brain–behavior correlations.

Use of imaging techniques continues to unfold with time and experience, and choosing either MRI or CT technique has been situationally determined. If neuropsychological correlations are made with acute bleeding (e.g., hemorrhages, aneurysms), then CT is the choice since it is more exact than an MRI scan within 72 hr of the insult. CT findings are successful in discriminating seizure types (Ardila, Montanes, Bernal, Serpa, & Ruiz, 1986). In chronic disease, an MRI scan has better resolution and is more anatomically descriptive months or years after the initial brain insult, and in areas where the likelihood of bone artifact is high on CT scans (e.g., posterior fossa regions). Preoperative three-dimensional MRI lesions can be more easily reconstructed than those observed on CT, making the task of selecting a surgical approach less burdensome for neurosurgeons. While lesions underlying language disturbances are visible by both CT and MRI techniques, the extent of lesions is inadequately defined with CT scans, but MRI scans show correspondences between subcortical and cortical lesions (DeWitt, Grek, Buonanno, Levine, & Kistler, 1985). Since neuropsychological measurements are most often made with outpatients during the chronic phase of the disease, the MRI may be the choice technique for brain–behavior correlations.

Other imaging techniques, such as PET, are functional measures that correlate with the severity of the pathological lesion, but the size of the hypometabolic region is generally larger than the area of pathological involvement as shown on histological examination of a resected specimen (Engel, Rausch, Lieb, Kuhl, & Crandall, 1981). Quite likely this enlargement is the result of metabolic changes surrounding a lesion (e.g., deafferentation), rather than the lesion itself. Moreover, PET scans often show metabolic depressions in adjacent, remote, or diaschisis areas (Heiss, Pawlik, Wagner, Ilsen, Herholz, & Wienhard, 1983). These extended metabolic disruptions represent brain dysfunctioning that correlate well with neuropsychological findings (Uzzell, 1989), reflecting behavioral disruptions associated with these outlying sites (Uzzell, Alves, & Alavi, 1990).

In terms of presurgical considerations, language disruption not predictably associated with classical areas (Broca's, Wernicke's, and connecting areas) requires correct identification, and studies of imaging and behavioral correlations provide assistance in this regard. Left hemisphere CT lesions outside the perisylvian region associated with aphasia (Naeser, Alexander, Helm-Estabrooks, Levine, Laughlin, & Geschwind, 1982; Vignolo, 1984) have been visualized as hypometabolic regions on PET scans (Metter, Jackson, Kempler, Riege, Hanson, Mazziotta, & Phelps, 1986). The most severe language deficits involved have mainly been localized in the posterolateral subcortical regions (Knopman, Selnes, Niccum, & Rubens, 1984; Kawahara, Sato, Muraki, Tanaka, Kaneko, & Uemura, 1986). Effective localization of non-classical language regions (as well as classical language regions) with neuropsychological and imaging correlations continues to challenge presurgical planning.

Lesion localization with PET is possible. Application of this dynamic technique has improved correlations between neuropathology and neuropsychological measures observed with static techniques, such as CT and MRI (Rao, Turski, Polcyn, Nickels, & Matthews, 1984; Uzzell, 1989; Ruff, Buchsbaum, Troster, Marshall, Lottenberg, Somers, & Tobias, 1989; Uzzell *et al.*, 1990). Deterrents against employing the PET technique include its high installational and operational costs. This has made a less expensive, poorer resolution, functional imaging technique, SPECT, more attractive. Preliminary correlations of deficit ratings of hypometabolic regions of the SPECT and neuropsychological findings of patients with partial seizures show better agreement in temporal and frontal regions than in parietal and occipital regions (Homan, Paulman, Devous, Walker, Jennings, & Bonte, 1989). Reports of correlations between metabolic imaging and neuropsychological findings are now sparse, but more are expected in the future.

Localizing lesions responsible for memory losses may be more complex than those for language dysfunctioning. Which neuronal structure(s) or what interconnection(s) are responsible for memory losses in resections of the anterior temporal lobe have not been unequivocally identified. Usually slightly larger resections are performed for treatment of intractable epilepsy in the right hemisphere (5–6 cm) than in the left hemisphere (4–5 cm) because of the greater preponderance of cases with language localized in the left hemisphere. Verbal memory declines following lateral, but not medial extent of left temporal lobe resections (Ojemann & Dodrill, 1985). In the case of limbic epilepsy, the hippocampal pyramidal cells of the end folium or Sommer's sector 3–5, which contains CA3 and CA1, are affected. Lately, the amygdala has been reported to be the neural structure most likely involved in intractable epilepsy (Vries, 1989), and its damage is associated with a poorer outcome for retention of verbal and nonverbal material (McMillan, Powell, Janota, & Polkey, 1987). Localizing neural structures responsible for memory losses is influenced by the variability in neural structures from one individual to another. It is well known neurosurgically that selective amygdalohippocampectomies and temporal lobectomies require modifications from patient to patient because of large individual variability of general and vascular anatomy of the brain (Ojemann & Dodrill, 1985; Wieser, 1986).

The special role attributed to the hippocampus for memory (Milner, 1972) has not always been supported after unilateral excision of the amygdala and hippocampus. Additional learning and memory deficits have not been observed 3 to 6 months postoperatively during testing with three series of materials: nonsense designs, drawings of common objects, and concrete nouns (Wieser, 1986). Verbal tasks (learning and memory of concrete nouns after a 30-min delay) and nonverbal tasks (learning and memory of nonsense designs after 30 min) tap left and right hemisphere functioning, respectively. As might be expected, learning and memory performances of the hemisphere opposite the side of surgery generally improve postoperatively, although ipsilateral hemispheric functioning shows improvement as well (Bornstein, McKean, & McLean, 1987). Again, the role of secondary effects has to be considered. Functional localized changes can result from secondary brain damage and intracranial hypertension (Uzzell, Obrist, Dolinskas, & Langfitt, 1986).

Neuropsychological Measurement Concerns

A second neurobiological issue relates to neuropsychological measurements. Questions about processes mediating behavioral changes raised during early studies remain unresolved, but may be answerable in the future. When studies of temporal lobectomies appeared, hypotheses were advanced relating short-term memory defects either to failures of storage or to inhibition mechanisms (Warrington & Weiskrantz, 1970; Milner, 1972; Warrington & Weiskrantz,

1968). Perhaps judgment should be suspended about process speculations until enough basic neuropsychological data have been reliably collected with improved techniques. Studies completed by many different investigators across many lesion locations and conditions with the latest neurobehavioral and imaging techniques can yield valid decisions about process judgments. Questions related to the differential sensitivity of neuropsychological instruments to various types of memory functioning need to be answered. There is a tendency for neuropsychologists to become complacent about tests, to ignore weaknesses, and not to be innovative. Questions about equivalency of Logical Memory and Visual Reproduction subtests from the Wechsler Memory Scale in measuring verbal and nonverbal recall, respectively, or equivalency of alternate forms (I and II) of the Visual Reproduction subtests limit inferences about memory-specific deficits of past studies. Changes found in the Wechsler Memory Scale–Revised address some of these issues. Continued modification and development of new tests that are administered to many patients under many different conditions are necessary to sharpen neurobehavioral measurements.

Comparability of memory disorders raises another neurobiological issue. For instance, are processes based on observed memory deficits of Korsakoff's patients similar to those based on recall abilities of patients with third ventricle tumors or missile injuries in the diencephalon? If the dorsomedial nucleus of the thalamus is responsible for the amnesia in Korsakoff's syndrome (Victor, Adams, & Collins, 1971), then is the dorsomedial nucleus damage responsible for memory losses in other conditions? Or the memory losses similar when input is remotely severed to the dorsomedial nucleus? Current evidence shows that lesions of cortical structures, subcortical nuclei, or white matter tracts surround the thalamus when memory deficits are present (Markowitsch, 1982; Metter, Riege, Hanson, Kuhl, Phelps, Squire, Wasterlain, & Benson, 1983; Brown, Kieran, & Patel, 1989). On the other hand, normal memory has been present in the face of medial thalamic damage, when that damage has been insufficient to cause amnesia, or the mamillothalamic tract has not been damaged (Kritchevsky, Graff-Radford, & Damasio, 1987) or electrically stimulated (Ojemann, 1971). Unique features of memory disruption after lesions to dorsomedial thalamus, mamillary bodies, or hippocampus have not been clearly established and are debatable (Squire, 1987). Refinement of lesion and functional correlations are needed.

Influence of Methodological Variables

A third neurobiological issue relates to methodological variables. In most neurosurgical cases examined neuropsychologically, timing is important. It is important to specify the time of the neuropsychological assessment, either preinjury or presurgical, and various postinjury or postsurgical examination times in research or clinical reports. The initial postsurgical neuropsychological examination can begin 3 to 4 days after surgery, if there are no secondary complications and the inpatient is oriented and medically stable. The duration of the examination is generally an hour or so each day for 3 to 4 days. Findings of these subacute examinations are most interesting, requiring a well-prepared and forbearing examiner. Recovery can be ascertained by comparing these subacute neuropsychological measurements with those made later during the chronic phase of the disease.

Other time considerations include: duration and frequency of seizures (if present), and patients' ages. Frequent and prolonged seizures with early age onset are associated with greater cognitive impairment. (Dikmen, Matthews, & Harley, 1975; Dikmen & Matthews, 1977). Older individuals have more difficulty and pose a greater surgical risk, perhaps due to less CNS reserve. Language and memory functioning, as well as lesion status vary with time. Dysfunctioning associated with one lesion during a given time period needs to be compared to that of another type of lesion in the same or different time period, in order to establish similar and dissimilar factors related to both lesions. More patients need to be examined neuropsychologically preinjury, presurgically, acutely (if possible), subacutely, and followed chronically, for broader and more complete understanding of brain–behavior relationships.

Brain trauma associated with a neurosurgical procedure has been minimized over the years with technical refinements including the previously mentioned installation of surgical microscopes in operating rooms and diagnostic radiology developments. Other factors, such as increased knowledge about the CNS, improved operating room lighting and sterile techniques, have lessened surgical trauma. Nevertheless, during surgery, prolonged periods of uncontrolled bleeding, persistent electrolyte imbalances, intracranial hypertension, and unforeseen neural findings can plague the surgeon. These secondary effects influence the neuropsychological examination, and discriminating between surgery and these secondary effects is a problem. Sometimes resections are sizable. Large lesions have a more negative outcome for adults than for children (Smith, 1981). Yet, arguments for increased recovery after large lesions have been made (Irle, 1987). Sensory losses may be present postoperatively. A permanent olfactory loss is a by-product of bifrontal approaches used to remove anterior skull base tumors since olfactory nerves are avulsed at the cribriform plate. Cranial nerve damage may or may not be transitory. An alert examiner needs to be aware of the postoperative effects of sensory and motor losses in the execution of higher cortical functional activities.

Neuropsychological measurements of neurosurgical cases require careful consideration of other influences, such as subject variables, practice effects, and medications. Subject variables include: emotional, interpersonal, and vocational adjustments, financial status, family support, and medical history, and influence outcome. If a patient is examined neuropsychologically various times pre- and postsurgically, then practice effects have to be considered. Practice effects tend to be ignored particularly in clinical situations, although attempts have been made to select tests with comparable, alternative forms that are sensitive to the disease or abnormality under investigation (Randt, Brown, & Osborne, 1980; Dodrill, 1982).

The influence of medications on cognitive functioning should not be underrated. These may be greater subacutely due to treatment of secondary insults and residual effects of postoperative anesthesia. Other kinds of medications vary with neurosurgical cases, but anticonvulsants are frequently encountered, and their influence on cognitive abilities varies with the kind of anticonvulsant prescribed (e..g, phenytoin has a greater influence than carbamazepine) (Trimble & Thompson, 1983; Dodrill, 1988). Neurochemical systems affecting cognitive abilities (Porch & Feeney, 1986; Cope, 1988) are reviewed elsewhere in this book, and the reader is advised to consult Chapter 17.

APPLICATION TO CLINICAL ASSESSMENT

Clinical neuropsychological assessment, in contrast to research, of acute inpatient neurosurgical cases can be fast-paced, and rather nontraditional at times because of the nature of neurosurgical services. Questions rapidly formulated are often addressed in a brief period prior to and/or following surgery and treatment. Comprehensive neuropsychological batteries cannot be administered because of time limitations and the delicate medical condition of patients undergoing many different kinds of diagnostic tests. Additionally, constitutional and medication factors affecting a patient's responses have to be considered. Aids in answering referral questions expeditiously have been the development of models from which to make inferences about clinical assessment data. The following inpatient case report illustrates the use of a comparative model to localize functioning within a brief preoperative time period.

A Focal Injury Case

D.T., a 60-year-old grandmother, developed uncontrolled right facial trembling 15 years prior to the hospital admission which was diagnosed as hemifacial spasm. Due to poor patient compliance, no diagnostic tests were performed. At the time of hospital admission, uncontrolled right facial spasm was observed followed by right facial fibrillation and an inability to speak. These events cleared rapidly.

The patient, who had completed 10 years of formal education before attending a clerical trade school for 1 year, had been employed as a clerk in an accounting office for 14 years. She had been married for 40 years, and she and her husband had two married sons, and four grandchildren.

On admission to the hospital a CT scan of the head revealed a calcified mass in the left Rolandic region which was consistent with oligodendroglioma, a slow-growing tumor. Since the CT characteristics of this type of tumor (calcification with little or no response to contrast enhancement) were unquestionable in this case, an MRI scan was not performed. The patient was placed on a daily dose of 400 mg of phenytoin. The neurosurgeon wanted an opinion about the effects of surgical removal of the tumor on language skills because of the tumor's location, and requested a neuropsychological examination. He did not want to subject the patient to a sodium amytal invasive procedure. Only a 1-hr period was available for the neuropsychological examination prior to surgery.

The theoretical approach taken for the neuropsychological assessment was based on a model of comparative functioning which seemed reasonable because of the focal nature of dysfunctioning observed in cases with tumors. The model's assumptions based on material-specific findings were that (1) verbal and nonverbal abilities would be equally intact, if D.T. had not developed a tumor, and (2) abnormalities of either verbal or nonverbal functioning correlated with the tumor location. Since the tumor lay in the left Rolandic region, there was a possibility that it encroached into Broca's area affecting expressive speech. An alternate hypothesis was that language functioning was localized in the right hemisphere, rather than in the left hemisphere.

Tests selected included: WAIS subtests (Comprehension, Similarities, Digit Span, Vocabulary, Picture Completion, and Block Design), Reitan–Indiana Aphasia Screening, Controlled Oral Word Association, Bender-Gestalt, Finger Tapping, Lateral Dominance, and clinical interview. Because of the limited time, tests to examine other measures of interest (such as memory, processing speed, and reasoning) were not included.

As shown in Table 15.1, preoperatively, verbal tasks consisting of age-corrected scores for Comprehension, Similarities, Digit Span, Vocabulary, and Controlled Oral Word Association were performed within the average to high-average range. D.T. had no difficulties naming, spelling, reading, writing, articulating, understanding, and solving arithmetic problems during the Aphasia Screening Test. On the other hand, age-corrected scores of the more nonverbal tests

TABLE 15.1. Neuropsychological Findings of D.T., Pre- and Postcraniotomy

Measure	Pre	Post 30 days
Comprehension	11	11
Similarities	10	10
Digit Span	10	10
Vocabulary	10	9
Picture Completion	7	7
Block Design	6	5
Mini-Mental Status Total	27	28
Controlled Oral Word Association	33	35
Finger Tapping (rate)		
Right hand	33	28
Left hand	30	28
Grip strength (kg)		
Right hand	12	10
Left hand	13	12

(Picture Completion and Block Design) were below those obtained with verbal tests. The cross drawn during the Aphasia Screening Test was disproportional, and several of the Bender-Gestalt designs were distorted. Grip strength, but not finger tapping, was reduced in the right hand. Seven behavioral tasks performed with the right hand indicated a preference for the use of that hand. All items on the Mini-Mental Status examination were performed accurately, except two items could not be recalled and the design copy was distorted.

Other factors had to be considered which might produce levels of inequality between verbal and nonverbal task performances, with dysfunctioning appearing on tasks requiring nonverbal skills. Situational factors during testing may have affected responses. However, D.T. had been cooperative, although apprehensive about impending surgery. There was no reason to suspect anxiety was greater during nonverbal tasks than during verbal tasks that could result in differential performances. Furthermore, D.T. had been well-adjusted both at work and at home. She denied the presence of any language disturbance, and none was observed during clinical interview and testing.

A second factor to consider was the effects of medication. Although memory, mental and motor speeds might have been influenced by phenytoin, memory and mental processing times were not measured, and motor speed (as reflected by finger tapping rate) did not seem to be affected. Perhaps this latter finding was related to the brief period that phenytoin had been taken.

The results suggested that language functioning was not localized in the left hemisphere, since dysfunctioning occurred during tasks requiring little verbal skill. D.T. was presumed to be one of the 5% of right-handers in the population with language functioning localized in the right hemisphere. This opinion was conveyed to the neurosurgeon, and surgery was performed followed by a postoperative neuropsychological examination.

Postoperatively, D.T. was examined at 30 days and the results were essentially unchanged from those obtained preoperatively (see Table 1). The minor reductions postoperatively in finger tapping and grip strength bilaterally may relate to inactivity during postoperative recovery and/or continued treatment with phenytoin during that time.

A Diffuse Injury Case

In complicated cases frequently seen in clinical practice, localizing lesions is extremely difficult, even when relying on the method of comparative functioning, as well as other methods. Brain–behavior correlations are often meager in such cases because of multiple determinants of brain damage and neuropsychological findings. For instance, localization is difficult following head trauma because of the presence of both diffuse and focal effects after injury. Secondary complications, such as elevated intracranial pressure, can occur, and produce brain damage. Furthermore, when a preexisting condition affecting cognitive abilities is present, then discriminating head trauma versus preexisting cognitive versus secondary complications in relationship to lesion localization is problematic. Additionally, the effects of medication on cognitive abilities further complicate the neuropsychological inferential process.

Since much recovery from head trauma is related to time postinjury, applying a successive neuropsychological examination model provides a framework from which to draw inferences, although this model has a degree of imprecision. Comparing the model of successive examinations with multiple imaging techniques improves the inferential process, but conclusions drawn remain imperfect because of the inexactness of radiological and behavioral measurements. The following head trauma patient with a premorbid learning disability illustrates the difficulty in localizing lesions in complicated cases.

W.C. was a 23-year-old left-handed automotive mechanic who sustained a head injury when a truck tire exploded sending him catapulting upward into the air. He was taken to the emergency room of a local hospital where he was markedly agitated and confused, inconsistently following commands and moving all extremities. He was given a Glasgow Coma Scale score of 9. Fractures of the left wrist, right finger, face, and orbits and periorbital edema and ecchymosis were present. Following a diagnosis of intracranial bleeding, he was transferred to a university hospital for treatment. Neurological examination on arrival revealed no spontaneous eye opening, or openings to painful stimulus. He did not attempt to speak, but localized pain in all four extremities. Corneal and oculocephalic reflexes were intact.

A CT scan of the head showed an inhomogeneous left lateral frontotemporal acute epidural hematoma with moderate left-to-right shift and effacement of left frontal horn. W.C. was taken immediately to the operating room where a left frontal craniotomy was performed, a right frontal intracranial monitoring device was inserted, and craniofacial plastic surgery was performed. When marked elevations of intracranial pressure (23–28 mm Hg) occurred that were unresponsive to mannitol and steroid therapy, the craniotomy site was reexplored and a 1-cm incision was made in the dura to evacuate cerebral spinal fluid that was under pressure. Thereafter, intracranial pressure stabilized within the normal range (0–10 mm Hg). A postoperative CT scan of the head showed changes in the left temporal area with compression of the left lateral ventricle.

One week following the accident, MRI of the head (as seen in the left panel of Fig. 15.1) showed a small temporal contusion beneath the residural epidural collection (as shown on the right side of the image), a small hemorrhagic contusion in the right superotemporal–opercular region with edema, and axonal shearing in the periventricular and corpus callosum regions. The right temporal contusion and axonal shearing injury had not been observed on previous CT scans. Neurological improvement was progressive, and orthopedic procedures were undertaken to repair fractures of the left wrist and right finger. He was discharged from the hospital 17 days after the injury. Neurological examination at the time of discharge revealed an alert mental status, grossly intact cranial nerves, as well as sensory and motor abilities. A daily dose of 300 mg of phenytoin was prescribed.

An ^{18}F-fluorodeoxyglucose PET scan completed 23 days postinjury showed

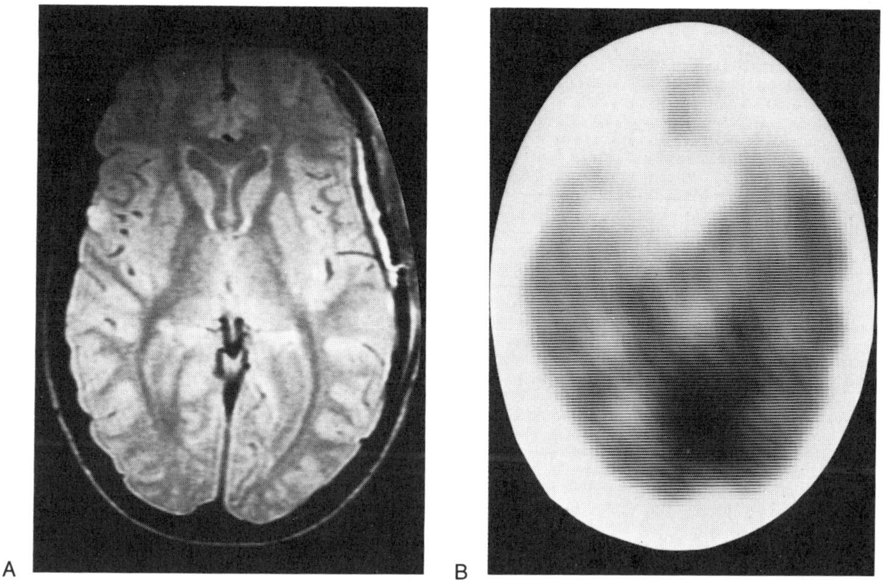

FIGURE 15.1. (A) An MRI section showing bitemporal contusion which was larger in the left hemisphere beneath the residual epidural collection (located on the right of the figure) and axonal shearing in the periventricular–corpus callosum regions. (B) A PET section showing inferior bifrontal hypometabolism which was larger in the left hemisphere (located on the left of the figure) following a head injury.

large metabolic depression in the inferior frontal regions which was more pronounced on the left side (see the right panel of Fig. 15.1). These areas of hypometabolism were possibly due to remote effects related to bitemporal contusions and/or axonal shearing injuries.

W.C.'s social history includes a two-year marriage with no children, and quitting public school during the tenth grade. He is the third of five children. His parents are divorced, with three sisters living with his father and one sister with his mother, while he and his wife live in an apartment. Prior to the injury, he had been repairing cars (which he enjoyed) in his father's body shop.

At age 15 years and 11 months he was labeled learning-disabled, and was administered a WISC-R as an aid in program planning, the scores of which are shown in Table 15.2 along with the WAIS scores obtained 33, 230, and 915 days postinjury. The neuropsychological examinations were conducted at these post-injury times at the request of the neurosurgeon. Although WISC-R and WAIS score comparisons may be somewhat imperfect, the scales are equivalent within the average range (Zimmerman & Woo-Sam, 1973). In this case the average Verbal and Performance IQ scores were obtained with the WISC-R and the final postinjury examination. Furthermore, WISC-R scores were the only available premorbid measures. As seen in Table 15.2, the WAIS scores were reduced at 33 and 290 days postinjury in comparison to the preinjury scores. By 915 days post-

TABLE 15.2. Neuropsychological Findings of W.C.

Measure	Pre	Post 33 days	Post 290 days	Post 915 days
Full Scale IQ	105	86	93	104
Verbal IQ	99	84	87	98
Performance IQ	111	91	93	112
Vocabulary	8	5	6	7
Arithmetic	10	4	7	11
Digit Span	10	10	9	10
Picture Completion	13	7	11	14
Picture Arrangement	12	10	9	13
Block Design	15	11	13	15
Memory Passages				
Immediate	—	2	7	7
30′ Delay	—	0	0	0
Visual Reproduction				
Immediate	—	—	5	12
30′ Delay	—	—	3	7
TPT Localization	—	—	2	5
Speech-Sounds Correct	—	—	45	48
Controlled Oral Word Association Frequency	—	—	19	25
Design Fluency Frequency	—	—	20	36
Grip strength (kg)				
Left hand	—	—	19	26
Right hand	—	—	11	17

injury, the WAIS scores had returned to the preinjury WISC-R levels, with Block Design, Picture Completion, and Picture Arrangement having elevated scores, while the Vocabulary score returned to its former lower level suggestive of an individual with a learning disability. Elevation of WAIS subtest scores over time that return to premorbid levels is a typical finding following moderate and mild head injuries.

During the 33-day postinjury examination period, many tests (Visual Reproduction, TPT, Speech-Sounds, Controlled Oral Word Association, Design Fluency, and grip strength) were not administered because of limited concentration and flexibility of both hands due to orthopedic casts. Grip strength when measured postinjury was reduced, particularly in the right (nonpreferred) hand. TPT Localization, Controlled Oral Word Association, and Design Fluency scores were elevated between 290 and 915 days postinjury, while those of Speech-Sounds, Memory Passages, and Visual Reproduction remained essentially unchanged, except for immediate Visual Reproduction recall score elevation which was not maintained during 30-min delayed recall. A TPT Memory score of seven was obtained during the second and third postinjury examinations. While these findings suggested that word and design fluency had improved by 915 days postinjury, recovery of auditory-verbal and visual short-term memory had not, even though the same form of the Wechsler Memory Scale had been administered at each test time.

The memory-specific deficits, as identified by a failure of 30-min delayed recall of Memory Passages and Visual Reproduction scores to elevate with time passage, might relate to the learning disability. Verbal encoding of Visual Reproduction designs is less likely in this case of a learning disability, although the immediate recall score elevation at 915 days postinjury may be due to practice effects and/or improvement. Memory deficits may also be related to phenytoin. However, memory losses, which were not noted premorbidly, were observed and reported by W.C., his wife and father in everyday life situations during the 915 days of follow-up. During the three postinjury examinations, W.C. was unable to spell or to discriminate left–right directions. These latter findings were reported by W.C., his wife and father to be present prior to the accident. Attributing Speech-Sounds Test difficulties solely to the head injury or learning disability is not possible since both affect performances of this test.

In the case of W.C. with a premorbid learning disability, sequential neuropsychological examinations and family and patient confirmations assisted in sorting out trauma-related memory-specific dysfunctioning that correlated with bitemporal contusions observed on MRI. However, the degree of the short-term memory deficits may relate to a premorbid learning disability, acute intracranial hypertension, and anticonvulsive medication. Frontal dysfunctioning observed on the PET was not discernible with the neuropsychological tests (Controlled Oral Word Association and Design Fluency) administered 290 and 915 days postinjury. The duration of the inferior frontal hypometabolism was unknown, since a PET scan was not repeated after 23 days.

SUMMARY

This chapter has reviewed the long-standing collaboration between neurosurgery and neuropsychology. The focus of these collaborations has been to correlate localized brain lesions primarily with two functions: language and memory. The intent of this chapter was to disclose strengths, as well as the pitfalls of neuropsychological assessment of neurosurgical patients. Correlations are complex, varying with lesion and remote lesion sites, time relative to onset, facets of language and speech, premorbid conditions, neuropsychological measurements, secondary complications, and medication regime. The introduction of the surgical microscope during the 1960s and diagnostic imaging developments during the 1970s and 1980s have improved surgical approaches. Nevertheless, unmanageable secondary complications are most destructive postoperatively, giving rise to additional brain damage that causes neuropsychological deficits.

Two models were presented for inferring dsyfunctioning from neuropsychological data collected from two neurosurgical patients. These models include comparing lateralized functioning attributed to each hemisphere and comparing functioning from successive measurements. While neither of these models is infallible, they provide a framework for guiding inferences. One case was representative of focal damage and was uncomplicated. Inferences from neuropsychological measurements were made more easily in this case than in the second case with diffuse damage, secondary complications, and significant premorbid factors. The latter complicated case precludes making decisive inferences about actions and interactions of the multiple determinants involved. By contrasting these two cases an awareness of both neurosurgical and neuropsychological limitations becomes apparent.

REFERENCES

Albert, M. L., Goodglass, H., Helm, N. A., Rubens, A. B., & Alexander, M. P. (1981). *Clinical aspects of dysphasia*. Berlin: Springer-Verlag.

Ardila, A., Montanes, P., Bernal, B., Serpa, A., & Ruiz, E. (1986). Partial psychic seizures and brain organization. *International Journal of Neuroscience, 30,* 23–32.

Benton, A. L. (1981). Aphasia: Historical perspectives. In M. J. Sarno (Ed.), *Acquired aphasia* (pp. 1–25). New York: Academic Press.

Benton, A. L., & Joynt, R. J. (1960). Early descriptions of aphasia. *Archives of Neurology, 3,* 205–221.

Berker, E. A., Berker, A. H., & Smith, A. (1986). Translation of Broca's 1865 report. Localization of speech in the third left frontal convolution. *Archives of Neurology, 43,* 1064–1074.

Bornstein, R. A., McKean, J. D. S., & McLean, D. R. (1987). Effects of temporal lobectomy for treatment of epilepsy on hemispheric functions ipsilateral to surgery: Preliminary findings. *International Journal of Neuroscience, 37,* 73–78.

Broca, P. (1863). Localisation des fonctions cerebrales: Diege du language articule. *Bulletin de la Societe d'Anthropologie, 4,* 200–203.

Broca, P. (1865). Du siege de la faculte du langage articule. *Bulletin de la Societe d'Anthropologie, 6,* 337–393.

Brown, G. G., Kieran, S., & Patel, S. (1989). Memory functioning following a left medial thalamic hematoma. *Journal of Clinical and Experimental Neuropsychology, 11,* 206–218.

Cope, D. N. (1988). Neuropharmacology and brain damage. In A.-L. Christensen & B. P. Uzzell (Eds.), *Neuropsychological rehabilitation* (pp. 19–38). Boston: Kluwer.

Cronin-Golomb, A. (1986). Figure-background perception in right and left hemispheres of human commissurotomy subjects. *Perception, 15,* 95–109.

Davis, R. A. (1987). Creativity in neurosurgical publications. *Neurosurgery, 20,* 652–663.

DeWitt, L. D., Grek, A. J., Buonanno, F. S., Levine, D. N., & Kistler, J. P. (1985). MRI and the study of aphasia. *Neurology, 35,* 861–865.

Dikmen, S., & Matthews, C. G. (1977). Effect of motor seizures frequency upon cognitive intellectual functions in adults. *Epilepsia, 18,* 21–30.

Dikmen, S., Matthews, C. G., & Harley, J. P. (1975). The effect of early versus late onset of major motor epilepsy upon cognitive intellectual function. *Epilepsy, 16,* 593–600.

Dodrill, C. B. (1982). Neuropsychology. In: J. Laidlaw & A. Richens (Eds.), *A textbook of epilepsy* (pp. 282–291). Edinburgh: Churchill Livingstone.

Dodrill, C. B. (1988). Effects of antiepileptic drugs on abilities. *Journal of Clinical Psychiatry, 49*(Suppl.), 31–34.

Engel, J., Jr., Rausch, R., Lieb, J. P., Kuhl, D. E., & Crandall, P. H. (1981). Correlation of criteria used for localizing epileptic foci in patients considered for surgical therapy of epilepsy. *Annals of Neurology, 9,* 215–224.

Friberg, L. (1989, May). Hemispheric dominance for language evaluated rCBF and Wada-test.

Preoperative evaluation before temporal lobe resection. Paper presented at the Fourth Nordic CBF Workshop, Faborg, Denmark.

Heiss, W.-D., Pawlik, G., Wagner, R., Ilsen, H. W., Herholz, K., & Wienhard, K. (1983). Functional hypometabolism of noninfarcted brain regions in ischemic stroke. *Journal of Cerebral Blood Flow and Metabolism, 3*(Suppl 1), S582–S583.

Hom, J., & Reitan, R. M. (1984). Neuropsychological correlates of rapid vs. slowly growing intrinsic cerebral neoplasms. *Journal of Clinical and Experimental Neuropsychology, 6,* 309–324.

Homan, R. W., Paulman, R. G., Devous, M. D., Walker, P., Jennings, L. W., & Bonte, F. J. (1989). Cognitive function and regional cerebral blood flow in partial seizures. *Archives of Neurology, 46,* 964–970.

Horsley, V., & Clarke, R. H. (1908). The structure and functions of the cerebellum examined by a new method. *Brain, 31,* 45–124.

Irle, E. (1987). Lesion size and recovery of function: Some new perspectives. *Brain Research Reviews, 12,* 307–320.

Jones-Gotman, M. (1986). Right hippocampal excision impairs learning and recall of a list of abstract designs. *Neuropsychologia, 24,* 659–670.

Kawahara, N., Sato, K., Muraki, M., Tanaka, K., Kaneko, M., & Uemura, K. (1986). CT classification of small thalamic hemorrhages and their implications. *Neurology, 36,* 165–172.

Knopman, D. S., Selnes, O. A., Niccum, N., & Rubens, A. B. (1984). Recovery of naming in aphasia. *Neurology, 34,* 1461–1470.

Kritchevsky, M., Graff-Radford, N. R., & Damasio, A. R. (1987). Normal memory after damage to medial thalamus. *Archives of Neurology, 44,* 959–962.

Lichtheim, L. (1885). On aphasia. *Brain, 7,* 433–484.

Markowitsch, H. J. (1982). Thalamic mediodorsal nucleus and memory: A critical evaluation of studies in animals and man. *Neurosciences and Biobehavioral Reviews, 6,* 351–380.

McMillan, T. M., Powell, G. E., Janota, I., & Polkey, C. E. (1987). Relationships between neuropathology and cognitive functioning in temporal lobectomy patients. *Journal of Neurology, Neurosurgery, and Psychiatry, 50,* 167–176.

Metter, E. J., Riege, W. H., Hanson, W. R., Kuhl, D. E., Phelps, M. E., Squire, L. R., Wasterlain, C. G., & Benson, D. F. (1983). Comparison of metabolic rates, language and memory in subcortical aphasias. *Brain and Language, 19,* 33–47.

Metter, E. J., Jackson, C., Kempler, D., Riege, W. H., Hanson, W. R., Mazziotta, J. C., & Phelps, M. E. (1986). Left hemisphere intracerebral hemorrhages studied by (F-18)-fluorodeoxyglucose PET. *Neurology, 36,* 1155–1162.

Miller, L., & Milner, B. (1985). Cognitive risk-taking after frontal or temporal lobectomy—II. The synthesis of phonemic and semantic information. *Neuropsychologia, 23,* 371–379.

Milner, B. (1971). Interhemispheric differences in the localization of psychological processes in man. *British Medical Bulletin, 27,* 272–277.

Milner, B. (1972). Disorders of learning and memory after temporal lobe lesions in man. *Clinical Neurosurgery, 19,* 421–446.

Milner, B. (1978). Clues to the cerebral organization of memory. In P. Buser & A. Rougeul-Buser (Eds.), *Cerebral correlates of conscious experience,* INSERM Symposium 6 (pp. 139–153). Amsterdam: Elsevier.

Milner, B., & Taylor, L. (1968). Lateralized suppression of dichotically presented digits after commissural section in man. *Science, 161,* 184–186.

Milner, B., & Taylor, L. (1972). Right-hemisphere superiority in tactile pattern-recognition after cerebral commissurotomy: Evidence for nonverbal memory. *Neuropsychologia, 10,* 1–15.

Naeser, M. A., Alexander, M. P., Helm-Estabrooks, N., Levine, H. L., Laughlin, S. A., & Geschwind, N. (1982). Aphasia with predominately subcortical lesion sites: Description of three capsular/putaminal aphasia syndromes. *Archives of Neurology, 39,* 2–14.

Ojemann, G. A. (1971). Alteration in nonverbal short term memory with stimulation in the region of the mamillothalamic tract in man, *Neuropsychologia, 9,* 195–201.

Ojemann, G. A. (1986). Mapping neuropsychological language parameters at surgery. *International Anaesthesiology Clinics, 24,* 115–131.

Ojemann, G. A., & Dodrill, C. (1985). Verbal memory deficits after left temporal lobectomy for epilepsy. *Journal of Neurosurgery, 62,* 101–107.

Penfield, W., & Jasper, H. (1954). *Epilepsy and the functional anatomy of the human brain.* Boston: Little, Brown.

Penfield, W., & Mathieson, G. (1974). Memory: Autopsy findings and comments on the role of hippocampus in experiential recall. *Archives of Neurology, 31,* 145–154.

Peterson, L. R., & Peterson, M. S. (1959). Short-term retention of individual verbal items. *Journal of Experimental Psychology, 58,* 193–198.

Petrucci, R. J., Buchheit, W. A., Woodruff, G. C., Karian, J. M., & DeFilipp, G. J. (1987). Transcallosal parafornicial approach for third ventricle tumors: Neuropsychological consequences. *Neurosurgery, 20,* 457–464.

Porch, B. E., & Feeney, D. M. (1986). Effects of antihypertensive drugs on recovery of aphasia. *Clinical Aphasiology, 16,* 309–314.

Randt, C. T., Brown, E. R., & Osborne, D. P. (1980). A memory test for longitudinal measurement of mild to moderate deficiencies. *Clinical Neuropsychology, 2,* 184–194.

Rao, N., Turski, P. A., Polcyn, R. E., Nickels, R. J., & Matthews, C. G. (1984). 18-F positron emission computed tomography in closed head injury. *Archives of Physical Medicine and Rehabilitation, 65,* 780–785.

Ruff, R. M., Buchsbaum, M. S., Troster, A. I., Marshall, L. F., Lottenberg, S., Somers, L. M., & Tobias, M. D. (1989). Computerized tomography, neuropsychology and positron emission tomography in the evaluation of head injury. *Neuropsychiatry, Neuropsychology, and Behavioral Neurology, 2,* 103–123.

Scoville, W. B., & Milner, B. (1957). Loss of recent memory after bilateral hippocampal lesions. *Journal of Neurology, Neurosurgery and Psychiatry, 20,* 11–21.

Signoret, J. L., Castaigne, P., Lhermitte, F., Abelanet, R., & Lavorel, P. (1984). Rediscovery of Leborgne's brain: Anatomical description with CT scan. *Brain and Language, 22,* 303–319.

Smith, A. (1981). Principles underlying human brain functions in neuropsychological sequelae of different neuropathological processes. In S. B. Filskov & T. J. Boll (Eds.), *Handbook of clinical neuropsychology* (pp. 347–405). New York: Wiley.

Smith, M. L., & Milner, B. (1984). Differential effects of frontal-lobe lesions on cognitive estimation and spatial memory. *Neuropsychologia, 22,* 697–705.

Sondhaus, E., & Finger, S. (1988). Aphasia and the CNS from Imhotep to Broca. *Neuropsychology, 2,* 87–110.

Sperry, R. W. (1961). Cerebral organization and behavior. *Science, 133,* 1749.

Squire, L. R. (1987). *Memory and brain.* New York: Oxford University Press.

Trimble, M. R., & Thompson, P. J. (1983). Anticonvulsant drugs, cognitive function, and behavior. *Epilepsia, 24,* (Suppl. 1), S55–S63.

Uzzell, B. P. (1989). Relationship between anatomical (CT, MRI) and functional (PET, neuropsychological) measurements. *Journal of Experimental and Clinical Neuropsychology, 11,* 67–68.

Uzzell, B. P., Obrist, W. D., Dolinskas, C. A., & Langfitt, T. W. (1986). Relationship of acute CBF and ICP findings to neuropsychological outcome in severe head injury. *Journal of Neurosurgery, 65,* 630–635.

Uzzell, B. P., Alves, W. M., & Alavi, A. (1990). Correlating PET and neuropsychological functioning following head injury. *Journal of Clinical and Experimental Neuropsychology, 12,* 388–389.

Victor, M., Adams, R. D., & Collins, G. H. (1971). *The Wernicke-Korsakoff Syndrome.* Philadelphia: F. A. Davis.

Vignolo, L. A. (1984). Aphasias associated with computed tomography scan lesions outside Broca's and Wernicke's areas. *Advances in Neurology, 42,* 91–98.

Vries, J. K. (1989). Localization of intractible epilepsy. Personal communication.

Wada, J. A. (1949). A new method for the determination of the side of cerebral dominance. A preliminary report on the intracarotid injection of sodium amytal in man. *Igaku to Seibutsugaku, 14,* 221–222.

Wada, J. A., & Rasmussen, T. (1960). Intracarotid injection of sodium amytal for the lateralization of cerebral speech dominance. *Journal of Neurosurgery, 17,* 266–282.

Wale, J., & Geffen, G. (1986). Hemispheric specialization and attention: Effects of complete and partial callosal section and hemispherectomy on dichotic monitoring. *Neuropsychologia, 14,* 483–496.

Warrington, E. K., & Weiskrantz, L. (1968). A study of learning and retention in amnesic patients. *Neuropsychologia, 6,* 283–291.

Warrington, E. K., & Weiskrantz, L. (1970). Amnesic syndrome: Consolidation or retrieval? *Nature, 228,* 628–630.

Wieser, H. G. (1986). Selective amygdalohippocampectomy: Indications, investigative technique and results. *Advances and Technical Standards in Neurosurgery, 13,* 39–133.

Wilkins, R. H., & Rengachary, S. S. (Eds.) (1985). *Neurosurgery.* New York: McGraw-Hill Book Company.

Zimmerman, I. L., & Woo-Sam, J. M. (1973). *Clinical interpretation of the Wechsler Adult Intelligence Scale.* New York: Grune & Stratton.

16

Psychoactive Drugs in the Psychotic and Affective Disorders

ALICE MEDALIA and JAMES GOLD

INTRODUCTION

The neuropsychological assessment of psychiatric patients is often complicated by the medications or treatments that are being administered. The clinician must discern whether impaired test performance reflects disease-related or iatrogenically induced cognitive deficit. In this chapter we review the literature investigating the effects of neuroleptics, antidepressants, and lithium on the neuropsychological test performance of psychiatric patients. For a review of the cognitive effects of these medications in normal subjects we refer the reader to Judd, Squire, Butters, Salmon, and Paller (1987). This review focuses on measures that are commonly used in the context of neuropsychological assessment. It is organized by medication and particular cognitive function or test that might be affected. At the end of each section we propose some clinical guidelines and theoretical hypotheses that can be generated on the basis of this literature.

Since the measurement of treatment effects is a complex endeavor, we will begin with a discussion of the methodological problems common to the bulk of studies reviewed. Incorporated in this discussion are some suggestions for future investigators.

ALICE MEDALIA • Departments of Psychiatry and Neurology, Albert Einstein College of Medicine, Bronx Municipal Hospital Center, Bronx, New York 10461. JAMES GOLD • Department of Psychology, National Institute of Mental Health, St. Elizabeths Hospital, Washington, D.C. 20032.

HANDBOOK OF NEUROPSYCHOLOGICAL ASSESSMENT: A Biopsychosocial Perspective, edited by Antonio Puente and Robert McCaffrey. Plenum Press, New York, 1992.

METHODOLOGICAL CONSIDERATIONS

Failure to Specify Treatment

Many studies fail to report the specifics of drug choice, dose, duration of treatment, as well as selection and dose of concurrent therapies and past drug history. These are serious omissions since drug regimes may not be comparable unless they are carefully controlled and uniform. Probably the most relevant pharmacologic variable in assessing drug-related neuropsychological performance is the CNS drug level, not the oral dose. Series of patients given uniform doses of lithium, antidepressants, or neuroleptics develop widely disparate clinical effects and blood levels in part due to variability in absorption and metabolism of drug (Meltzer, Kane, & Kolakowska, 1983). Obviously, older studies did not control for these dimensions as our knowledge of them is quite recent.

The Selection of Tasks

Some of the discrepancies in the literature arise because of differences in the way a cognitive function is defined and measured. For example, memory has been examined using a variety of recall and recognition tasks, some of which measure immediate and others of which measure delayed learning. Since these tasks are not necessarily comparable in the level of difficulty or type of memory required, it is hard to generalize across studies. Also at issue are the validity and reliability of measures and the magnitude of expected practice effects when a test–retest design is utilized. The failure to find improvement on retest is not necessarily evidence of a nonsignificant drug effect on performance. In fact, an expectable practice effect may not have appeared which does represent a drug-related performance deficit.

The Selection of Patients

In many of these studies, subjects of widely varying diagnoses or diagnostic subgroups were often grouped together simply as psychiatric, schizophrenic, or affective patients with no diagnostic criteria being stated. Furthermore, much of the literature predates the DSM-III and the RDC. Since contemporary diagnostic practice has changed so dramatically, the applicability of many of these studies to current clinical populations is at best uncertain.

Other patient variables, such as age and educational background, are often poorly controlled. Further, the majority of studies reviewed have been conducted in tertiary care settings, raising the possibility of a selection bias favoring patients who have more chronic and treatment-resistant illnesses.

The Question of Controls and Design

Many studies utilized inadequate control groups including post hoc comparisons of medicated versus unmedicated patients when treatment was not randomly assigned. Many other researchers simply reported correlations of oral drug dose with test performance, a method that does not address the fact that oral dose does not bear a linear relationship with CNS drug level.

Those studies utilizing test–retest designs with baseline testing preceding initiation of drug treatment or changes in medication schedule (such as dose, the addition of anti-Parkinson medications) allow each subject to serve as his/her own control and eliminate the severe problem of the heterogeneity of cognitive performance among patients with severe psychiatric illnesses. Clearly, such a design is most practical for samples of acute admission patients who are often medication-free until a diagnostic assessment is made.

To summarize, standardization of diagnostic and treatment variables, selection of tasks with known reliability and validity, use of proper controls, and test–retest designs are essential for methodologically sound research on drug effects.

NEUROLEPTICS

Within psychiatry, neuroleptics are most commonly used to treat the psychotic symptoms of patients with schizophrenia. Many studies have shown neuroleptics to be highly effective in managing the positive symptoms of patients with schizophrenia. In contrast, there are fewer investigations of the effects of these drugs on cognitive functioning. The delineation of these effects is of clear importance as it bears on clinical practice, interpretation of research findings, and theoretical understanding of schizophrenia.

This section reviews the literature investigating the effects of neuroleptics on neuropsychological test performance of patients with schizophrenia. We examine the evidence for medication effects on motor coordination, visual motor integration, IQ, planning, and aspects of attentional functioning. For an expanded review of the effects of neuroleptics on the test performance of patients with schizophrenia, we refer the reader to Medalia, Gold, & Merriam (1988).

Planning

Maze tests are commonly used as measures of foresight and planning although motor and perceptual skills are also required. Performance on mazes is often impaired in patients with frontal lobe damage (Riddle & Roberts, 1978). The original work examining drug effects on maze performance was done by Porteus (1957) and Porteus and Barclay (1957) who did two test–retest studies using heterogeneous samples of "psychotic" patients. In two independent samples, Porteus found significant decrements in maze performance following 6 weeks of treatment with 300 mg chlorpromazine despite concurrent improvement in ward behavior. Furthermore, he reported increasing deficit with longer duration of treatment. He also noted that the performance of medicated patients was marked by perseverative errors, a tendency also found among leukotomized patients.

Nonsignificant trends toward drug-induced decrement on maze performance were reported by two research groups using test–retest placebo-control designs with 30 days of drug treatment (Judson & MacCasland, 1960; Mason-Browne & Borthwick, 1957). Three studies that either did not specify treatment or used small heterogeneous samples did not find a drug effect on maze performance (Aaronson, 1963; Small, Small, Milstein, & Moore, 1972; Petrie & Le Beau, 1956).

This group of older studies raises the possibility of a drug-related impairment: none report positive effects while several mention either significant negative effects or trends. The possibility of such an impairment is interesting in light of speculation that the frontal lobes are affected by the impact of neuroleptics on mesocortical dopaminergic pathways (Goldberg, 1985).

Studies of Intelligence

Patients with schizophrenia often perform more poorly than normals and psychiatric control groups on intelligence measures (Heaton & Crowley, 1981; Aylward, Walker, & Bettes, 1984). The extent to which medications influence this finding has been experimentally examined in 11 studies, all of which used the Wechsler Bellevue or Wechsler Adult Intelligence Scale to measure intelligence.

Six studies report positive medication effects. However, one study employed mixed organic and psychiatric subject groups (Finn, Nadolski, Guy, & Gross, 1955), another involved the concurrent use of ECT (Kovitz, Carter, & Addison, 1955), and one gave no statistical analysis (Petrie & Le Beau, 1956). Both Gilgash (1961) and Castner, Covington, and Nickols (1958) report improvements primarily on Performance measures. The Gilgash study used catatonic patients; perhaps chlorpromazine enhanced psychomotor speed leading to higher Performance IQs. More recently, Depue, Dubicki, and McCarthy (1975) reported significant positive effects of phenothiazines in a subgroup of "active" as opposed to "withdrawn" schizophrenics.

Several studies, including the previously cited study by Judson and MacCasland (1960), report no effect of medication on IQ beyond practice effects. Abrams (1958) found only practice effects after 4 months of treatment with moderate doses of chlorpromazine in a test–retest placebo-controlled study of chronic patients. Gibbs, Wilkins, and Lauterbach (1957) report similar practice effects in both their placebo and chlorpromazine groups who were tested at 6-week intervals. Pearl (1962) found that phenothiazines had little overall effect on the intellectual functioning of chronic schizophrenics. More recently, Gold and Hurt (1990) found a 6-point IQ increase following 26 days of haloperidol treatment, an increase consistent with expectable practice effects.

All these studies report a numeric increase in IQ scores. However, in at least half of them the increase is at the level expected on the basis of practice. Of note, Gold and Hurt (1990) observed that neuroleptics did improve the amount of thought disorder present on the WAIS itself. Thus, despite clear evidence of clinical improvement in their sample, the cognitive benefit was modest and likely attributable to practice. The weight of evidence from both the older placebo-controlled studies and the most recent study in the area suggests that neuroleptics do not affect IQ performance.

Attention

The literature on attentional deficits in schizophrenic patients is quite vast and we refer the reader to Neuchterlein and Dawson (1984) for an overview of recent information processing research. Our review focuses on two measures of attention: reaction time and the Continuous Performance Test.

Reaction Time

In one of the most widely cited studies, Spohn, LaCoursiere, Thompson, and Coyne (1977) found a positive effect of medication on one of four RT indices: reaction time in a series of regular short preparatory intervals. They found that this measure was also correlated with improvement in ward behavior, suggesting a relationship between attentional dysfunction and symptomatic state.

However, a more recent study by the same research group (Spohn, Coyne, LaCoursiere, Mazur, & Hayes, 1985) pointed toward a negative impact of medication, possibly mediated by extrapyramidal syndrome (EPS). They studied 84 RDC chronic schizophrenics who were receiving a variety of neuroleptics and anti-Parkinson medications. Significant correlations were found between high neuroleptic dose, ratings of abnormal involuntary movements, and reaction time (RT) slowing, but there was no effect of drug or tardive on RT crossover. In this study, dose was not randomly assigned.

The relationship between extrapyramidal dysfunction and RT has also been reported by Weaver and Brooks (1961). They found that withdrawing anti-Parkinson medications from 14 chronic patients on neuroleptics, had a negative effect. In another study of 26 chronic patients, Brooks and Weaver (1961) found that the withdrawal of chlorpromazine led to both symptomatic exacerbation and RT slowing which was reversed by the introduction of trifluoperazine and further improved when anti-Parkinson medication was added to the drug regime. Strauss, Lew, Coyle, and Tune (1985) also found a positive relationship between EPS ratings and RT slowness in a sample of 28 outpatient DSM-III chronic, undifferentiated schizophrenics.

The majority of reports using samples of chronic patients have not found significant neuroleptic effects on RT (Pearl, 1962; Serafetinides, Collins, & Clark, 1972; Heilizer, 1959; Pugh, 1968; Lloyd & Newbrough, 1964; Held, Cromwell, Frank, & Fann, 1970; Strauss *et al.*, 1985). Studies of more acute populations have yielded contradictory results. Rosofsky, Levin, and Holzman (1982) studied a sample of 17 normals and 86 psychiatric patients (including 48 DSM-II schizophrenics). They found a significant correlation between drug dose and RT slowing. The largest study of this question was performed by Schooler and Goldberg (1972) utilizing a sample of 289 acute admission schizophrenics. They tested RT before and after 5, 13, and 26 weeks of treatment with a variety of phenothiazines. They found significant improvement of RT after 5 weeks of treatment, with no further improvement with continuing treatment. The cross-over pattern was most evident at pretreatment testing and was somewhat attenuated in later testings.

While this literature is marked by contradictory reports, we suggest the following summary. The core schizophrenic deficits revealed by RT measures, particularly the phenomenon of RT cross-over, are not significantly affected by medication. When RT decrements are found, they are likely to be the result of EPS. RT improvement in response to treatment is more likely to occur in acute than chronic patients.

Continuous Performance Test

The CPT is a widely used task that is thought to measure sustained attention or vigilance. The subject is required to look at a continuous series of briefly presented stimuli (typically single letters or numbers) and press a response button when a predesignated stimulus is perceived. Deficits in CPT performance have been found in populations at high risk for schizophrenia, acutely ill patients, and patients who are in a relatively remitted state, suggesting that the test taps an area of core schizophrenic deficit rather than simply a psychotic state-related dysfunction (Neuchterlein & Dawson, 1984).

Two studies suggest that medication improves performance on the CPT. Spohn *et al.* (1977) found that in their drug treated group, percent omission errors declined over the period of treatment whereas they increased in the placebo group. In addition, they found that this improved CPT performance was correlated with improvements in clinical state. Orzack, Kornetsky, and Freeman (1967) administered carphenazine (400 mg daily) to 18 hospitalized chronic schizophrenics who had been drug-free for 1 month. CPT scores significantly improved over the 12-week treatment period, an improvement that was correlated with clinical improvement on the Lorr Rating Scale.

In a review article about his work with the CPT, Kornetsky (1972) concluded that the CPT is impaired in 40–45% of testable patients and that chronic administration of phenothiazines improves CPT scores while acute administration impairs performance, findings that other researchers have not consistently replicated. Serafetinides and Clark (1973) studied the acute effects of a variety of neuroleptics administered to a sample of 43 chronic schizophrenics who had been medication-free for 12 weeks. They failed to find evidence of acute impairment by comparing results of testing prior to drug ingestion with a retest 4 hr later. In their larger study of 57 patients, Serafetinides *et al.* (1972) found that 12 weeks of medication did not affect CPT performance.

In three different studies of RDC schizophrenics, Walker reported no difference in the CPT scores of medicated versus unmedicated patients (Walker, 1981; Walker & Green, 1982; Walker & Shaye, 1982). Treatment was not randomly assigned in any of these studies and in the second cited study there were only five unmedicated patients.

Summarizing across studies, we find contradictory data concerning both acute performance deficits and drug-related improvements in CPT performance. Nevertheless, because of its methodological advantages we would tend to give some weight to the study by Spohn *et al.* (1977), which did find neuroleptic-related CPT improvement. Neuroleptic-related improvement of attention has been demonstrated in studies using other types of attentional measures such as span of apprehension (Spohn *et al.*, 1977; Marder, Asarnow, & Van Putten, 1984) and susceptibility to auditory and visual distraction (Oltmanns, Ohayon, & Neale, 1979; Spohn *et al.*, 1985). These data provide some converging evidence that is consistent with the Spohn *et al.* (1977) findings of CPT improvements with medication.

Memory

Researchers have consistently reported that patients with schizophrenia display memory deficits when compared to other psychopathological populations and to normals (Koh, 1978; Koh, Grinker, Marasarz, & Forman, 1981). The role of medication in these deficits has been the topic of several studies. Research in this area has benefited from the recent technologies that make it possible to obtain CNS levels for anticholinergics and neuroleptics.

Nonverbal Memory

Only five studies report on the use of visual memory tasks. Pearl (1962) found that prochlorperazine was the only of four phenothiazines to effect a change on Benton Visual Retention performance. He stated that with the number of *t* tests made, this could have been a chance finding. Castner *et al.* (1958) report a nonsignificant positive trend on the Graham Kendall. Lloyd and Newbrough (1964) found a nonsignificant trend toward performance decrement when they presented the Graham Kendall tachistoscopically, a technique that alters the task by increasing attentional demands.

Koh *et al.* (1981) studied a sample of 32 psychiatric patients (including 16 patients with schizophrenia) and 16 normals using a facial recognition test. Patients who were treated with low doses of neuroleptics performed at slightly lower levels than nonmedicated patients; a comparison confounded by nonrandom assignment of treatment.

Perlick, Stastny, Katz, Mayer, and Mattis (1986) administered the Benton Revised Visual Retention Test to 17 patients with schizophrenia and found a nonsignificant correlation between neuroleptic and anticholinergic levels and task performance.

Verbal Memory

The effects of medication on verbal memory have been assessed using a variety of tasks, including list learning, paragraph recall, and paired associate learning. We review here only those studies that discriminated between the effects of neuroleptics and anticholinergics. For a review of the older studies that did not have the benefit of technology to obtain CNS levels for neuroleptics and anticholinergics, we refer the reader to Medalia *et al.* (1988).

Calev, Venables, and Monk (1983) found chronic schizophrenic subjects to be impaired on recognition and recall but did not observe a significant correlation between phenothiazine dose and memory. Also, there was no difference between the subjects who were taking anti-Parkinson medication and those who were not. Later, Calev (1984) used recognition and recall tasks matched for difficulty and found that patients with schizophrenia taking neuroleptics and anticholinergics had poorer recall compared to recognition, and worse recall than that of patients taking only neuroleptics. Calev noted that this finding may have been confounded in that patients receiving anticholinergics appeared to be more disturbed. Still, his results raise the possibility that the pattern of superior recognition compared to recall, thought to characterize patients with schizophrenia (Koh, 1978), may be the result of an anticholinergic effect rather than a feature of schizophrenic pathology *per se*.

Tune, Strauss, Lew, Breitlinger, and Coyle (1982) analyzed the serum neuroleptic and anticholinergic levels of 24 medicated RDC outpatients with chronic schizophrenia and found no correlation between neuroleptic levels and symptom severity ratings, vocabulary scores, or recall of a ten-word list. However, anticholinergic level was highly negatively correlated with recall ($r = -0.51$).

Perlick *et al.* (1986) correlated anticholinergic and neuroleptic levels with performance of 17 patients with chronic schizophrenia on several tasks including list recall and recognition and paired associate learning. Serum anticholinergic level correlated inversely with recall but not recognition of a verbal list. There was no significant correlation between drug and verbal paired associate learning. Serum neuroleptic levels did not significantly affect list recall. This study is particularly interesting because the majority of anticholinergic activity arose from the neuroleptic medications and not from antiparkinsonian agents.

The weight of more recent evidence is toward a negative drug effect on memory functioning, particularly on verbal recall. This negative effect appears to be traceable to anticholinergic activity. In studies specifically addressing the effects of anticholinergic activity on the memory of patients with schizophrenia, drugs with high anticholinergic properties (benztropine, trihexyphenidyl) caused considerable decrement in short-term recall (Hitri, Craft, Fallon, Sethi, & Sinha, 1987; Fennig, Levine, Naisberg, & Elizur, 1986). Since many neuroleptics possess intrinsic antimuscarinic activity, memory impairment on the anticholinergic basis may be seen even in the absence of additional anti-Parkinson medication.

Motor Functioning

A number of studies have examined drug effects on psychomotor functioning, although only three of them utilized modern diagnostic criteria when selecting their subjects.

Purdue Pegboard and Assembly

The Purdue Pegboard consists of a board with small holes into which the subject is to rapidly place pegs. Two studies report that neuroleptics significantly impair Purdue performance (Pearl, 1962; Rosofsky *et al.*, 1982). Serafetinides and Clark (1973) note that single doses (50 mg clopenthixol or 200 mg chlorpromazine) produce acute Purdue decrements compared to Haldol and placebo. None of these studies report on the use of anti-Parkinson medication. Weaver and Brooks (1961) and Brooks and Weaver (1961) found that performance improved with a switch from neuroleptic to placebo, even in the face of concurrent symptomatic exacerbation. They further demonstrated the positive impact of anti-Parkinson medications on EPS and Purdue deficits. Two studies found no evidence of drug effects on Purdue performance (Heilizer, 1959; Serafetinides *et al.*, 1972). One study (Clark, Ray, & Ragland, 1963) found that scores increased after 16 weeks of treatment and stayed at that level after patients were drug-free for 1 year.

Pursuit Rotor

This task requires the subject to keep a stylus in contact with a target that is embedded in a revolving turntable. Weaver and Brooks (1961) and Brooks and Weaver (1961) found that performance was impaired with increasing EPS and improved when anticholinergic therapy controlled the Parkinson symptoms. Of interest, peak motor performance coincided with increased psychiatric symptomatology, suggesting that neuroleptic-induced EPS creates more motor interference than the psychotic symptoms. Kornetsky, Pettit, Wynne, and Evarts (1959) found that 200 mg of chlorpromazine led to an acute impairment in 12 patients with chronic schizophrenia. Retesting after 2 weeks found a nonsignificant decrement. Whitehead and Thune (1958) found no effect on drug and placebo groups after 2 months of treatment.

Finger Tapping

Eight studies found that neuroleptics did not affect tapping speed (Shatin, Rockmore, & Funk, 1956; Serafetinides *et al.*, 1972; Tourlentes, Hunsiker, & Hurd, 1958; Pugh, 1968; Fredericks & Finkel, 1978; Howard, Hogan, & Wright, 1975; Small *et al.*, 1972; Goode, Manning, Middleton, & Williams, 1981). Pearl (1962) found that tapping rate was improved by perphenazine compared to chlorpromazine, prochlorperazine, and placebo. Three studies found evidence of a decrement. Kornetsky *et al.* (1959) found a significant acute decrement with 200 mg chlorpromazine and a nonsignificant decrement after 2 weeks of treatment. Rosofsky *et al.* (1982) found that slower speed correlated with drug dose. Weaver and Brooks (1961) reported that tapping was impaired by increased EPS but presented no data.

Grip Strength

Shatin *et al.* (1956) found that chlorpromazine led to a nonsignificant increase after 11 days of treatment. Rosofsky *et al.* (1982) did not find a significant correlation between drug dose and grip strength.

Summary of Studies on Motor Performance

Antipsychotics are most likely to impair Purdue and Pursuit Rotor performance but have little effect on other motor tasks. The impairment on the Purdue and Pursuit Rotor appears to be strongly influenced by neuroleptic-induced EPS.

Visual–Motor Coordination

Included in this section are studies utilizing the Bender Gestalt Test, the Trail Making Test, and Digit Symbol Substitution Tests.

Bender-Gestalt

Three older studies examined the effect of chlorpromazine on Bender-Gestalt performance. Heilizer (1959) and Judson and MacCasland (1960) reported no drug effect on performance and Winter and Frederickson (1956) reported a nonsignificant negative effect.

Trail Making

Simon (1967) reported that neuroleptic dose and Trail Making performance were not correlated and that there was no effect of drug withdrawal on performance of patients with chronic schizophrenia. However, examination of the raw data demonstrates that the two groups (on drug/off drug) were poorly matched on baseline performance and there is suggestive evidence of a drug-related impairment which is not significant due to the tremendous variability within groups.

Digit Symbol Substitution Tests

The majority of studies did not find a significant drug effect (Killian, Holzman, Davis, & Gibbons, 1984; Pearl, 1962; Orzack *et al.*, 1967; Spohn *et al.*, 1977; Serafetinides *et al.*, 1972; Mason-Browne & Borthwick, 1957; Shatin *et al.*, 1956; Gold & Hurt, 1990). The study by Kornetsky *et al.* (1959) found that chronic administration of antipsychotics did not impair performance whereas acute administration did. Scores declined from baseline 90 min after administration of 200 mg chlorpromazine.

Four studies, all of which have methodological or interpretive problems, found a positive effect (Ray, Ragland, & Clark, 1964; Spiegal & Spiegal, 1967; Castner *et al.*, 1958; Serafetinides & Clark, 1973).

A summary of the studies of visual–motor coordination suggests that neuroleptics probably do not significantly affect the visual–motor coordination required for the Bender Gestalt, Trail Making, and Digit Symbol tasks.

Clinical Implications

This review suggests that various cognitive functions are differentially affected by neuroleptics. There is evidence that these medications may impair planning ability, fine motor coordination, and memory. Patients on neuroleptics are most likely to have difficulty on the following tests of these functions: Porteus Maze, Purdue Pegboard, Pursuit Rotor, and tests of verbal or nonverbal recall. There is less evidence of significant medication effects on visual–motor integration, attention, and IQ. The few studies of acute medication effects on schizophrenic cognition suggest that motor and visual–motor skills are the ones most likely to be compromised acutely.

The finding of a drug-related impairment in fine motor coordination is hardly surprising. The appearance of motor deficits related to disruption of dopaminergic transmission is not specific to schizophrenia, and occurs in all neuroleptic-treated populations. Similarly, the finding of memory impairment subsequent to muscarinic blockade is not unique to schizophrenia. Thus, the memory and motor deficits induced in patients with schizophrenia by medication conform with what is well known from other areas of psychopharmacology.

Impairment on maze task performance was reported in several older studies. This finding is intriguing since maze tasks are construed as tests of executive planning and are often linked to frontal lobe integrity. The frontal lobes receive extensive dopaminergic innervation from the mesocortical system and it is conceivable that neuroleptics interfere with this system sufficiently to elicit a subtle toxic effect on planning skills. Although speculative, this interpretation of the literature supports Goldberg's (1985) hypothesis that there are iatrogenic frontal effects of neuroleptics on the basis of dopaminergic blockade in the mesocortical projections. Since cognitive impairment may also derive from inherent frontal lobe dysfunction independent of medication, the relative contribution of integral and iatrogenic frontal lobe dysfunction to schizophrenia needs to be delineated.

Implications for an Understanding of Schizophrenia

Years of clinical documentation and research indicate that schizophrenia is characterized by both psychotic symptoms and impairment of basic cognitive abilities. The impact of medication on cognitive functioning and psychosis may help to clarify the relationship of these two symptoms. We did not find strong evidence that medication improves performance on traditional neuropsychological measures, while it is clear from clinical efficacy studies not reviewed here (see Baldessarini, 1977) that medication often proves effective in the management of active, psychotic symptoms. There is evidence that neuroleptics improve some aspects of cognitive functioning, particularly those skills, like proverb interpretation, that are related to thought disorder. Performance on tasks that require organized verbal expression may improve with medication, reflecting overall changes in symptomatic state. However, on the more structured neuropsychological instruments, such changes have rarely been reported. This argues against a model that posits that psychosis causes the cognitive deficits through a form of interference or distraction. It also challenges the model that cognitive deficits underlie psychosis, i.e., that faulty information processing is the foundation for the deranged thinking and beliefs that are evident in florid psychotic symptoms. Certainly, at the height of an acute psychosis, cognitive processes may be disrupted and then improve with symptom remission. However, cognitive functions remain relatively impaired throughout the patients' life span, whereas psychotic symptoms may fluctuate or remit. If psychotic symptoms arise from subtle cognitive failures, it is hard to imagine that the amelioration of symptoms would not either require, or partially involve, the amelioration of cognitive deficits as well. Nevertheless, the fact is that cognitive impairment, as commonly measured, is a relatively stable feature of schizophrenic pathology.

These very factors that argue against the first two models give support to a third alternative, that cognitive dysfunction and psychosis are largely independent dimensions of schizophrenic pathology, dimensions whose course and response to treatment may be different but are nevertheless the result of a common etiology. Although schizophrenic cognitive dysfunction is heterogeneous and many functions are disrupted by active psychosis, many of these patients remain cognitively impaired throughout their lives, independent of fluctuations in the psychotic process. Furthermore, impairment in cognitive processes such as IQ and attention often predates psychosis, suggesting that these processes are independent in their onset. Although this view is speculative and requires support from prospective research, the finding that medications have little effect on neuropsychological test performance coupled with the evidence (Baldessarini, 1977) that medications ameliorate psychotic symptoms, lend support to this model.

ANTIDEPRESSANTS

There are two major classes of drugs that are used to treat the symptoms of depression: tricyclics and monoamine oxidase inhibitors (MAO-I). These medications might be expected to have different cognitive effects as many of the tricyclics have anticholinergic properties not seen with the MAO-Is (Clemmesen, 1988). Unfortunately, this possibility cannot be addressed on the basis of the available literature, and thus our discussion of these two classes of medication has been combined.

Methodological problems most salient in this group of studies concern failures to consider anticholinergic toxicity or to adequately delineate subjects' clinical state. Some depressed patients present with such profound cognitive disturbances that they are considered to have a pseudodementia; others have no cognitive disturbance at all. Furthermore, lack of delineation of the psychiatric features of the group (e.g., presence of concomitant psychosis, anxiety, or other features) contributes to the contradictory nature of this clinical literature.

Studies of Intelligence

There have been two reports of tricyclic-related improvements in IQ among depressed children, particularly dramatic among children with melancholic depressions (Staton, Wilson & Brumback, 1981; Wilson & Staton, 1984). However, the results with adult samples suggest very little impact of pharmacological treatment on measures of IQ. Donnelly, Murphy, Goodwin, and Waldman (1982) reported significant gains on retesting following treatment with a variety of antidepressants. However, the extent of the improvement was four Full Scale IQ points, an amount of change expected on the basis of practice alone. WAIS IQ gains consistent with practice effects have also been reported following imipramine treatment (Kendrick & Post, 1967). Similarly, Killian, Holzman, Davis, and Gibbons (1984) reported that a group of depressed patients treated for 4 weeks with antidepressants demonstrated no gains on four WAIS subtests beyond that achieved by the continuously treated control group. Wittenborn, Plante, Burgess, and Maurer (1961*b*) reported no performance differences between placebo, ECT, and imipramine-treated patients on the Similarities, Digit Symbol, or DAT Numerical Ability Test. Another study by this group found that iproniazid, a MAO-I, did improve Similarities and DAT Numerical Ability compared to placebo and ECT groups (Wittenborn, Plante, Burgess, & Livermore, 1961*a*).

Several reports raise the possibility of negative medication effects. Howard *et al.* (1975) reported a negative correlation of tricyclic dose and WAIS performance in a sample of "neurotic depressives." Legg and Stiff (1976) reported that placebo patients demonstrated greater improvements on retesting than patients treated with imipramine or chlorpromazine. Similarly, Friedman, Granick, Cohen, and Cowitz (1966) reported superior performance by placebo patients on the Similarities subtest compared with imipramine-treated patients, with no differences between the groups on Picture Completion or Digit Symbol. The majority of studies suggest that antidepressant treatment has minimal effect on IQ in adult depressed samples.

Halstead–Reitan and Luria–Nebraska Neuropsychological Batteries

Fromm-Auch (1983) has done the most comprehensive study in this area, examining a group of 33 patients prior to the beginning of treatment and upon symptomatic remission with an extended Halstead–Reitan Battery. The majority of patients were treated with tricyclics while approximately one fourth received MAO-Is. Based upon blind clinical evaluation of test results, 56% of patients were rated as abnormal prior to treatment while 36% were still considered abnormal following treatment. Paradoxically, this study suggests both significant change as well as persisting cognitive dysfunction in a significant number of patients. It appears that the TPT, Category Test, and Memory for Designs were the tasks most positively affected by treatment (Fromm & Schopflocher, 1984). The authors did not report any comparisons of the different drugs employed in the study. Wilson and Staton (1984) reported treatment-related improvements on both the Category Test and Trails B among depressed children. Similar findings of improvement of Category Test performance following symptomatic remission have been reported by Donnelly, Waldman, Murphy, Wyatt, and Goodwin (1980) and by Savard, Rey, and Post (1980) although the latter study reported that a subgroup of relatively older bipolar patients continued to score in the impaired range on retesting. Elwan, Souief, Hassan, and Allam (1976) reported no effect of amitriptyline on Trails B performance. Bellini, Gambini, Palladino, and Scarone (1988) reported no difference in Luria–Nebraska performance between patients on and off tricyclics in a study where treatment was not randomly assigned. Howard *et al.* (1975) reported a negative correlation of tricyclic dose and sensory perceptual and motor measures from the Halstead in their subsample of older patients. Overall, the literature suggests that clinically effective antidepressant treatment may facilitate performance on portions of the Halstead–Reitan Battery, at least in a subgroup of patients.

Attention

Reaction time and vigilance are the two most commonly studied aspects of attentional functioning outside of simple measures of digit span. Three studies have found a relationship between improvement in depressive symptoms with antidepressant treatment and better performance on measures of auditory signal detection, choice reaction time, and a computerized version of Digit Symbol (Malone & Hemsley, 1977; Seppala, Linnoila, & Mattila, 1978; Rogers, Lees, Smith, Trimble, & Stern, 1987). However, the majority of studies have not found any effect of tricyclic treatment on RT (Friedman *et al.*, 1966; Glass, Uhlenhuth, Hartel, Matuzas, & Fischman, 1981; Legg & Stiff, 1976; Lovett Doust, Lewis, Miller, Sprott, & Wright, 1959; Pishkin, 1962). There are three reports of negative effects of medication on attentional measures including auditory vigilance and RT (Amin, Khan, & Lehman, 1980; Friedman *et al.*, 1966; Lovett Doust *et al.*, 1959). On balance, it appears that antidepressant treatment does not have a major impact on attentional performance.

Motor Functioning

The majority of studies that have examined antidepressant effects on motor functioning have reported no effect of treatment on either Finger Tapping or Digit Symbol performance (Glass *et al.*, 1981; Legg & Stiff, 1976; Kendrick & Post,

1967; Killian *et al.*, 1984; Snow & Rickels, 1964; Wilson & Staton, 1984; Wittenborn *et al.*, 19611,b). Positive effects of imipramine have been noted on tapping and hand dynameter (Friedman *et al.*, 1966), and Kenning, Richardson, and Tucker (1960) reported nonsignificant positive trends on tapping, dotting, and Digit Symbol. Negative effects of imipramine on tapping were reported by Amin *et al.* (1980). Seppala *et al.* (1978) reported that doxepin impaired performance on a simulated driving task while chlorimipramine had no effect. Raskin, Friedman, and DiMascio (1983) reported that patients on placebo performed better than imipramine- and phenelzine-treated patients on a battery of motor and graphomotor tasks. In summary, there is little evidence that antidepressant treatment facilitates motor performance. Rather, the bulk of evidence points to the lack of a medication effect.

Memory

The impact of antidepressant treatment on memory performance has been examined in eight studies. Unfortunately, none of them considered the anticholinergic effects of antidepressant treatment. Three studies found a drug-related improvement in memory functioning. Sternberg and Jarvik (1976) reported that imipramine and amitriptyline enhanced memory performance in a sample of endogenous depressives treated with tricyclic doses ranging from 150 to 350 mg a day. In this study, clinical improvement and memory improvement were strongly related. Glass *et al.* (1981) reported improved performance on a Sternberg memory scanning task in a placebo-controlled multiple cross-over design. This improvement in error rate could also reflect an improvement in sustained attention. Amin *et al.* (1980) reported improved short-term memory with imipramine.

Two studies suggest that memory is unaffected by antidepressants. Henry, Weingartner, and Murphy (1973) found no effect of imipramine on several laboratory measures of memory although their sample size of six suggests their results should be regarded with caution. Kendrick and Post (1967) reported no effect of 12 weeks of imipramine treatment on synonym learning or the Inglis Paired Associate learning tests.

Four studies suggest a drug-related decrement in memory performance. In two studies, placebo patients outperformed patients treated with a variety of antidepressants (Legg & Stiff, 1976; Raskin *et al.*, 1983). Another study found memory improvement in patients treated with ECT that was not found in patients treated with amitriptyline (Cawley, Post, and Whitehead, 1973). Calvev, Ben Tzvik, Shapira, Drexler, Carasso, and Lerer (1989) reported a decline from pretreatment baseline in delayed recall of paired associates in a group of ten patients treated with 200 mg imipramine for 3 weeks. They observed no medication effect on measures of visual recall or remote memory. Of interest, this group had no clinical symptomatic benefit from treatment at the time of the second testing.

This group of studies is nearly evenly divided between positive, negative, and no-effect findings, defying easy summary. However, in our view the studies of Sternberg and Jarvick (1976), Glass *et al.* (1981), and Calev *et al.* (1989) should be weighted most heavily on methodological grounds. Two studies suggest memory enhancement, perhaps on the basis of an improvement in clinical state. In the other study, there was no clinical improvement and memory scores declined. Possibly, when antidepressants lead to improved mood, this has a beneficial effect on memory that outweighs the deleterious effects of anticholinergics on memory. This topic deserves additional investigation given the importance of memory function in the differential diagnosis of dementia and depression in elderly patients.

Clinical Implications

This literature has several implications for clinical assessment. Most studies suggest rather minimal effects of antidepressant medications on IQ, attention, and motor skills. There are some data suggesting enhanced performance on the Halstead–Reitan battery for a subgroup of patients, with particular enhancement on the Category Test. However, the literature on memory is too contradictory to yield conclusions. There are some reports of negative medication effects across a variety of cognitive functions. To the extent negative effects exist, they are likely to be the result of the anticholinergic properties of the tricyclics although it should be pointed out that this notion is entirely speculative as the issue has not been directly researched. It seems likely that the cognitive impairments related to anticholinergic mechanisms are outweighed by the cognitive enhancing effect of symptomatic remission for most patients.

The existence of negative effects raises the possibility of a false-positive diagnosis of "brain damage" on the basis of impaired neuropsychological test performance. As a first step to assess this possibility, anticholinergic side effects should be assessed including drowsiness, dry mouth, and blurred vision. If such symptoms are present, retesting following either a dose reduction or change in medication is probably indicated. Testing should generally be delayed until patients have had an opportunity to accommodate to the initiation of drug treatment or to major changes in dose, as side effects are frequently most pronounced early in treatment. In the assessment of elderly patients where a differential diagnosis of dementia versus depression is in question, the issue of negative medication effects needs to be carefully considered as elderly patients are often extremely sensitive to relatively small doses and polypharmacy is common (Kendrick & Moyes, 1979).

Implications for an Understanding of Depression

Impairment of a variety of cognitive functions frequently occurs in depressive illnesses. For example, impairment of concentration is a central symptom of depression which is included in the DSM-III-R as one of the criteria for the disorder. The relative contribution of state, trait, and iatrogenic factors to these cognitive deficits is a matter of controversy. Several studies have reported that the severity of depressive symptoms correlates with the degree of impairment of reaction time, perceptual–motor speed, abstracting ability, and memory (Byrne, 1976; Cohen, Weingartner, Smallberg, Pickar, & Murphy, 1982; Silberman, Weingartner, & Post, 1983; Weckowicz, Tam, Mason, & Bay, 1978). Also, there are reports documenting a relationship between the improvement of symptomatic state and changes in cognitive functioning (Jones, Henderson, & Welch, 1988; Sternberg & Jarvik, 1976). Such evidence suggests that cognitive impairment is primarily a function of the depressed state and varies with the severity of the mood disturbance.

Some studies, however, have failed to find such direct linear relationships between symptom severity and cognitive performance (Coughlan & Hollows, 1984; Kopelman, 1986). Furthermore, there is some evidence that cognitive impairment may persist beyond the acute symptomatic episode in a subgroup of depressed patients (Braff, Glick, Johnson, & Zisouk, 1988; From-Auch, 1983). This subgroup has not been well characterized although there is evidence that persistent cognitive impairment may be more frequently observed in older bipolar patients (Savard *et al.*, 1980).

The literature on antidepressants and neuropsychological test performance suggests that these medications have minimal effects on cognition. This research literature is at odds with our clinical experience. In the midst of a depressive episode, many patients are unable to work due to severe concentration deficits. Yet, many depressed patients are able to return to their former employment following treatment of their symptoms. One must assume that a significant improvement of attention and concentration must take place in order for patients to be able to function in a competitive employment situation.

Several methodological issues may account for the discrepancy between the research literature and clinical experience. First, patients are likely to vary in the extent to which they present with cognitive impairments and those with the most severe forms of cognitive dysfunction may never be studied as they are essentially untestable. By looking only at patients with mild impairment, researchers minimize opportunities to see a change in cognitive functioning. Second, the time course for recovery of cognitive symptoms may be much longer than that for affective symptoms. Longer retest intervals might reveal that at least in a subgroup of patients, cognitive symptoms eventually improve.

LITHIUM

Lithium's efficacy as a treatment for bipolar affective disorders is generally accepted. Although affective symptoms typically improve, patients may complain of a variety of side effects including decreased cognitive functioning (Schou, 1968; Bajor, 1977; Coppen, 1978; McCreadie & Morrison, 1985; Preodor, Wolpert, Ostrow, Holinger, & Wolpert, 1977). Reports of these subjective complaints have spurred research on the effects of lithium on cognitive functioning.

Memory, attention, and perceptual–motor skills are the cognitive functions typically examined in the literature and will be the focus here.

In addition to the general methodological issues discussed previously, two problems are salient in this group of studies. Most important, lithium is potentially toxic and it is thus crucial to consider signs of toxicity as a variable to be statistically covaried with the cognitive function under investigation. Unfortunately, most studies simply specify range of blood level in the treated group and then proceed to compare patients on with those off lithium. Another issue concerns the delineation of clinical state. Affective disorders encompass a number of subgroups that differ according to their characterization as unipolar or bipolar, according to severity of symptoms, and the coexistence of other symptoms like psychosis or anxiety. Since affective states themselves have been associated with cognitive dysfunction, it is important for clinical characteristics to be carefully delineated if the question of state versus trait versus iatrogenic cognitive disorder is to be addressed.

Memory

The effect of lithium on memory has been the subject of most of the investigations on cognitive side effects. Six studies report that lithium has no effect on memory. Henry *et al.* (1973) found that impaired performance on verbal list learning tests was associated with degree of depression and mania, but was unaffected by lithium treatment ($N = 12$). Telford and Worrall (1978) tested seven stable affectively disordered patients while on lithium (average level = 0.83) and after 2 weeks off the drug. They reported that stopping lithium had no effect on ratings of mood, attention (PASAT), or memory (Wechsler Memory Scale Logical Memory and Visual Reproductions). Marusarz, Wolpert, and Koh (1981) found that their six bipolar patients who were drug-free 1 month performed comparably on verbal list recall tasks to the seven, sicker bipolar patients on maintenance lithium. Smigan and Perris (1983) tested 30 affectively disordered patients before treatment and again after 4 and 12 months of lithium therapy. Four tests—the 30 Word Pair Test, 30 Person-Data Test, 30 Figure Test, and 30 Face Test—were used with an immediate and delayed response format. Application of the Bonferroni statistic shows that immediate recognition of 30 faces improved over the testing sessions; other changes were nonsignificant.

Two studies reporting "no effect" examined the impact of treatment duration on memory. Ghadirian, Engelsmann, and Amanth (1983) administered the Wechsler Memory Scale (WMS) and Benton Visual Retention Test (BVRT) once to 30 stable bipolar patients, some of whom were treated less than and some more than 10 months. They found that age but not duration of treatment correlated with performance on memory tests. In a follow-up study (Engelsmann, Katz, Ghadirian, & Schachter, 1988) 18 of the patients tested in the first study were retested 6 years later. Scores on the WMS and BVRT remained stable but again age was found to correlate with performance.

Six studies found evidence of a lithium-related memory impairment. Kusumo and Vaughan (1977) compared 13 affectively disordered patients with 13 normals on several tasks including a Peterson short-term memory test and immediate and delayed paired associate learning. Patients on lithium performed worse at the 15-sec delay of the Peterson short-term memory task; other group comparisons were nonsignificant. Rapp and Thomas (1979) attempted to replicate these findings by comparing 10 normals and 10 affectively disordered patients on lithium and found similar results with the Peterson short-term memory task. In addition, they found that the drug-treated group did worse on the long-term memory paired associate learning task. These studies would have benefitted from more careful subject recruitment—although patients did not have ECT within the last 6 weeks, the memory impairments subsequent to ECT can last up to 6 months.

Two studies used the Buschke list learning paradigm to examine lithium effects on storage and retrieval. Reus, Targum, Weingartner, and Post (1979) compared 17 stable outpatient bipolar patients on lithium with 7 who were not on lithium and found that the lithium group recalled less on each trial and was more inconsistent in retrieving words from long-term storage. Shaw, Stokes, Mann, and Manevitz (1987), in perhaps the most methodologically sound study of lithium and memory, tested affectively disordered patients on placebo and on lithium. Long-term storage and long-term retrieval improved when patients were on placebo and then worsened when they were on lithium. Immediate recall also improved on placebo but did not worsen when patients were put back on lithium.

Squire, Judd, Janowsky, and Huey (1980) used a sophisticated double-blind cross-over design which allowed patients to be tested on placebo and lithium and found that higher lithium levels correlated with poorer performance on memory tasks. Scores on the various verbal and nonverbal recall tasks did not change from the placebo to lithium conditions. Caution must be used in generalizing these findings to the affectively disordered population since 13 of the 16 patients were alcoholics.

Christodoulou, Kokkevi, Lykouras, Stefanis, and Papadimitriou (1981) tested 15 affectively disordered patients while on lithium and again 15 days after it had been discontinued. Use of the Bonferroni statistics shows that performance on the immediate and delayed version of the BVRT significantly improved once lithium was discontinued. Scores on the Rey Verbal Learning Test and Digit Span backwards improved nonsignificantly during the placebo condition. Recall on a paired associated learning task was virtually the same during the lithium and placebo conditions.

In summary, this literature does not support the presence of positive lithium effects on memory and gives some evidence for a negative effect. It does not appear that duration of lithium treatment is associated with memory deficit. Although six studies reported no effect and six reported negative effects, suggesting that this remains a controversial area, we would put the greatest weight on the findings of Shaw *et al.* (1987) who conducted the most methodologically sophisticated study of affectively disordered patients. They found a lithium-related impairment in long-term storage and retrieval.

Attention

There are four studies with affectively disordered patients that address this issue. Elass, Mellerup, Rafaelsen, and Theilgaard (1981) compared auditory RT performance of 22 lithium-treated bipolar patients with that of 20 normal controls and 19 bipolars not on lithium (although 12 were on other psychotropics). Patients treated with lithium showed longer RTs than either of the other groups. All groups had slower RTs in the morning than the afternoon or night. Muller-Oerlinghausen, Bauer, Girke, Kanowski, and Goncalves (1977) found vigilance deficits in both lithium-treated bipolar patients and normal controls. Telford and Worrall (1978) found no effect of lithium on seven bipolar patients' performance of the Paced Serial Addition Task. Joffe, MacDonald, and Kutcher (1988) found no effect of lithium or carbamazepine on a letter cancellation test. These studies suggest that lithium may compromise attention as measured by RT and vigilance.

Visual–Motor Skills

Tremor is a common side effect of lithium and it is reasonable to expect that treated patients might be slower on timed visual–motor tasks. Surprisingly, no study has correlated degree of tremor with visual–motor performance. Four studies have measured visual–motor skills, usually with the Digit Symbol subtest of the WAIS. All report a lithium-related decrement in visual–motor performance.

Squire *et al.* (1980) reported that subjects were significantly slower on a digit symbol substitution test during the lithium condition. Trailmaking A performance was marginally different during the placebo and lithium conditions. Serum lithium levels did not correlate with performance on either test.

Demers and Heninger (1971) reported that therapeutic ranges of lithium were associated with neuromuscular symptoms and a decline in Digit Symbol scores but no change on the Bender-Gestalt. Digit Symbol scores improved and neuromuscular symptoms subsided at the time when lithium was stopped. Their sample included six patients with a history of bipolar disorder.

Loo, Bonnel, Etevenon, Benyacoub, and Slowen (1981) found that lithium-treated outpatient bipolar patients performed worse than nonbipolar psychiatric outpatients on Digit Symbol. Shaw *et al.* (1987) looked at finger tapping, a more purely motor task, and found that the scores of affectively disordered patients improved during the placebo condition and then worsened during the lithium phase.

These studies strongly suggest that lithium has an adverse effect on visual–motor performance. There is some evidence that the neuromuscular effects of lithium are associated with the decline in test performance, although no formal statistical analysis of this association has been done.

Miscellaneous Cognitive Tests

Lithium does not appear to have an effect on Block Design performance (Telford & Worrall, 1978), on Porteus Maze or Trailmaking B performance (Squire *et al.*, 1980).

Clinical Implications

There is convincing evidence that lithium causes affectively disordered patients to be slower on visual–motor tasks like Digit Symbol. There is also some evidence that lithium may impair attention and long-term storage and retrieval. Performance on tests like Block Design, Porteus Maze, and Trailmaking B seems to be unaffected. Clinicians examining patients on lithium should be careful to observe for signs of toxicity and tremor. In addition to objectively testing cognitive functions, clinicians should encourage patients to describe any changes in cognitive functioning. Patients may perform adequately on tests of memory but subjectively experience a memory deficit. Such complaints are a major factor in medication noncompliance.

Implications for an Understanding of Bipolar Illness

Lithium is used to stabilize the mood of bipolar patients. The studies of its effects on cognitive functioning suggest that it also has the effect of slowing performance on certain tasks. It may be that this is simply a motor slowing, although it could also exert effects by slowing information processing. Judd and his colleagues (Judd, Hubbard, Janowsky, Huey, & Takahashi, 1977; Judd, 1979) have been particularly interested in this issue and have argued that one of the mechanisms by which lithium exerts an antimanic effect is through slowing of central cognitive processing. Although there are insufficient data to make a convincing argument on behalf of this hypothesis, we do believe that the literature showing lithium-related impairments on visual–motor tasks, memory, and rate of information processing makes this a worthwhile area for future investigation.

SUMMARY

The medications commonly administered to schizophrenic and affectively disordered patients often provide dramatic relief of their psychiatric symptoms. This chapter has reviewed the evidence for their impact on neuropsychological test performance. Neuroleptics can negatively affect memory, fine motor coordination, and planning ability but do not have clear or large effects on other aspects of test performance. Antidepressants are not associated with significant changes in test performance, although the literature in this area has sufficient methodological problems that caution must be exercised in accepting this conclusion. Lithium can impair visual–motor speed, memory, and possibly attention. Clinicians assessing cognitive functioning in psychiatric patients would be well advised to document the potential impact of medications on test results. The study of the effects of medications on neuropsychological test performance continues to be an important area of investigation that has bearing on clinical practice, the interpretation of research and assessment findings, as well as the theoretical understanding of the underlying disease process.

REFERENCES

Aaronson, B. S. (1963). The comparative sensitivity of the qualitative and quantitative Porteus Maze scores to drug effects. *Journal of Clinical Psychology, 19,* 184–185.

Abrams, J. (1958). Chlorpromazine in the treatment of chronic schizophrenia. *Diseases of the Nervous System, 19,* 20–28.

Amin, M. M., Khan, P., & Lehman, H. E. (1980). The differential effects of viloxazine and imipramine on performance tests: Their relationship to behavioral toxicity. *Psychopharmacology Bulletin, 16,* 57–60.

Aylward, E., Walker, E., & Bettes, B. (1984). Intelligence in schizophrenia: Meta-analysis of the research. *Schizophrenia Bulletin, 10,* 430–459.

Bajor, G. F. (1977). Memory loss with lithium. *American Journal of Psychiatry, 134,* 588.

Baldessarini, R. J. (1977). *Chemotherapy in psychiatry.* Cambridge, Mass.: Harvard University Press.

Bellini, L., Gambini, O., Palladino, F., & Scarone, S. (1988). Neuropsychological assessment of functional central nervous system disorders. I. Hemispheric functioning characteristics in schizophrenia and affective illness. *Acta Psychiatrica Scandinavica, 78,* 242–246.

Braff, D. L., Glick, I. D., Johnson, M. H., & Zisook, S. (1988). The clinical significance of thought disorder across time in psychiatry patients. *Journal of Nervous and Mental Disease, 176,* 213–220.

Brooks, G., & Weaver, L. (1961). Some relations between psychiatric and psychomotor behavior changes associated with tranquilizing medications. *Comprehensive Psychiatry, 2,* 203–210.

Byrne, D. G. (1976). Choice reaction times in depressive states. *British Journal of Social and Clinical Psychology, 15,* 149–156.

Calev, A. (1984). Recall and recognition in mildly disturbed schizophrenics: The use of matched tasks. *Psychological Medicine, 14,* 425–429.

Calev, A., Venables, P. H., & Monk, A. F. (1983). Evidence for distinct verbal memory pathologies in severely and mildly disturbed schizophrenics. *Schizophrenia Bulletin, 9,* 247–264.

Calev, A., Ben Tzvi, E., Shapira, B., Drexler, H., Carasso, R., & Lerer, B. (1989). Distinct memory impairments following electroconvulsive therapy and imipramine. *Psychological Medicine, 19,* 111–119.

Castner, C. W., Covington, C. M., & Nickols, J. E. (1958). The effects of a Thorazine-centered treatment program with psychological evaluations. *Texas Report of Biological Medicine, 16,* 21–30.

Cawley, R. H., Post, F., & Whitehead, A. (1973). Barbiturate tolerance and psychological functioning in elderly depressed patients. *Psychological Medicine, 3,* 39–52.

Christodoulou, G. N., Kokkevi, A., Lykouras, E. P., Stefanis, C. N., & Papadimitriou, G. N. (1981). Effects of lithium on memory. *American Journal of Psychiatry, 138,* 847–848.

Clark, M. L., Ray, T. S., & Ragland, R. E. (1963). Chlorpromazine in chronic schizophrenic women: Rate of onset and rate of dissipation of drug effects. *Psychosomatic Medicine, 3,* 212–217.

Clemmesen, L. (1988). Anticholinergic side-effects of antidepressants: Studies of the inhibition of salivation. *Acta Psychiatrica Scandinavica Supplement 345, 78,* 90–93.

Cohen, R. M., Weingartner, H., Smallberg, S. A., Pickar, D., & Murphy, D. L. (1982). Effort and cognition in depression. *Archives of General Psychiatry, 39,* 593–597.

Coppen, A. (1978). Lithium and memory impairment. *Lancet, 1,* 448.

Coughlan, A. K., & Hollows, S. E. (1984). Use of memory tests in differentiating organic disorder from depression. *British Journal of Psychiatry, 145,* 164–167.

Demers, R. G., & Heninger, G. R. (1971). Visual-motor performance during lithium treatment: A preliminary report. *Journal of Clinical Psychopharmacology, 11,* 274–279.

Depue, R. A., Dubicki, M. D., & McCarthy, T. (1975). Differential recovery of intellectual, associational, and psychophysiological functioning in withdrawn and active schizophrenics. *Journal of Abnormal Psychology, 84,* 325–330.

Donnelly, E. F., Waldman, I., Murphy, D. L., Wyatt, R. J., & Goodwin, F. K. (1980). Primary affective disorder: Thought disorder in depression. *Journal of Abnormal Psychology, 89,* 315–319.

Donnelly, E. F., Murphy, D. L., Goodwin, F., & Waldman, I. (1982). Intellectual function in primary affective disorder. *British Journal of Psychiatry, 140,* 633–636.

Elass, P., Mellerup, E. T., Rafaelsen, O. J., & Theilgaard, A. (1981). Effect of lithium on reaction time—A study of diurnal variations. *Psychopharmacology, 72,* 279–282.

Elwan, O., Souief, M., Hassan, M. A., & Allam, M. (1976). Psychometric assessment of the therapeutic efficacy of antidepressant agents. *Journal of International Medical Research, 4,* 118–124.

Engelsmann, F., Katz, J., Ghadirian, A. M., & Schachter, D. (1988). Lithium and memory: A long-term follow-up study. *Journal of Clinical Psychopharmacology, 8,* 207–212.

Fennig, S., Levine, Y., Naisberg, S., & Elizur, A. (1986). The effect of trihexyphenidyl (Artane) on memory in schizophrenic patients. *Progress in Neuro-Psychopharmacology & Biological Psychiatry, 11,* 71–78.

Finn, M. H. P., Nadolski, F., Guy, W., & Gross, M. (1955). Clinical, psychological, and myoneural changes in psychotic patients under oral Serpasel medication. *Journal of Nervous and Mental Disease, 122,* 458–467.

Fredericks, R. S., & Finkel, P. N. (1978). Schizophrenic performance on the Halstead–Reitan Battery. *Journal of Clinical Psychology, 34,* 26–30.

Friedman, A. S., Granick, S., Cohen, H. W., & Cowitz, B. (1966). Imipramine (Tofranil) vs. placebo in hospitalized psychotic depressives. *Journal of Psychiatry Research, 4,* 13–36.

Fromm, D., & Schopflocher, D. (1984). Neuropsychological test performance in depressed patients before and after drug therapy. *Biological Psychiatry, 19,* 55–71.

Fromm-Auch, D. (1983). Neuropsychological assessment of depressed patients before and after drug therapy: Clinical profile interpretation. In P. Flor-Henry & J. Gruzelier (Eds.), *Laterality and psychopathology* (pp. 83–102). Amsterdam: Elsevier.

Ghadirian, A. M., Engelsmann, F., & Amanth, J. (1983). Memory functions during lithium therapy. *Journal of Clinical Psychopharmacology, 3,* 313–315.

Gibbs, J. J., Wilkens, B., & Lauterbach, C. G. (1957). A controlled clinical psychiatric study of the drug chlorpromazine. *Journal of Clinical and Experimental Psychopathology, 18,* 269–283.

Gilgash, C. A. (1961). Thorazine therapy with catatonic schizophrenics in relation to Wechsler verbal and performance subtest comparison. *Journal of Clinical Psychology, 17,* 95.

Glass, R. M., Uhlenhuth, E. H., Hartel, F. W., Matuzas, W., & Fischman, M. W. (1981). Cognitive dysfunction and imipramine in outpatient depressives. *Archives of General Psychiatry, 38,* 1048–1051.

Gold, J., & Hurt, S. (1990). The effects of haloperidol on thought disorder and IQ in schizophrenia. *Journal of Personality Assessment, 54,* 390–400.

Goldberg, E. (1985). Akinesia, tardive dysmentia, and frontal lobe disorders in schizophrenia. *Schizophrenia Bulletin, 11,* 255–263.

Goode, D. J., Manning, A. A., Middleton, J. F., & Williams, B. (1981). Fine motor performance before and after treatment in schizophrenic and schizoaffective patients. *Psychiatry Research, 5,* 247–255.

Heaton, R. K., & Crowley, T. J. (1981). Effects of psychiatric disorders and their somatic treatment on neuropsychological test results. In S. B. Filskov & T. B. Boll (Eds.), *Handbook of clinical neuropsychology* (pp. 481–525). New York: Wiley.

Heilizer, F. (1959). The effects of chlorpromazine on psychomotor and psychiatric behavior of chronic schizophrenic patients. *Journal of Nervous and Mental Disease, 128,* 358–364.

Held, J. M., Cromwell, R. L., Frank, E. T., Jr., & Fann, W. E. (1970). Effects of phenothiazines on reaction time in schizophrenics. *Journal of Psychiatric Research, 7,* 209–213.

Henry, G. M., Weingartner, H., & Murphy, D. L. (1973). Influence of affective states and psychoactive drugs on verbal learning and memory. *American Journal of Psychiatry, 130,* 966–971.

Hitri, A., Craft, R. B., Fallon, J., Sethi, R., & Sinha, D. (1987). Serum neuroleptic and anticholinergic activity in relationship to cognitive toxicity of antiparkinsonian agents in schizophrenic patients. *Psychopharmacology Bulletin, 23*, 33–37.

Howard, M. L., Hogan, T. P., & Wright, M. W. (1975). The effects of drugs on psychiatric patients' performance on the Halstead–Reitan Neuropsychological Test Battery. *Journal of Nervous and Mental Disease, 161*, 166–171.

Joffe, R. T., MacDonald, C., & Kutcher, S. P. (1988). Lack of differential cognitive effects of lithium and carbamazepine in bipolar affective disorder. *Journal of Clinical Psychopharmacology, 8*, 425–428.

Jones, B. P., Henderson, M., & Welch, C. A. (1988). Executive functions in unipolar depression before and after electroconvulsive therapy. *International Journal of Neuroscience, 38*, 287–297.

Judd, L. L. (1979). Effect of lithium on mood, cognition and personality function in normal subjects. *Archives of General Psychiatry, 36*, 860–865.

Judd, L. L., Hubbard, B., Janowsky, D. S., Huey, L. Y., & Takahashi, K. I. (1977). The effect of lithium carbonate on the cognitive functions of normal subjects. *Archives of General Psychiatry, 34*, 355–357.

Judd, L. L.., Squire, L. R., Butters, N., Salmon, D. P., & Paller, K. A. (1987). Effects of psychotropic drugs on cognition and memory in normal humans and animals. In H. Y. Meltzer (Ed.), *Psychopharmacology: The third generation of progress* (pp. 1467–1475). New York: Raven Press.

Judson, A. J., & MacCasland, B. W. (1960). The effects of chlorpromazine on psychological test scores. *Journal of Consulting Psychology, 24*, 192.

Kendrick, D. C., & Moyes, I. C. A. (1979). Activity, depression, medication and performance on the Revised Kendrick Battery. *British Journal of Social and Clinical Psychology, 18*, 341–350.

Kendrick, D. C., & Post, F. (1967). Differences in cognitive status between healthy, psychiatrically ill, and diffusely brain-damaged elderly subjects. *British Journal of Psychiatry, 113*, 75–81.

Kenning, I. S., Richardson, N. L., & Tucker, F. G. (1960). The treatment of depressive states with imipramine hydrochloride. *Canadian Psychiatric Association Journal, 5*, 60–64.

Killian, G., Holzman, P., Davis, J. M., & Gibbons, R. (1984). Effects of psychotropic medication on selected cognitive and perceptual measures. *Journal of Abnormal Psychology, 93*, 58–70.

Koh, S. D. (1978). Remembering of verbal materials by schizophrenic young adults. In S. Schwartz (Ed.), *Language and cognition in schizophrenia* (pp. 59–99). Hillsdale, N.J.: Erlbaum.

Koh, S. D., Grinker, R. R., Sr., Marasarz, T. Z., & Forman, P. L. (1981). Affective memory and schizophrenic anhedonia. *Schizophrenia Bulletin, 7*, 292–307.

Kopelman, M. D. (1986). Clinical tests of memory. *British Journal of Psychiatry, 148*, 517–525.

Kornetsky, C. (1972). The use of a simple test of attention as a measure of drug effects in schizophrenic patients. *Psychopharmacologia, 24*, 99–106.

Kornetsky, C., Pettit, M., Wynne, R., & Evarts, E. V. (1959). A comparison of the psychological effects of acute and chronic administration of chlorpromazine and secobarbital in schizophrenic patients. *Journal of Mental Science, 105*, 190–198.

Kovitz, B., Carter, J. T., & Addison, W. P. (1955). A comparison of chlorpromazine and reserpine in chronic psychosis. *A.M.A. Archives of Neurology and Psychiatry, 74*, 467–471.

Kusumo, K. S., & Vaughn, M. (1977). Effects of lithium salts on memory. *British Journal of Psychiatry, 131*, 453–457.

Legg, J. S., & Stiff, M. P. (1976). Drug related test patterns of depressed patients. *Psychopharmacology, 50*, 205–210.

Lloyd, D. N., & Newbrough, J. R. (1964). Sensory changes with phenothiazine medication in schizophrenic patients. *Journal of Nervous and Mental Disease, 139*, 169–175.

Loo, H., Bonnel, J., Etevenon, P., Benyacoub, J., & Slowen, P. (1981). Intellectual efficiency in manic–depressive patients treated with lithium. *Acta Psychiatrica Scandinavica, 64*, 423–430.

Lovett Doust, J. W., Lewis, D. J., Miller, A., Sprott, D., & Wright, R. L. D. (1959). Controlled assessment of antidepressant drugs, including Tofranil. *Canadian Psychiatric Association Journal, 4*, S190–194.

Malone, J. R. L., & Hemsley, D. R. (1977). Lowered responsiveness and auditory signal detectabilty during depression. *Psychological Medicine, 7*, 717–722.

Marder, S. R., Asarnow, R. F., & Van Putten, T. (1984). Information processing and neuroleptic response in acute and stabilized schizophrenic patients. *Psychiatry Research, 13*, 41–49.

Marusarz, T. Z., Wolpert, E. A., & Koh, S. D. (1981). Memory processing with lithium carbonate. *Journal of Clinical Psychiatry, 42*, 190–192.

Mason-Browne, N. O., & Borthwick, J. W. (1957). The effects of perphenazine (Trilafon) on modification of crude consciousness. *Diseases of the Nervous System, 18*, 300–306.

McCreadie, R. G., & Morrison, D. P. (1985). The impact of lithium in south-west Scotland. I. Demographic and clinical findings. *British Journal of Psychiatry, 146*, 70–80.

Medalia, A., Gold, J., & Merriam, A. (1988). The effects of neuroleptics on neuropsychological test results of schizophrenics. *Journal of Clinical Neuropsychology, 3*, 249–271.

Meltzer, H. Y., Kane, J. M., & Kolakowska, T. (1983). Plasma levels of neuroleptics, prolactin levels, and clinical response. In J. T. Coyle & S. J. Enna (Eds.), *Neuroleptics: Neurochemical, behavioral, and clinical perspectives* (pp. 255–280). New York: Raven Press.

Muller-Oerlinghausen, B., Bauer, H., Girke, W., Kanowski, S., & Gonclaves, N. (1977). Impairment of vigilance and performance under lithium-treatment. Studies in patients and normal volunteers. *Pharmakopsychiatrie-Neuropsychopharmakologie, 10*, 67–78.

Neuchterlein, K. H., & Dawson, M. E. (1984). Information processing and attentional functioning in the developmental course of schizophrenic disorders. *Schizophrenia Bulletin, 10*, 160-›03.

Oltmanns, T. F., Ohayon, J., & Neale, J. M. (1979). The effect of medication and diagnostic criteria on distractibility in schizophrenia. *Journal of Psychiatric Research, 14*, 81–91.

Orzack, M. H., Kornetsky, C., & Freeman, H. (1967). The effects of daily administration of carphenazine on attention in the schizophrenic patient. *Psychopharmacologia, 11*, 31–38.

Pearl, D. (1962). Phenothiazine effects in chronic schizophrenia. *Journal of Clinical Psychology, 18*, 86–89.

Perlick, D., Stastny, P., Katz, I., Mayer, M., & Mattis, S. (1986). Memory deficits and anticholinergic levels in chronic schizophrenia. *American Journal of Psychiatry, 143*, 230–232.

Petrie, A., & Le Beau, J. (1956). Psychological changes in man after chlorpromazine and certain types of brain surgery. *Journal of Clinical and Experimental Psychopathology, 17*, 170–179.

Pishkin, V. (1962). CPT and VCRT performances as functions of imipramine and nialamide. *Journal of Clinical Psychology, 18*, 83–86.

Porteus, S. D. (1957). Maze test reactions after chlorpromazine. *Journal of Consulting Psychology, 21*, 15–20.

Porteus, S. D., & Barclay, J. E. (1957). A further note on chlorpromazine: Maze reactions. *Journal of Consulting Psychology, 21*, 297–299.

Preodor, D., Wolpert, G. Y., Ostrow, D., Holinger, P., & Wolpert, E. A. (1977). Memory loss with lithium treatment. *American Journal of Psychiatry, 134*, 1047–1048.

Pugh, L. A. (1968). Response time and electrodermal measure in chronic schizophrenia: The effects of chlorpromazine. *Journal of Nervous and Mental Disease, 146*, 62–70.

Rapp, M. S., & Thomas, M. R. (1979). Lithium and memory loss. *Canadian Journal of Psychiatry, 24*, 700–701.

Raskin, A., Friedman, A. S., & DiMascio, A. (1983). Effects of chlorpromazine, imipramine, diazepam, and phenelzine on psychomotor and cognitive skills of depressed patients. *Psychopharmacology Bulletin, 19*, 649–652.

Ray, T. S., Ragland, R. E., & Clark, M. L. (1964). Chlorpromazine in chronic schizophrenic women: Comparison of different effects on various psychological modalities during and after treatment. *Journal of Nervous and Mental Disease, 138*, 348–353.

Reus, V., Targum, S. D., Weingartner, H., & Post, R. M. (1979). Effect of lithium carbonate on memory processes of bipolar affectively ill patients. *Psychopharmacology, 63*, 39–42.

Riddle, M., & Roberts, A. H. (1978). Psychosurgery and the Porteus Maze Tests. *Archives of General Psychiatry, 35*, 493–497.

Rogers, D., Lees, A. J., Smith, E., Trimble, M., & Stern, G. M. (1987). Bradyphrenia in Parkinson's disease and psychomotor retardation in depressive illness. *Brain, 110*, 761–776.

Rosofsky, I., Levin, S., & Holzman, P. S. (1982). Psychomotility in the functional psychosis. *Journal of Abnormal Psychology, 91*, 71–74.

Savard, R. J., Rey, A. C., & Post, R. M. (1980). Halstead–Reitan Category Test in bipolar and unipolar affective disorders. *Journal of Nervous and Mental Disease, 168*, 297–304.

Schooler, N. R., & Goldberg, S. C. (1972). Performance tests in a study of phenothiazines in schizophrenia: Caveats and conclusions. *Psychopharmacologia, 24*, 81–98.

Schou, M. (1968). Lithium in psychiatric therapy and prophylaxis. *Journal of Psychiatric Research, 6*, 67–95.

Seppala, T., Linnoila, M., & Mattila, M. J. (1978). Psychomotor skills in depressed outpatients treated with L-tryptophan, doxepin or chlormipramine. *Annals of Clinical Research, 10*, 241–221.

Serafetinides, E. A., & Clark, M. L. (1973). Psychological effects of single dose antipsychotic medication. *Biological Psychiatry, 7*, 263–267.

Serafetinides, E. A., Collins, S., & Clark, M. L. (1972). Haloperidol, clopenthixol, and chlorpromazine in chronic schizophrenia. *Journal of Nervous and Mental Disease, 154*, 31–42.

Shatin, L., Rockmore, L., & Funk, I. C. (1956). Response of psychiatric patients to massive doses of Thorazine: II. Psychological test performance and comparative drug evaluation. *Psychiatric Quarterly, 30*, 402–416.

Shaw, E. D., Stokes, P. E., Mann, J. J., & Manevitz, A. Z. A. (1987). Effects of lithium carbonate on the memory and motor speed of bipolar outpatients. *Journal of Abnormal Psychology, 96*, 64–69.

Silberman, E. K., Weingartner, H., & Post, R. M. (1983). Thinking disorder in depression. *Archives of General Psychiatry, 40*, 775–780.

Simon, S. H. (1967). Effects of tranquilizers on the Trail Making Test with chronic schizophrenics. *Journal of Consulting Psychology, 31*, 322–323.

Small, I. F., Small, J. G., Milstein, V., & Moore, J. E. (1972). Neuropsychological observations with psychosis and somatic treatment. *Journal of Nervous and Mental Disease, 155*, 6–13.

Smigan, L., & Perris, C. (1983). Memory functions and prophylactic treatment with lithium. *Psychological Medicine, 13*, 529–536.

Snow, L. H., & Rickels, K. (1964). The controlled evaluation of imipramine and amitriptyline in hospitalized depressed psychiatric patients. *Psychopharmacologia, 5*, 409–416.

Spiegal, D. E., & Spiegal, P. K. (1967). The effects of carphenazine, trifluoperazine, and chlorpromazine on ward behavior, physiological functioning, and psychological test scores in chronic schizophrenic patients. *Journal of Nervous and Mental Disease, 144*, 111–116.

Spohn, H. E., LaCoursiere, R. B., Thompson, K., & Coyne, L. (1977). phenothiazine effect son psychological and physiological dysfunction in chronic schizophrenics. *Archives of General Psychiatry, 34*, 633–644.

Spohn, H. E., Coyne, L., LaCoursiere, R., Mazur, D., & Hayes, K. (1985). Relation of neuroleptic dose and tardive dyskinesia to attention, information-processing, and psychophysiology in mediated schizophrenics. *Archives of General Psychiatry, 42*, 849–859.

Squire, L. R., Judd, L. L., Janowsky, D. S., & Huey, L. Y. (1980). Effects of lithium carbonate on memory and other cognitive functions. *American Journal of Psychiatry, 137*, 1042–1046.

Staton, R. D., Wilson, H., & Brumback, R. A. (1981). Cognitive improvement associated with tricyclic antidepressant therapy. *International Journal of Neuroscience, 24*, 307–312.

Sternberg, D. E., & Jarvik, M. E. (1976). Memory functions in depression. *Archives of General Psychiatry, 33*, 219–224.

Strauss, M., Lew, M., Coyle, J., & Tune, L. (1985). Psychopharmacologic and clinical correlates of attention in chronic schizophrenia. *American Journal of Psychiatry, 142*, 497–499.

Telford, R., & Worrall, E. P. (1978). Cognitive functions in manic–depressives: Effects of lithium and physostigmine. *British Journal of Psychiatry, 133*, 424–428.

Tourlentes, T. T., Hunsiker, A. L., & Hurd, D. E. (1958). Chlorpromazine and communication processes. *Archives of Neurology and Psychiatry, 79*, 468–472.

Tune, L., Strauss, M., Lew, M., Breitlinger, E., & Coyle, J. T. (1982). Serum levels of anticholinergic drugs and impaired recent memory in chronic schizophrenic patients. *American Journal of Psychiatry, 139*, 1460–1462.

Walker, E. (1981). Attentional and neuromotor functions of schizophrenics, schizoaffectives, and patients with other affective disorders. *Archives of General Psychiatry, 38*, 1355–1358.

Walker, E., & Green, M. (1982). Motor proficiency and attentional task performance of psychotic patients. *Journal of Abnormal Psychology, 91,* 261–268.

Walker, E., & Shaye, J. (1982). Familial schizophrenia: A predictor of neuromotor and attentional abnormalities in schizophrenia. *Archives of General Psychiatry, 39,* 1153–1156.

Weaver, L. A., & Brooks. G. W. (1961). The effects of drug-induced Parkinsonism on the psychomotor performance of chronic schizophrenics. *Journal of Nervous and Mental Disease, 133,* 148–154.

Weckowicz, T. E., Tam, C. N. I., Mason, J., & Bay, K. S. (1978). Speed in test performance in depressed patients. *Journal of Abnormal Psychology, 87,* 578–582.

Whitehead, W. A., & Thune, L. E. (1958). The effects of chlorpromazine on learning in chronic psychotics. *Journal of Consulting Psychology, 22,* 379–383.

Wilson, H., & Staton, R. D. (1984). Neuropsychological changes in children associated with tricyclic antidepressant therapy. *International Journal of Neuroscience, 24,* 307–312.

Winter, W. D., & Frederickson, W. (1956). The short-term effects of chlorpromazine on psychiatric patients. *Journal of Consulting Psychology, 20,* 431–434.

Wittenborn, J. R., Plante, M., Burgess, F., & Livermore, N. (1961*a*). The efficacy of electroconvulsive therapy, iproniazid and placebo in the treatment of young depressed women. *Journal of Nervous and Mental Disease, 133,* 316–332.

Wittenborn, J. R., Plante, M., Burgess, F., & Maurer, H. (1961*b*). A comparison of imipramine, electroconvulsive therapy and placebo in the treatment of depressions. *Journal of Nervous and Mental Disease, 135,* 131–137.

17

Neuropsychological Toxicology

DAVID E. HARTMAN

INTRODUCTION

The field of neuropsychological toxicology is a relatively recent offshoot of clinical neuropsychology that unites a variety of neuropsychological studies concerned with endogenous or exogenous toxin exposure. The substances capable of investigation by psychometric neuropsychological methods are as familiar as alcohol, and as obscure as aliphatic hydrocarbons. Some, like alcohol, lead, or toluene, have been the subjects of frequent investigation. Alternatively, little is known about the neuropsychological effects of other neurotoxicants, including allergens, biological toxins, many pharmaceuticals, industrial wastes, or even many commonly abused drugs, e.g., cocaine, PCP. The common thread tying these substances to a field called *neuropsychological toxicology* is that each substance is capable of inducing nervous system impairment, and those impairments can be detected by neuropsychological measures.

What sets neuropsychological toxicology somewhat apart from conventional neuropsychology is its explicit link with neurochemistry, toxicology, and occupational medicine; these are the interconnected net of specialties that support this new behavioral science. In neuropsychological toxicology, neuropsychologists have a common vocabulary to discuss an enormous range of substances capable of causing behavior change and amenable to investigation, including metals, solvents, pesticides, and abused or prescription drugs.

A complete enumeration of neurotoxic industrial substances, mixtures, and compounds is not known, primarily because the capacity of industry to produce new materials has far outstripped the ability of researchers to test them. According to Landrigan, Kreiss, Xintaras, Feldman, and Heath (1980) there are "[m]ore than 1000 new compounds . . . developed each year in addition to the

DAVID E. HARTMAN • Department of Psychiatry, Cook County Hospital, University of Illinois Medical Center, Chicago, Illinois 60612-9985.

HANDBOOK OF NEUROPSYCHOLOGICAL ASSESSMENT: A Biopsychosocial Perspective, edited by Antonio E. Puente and Robert J. McCaffrey. Plenum Press, New York, 1992.

approximately 40,000 chemicals and 2,000,000 mixtures, formulations and blends already in industrial use" (p. 43). Any of the hundreds of prescription or abused drugs that affect consciousness or affect must be added to the total of neurotoxic substances.

Similarly large numbers of medical patients are at cognitive risk from legitimate intake of pharmaceuticals. Many common prescription drugs, including steroids, tranquilizers, oncology medications, and others, cause detectable deficits in neuropsychological function; some severe enough to contraindicate or constrain their use.

Added to that total are more than 18 million problem drinkers in the United States alone. Constant and voluntary exposure to ethanol can be a subtle or severe assault upon the nervous system, and costs U.S. society an estimated $43 billion a year. Drug abusers make up a fourth large and disparate group who voluntarily expose themselves to brain-damaging substances. A 1987 survey of high school seniors found that almost 7% had used intoxicating inhalants (e.g., glue sniffing) and in certain Mexican communities these deadly neurotoxins are used *daily* by 22% of minors (Crider & Rouse, 1988). Drug abuse causes economic losses of at least $10 billion each year in the United States (Rufener *et al.*, 1977).

Thus, the real world contains a large cohort of neurotoxic exposure victims, both involuntary and voluntary, and there remains a "great need for the systematic development of longitudinal studies of the natural history and progression of CNS changes accompanying toxic exposure" (White & Feldman, 1987, p. 396). The demand for such studies is impelled by more than abstract curiosity. Millions of workers are exposed to *known* neurotoxins, while untold numbers work with industrial substances that have not even been tested for neurotoxicity. Neuropsychological methods are needed to track acute and longitudinal changes of cognitive function in these individuals, both for diagnostic and for rehabilitative purposes. The need for neuropsychological techniques is impelled by both real world concerns about the cognitive functioning and safety of exposed individuals as well as epidemiology, although the huge numbers of exposure victims provide an immediate mandate to proceed with human studies.

Despite large numbers of individuals exposed to this enormous chemical cornucopia, concerted neuropsychological investigations of neurotoxicants began quite recently, reflecting increased interest and coordinated effort among the disciplines of neuropsychology, neurology, and industrial medicine. While progress has been rapid during the past decade, significant knowledge gaps remain at all levels of investigation, from the biochemical to the neuropsychological. There is frustration that progress has been

> surely too slow with respect to the needs of our society where the great majority of occupational and environmental chemicals . . . are primarily neurotoxic. [Maroni & Barbieri, 1989]

Explaining the Delayed Collaboration of Neuropsychology and Toxicology

Given such a vast array of substances and individuals potentially affected, it seems curious that neuropsychologists would have ignored or failed to understand the need for relevant investigations until quite recently. The omission is more understandable when interpreted against the background of neuropsychology's historical development.

First, the historical concerns of neurology influenced neuropsychological areas of investigation. It is not surprising that modern neuropsychologists followed their neurological forebears in analyzing localizable cortical damage. From the arbitrary localization schemas of Gall and Spurzheim in the 19th century, neuroanatomists were led by Paul Broca, Carl Wernicke, and especially by the English neurologist John Hughlings Jackson into ever more subtle and complex theories of cortical localization and its relation to behavior. Alexander Luria, perhaps the most creative and influential systematizer in modern clinical neuropsychology, contributed to this effort.

> The neuropsychologist who is confronted by [disturbances in functional brain systems] must first ascertain what factors are actually involved in the particular mental activity and what *structures* of the brain constitute its neuronal basis. These two problems can only be solved by comparison of all the symptoms which arise in *lesions of one strictly localized focus* in the cortex (or subcortex) . . . and by a thorough analysis of the character of a disturbance of this system by *brain lesions in different locations* . . . [italics added] [Luria, 1973, p. 39]

Neuropsychology might have developed a tradition of neurotoxic investigation as early as the beginning of the 20th century, but abandoned these diffuse disorders after it became enamored by higher cortical function localization in the 1950s. During the first third of the 20th century, mental function *deterioration* and not localization was the dominant paradigm in neuropsychology (e.g., Babcock, 1930). Psychologists were applying the tools of Wundt, Cattell, and the mental testing movement to the study of abnormal or deteriorated mental states. Many of those investigations were of cognitive functions under artificially induced states of neurotoxic impairment. For example, cognitive tests were performed with subjects under the influence of alcohol, paraldehyde, trional, bromide of sodium, and caffeine (Hoch, 1904). Carbon monoxide exposure was also the subject of investigation.

Such rudimentary neuropsychological explorations of acute neurotoxicity might have blossomed into more elaborate neuropsychological investigations were it not for an alteration in neuropsychological canon in the latter half of the 20th century.

Beginning with Ward Halstead, neuropsychology was strongly propelled toward behavioral analysis of higher cortical localization of brain injury. Halstead was a vocal proponent of using mental testing apparatus for the purpose of localization, lateralization, and lesion detection. As Matarazzo (1972) relates,

> Apparently so sure was Halstead that the psychological assessment techniques he and others were developing could help in effectively differentiating the brain-damaged individual from the patient who was not brian-damaged that he soon began to concentrate his research efforts, instead, on attempting to localize more precisely such lesions within the brain. [p. 384]

Parsons's reminiscence of Halstead's 1951 talk at Worcester State Hospital corroborates Matarazzo:

> The results of his research, [Halstead] averred, enabled him to predict lesions in the brain with great accuracy. . . . Afterwards, most of us shook our heads and said that it was too good to be true, that brain functions were not as localizable as he was portraying them. . . . [1986, p. 156]

Dr. Halstead's most famous graduate student, Ralph Reitan, is similarly cited for his contributions toward lateralizing and localizing brain damage. Initial studies began by discriminating the presence or absence of brain damage (Reitan, 1955), and were followed by investigations into the "lateralization, localization, nature, and type of lesion" (Reitan, 1964, cited in Parsons, 1970, p. 6). When Parsons visited Reitan in 1957, he found Reitan "busily concerned with identification of the lesion, lateralization, localization, and ultimately the prediction of the type of lesion" (1986, p. 157). Russell, Neuringer, and Goldstein (1970) indicated that "much of Reitan's later work . . . has been devoted to the study of localized brain damage, especially lateralization" (1970, p. 24).

Such assiduous emphasis on localization, lateralization, and lesion detection helped steer neuropsychological interest toward analysis of focal lesion states and consign everything else to a wastebasket of "diffuse" disorders. Emphasis on higher cortical function and localization of behavioral abnormalities also produced an understandable spate of research in topics that fit the model. Open and closed head injury, brain tumor, cerebrovascular accident, arteriovenous malformations, focal seizure disorders, and other types of lateralizable, localizable cortical injuries could be analyzed in their relationship to behavioral abnormalities. Brain damage without clearly defined lesion states (e.g., alcohol) was analyzed according to the same criteria, i.e., whether the lesion was diffuse or focal, lateralized to a particular hemisphere, and whether or not it caused discernible brain lesions.

This emphasis on what I have termed the *3L*'s in neuropsychology (localization, lateralization, and lesion detection) had both positive and negative consequences for the field. On one hand, the *3L* worldview encouraged validation of neuropsychological methods in general, and defined important neurobehavioral sequelae for many disorders of higher cortical function.

Just as inevitably, however, *3L* philosophy gave psychologists no conceptual basis upon which to investigate (or even find interesting) lesions that did not have a discrete cortical locus. Neurochemical and toxicological diseases in particular, because of their subtle and diffuse effects, did not fit easily within the "3L" *zeitgeist*. Neither did drug effects, Parkinson's disease, or psychiatric disorders triggered by abnormal neurochemical states.

Thus, neuropsychological analysis of neurotoxic syndromes had a promising beginning in the first decade of the 20th century when analysis of mental function and nonspecific deteriorations were subjects of interest. When neuropsychologists shifted their interest to behavioral correlates of higher cortical function during the 1950s–1970s, the result was relatively less interest in diffuse lesions or extracortical injuries.

Neuropsychology's rediscovery of neurotoxicity began with pioneering studies in Scandinavia (e.g., Hanninen, 1971). While some early investigations suffered from methodological insufficiencies, increasing numbers and quality of available studies have had a profound influence on neuropsychology, expanding both its perspective and its utility. The price of this expansion was the acceptance of a neuroscientific outlook that transcends *3L* neuropsychology. While knowledge of structural brain abnormalities caused by various toxins is important (see Table 17.1), localizable brain aberration is but one route to neuropsychological impairment. Other factors capable of influencing neuropsychological performance include general systemic health factors, neurochemical integrity, neuroendocrine function, pharmacology, and the type of toxic effects exerted by the toxicant under study. The emphasis is clearly more holistic than *3L* neuropsychology since

> . . . [A]scertaining how an organism responds to toxic insult . . . often requires correlating *biochemical* endpoints to observed *behavioral*, *morphological*, *pharmacological and/or physiological* changes. [italics added] [Mailman & Lewis, 1987, p. 132]

Neuropsychologists participate in this multidisciplinary diagnostic effort by measuring the cognitive, affective, and neurobehavioral correlates of biochemical and pharmacological lesions caused by toxic insult. In order to do so, it is necessary to have some basic understanding of the mechanisms underlying neurotoxic damage.

Basic Knowledge

Any new field of inquiry requires its own basic vocabulary and neuropsychological toxicology is no different in this regard than any other subspecialization of clinical neuropsychology. In addition to the highly summarized material provided here, neuropsychologists without backgrounds in the field will find it useful to peruse general introductions of neurotoxic effects in books by Goetz (1985) and Hartman (1988*b*). The former does not review neuropsychological investigations but provides useful clinical and biological data. The latter reviews neuropsychological methodology, research, and case studies in neuropsychological toxicology. Other useful texts for basic toxicology and biochemistry include *Experimental and Clinical Neurotoxicology* (Spencer & Schaumburg, 1980), *Cognitive Neurochemistry* (Stahl, Iversen, & Goodman, 1987), and *Toxicology: The Basic Science of Poisons* (Klaassen, Amdur, & Doull, 1986). Basic principles of neurochemistry and neuroscience are available in *Principles of Neural Science*

TABLE 17.1. Nervous System Loci for Selected Neurotoxins[a]

Cortical gray matter	Subthalamus	Schwann cells
Azide	Azide	Acrylamide
Barbiturate	Carbon monoxide	Carbon disulfide
Carbon disulfide	Manganese	DDT
Cyanide	Internal capsule	Iminodipropionitrile
Lead	Azide	Isoniazide
Mercury	Carbon monoxide	Lead
Methyl bromide	Corpus callosum	Vinca alkaloids
Nitrogen trichloride	Azide	Sensory N. thalamus
Hippocampus	Carbon monoxide	Acetylpyridine
Acetylpyridine	Cyanide	Glutamate
Azide	Hexachlorophene	Lead
Barbiturate	Isoniazide	Mercury (organic)
Carbon monoxide	Lead	Anterior horn
Cyanide	Malononitrile	Carbon disulfide
Caudate/putamen	Triethyltin	Cyanide
Barbiturate	Optic chiasm	Iminodipropionitrile
Carbon disulfide	Barbiturate	Isoniazide
Cyanide	Carbon monoxide	Lead
Malononitrile	Cyanide	Vinca alkaloids
Manganese	Hexachlorophene	Hypothal. Vent. N.
Nitrogen trichloride	Isoniazid	Glutamate
Globus pallidus	Lead	Gold thioglucose
Carbon monoxide	Malononitrile	Mammillary bodies
Cyanide	Triethyltin	Nitrogen trichloride
Gold thioglucose		Tegmentum
Manganese		Azide
Methyl bromide		Cyanide
		Nitrogen trichloride

[a]After Northon (1986)

(Kandel & Schwartz, 1985). A third source of material is the extensive government data base of toxic substance effects available from OSHA (Occupational Safety and Health Administration), NIOSH (National Institute of Occupational Safety and Health), and NIDA (National Institute for Drug Abuse). Readings, coupled with actual patient examinations give the interested neuropsychologist an adequate perspective concerning neurotoxic effects on neuropsychological function. Failure to acquire such knowledge inevitably impairs credibility, as was the case in a skeptical evaluation of the field by a neuropsychologist who admitted that he had never heard of solvent-induced dementia (Bieliauskas, 1990).

BIOLOGICAL RATIONALE FOR NEUROPSYCHOLOGICAL TOXICOLOGY

Such skepticism sometimes results from difficulty bridging the gap between the toxicology laboratory and the realm of clinical neuropsychology. Most neuropsychologists have no background in biochemistry or toxicology, and many practitioners would argue that a detailed background in these areas has never been necessary for competence in the field. As has been argued earlier in this chapter, however, the sheer numbers of potential neurotoxicants in the natural and industrial environments provide a mandate to proceed with clinical and research investigations. Thus, it has *become* necessary for neuropsychologists to adapt and strengthen their own discipline by acquiring a working knowledge of modern neuroscience as it applies to neurotoxic exposure effects.

The information presented in this chapter emphasizes the need for a psychobiological rationale to understanding neurotoxic exposure. Readers who find the information presented in this chapter too rudimentary share the author's frustration at the lack of research bridging the gap between basic theory and neuropsychological function. This audience is urged to survey the relevant occupational medicine, neurological, and psychiatric literature on toxic exposure, to provide some of the multidisciplinary perspective that is required.

Alteratively, those who feel daunted by the scope of new knowledge acquisition may be reassured by the knowledge that toxicological and neurochemical variables are only two of the many factors contributing to a neuropsychological end-state. The neuropsychologist with clinical expertise in the social, personality, and cognitive components of behavior already has many of the prerequisites needed for participation in neuropsychological toxicology.

Neurobiology and Neurotoxicity

Environmental and naturally occurring neurotoxins are coming to be viewed as capable of damaging chemical transmission of nerve impulses in the central and peripheral nervous system. The central nervous system is protected from damage by the blood–brain barrier, possibly including glial and endothelial cells. The peripheral nervous system is not so completely protected; however, both central and peripheral nervous systems are at risk from neurotoxic damage from several types of injury. *Anoxia* is one of the principal mechanisms of damage; neurons are especially sensitive to oxygen deprivation and need as much as ten times the oxygen of nearby glial cells (Ruscak, Ruscakova, & Hager, 1968).

Norton (1986) described three types of anoxia from neurotoxic exposure:

- *Anoxic anoxia*: from inadequate oxygen supply in the presence of adequate blood flow. Carbon monoxide poisoning is a common example, since oxygen is preferentially replaced in the hemoglobin molecule by unusable CO.
- *Ischemic anoxia*: any loss of oxygen caused by decrease in arterial blood flow. Any substance capable of causing hypotension or interfering with cardiac function may indirectly cause nervous system damage via ischemic anoxia. Cyanide's capability of causing hypotension is an example.
- *Cytotoxic anoxia*: is the result of direct interference with cell metabolism while oxygen and blood supply remain normal. Cyanide is also a culprit in cytotoxic anoxia, causing damage to both gray and white matter.

Each type of anoxia in turn is capable of gradually increasing cellular damage, via loss of mitochondrial granules and edema. Cerebral edema, in turn, further worsens hypoxia and results in accumulation of lactate, ammonia, and inorganic phosphates.

Synaptic Damage from Neurotoxicants

In the synapse, degradation of neurotransmission can occur at any level of *presynaptic* process, including transmitter synthesis, storage, release, and termination of neurotransmitters (Atchison, 1989). Neurotoxicants may also affect the nerve on the *receptor* end of the synapse, including transmitter binding to the receptor cell; "activation of the receptor associated ionic channel, and degradation of chemical transmitter" (Atchison, 1989, p. 393). Lead has a direct effect on synaptic action by presynaptic block of the end-plate potential and may also interfere with enzyme inhibition at several sites (Goetz, 1985).

Cellular Damage from Neurotoxicants

Central and peripheral nervous system structures appear to be differentially sensitive to toxic damage (O'Callaghan, 1989). In animal studies, it is possible to measure differential responses of nervous system cells to toxic damage by measuring the proteins unique to each type of cell. *Trimethyl tin*, for example, causes extensive damage to certain areas of the rat hippocampus and cell protein degradations unique to those areas can be observed (O'Callaghan, 1989). One of the principal neurotoxic effects of *mercury* is said to be related to that metal's inhibition of protein and RNA synthesis. *Toluene*, in rat brain studies, produces a 50% reduction of catecholaminergic neurons after 4 weeks of exposure to 250 and 1000 ppm toluene (Bjornaes & Naalsund, 1988). Human studies have corroborated similar cellular damage. For example, Rosenberg, Spitz, Filley, Davis, and Schaumberg (1988) performed magnetic resonance imaging (MRI) scans of 11 chronic toluene abusers. Three subjects had abnormal MRIs with "diffuse, cerebral, cerebellar, and brainstem atrophy" that ranged in severity from mild to marked. Ventricular dilation was also seen, and other MRI findings suggested severe white matter damage. No improvement was observed on repeated MRI scans over an 18-month follow-up period, suggesting that toluene-induced physical injury to the brain may be irreversible.

Subcellular components are also differentially sensitive to neurotoxic damage. Nissl substance, a structure with high ribosome content, has been shown to be destroyed by methyl mercury. The small numbers of ribosomes in cerebellar and cerebrocoritical neurons may explain why those areas are so easily affected by mercury poisoning. Chronic heroin intoxication has also been shown to affect Nissl substance in primate studies (Hirano & Llena, 1980). This suggests that Nissl substance-damaging neurotoxicants may affect the cells' ability to synthesize protein and thus regenerate or repair itself. Other structures of the cell known to be differentially affected by neurotoxicants include mitochondria (LSD-25, heroin), neurofibrils (aluminum, colchicine, vinca alkaloids), and the synapse (glutamate, organic mercury) (Hirano & Llena, 1980).

Damage to various components of white matter has also been tied to specific neurotoxins, including acrylamide, alcohol, triethyl tin, *n*-hexane, methyl *n*-butyl ketone, 2,5-hexanedione, arsenic, carbon disulfide, and tri-ortho-cresyl phosphate (Hirano & Llena, 1980). White matter is vulnerable to a variety of neurotoxicity-related effects, including ischemia with ensuing demyelination or direct toxic injury to the underlying axon.

While subcellular damage as a function of neurotoxicants may seem rather far from the neuropsychologist's domain, knowledge of neurotoxin-specific cell damage has two benefits. First, it takes neurotoxic exposure out of the mystical realm of "diffuse" disorders. Second, detailed knowledge of the neurostructural basis of toxin exposure cannot help but increase understanding of the behavioral impairment that ensues.

Neurochemical Damage from Neurotoxicants

Neurochemical damage is perhaps the most interesting frontier in neuropsychology. A wide range of clinical syndromes are better understood by the damage they exert on neurochemical tracts rather than on structure in the way that neuropsychologists typically think of the term (e.g., lobes, sulci, hemisphere). Parkinson's disease, for example, is a clinical syndrome where dopaminergic neurons from the pigmented nuclei of the substantia nigra and locus coeruleus are selectively and severely damaged. These nuclei project to the striatum, the limbic system (nucleus accumbens, olfactory tubercle, and amygdala) as well as the frontal cortex (Cote & Crutcher, 1985). Among other symptoms, Parkinson's "profoundly disrupts" the motor act control mechanisms of the prefrontal cortex (Goldman-Rakic, 1987). Without understanding the cognitive neurochemistry of Parkinson's the neuropsychologist is left to explain a diffuse and apparently unconnected set of deficits, including impaired voluntary movement, flattened affect, and eventual dementia. In linking Parkinson's to specific correlates of neurochemical lesion, however, the relationship of behavior to brain damage is far more consistent and interpretable. Goldman-Rakic (1987) argues that catecholamine impairments in dopamine and norepinephrine systems may explain a variety of behavioral disorders. By extension, neuropsychological deficits resulting from a wide range of disorders, including those from neurotoxicants, may be rendered more understandable via an analysis of cognitive neurochemistry.

Solvent exposure is a particular case in point. Heretofore, clinical neuropsychologists attempting to explain how highly lipophilic substances like solvents affect the nervous system could find no markers to structurally "localize" their effects. This led to rather uninteresting characterizations of industrial solvent toxicity as a "diffuse" problem.

Reconceptualizing the systemic nervous effects of solvents and other neurotoxicants as *neurochemical* toxins would allow subsequent neurobehavioral comparison based on neurotransmitter systems rather than physical topographic damage. Recent evidence suggests that many common neurotoxins act upon brain neurochemistry to produce neurotoxic abnormalities in cognition, affect, or behavior. For example, many common *solvents* "recognize dopamine as a selectively vulnerable target suggest[ing] that dopamine depletion . . . may have a role in solvent toxicity to the CNS" (Mutti & Franchini, 1987, p. 722) and may explain certain reversible impairments in human vigilance, psychomotor speed, and mood (Mutti, Falzio, Romanelli, Bocchi, Ferroni, & Franchini, 1988). Freed and Kandel (1988) reviewed animal and human data suggesting that selective attention is mediated by the locus coeruleus and its principal neurotransmitter, norepinephrine (NE). When dopamine-β-hydroxylase (an enzyme involved in the production of NE) is inhibited, the result is a transient amnesia related to changes in NE levels. Inhibition of β-hydroxylase is also one consequence of carbon disulfide exposure, a highly neurotoxic solvent (Costa, 1988). It is possible that further investigations of solvents may produce useful correlations between neurotransmitter dysfunction and neuropsychological impairment.

Many *pesticides* inhibit the normal degradation of neurotransmitters as a principal neurotoxic effect. For example, organophosphates and carbamates inhibit (possibly irreversibly) the enzyme acetylcholinesterase, whose function would ordinarily be to break down acetylcholine. The toxic effects of these pesticides, then, are due to the overstimulation of the cholinergic system by an excess amount of acetylcholine. Disorders of other neurochemical pathways have also been implicated in *organophosphate* pesticide exposure, including noncholinergic systems involving biogenic amines, glutamic acid, γ-aminobutyric acid, cyclic nucleotides, and others. These systems "may play important roles in the initiation, continuation and disappearance of organophosphorus cholinesterase inhibitor-induced neurotoxicity" (Ho, 1988, p. 151).

Much has been learned from the psychiatric literature about the behavioral consequences of cholinergic abnormalities. For example, anticholinergic drugs may cause delirium, agitation, and can cause a toxic psychosis that mimics dementia. Memory deficits are common consequences of neuroleptic medications with anticholinergic effects as well as the antiparkinsonian drugs with which they are often paired (e.g., Tune, Strauss, Lew, Breitlinger, & Coyle, 1982; Perlick, Stastny, Katz, Mayer, & Mattis, 1986). Both types of medications have anticholinergic properties (Hartman, 1988*b*). Since cognitive impairment over time cannot be tied to serum anticholinergic level, the use of neuropsychological tests may provide important information about the clinical extent of cholinergic impairment long after initial biochemical markers have ceased to be diagnostic.

Viewing neurotoxicants as neurochemical toxins may also facilitate insight into nonindustrial neuropsychological abnormalities. Attention deficit disorder, long considered the most nebulous of neuropsychological deficits from a structural viewpoint, becomes a more interesting target of investigation when viewed as an abnormality of noradrenergic or dopaminergic metabolism (Oades, 1987; Freed & Kandel, 1988). Even classically "functional" conditions like posttraumatic stress disorder may prove to have neurochemical substrates

(Kolb, 1987). Analysis of system neurochemistry in these disorders may generate useful neuropsychological hypotheses and help direct subsequent investigations of those systems.

Neurochemical abnormalities do not have to involve direct destruction of neurotransmitter systems to produce neurotoxic damage. Impairments may be produced via general inhibition of metabolic processes. *Lead*, for example, is capable of disrupting brain enzymes, including Na, K-ATPase, which is indirectly responsible for maintaining cellular fluid balance and action potentials (Bertoni & Sprenkle, 1988). Disruption of this enzyme, then, could allow the cerebral edema seen in severe lead poisoning. Bertoni and Sprenkle (1988) traced the effects of acute lead injection into animal subjects. One lead injection produced generalized decreases in cerebral glucose metabolism. Significant reductions were also discovered in local cerebral metabolism in the medial geniculate bodies, inferior colliculus, and the sensory cortex. The auditory cortex appeared to be particularly at risk, a finding that has also been seen in a 5-year electrophysiological study of children by Otto, Robinson, Baumann, Schroeder, Mushak, Kleinbaum, and Boone (1985). The authors suggested that lead exposure shows preferential neurotoxicity in areas of highly active glucose metabolism, Na, K-ATPase activity, or high synaptic densities.

One of the most striking cases of toxin-induced neurochemical damage comes from the victims of 1-methyl-4-phenyl-1,2,3,6-tetrahydropyridine (MPTP). Northern California users of this inaccurately distilled "designer-drug" heroin analogue developed parkinsonian symptoms after MPTP destroyed dopaminergic neurons in the substantia nigra and possibly the locus coeruleus. Neuropsychological consequences of MPTP were similar to those found in idiopathic Parkinsonism, including perceptual motor and frontal lobe dysfunction (Stern & Langston, 1985). The exact neurochemical etiology of this process remains unclear, but Bleecker (1988) speculated that a conversion product of MPTP called MPP^+ (1-methyl-4-phenylpyridinium ion) is produced by the glial cells via monoamine oxidase (MAO) B. Rodent studies have shown that aged animals produce greater quantities of MAO through increased numbers of glial cells and this process may explain why older animals are more susceptible to Parkinson's. It remains to be determined whether MPTP Parkinson's is produced by a similar etiology.

The severe neurotoxicant effects of MPTP may prove especially relevant to neuropsychological toxicologists concerned with industrial poisonings. At the Third International Symposium on Neurobehavioral Methods in Occupational and Environmental Health, Spencer (1988) presented positron emission tomography (PET) scans from several victims of MPTP poisoning. One patient in particular did not display parkinsonian symptoms, but showed drastically reduced levels of brain dopamine on PET scan. Spencer hypothesized there may be many patients like this not-yet-parkinsonian subject; exposed to substances less immediately destructive than MPTP, but still capable of causing insidious neurochemical damage. Slow depletion of an individual's function neurochemical reserves may occur during decades of workplace neurotoxic exposure.

Like the victim of MPTP who remains clinically aparkinsonian, these workers live on borrowed time; taking years to develop a parkinsonian symptom profile—by which time the symptom is no longer seen to be related to neurotoxic damage. This possibility has also been discussed by Silbergeld (1982).

Bleecker (1988) has proposed that parkinsonism may be a "final common pathway for many neurotoxic substances" besides MPTP, including carbon monoxide, manganese, and carbon disulfide. While the disease state itself may show a limited range of clinical expression, neurotoxic damage may occur in a number of anatomical structures.

The chronic and insidious influence of neurotoxic exposure may not be limited to parkinsonian symptoms. Support for Spencer's conjecture comes from an intriguing case–control study of long-term occupational exposure by Freed and Kandel (1988). The authors examined 150 patients diagnosed with Alzheimer's disease for history of chronic exposure to metals and/or solvents in the workplace. They found that 55 of the 150 (37%) "met the operational definition for long-term occupational exposure," while only 7 of 57 (12%) of nondemented controls had similar exposure histories (Freed & Kandel, 1988, p. 397). While these results obviously require a larger and more diverse subject population to constitute a valid epidemiological study, the numbers obtained by Freed and Kandel strongly indicate the need for research follow-up of this important question.

Neurosensory Damage from Neurotoxicants

Several studies have suggested that some neurotoxicants, most notably alcohol and industrial solvents, have selective effects within the sensory and motor neural systems. Central demyelination and peripheral neuropathies are probably responsible for symptom formation. For example, ototoxicity has been reported in one study (Arlien-Soberg, Bruhn, Tyldensted, & Melgaard, 1979) while damage to the vestibular apparatus was discovered in another study (Arlien-Soberg, Zilstorff, Grandjean, & Milling-Pedersen, 1981). Postural sway in children as an index of proprioceptive function, was found to be significantly related to blood lead levels in the second year of life (Bhattacharya, Shukla, Bornschein, Dietrich, & Kopke, 1988). A wide variety of sensory examinations have been suggested as being useful in neurotoxic exposure, including vibration, temperature, pain, hearing, and smell (Nylen, 1985). More complex neuropsychological tests have also been suggested as being capable of detecting nervous system dysfunction of neurotoxic etiology, including event-related evoked potentials (e.g., P-300) (Nylen, 1985; Dyer, 1990).

Several recent studies have suggested that subtle dysfunction of sensory apparatus is produced by solvent exposure. One such investigation compared workers in a University of Quebec printshop with a mixed group of non-solvent-exposed controls (Braun, Daigneault, & Gilbert, 1989). Groups were compared on a variety of neuropsychological tests, including trail-making, Wisconsin

Card Sorting, Rey Memory, finger tapping, grooved pegboard, and others, as well as on the Lanthony D-15 desaturated color panel. The latter consists of 15 pale pastel-colored disks that subjects are required to arrange along a chromatic continuum. Printers showed significantly impaired fine color discrimination or "dyschromatopsia" compared to controls. These were printers who worked in a relatively modern and well-ventilated "shop" and did not display neuropsychological abnormalities on any of the other tests. Results are consistent with Mergler, Blain, and Lagace's (1987) study where 80% of highly exposed solvent workers and 23% of moderately exposed workers showed chromatic discrimination loss. The results were not related to age-related lens opacification and ocular examination suggested no major damage, leading the authors to infer that chromatic discrimination difficulties had a neural rather than an ocular basis.

Ophthalmotoxic effects of certain solvents, including methanol, ethanol, carbon disulfide, and methyl chloride, are well known and have been suggested to reflect retinal damage, and in more severe cases, damage to the optic nerve. These studies and others obtaining similar results (e.g., Mergler & Blain, 1987; Mergler, Belanger, de Grosbois, & Vachon, 1988) suggest that a simple test of desaturated color perception provides an early warning of solvent exposure damage. In addition, investigations of lead (Schuttmann, Bohn, & Hager, 1971), cyanide (Heaton, 1962), and thallium (Bahiga, Kotb, & El-Dessoukey, 1978) suggest that exposure to metals may also degrade visual pathway or retinal function, and thus be amendable to sensory investigation.

Exposure to metals may also degrade sensory and motor pathways. Exposure to lead, mercury, and certain pesticides may also damage these systems (Norton, 1986).

In aggregate, the subtle sensory abnormalities observed in these studies strongly indicate the need for inclusion of sensory testing in neuropsychological toxicology batteries. Toxicological characteristics of many neurotoxic substances suggest that sensory and motor functions should receive increased attention and test development by clinical neuropsychologists.

Indirect Neurotoxic Effects

The capability of a substance to cause brain damage does not assume that its primary locus of effect lies inevitably in the brain. Tarter, Van Thiel, and Edwards (1988) have cogently outlined how damage to various body systems, including pulmonary, renal, cardiac, and others, may indirectly cause neuropsychological impairment. An example of probable brain damage/neurotoxicity that appears to begin in the pulmonary system is the herbicide *paraquat*, a widely used commercial product that caused 1300 poisoning deaths in Japan alone (Crome, 1986, cited in Hughes, 1988). Cases of paraquat poisoning are often associated with suicide attempts or accidental ingestion of a 20% paraquat solution. Ingestion causes severe lung damage (pulmonary fibrosis) and the brain is severely affected by edema, possibly as a result of hypoxia and inflammation and hemorrhage of small cerebral blood vessels (Hughes, 1988).

Lead and mercury are two other well-known neurotoxins whose additional destructive preference for renal tissue may aggravate neurotoxic damage and serve to remind the reader that any neurotoxicant capable of damaging the kidneys, heart, or other system may also cause neuropsychological damage through a variety of mechanisms, including lowering the amount of brain blood, oxygen, or nutrients, or by allowing toxic waste products to circulate in the brain (Hartman, 1988*b*).

Neuropsychological Effects of Neurotoxic Exposure

Toxicology does not give neuropsychologists a one-to-one correspondence between damage of the sort mentioned above, and neuropsychological impairments. there are many unanswered questions about the effects of individual difference variables, the interactive effects of age, health history, substance abuse, and synergistic effects of multiple exposure, that have not been adequately investigated. Large-scale research investigations may not, in any case, answer clinical questions for each individual, and a thorough multisystem evaluation on a case-by-case basis remains the most effective clinical procedure.

The variance attributable to demographic, educational, and health-related factors does not eliminate the possibility of attributing general types of neuropsychological deficits to exposure to neurotoxic substances. Table 17.2 lists patterns of neuropsychological deficits commonly noted in exposure to representative neurotoxins.

CLINICAL ASSESSMENT ISSUES

Clinical Neuropsychological Evaluations for Neurotoxic Exposure

Neuropsychological evaluation of possible neurotoxic exposure should take place as part of a multidisciplinary investigation. Medical, psychological, occupational, and educational data are required as is information concerning age and premorbid capabilities. Clinicians attempting to fit neuropsychological data into this information array must take special care in the examination. The clinician lacks the luxuries of the researcher or epidemiologist, including a large control population for comparison, and rarely has the kind of strong cause–effect data that are an explicit parameter of animal research. Lacking these prerequisites, the neuropsychological examination must be extensive, flexible, and above all, cautious in both procedure and conclusion; it is necessary to consider neurotoxic exposure as just one possibility in a massive rule-out of other physical, psychological, and mixed-etiology disorders.

Hänninen (1988) and Hartman (1988*b*) have discussed some of the variables required by such an enterprise, including those listed in Table 17.3.

TABLE 17.2. Neuropsychological Effects of Exposure to Common Neurotoxins[a]

Agent	Effects	Major uses/exposure sources
Arsenic	Memory impairment; CNS, PNS, and affect impairments; motor and visuomotor impairments; impairments secondary to cardiotoxicity	Pesticides, pigments Electroplating industry Seafood Smelters Semiconductor manufacturing
Carbon monoxide	Impaired arousal, vigilance, attention, motor speed, and coordination; visuospatial and visuomotor impairments	
Lead	Memory impairments; impairments in cognitive efficency and flexibility; visuospatial deficits; lowered IQ; dementia. Hyperactivity and retardation in children. Hallucinations and seizures from orgnolead. Depression; organic affective syndrome	Solder Leaded paint Moonshine Insecticides Auto body shops Battery manufacturing Foundries, smelters Drinking water from lead pipes
Mercury	Fine motor coordination, possible organic affective syndrome, e.g., "erethism," visuomotor impairments	Thermometers and scientific instruments Dental amalgam Electroplating industry Photography Feltmaking Textiles Pigments Taxidermy
Organic solvents (mixtures)	Memory, attention, visuospatial, and cognitive efficiency impairments; impaired fine motor coordination, organic affective syndrome	Dry cleaning fluid Semiconductor industry Degreasing Paint removing, gluing, lacquers, rubber solvents Adhesive in shoe and book industry Auto and aviation fuels
Organophosphates	Memory impairments, lowered arousal and attention. Organic affective syndrome; fine motor coordination and visuomotor impairments	Pesticides Agricultural industry

[a]After Hartman and Hessl (in press).

Test Administration

The complexity and subtlety of these issues virtually mandate that the *entire* examination be *personally conducted* by the expert neuropsychologist. The practice of using paraprofessional technicians, while apparently endorsed by a faction of American neuropsychologists (DeLuca, 1989), is strongly discouraged for neurotoxicity evaluations. Individual response profile variability in neurotoxic effects, the need for flexible administration of additional tests, and the

TABLE 17.3. Required Contextual Information for Neuropsychological Toxicology Evaluation

1. Detailed knowledge of the exposure agent, its site of action in various organ systems, and whether patient behavior is consistent with the actions of that agent
2. Exposure history, including the duration and intensity of exposure
3. Premorbid personality of the subject, including interpersonal and marital functioning
4. Use of prescription and abused drugs, and alcohol
5. Occupational history and interpersonal adjustment to work, including relationships with co-workers and authorities

considerable difficulties involved in separating neurotoxic abnormalities from functional deficits (or even deliberate attempts to malinger) all require direct, hands-on participation in the assessment by an expert clinician at all points in the evaluation.

Test Selection

A work group of scientists and clinicians were assembled in 1985 to recommend neuropsychological test procedures for solvent intoxication syndromes (Cranmer & Golberg, 1986). Rather than recommending a fixed battery, like the Halstead–Reitan or the World Health Organization (WHO) neuropsychological battery, the workshop participants recommended that a range of neuropsychological functions be evaluated in the context of a flexible battery. Their recommendations have applicability for general neurotoxic evaluation, and include recommendations for the *minimum* categories of tests listed in Table 17.4.

Taking the research of Mergler *et al.* (1987) and others into account, the

TABLE 17.4. Recommendations for Test Selection for Neurotoxic Assessments

Function	Representative tests
Psychomotor	Grooved pegboard, finger tapping, Santa Ana Pegboard Test
Sustained attention/concentration	Digit Symbol, Trailmaking, computerized attentional tasks
Verbal and nonverbal memory	Bushke Selective Reminding Test, Wechsler Memory Scale-Revised (WMS-R) and original WMS with Russell revision
Verbal learning	WMS, WMS-R Rey Auditory Verbal Learning Test, WMS Associate Learning
Visuoconstructive abilities	Block Design, (WAIS-R subtest) Tactual Performance Test
Concept formation	Category Test, Wisconsin Card Sorting Test
Stanardized evaluation of personality and affect	Profile of Mood States, MMPI-2

inclusion of several sensory tests like the Lanthony D-15 panel or the more complete Farnsworth–Munsell 100 Hue test (Farnsworth, 1957). Tests of vibration (e.g., the Vibratron) and olfaction (e.g., the University of Pennsylvania Smell Identification Test) may also prove important additions to future neuropsychological toxicology batteries.

PROBLEMS AND PROSPECTS

Investigation of New Populations

Neuropsychologists who typically make their homes in academia, psychiatry departments, or rehabilitation settings may have little familiarity with industrial and medical populations commonly at risk for neurotoxicant exposure. Similarly, hospital research in pharmacotherapeutics often lacks neuropsychological input, and government testing has been more typically concerned with the cancer-causing properties of proposed medications than their subtle neurotoxic effects. Only an active outreach by neuropsychologists will serve to encourage the multidisciplinary research and clinical practice that is so badly needed.

Political Impediments

Neuropsychologists must also be sensitive to the political and legal constraints in the United States that have served to limit or impede productive neuropsychological research in neurotoxicology. Unlike the Scandinavian countries where medicine, law, and business enjoy a less adversarial relationship, U.S. labor–management conflicts have caused employees to be suspicious of any management attempt to detect worker impairment. This sensitivity has been aggravated by recent attempts in many industries to mandate drug testing. Management may be no more enthusiastic than labor for neuropsychological studies to proceed, since workers found to be impaired by neurotoxicants could then litigate against the company for expensive damage awards.

Limitations and Cautions

One objection frequently raised concerning the use of neuropsychological methods is that neuropsychological testing results often cannot be interpreted as a function of basic scientific knowledge about neurotoxicity. Individual differences in subject response, lack of clear neuropathological understanding of neurotoxicants, and variabilities in skills, personality, and premorbid factors all conspire to make neuropsychological evaluation of neurotoxicity an occasionally difficult and ambiguous exercise.

The diagnostic complexity of this multidisciplinary field has led some critics to incorrectly attribute toxic effects to unrelated psychiatric disorder (e.g.,

Bieliauskas, 1990) or to argue against the use of neuropsychological methods for human clinical diagnosis. There is certainly no disputing that neuropsychology lacks a carefully worked out matrix of correlations between neurochemical/toxicological nervous system abnormalities and psychometric test results. It is also certainly the case that humans are far more difficult subjects of investigation than laboratory rats. Humans arrive for clinical evaluation with their uncontrollable variability. Age, education, general health, premorbid personality status, and substance abuse are just a few major sources of variance. There is no doubt that humans are quite varied and occasionally difficult to investigate with neuropsychological methods. However, in fairness to neuropsychological toxicology, these are common difficulties in neuropsychology generally, and are not specific to analysis of toxic effects. There is no substitute for careful data evaluation and a cautious, conservative approach.

Clinical and Research Problems

The accuracy of clinical or research study of neurotoxic effects can be improved with awareness of potential assessment biases in the neuropsychological status of those individuals exposed to neurotoxic substances. While these biases are most likely to be observed in group design research, the clinician responsible for case-by-case diagnosis must also understand the possible influences of bias and individual differences in response to neurotoxicants.

Bias Effects in Neuropsychological Assessment

The "Healthy Worker," the "Exploited Worker," and the Malingering Worker. The evaluation of neurotoxicity is complicated from neurobiological as well as neuropsychological perspectives by the problem of individual difference variability in subject response to neurotoxic substances. Systematic biases in neurotoxic sensitivity may be introduced by what has been termed the "healthy worker effect." This phenomenon involves the observation that employed workers will, on average, be healthier than the general population. Healthy workers do not, by definition, include the unemployed, retirees, the aged, the chronically ill, and other groups who will show higher mortality and poorer health than the working population. Similarly, workers with exposure to neurotoxins may self-select for tolerance to those substances. Employees who show initial sensitivity to solvents or metals, for example, become ill and either voluntarily leave or are terminated from employment due to incapacity. Those who remain at work are presumably a select group with decreased sensitivity to a given neurotoxin. Unfamiliarity with this effect may lead to a conclusion that a particular neurotoxin has minimal effects in a working population, a possible *underestimate* of a true effect.

A bias that may skew neuropsychological tests toward *overestimates* of neurotoxicity might be termed the "exploited worker effect." Those employees with the lowest level of premorbid intellectual function also may be the most likely to be taken advantage of and assigned to dangerous exposure employment. These workers would be the least knowledgeable and least able by virtue of their low skills to find a safer job. Neuropsychological evaluations in a population of such workers exploited for their minimal skills could show impairments resembling neurotoxic damage that are actually related to *premorbid* capabilities.

Another potential area of bias is the inclusion of subjects who are currently litigating damage awards for neurotoxic poisoning. It is important for both clinical and research neuropsychologists to be sensitive to this source of variance in their neuropsychological assessments. Where there is potential for monetary or psychological secondary gain, inclusion of tests for neuropsychological malingering (e.g., Binder & Pankratz, 1987; Hisock & Hisock, 1989) is strongly advised.

Individual Differences. Neuropsychological assessments are further complicated by *individual differences* in patient response to neurotoxic substances. Such interindividual variation can be caused by multiple and in many cases, little-researched factors. These include age, diet, health status, weight, immunocompetence, alcohol, drug, or prescription medication use, smoking, and genetic constitution (Vesell, 1987). Any single or interactive combination of these variables may determine why some individuals become ill and others do not when exposed to toxic substances. There is little research available on most of these factors to aid individual clinical diagnoses. However, neuropsychological measures may become useful and important dependent variables in the rapidly developing fields of "ecogenetics" and pharmacogenetics, two offshoots of toxicology concerned with the influence of genetics on environmental toxin or drug response.

For example, Wilson (1988) has reported substantial individual differences in response on psychophysiological tests to acute alcohol ingestion, suggesting the utility of neuropsychological tasks as dependent measures of genetic or biochemical individuality to toxic substances. Genetic variability may be more complex than simply predisposing subjects toward different biochemical responses to toxins. As Pickens and Svikis (1988) point out, nonpharmacological genetic variation may also influence drug-taking response. Some of these variations could include predisposition to sociopathy or high-stimulation risk-taking. Genetic variation could also produce individuals who are not protected from toxic substance damage. For example, subjects predisposed toward severe hangovers after drinking alcohol may shun the intoxicant, while those whose genetic makeup does not include the "protective" function of a hangover may consume more intoxicants, or be able to tolerate excessive workplace toxin exposure. Neuropsychological methods have already begun to be employed in the investigation of alcoholism-prone families, with intriguing results (e.g., Schaeffer, Parsons, & Yohman, 1984; Tarter, Hegedus, Goldstein, Shelly, & Atterman, 1984). perhaps the understanding of such studies will eventually be enhanced with data from a pharmacogenetic perspective.

CONCLUSIONS

Neuropsychologists can use information of the type presented here to further their own studies in neuropsychological toxicology, thereby becoming the interdisciplinary researchers and clinicians demanded by the field. According to Costa (1988),

> An ideal approach to the study of neurotoxicity is to combine the appropriate neurochemical techniques with *tests that assess those behaviors affected* by the neurochemical changes observed. [italics added]

Neuropsychologists are well trained to provide behavioral assessments of the sort advocated by Costa. It will remain their task to identify the behavioral tests and patterns of test abnormality that point to neurochemical lesion or other nonfocal lesion state. This exploration is already beginning and can be seen in the search of Stern and Langston (1985), Tarter *et al.* (1988), and many others who have linked neuroscience to neuropsychology. Integrating modern neuroscience, neurochemistry, and toxicological data with behavioral analysis of neurotoxin exposure should reveal much about brain–behavior relationships as neuropsychologists expand their field away from anachronistic structural localization models into the multidimensional arena of neuroscience. With increased attention to the psychobiological foundations of behavior, neuropsychological toxicology can be at the forefront of a new and exciting role for psychology in the clinic, the classroom, the laboratory, and the world at large.

REFERENCES

Arlien-Soberg, P., Bruhn, P., Tyldensted, C., & Melgaard, B. (1979). Chronic painters syndrome. Chronic toxic encephalopathy in house painters. *Acta Neurologica Scandinavica, 60,* 149–156.

Arlien-Soberg, P., Zilstorff, K., Grandjean, B., & Milling-Pedersen, L. (1981). Vestibular dysfunction in occupational chronic solvent intoxication. *Clinical Otolaryngology, 6,* 285–293.

Atchison, W. J. (1989). Effects of neurotoxicants on synaptic transmission: Lessons learned from electrophysiological studies. *Neurotoxicology and Teratology, 10,* 393–416.

Babcock, H. (1930). An experiment in the measurement of mental deterioration. *Archives of Psychology, 117,* 1–61 [whole issue].

Bahiga, L. M., Kotb, N. A., & El-Dessoukey, E. A. (1978). Neurological syndromes produced by some toxic metals encountered industrially or environmentally. *Zeitschrift fur Ernahrungswissen Schaft, 17,* 84–88.

Bertoni, J. M., & Sprenkle, P. M. (1988). Lead acutely reduces glucose utilization in the rat brain especially in higher auditory centers. *NeuroToxicology, 9,* 235–242.

Bhattacharya, A., Shukla, R., Bornschein, R., Dietrich, K., & Kopke, J. E. (1988). Postural disequilibrium quantification in children with chronic lead exposure: A pilot study. *NeuroToxicology, 9,* 327–340.

Bieliauskas, L. (1990). Review of neuropsychological toxicology and neurotoxins in clinical practice. *The Clinical Neuropsychologist, 4,* 86–93.

Binder, L. M., & Pankratz (1987). Neuropsychological evidence of a factitious memory complaint. *Journal of Clinical and Experimental Neuropsychology, 9,* 167–171.

Bjornaes, S., & Naalsund, L. U. (1988). Biochemical changes in different brain areas after toluene inhalation. *Toxicology, 49,* 367–374.

Bleecker, M. (1988). Parkinsonism: A clinical marker of exposure to neurotoxins. *Neurotoxicology and Teratology, 10*, 475–478.

Braun, C. M. J., Diagneault, S., & Gilbert, B. (1989). Color discrimination testing reveals early printshop neurotoxicity better than a neuropsychological test battery. *Archives of Clinical Neuropsychology, 4*, 1–13.

Costa, L. G. (1988). Interactions of neurotoxicants with neurotransmitter systems. *Toxicology, 49*, 359–366.

Cote, L., & Crutcher, M. D. (1985). Motor functions of the basal ganglia and diseases of transmitter metabolism. In E. R. Kandel & J. H. Schwartz (Eds.), *Principles of neural science* (pp. 523–535). Elsevier.

Cranmer, J. M., & Goldberg, L. (Eds.). (1986). Proceedings of the Workshop on Neurobehavioral Effects of Solvents. *NeuroToxicology, 7*(4), 1–95.

Crider, R. A., & Rouse, B. A. (1988). Inhalant overview. In R. A. Crider & B. A. Rouse (Eds.), *Epidemiology of inhalant abuse: An update* (pp. 1–7). NIDA Research Monograph 85, DHHS 88-1577.

Crome, P. (1986). Paraquat poisoning. *Lancet, 1*, 333–334.

DeLuca, J. W. (1989). Neuropsychology technicians in clinical practice: Precedents, rationale, and current deployment. *The Clinical Neuropsychologist, 3*, 3–21.

Dyer, R. S. (1990). Evoked potentials: Physiological methods with human applications. In B. L. Johnson (Ed.), *Advances in Neurobehavioral Toxicology*, (pp. 165–174). Chelsea, MI: Lewis Publishers.

Farnsworth, D. (1957). *The Farnsworth–Munsell 100 Hue test manual*. Baltimore: Macbeth Corp.

Freed, D. M., & Kandel, E. (1988). Long-term occupational exposure and the diagnosis of dementia. *NeuroToxicology, 9*, 391–400.

Goetz, C. G. (1985). *Neurotoxins in clinical practice*. New York: Spectrum Publications.

Goldman-Rakic, P. S. (1987). Circuit basis of a cognitive function in non-human primates. In S. M. Stahl, S. D. Iversen, & E. C. Goodman (Eds.), *Cognitive neurochemistry* (pp. 90–110). New York: Oxford University Press.

Hänninen, H. (1971). Psychological picture of manifest and latent carbon disulphide poisoning. *British Journal of Industrial Medicine, 28*, 374–381.

Hänninen, H. (1988). The psychological performance profile in occupational intoxications. *Neurotoxicology and Teratology, 10*, 485–488.

Hartman, D. E. (1988*a*). Neuropsychology and the neurochemical lesion: Evolution, applications and extensions. *NeuroToxicology, 9*(3), 401–404.

Hartman, D. E. (1988*b*). *Neuropsychological toxicology. Identification and assessment of human neurotoxic syndromes*. Elmsford, N.Y.: Pergamon Press.

Hartman, D. E., & Hessl, S. (in press) Adverse effects of pollutant exposure: Neurobehavioral disorders. In A. Tarcher (Ed.), *Principles and practice of environmental medicine*. New York: Plenum Press.

Heaton, J. M. (1962). Chronic cyanide poisoning and optic neuritis. *Transactions of the Ophthalmological Society of the United Kingdom, 82*, 263–269.

Hirano, A., & Llena, J. F. (1980). The central nervous system as a target in toxic-metabolic states. In P. S. Spencer & H. H. Schaumburg (Eds.), *Experimental and clinical neurotoxicology* (pp. 24–34). Baltimore: Williams & Wilkins.

Hisock, M., & Hisock, C. K. (1989). Refining the forced-choice method for the detection of malingering. *Journal of Clinical and Experimental Neuropsychology, 11*, 967–974.

Ho, I. K. (1988). Interactions in neurotoxicology. *Neurotoxicology, 9*, 151–152.

Hoch, A. (1904). A review of some psychological and physiological experiments done in connection with the study of mental diseases. *Psychological Bulletin, 1*, 241–257.

Hughes, J. T. (1988). Brain damage due to paraquat poisoning: A fatal case with neuropathological examination of the brain. *NeuroToxicology, 9*, 243–248.

Kandel, E. R., & Schwartz, J. H. (Eds.). (1985). *Principles of neural science* (2nd ed.). Amsterdam: Elsevier.

Klaassen, C. D., Amdur, M. O., & Doull, J. (Eds.). (1986). *Toxicology: The basic science of poisons*. New York: Macmillan Co.

Kolb, L. C. (1987). A neuropsychological hypothesis explaining post-traumatic stress disorders. *American Journal of Psychiatry, 144*, 989–995.

Landrigan, P. J., Kreiss, K., Xintaras, C., Feldman, R. G., & Heath, C. W., Jr. (1980). clinical epidemiology of occupational neurotoxic disease. *Neurobehavioral Toxicology, 2*, 43–48.

Luria, A. (1973). *The working brain*. New York: Basic Books.

Mailman, R. B., & Lewis, M. H. (1987). Neurotoxicants and central catecholamine systems. *Neurotoxicology, 8*(1), 123–140.

Maroni, M., & Barbieri, F. (1989). Biological indicators of neurotoxicity in central and peripheral toxic neuropathies. *Neurotoxicology and Teratology, 10*, 479–484.

Matarazzo, J. D. (1972). *Wechsler's measurement and appraisal of adult intelligence*. Baltimore: Williams & Wilkins.

Mergler, D., & Blain, L. (1987). Assessing color vision loss among solvent-exposed workers. *American Journal of Industrial Medicine, 12*, 195–203.

Mergler, D., Blain, L., & Lagace, J. P. (1987). Solvent-related color vision loss: An indicator of neural damage? *International Archives of Occupational and Environmental Health, 59*, 313–321.

Mergler, D., Belanger, S., de Grosbois, S., & Vachon, N. (1988). Chromal focus of acquired chromatic discrimination loss and solvent exposure among printshop workers. *Journal of Toxicology, 49*, 341–348.

Mutti, A., & Franchini, I. (1987). Toxicity of metabolites to dopaminergic systems and the behavioral effects of organic solvents. *British Journal of Industrial Medicine, 44*, 721–723.

Mutti, A., Falzio, M., Romanelli, M. C., Bocchi, C., Ferroni, C., & Franchini, I. (1988). Brain dopamine as a target for solvent toxicity: Effects of some monocyclic aromatic hydrocarbons. *Toxicology, 49*, 77–82.

Norton, S. (1986). Toxic responses of the central nervous system. In C. D. Klaassen, M. O. Amdur, & J. Doull (Eds.), *Toxicology: The Basic science of poisons* (pp. 359–386). New York: Macmillan Co.

Nylen, P. R. (1985). Neurophysiological methods. *Scandinavian Journal of Work Environment and Health, 2* (Suppl. 1), 95–96.

Oades, R. D. (1987). Attentional deficit disorder with hyperactivity (ADDH): The contribution of catecholaminergic activity. *Progress in Neurobiology, 29*, 365–391.

O'Callaghan, J. P. (1989). Neurotypic and gliotypic proteins as biochemical markers of neurotoxicity. *Neurotoxicology and teratology, 10*, 445–452.

Otto, D., Robinson, G., Baumann, S., Schroeder, S., Mushak, P., Kleinbaum, D., & Boone, L. (1985). 5-year follow-up study of children with low-to-moderate lead absorption: Electro-physiological evaluation. *Environmental Research, 38*, 168–186.

Parsons, O. (1970). Clinical neuropsychology. *Current Topics in Clinical and Community Psychology, 2*, 1–60.

Parsons, O. (1986). Overview of the Halstead–Reitan Battery. In T. Incagnoli, G. Goldstein, & C. J. Golden (Eds.), *Clinical application of neuropsychological test batteries* (pp. 155–192). New York: Plenum Press.

Perlick, D., Stastny, P., Katz, I., Mayer, M., & Mattis, S. (1986). Memory deficits and anticholinergic levels in chronic schizophrenia. *American Journal of Psychiatry, 143*, 230–232.

Pickens, R. W., & Svikis, D. S. (1988). Genetic vulnerability to drug abuse. In R. W. Pickens & D. S. Svikis (Eds.), *Biological vulnerability to drug abuse* (pp. 1–8). NIDA Research Monograph 89, DHHS Publ. (ADM)88-1590.

Reitan, R. (1955). Certain differential effects of left and right cerebral lesions in human adults. *Journal of Comparative and Physiological Psychology, 48*, 474–477.

Rosenberg, N. L., Spitz, M. C., Filley, C. M., Davis, K. A., & Schaumberg, H. H. (1988). Central nervous system effects of chronic toluene abuse—Clinical, brainstem evoked response and magnetic resonance imaging studies. *Neurotoxicology and Teratology, 10*, 489–495.

Rufener, B. L., et al. (1977). *Management effectiveness measures for NIDA drug abuse treatment programs, Volume II: Costs to society of drug abuse*. NIDA, Contract 271-75-1016.

Ruscak, M., Ruscakova, D., & Hager, H. (1968). The role of the neuronal cell in the metabolism of the rat cerebral cortex. *Physiologica Bohemoslov, 17*, 113–121 [translation].

Russell, E. W., Neuringer, C., & Goldstein, G. (1970). *Assessment of brain damage: A neuropsychological key approach*. New York: Wiley–Interscience.

Schaeffer, K. W., Parsons, O. A., & Yohman, J. R. (1984). Neuropsychological differences between male familial and nonfamilial alcoholics and non-alcoholics. *Alcoholism: Clinical and Experimental Research, 8* 347–351.

Schuttmann, W., Bohn, E., & Hager, G. (1971). Neuritis of the optic nerve as a monosymptomatic form of lead poisoning. *Zeitschrift fur die gesamte Hygiene und ihre Grenzebiete, 17*, 342–348.

Silbergeld, E. (1982). Current status of neurotoxicology, basic and applied. *Trends in Neuroscience*, 291–294.

Spencer, P. (1988). Introductory address. Presented at the Third International Symposium on Neurobehavioral Methods in Occupational and Environmental Health. Washington, D.C.: World Health Organization.

Spencer, P., & Schaumburg, H. H. (1980). *Experimental and clinical neurotoxicology*. Baltimore: Williams & Wilkins.

Stahl, S. M., Iversen, S. D., & Goodman, E. C. (Eds.). (1987). *Cognitive neurochemistry*. New York: Oxford University Press.

Stern, Y., & Langston, J. W. (1985). Intellectual changes in patients with MPTP-induced parkinsonism. *Neurology, 35*, 1506–1509.

Tarter, R. E., Hegedus, A. M., Goldstein, G., Shelly, C., & Alterman, A. (1984). Adolescent sons of alcoholics: Neuropsychological and personality characteristics. *Alcohol: Clinical and Experimental Research, 8*, 216–222.

Tarter, R. E., Van Thiel, D. H., & Edwards, K. L. (1988). *Medical neuropsychology*. New York: Plenum Press.

Tune, L. E., Strauss, M. E., Lew, M. F., Breitlinger, E., & Coyle, J. T. (1982). Serum levels of anticholinergic drugs and impaired recent memory in chronic schizophrenic patients. *American Journal of Psychiatry, 139*, 1460–1461.

Vesell, E. S. (1987). Pharmacogenetic perspectives on susceptibility to toxic industrial chemicals. *British Journal of Industrial Medicine, 44*, 505–509.

White, R. G., & Feldman, R. H. (1987). Neuropsychological assessment of toxic encephalopathy. *American Journal of Industrial Medicine, 11*, 395–398.

Wilson, J. R., (1988). Individual differences in drug response. In R. W. Pickens & D. S. Svikis (Eds.), *Biological vulnerability to drug abuse* (pp. 93–107). NIDA Research Monograph 89, DHHS Publ. (ADM)88-1590.

IV

Epilogue

18

Overview, Limitations, and Directions

ROBERT J. MCCAFFREY and ANTONIO E. PUENTE

INTRODUCTION

There is little doubt that individuals with brain injuries constitute a significant segment of our health care population. Of growing concern is the percentage of these patients who are chronic and unresponsive to rehabilitative efforts. Hence, little question should exist as to the importance of addressing the concerns of this population. Traditionally, behavioral or psychological issues have almost always been considered nonexistent or unimportant in addressing brain injury. Fortunately, this erroneous and incomplete approach has evolved to include behavior and, thus, clinical neuropsychology (Puente, 1989).

The inclusion of behavior in the understanding of the effects of brain injury has assumed a belief that behavior is unidimensional and not affected by contextual variables. Specifically, the current understanding of the effects of brain injury on behavior does little to place the patients and their injury in a larger contextual environment. Costa (1988) has argued that while neuropsychological tests are sensitive to brain dysfunction, they are not dysfunction-specific. Costa addresses the need for more research to deal with this lack of specificity. This observation is a function of the need to develop more comprehensive understanding of syndromes and measurement devices. This approach is, however, not enough. For example, new studies call into question the validity of current neuropsychological understanding (Faust & Ziskin, 1988). While one may cogently argue that such criticisms are not only unfair but downright

ROBERT J. MCCAFFREY • Department of Psychology, The University at Albany, State University of New York, Albany, New York 12222. ANTONIO E. PUENTE • Department of Psychology, University of North Carolina at Wilmington, Wilmington, North Carolina 28403-3297.

HANDBOOK OF NEUROPSYCHOLOGICAL ASSESSMENT: A Biopsychosocial Perspective, edited by Antonio E. Puente and Robert J. McCaffrey. Plenum Press, New York, 1992.

misguided (Matarazzo, 1990), the questions are not without foundation. We believe that the question of validity can be best answered by placing the patient's behavior in the context of a wide range of biopsychosocial variables rather than by developing more "specific" tests, as Costa (1988) has suggested. To do otherwise would continue to produce an incomplete understanding of brain function.

This logical orientation has been interwoven into related disciplines. For example, Moccaci (1984) has argued that social, cultural, and related factors are taken into account when understanding basic psychological processes but tend to be neglected when considering neuropsychological factors. Moccaci cites extensive evidence on how cultural variables affect hemispheric processing and also suggests that neuropsychological approaches to the understanding of brain function need to address these contextual variables.

SCOPE AND LIMITATIONS OF THE PRESENT VOLUME

First and foremost, this volume is not intended as a replacement or competition for such excellent treatises in neuropsychological assessment as Lezak's *Neuropsychological Assessment* (1988), Franzen's *Reliability and Validity in Neuropsychological Assessment* (1989), and others. Indeed, it would seem foolish to attempt to supercede the work of these authors since they present an excellent overview of several major aspects of assessment. The orientation of these contributions, however, has typically been psychometric in origin with the most powerful and useful knowledge being that of the instrument itself.

Other texts focus on understanding a specific behavioral problem. For example, Squires (1987) places critical importance on understanding memory disorders rather than on the tests that measure such impairments. Again, Squires and others have done an admirable job in presenting their approach to the understanding of brain dysfunction.

Unfortunately, knowledge of the syndrome and the tests used to measure the signs and symptoms of the disorder is not enough to adequately assess brain dysfunction. Technical expertise is no replacement for clinical sensitivity. Missing in these two orientations (i.e., tests and syndrome knowledge) is the importance of understanding the patients in their context whether it be biological, demographic, psychological, social, and/or environmental. Placing the patients in the context of their life's situation increases the validity of our neuropsychological understanding. To do otherwise, undermines the ultimate criterion in clinical neuropsychology—accurate understanding of neuropsychological function and dysfunction.

This volume is not meant to replace or supercede existing neuropsychological knowledge but to supplement our existing knowledge base. This compendium of contributions adds and enhances to this existing body of knowledge with an understanding of the tests and syndromes as a prerequisite to the application of the information found in this book. After all, the major direction of each chapter is how specific variables affect performance on neuropsychological tests.

OVERVIEW

The present volume represents an attempt on the part of scientists and practitioners to address the role of fundamental biopsychosocial variables in both basic research and the clinical application of neuropsychology. The importance of considering constitutional and demographic factors was addressed in Part I. The importance of considering the subject/patient in the context of his or her developmental period across the life span was addressed by considering many populations—perinatal and infants, children, adults, and geriatric. Emory *et al.* outlined the significance of considering perinatal factors in the neuropsychological assessment of both infants and older children. Moreover, the possible link between perinatal complications in the offspring of individuals at genetic risk for the development of forms of psychopathology, such as schizophrenia, underscores the importance of assessing for these types of factors. The chapter on childhood factors underscores the importance of developing both assessment procedures and instruments that are specific to the child's developmental period. Children should not be viewed as downward extensions of adults. Along these same lines, the chapter on adult development and aging highlights the importance of differentiating normal cognitive changes from those associated with disease processes and/or affective states. An important factor is the need to consider the patient relative to appropriate norms. For example, it would be inappropriate to compare patients with chronic medical illnesses to healthy, older adults. Such a comparison could conceivably result in a significant misdiagnosis.

A consideration of sex and gender differences is an important endeavor in neuropsychological assessment in its own right. The importance of including these types of variables in both neuropsychology and related areas has recently been highlighted by the National Institute of Health's policy indicating the inclusion of females in studies.

The study of handedness and the lateralization of hemispheric functioning provides an opportunity to study the brain's organization of cognitive functioning. Knowledge of factors associated with lateralization of functioning is especially important when designing an implementing remediation and rehabilitation program following insults to the brain.

The role of bilingualism as an important variable in both basic and applied neuropsychological assessment is an important issue as outlined by Manuel-Dupont *et al.* and is one that is likely to continue to demand the attention of clinical neuropsychologists as the population of bilingual citizens in the United States increases. Coupled closely with the issue of bilingualism is the role of sociocultural factors in basic and applied clinical neuropsychology. As detailed by Ardila *et al.*, this issue goes to the heart of understanding patients in the context of their life and underscores the importance of developing norms based on diverse populations, in order not to confound sociocultural factors with neuropsychological dysfunction. In fact, the impending revisions of the *Ethical Principles of Psychologists* highlight the importance of understanding the patient in the context of his or her life.

Part II dealt with psychopathological factors as they are likely to influence the evaluation of patients with known or suspected CNS dysfunction. Research into the neuropsychological bases of the anxiety, depressive, and schizophrenic disorders is important since it is likely to increase our understanding of the underlying physiological bases of these disorders. The role of neuropsychological assessment in evaluating these types of disorders is not only useful in terms of differential diagnosis of psychopathological factors from underlying organic factors but is also useful in providing behavioral correlates of changes associated with other assessment procedures such as neurological exams, neuroimaging, basic biology, and other variables. As highlighted by Orsillo and McCaffrey, subject selection factors, changes in the DSM-III's diagnostic criteria, and a failure on the part of the investigators to provide detailed descriptions of patient samples (e.g., handedness, coexisting medical conditions) may have contributed to the discrepancies reported in both the clinical and research literature. In addition, the failure to evaluate and/or control for other variables appears to have added to the contradictory findings, especially with regard to the results of PET scans with panic disordered patients. Specifically, Mountz, Modell, Wilson, Curtis, Lee, Schmaltz, and Kohl (1989) found that hyperventilation, a correlate of state anxiety, has a profound influence on changes in patients' PET scans. The importance of understanding both the neuropsychology of depressive disorders and the interaction of depressed states with various underlying medical conditions was highlighted by Newman and Sweet. Their review indicating that magnetic resonance imaging studies have localized structural changes in the brains of patients with affective disorders highlights the importance of consideration of the role of depressive deficits in both basic and routine clinical neuropsychological assessment.

Neuropsychology had a great deal to contribute to the scientific investigation of schizophrenia. While there is little evidence to indicate that patients with the diagnosis of schizophrenia share a common organic impairment, Walker *et al.* note that the neuropsychological performance profiles may be related to the symptom profiles of patients with the diagnosis of schizophrenia.

The practicing clinical neuropsychologist is also likely to be called upon to assist in the evaluation of patients where a suspected pseudoneurological disorder may be present. The differential diagnosis of neurological versus pseudoneurological has important implications in terms of care and treatment of individual patients as outlined by Horton. Another area of increasing importance for the practicing neuropsychologist is the detection of deception and malingering in patients who have sustained some form of CNS trauma. While the detection of deception for possible secondary gain is an important factor in the care and treatment of the individual patient, Binder also notes that this area is one that has important implications in terms of providing forensic neuropsychological services.

Part III focused on biological and environmental factors. Biological and environmental factors present a set of important variables to be considered when evaluating diverse groups of medical patients. The chapter on peripheral motor and sensory disorder by Delay and Isaac highlights the importance of a thorough working knowledge of both the peripheral as well as central nervous system when interpreting a patient's complaints and neuropsychological profile. The chapter on cardiovascular and somatic disorders by Lorig reviews a number of medical conditions that are likely to be important factors in the neuropsychological evaluation of patients in a medical setting. Uzzell's chapter provides a pertinent overview of the sequelae associated with neurosurgical interventions.

The abuse of psychoactive substances is a major health problem in the United States and, as such, is likely to be a confounding factor in the neuropsychological assessment of patients who have sustained trauma to the CNS from motor vehicle accidents. In addition, the abuse of psychoactive substances is also an important issue in the designing and implementation of substance abuse treatment services. As such, the clinical neuropsychologist may be called upon not only to evaluate patients with a history of substance abuse but also to provide treatment recommendations and long-term postcare recommendations.

The growing concern over the environment and presence of neurotoxins in the environment, especially the workplace, has led to the emergence of the field of neuropsychological toxicology. As outlined by Hartman, the area of neuropsychological toxicology is likely to continue to show considerable growth both in terms of basic research and also in terms of medicolegal issues. Given that the area of neuropsychological toxicology is relatively new, a great deal of basic research needs to be conducted. The application of clinical neuropsychological assessment techniques and procedures is expected to have a profound and important impact in evaluating the impact of neurotoxins in our environment.

There are many variables that affect performance on a neuropsychological test. This book was intended as a comprehensive presentation of the major variables involved with the assessment of brain dysfunction using clinical neuropsychological tests. Nevertheless, other variables could be playing a (*potentially significant*) role in this situation. Additional clinical experience and research should uncover these variables.

Some of these variables are obvious and have been addressed in limited fashion within several of our chapters and in previous contributions. For example, Tarter, Van Thiel, and Edwards's (1988) edited volume *Medical Neuropsychology* presented the interface between a variety of medical disorders (e.g., renal failure) and neuropsychological performance. In the present book, several contributors address these and related issues to some extent (e.g., see Delay and

Isaac). Thus, the medical status of the patient plays a critical role in mediating neuropsychological performance. Other variables may be even more obvious. Reynolds and Fletcher-Janzen's (1989) *Handbook of Clinical Child Neuropsychology*, for example, outlines in detail how developmental factors affect neuropsychological function. In this volume, three separate chapters address developmental issues across the life span.

A number of other variables are much less obvious and are less understood. Some of these variables are biological. For example, race probably plays a more significant role in brain function and dysfunction than commonly thought. Unfortunately, sociopolitical issues have clouded the necessary research that needs to be performed. If one draws from recent sociopsychological literature (Jones, in press), it may be that within-race differences may actually be larger than between-race differences if critical confounding variables (e.g., socioeconomic status) are held constant. Regardless, the question of race and other biological variables needs to be empirically addressed.

Other variables equally ignored include demographic factors and longstanding personality traits and disorders. Matthews in this volume discusses sex differences in a variety of tasks. However, the issues of gender and sexual orientation, while difficult to address, may be as important as biological sex. Though yet unpublished, Henninger-Pechsted (personal communication, 1990) has been examining the role of hemispheric dominance in multiple personality disorders. One of her basic assumptions includes the role of the dominant hemisphere in modulating undesirable affect resulting from early traumatic experiences.

Other variables may be even more speculative than those previously considered in this section. These include a host of other biological (e.g., metabolic rate), demographic (e.g., religion), and other personality (e.g., Axis II disorders) variables. Until such knowledge is more commonly available, caution should be used before ruling out the importance of any of these variables in understanding neuropsychological deficits.

In anticipation of this body of knowledge, we welcome suggestions and directions on how these and other variables manifest themselves in neuropsychological functions.

SCIENTIFIC MODEL OF CLINICAL NEUROPSYCHOLOGY

The primary goal of the neuropsychologist is to conduct a scientifically correct but clinically sensitive evaluation of a broad spectrum of patients. As such, the clinical neuropsychologist must have an appreciation and an understanding of the basic issues surrounding the diversity of both patients and medical/psychiatric disorders. The most recent draft of the Ethical Principles of the American Psychological Association emphasizes the importance of understanding the patient in the context of his/her life. The performance of scientifically correct but clinically sensitive evaluations incorporating diversity issues poses a unique challenge to the clinical neuropsychologist. In this regard, the role of the clinical neuropsychologist must go beyond the level of assessor only. Increasingly, clinical neuropsychologists are in positions in which they are asked to make predictions and/or provide treatment/rehabilitation options on issues for which there is a limited scientific basis upon which to draw. This challenge must be addressed by both the individual practitioner and the field in general.

METHODOLOGICAL ISSUES: CONFLICTUAL FINDINGS

At the present time, there are a number of areas in clinical neuropsychology in which there are conflictual research reports. The presence of conflictual findings ought not to be viewed as a source of irritation but rather as representing a challenge to the field. Specifically, there are a number of factors that are either known or presumed to be important mediating variables in clinical neuropsychology. In fact, the intent of the present volume was to begin the process of considering these potentially important variables in general clinical neuropsychological assessment. Included among these mediating variables are subject selection factors, diagnostic criteria, education, IQ, cultural factors, learning disabilities, and developmental disabilities. While basic research into each of these issues has been—and is being—conducted, our knowledge of the impact of these factors is far from complete. Thus, it should come as no surprise that conflictual results are often found in both the basic and clinical research literature. For example, Orsillo and McCaffrey in their review of the anxiety disorder literature note that there have been marked discrepancies in terms of the criteria used in arriving at the diagnosis for various anxiety disorders. In addition, investigators in this field often have failed to obtain basic information associated with such important factors such as handedness and the role of state versus trait anxiety. The conflictual findings based on the use of PET scans to evaluate the neurophysiology of panic disorders appear to be related to the failure to control for the presence of hyperventilation (Mountz *et al.*, 1989).

In the clinical domain, there are also often reports of contradictory findings. For example, the efficacy of attention-remediation training in patients who have suffered a traumatic brain injury is an applied area of clinical neuropsychology in which contradictory findings are the norm (see McCaffrey & Gansler, in press, for review). The attention-remediation studies often assume that traumatically brain-injured patients represent a homogeneous population based on some set of post-TBI criteria. Moreover, basic variables such as the extent and duration of coma, time since TBI, handedness, medication regimens, concurrent medical conditions, and other variables are often not reported. In terms of evaluating the efficacy of the treatment intervention, factors such as the role of spontaneous recovery of function are often not considered. The presence of discrepant research findings highlights the importance of both considering and investigating basic biopsychosocial variables in both basic research and the clinical application of neuropsychology.

FUTURE ROLES IN APPLICATIONS OF CLINICAL NEUROPSYCHOLOGY

The statement that "psychology has a long past, but only a short history" is attributed to Ebbinghaus (Boring, 1950). In many ways, this statement is equally applicable to the area of clinical neuropsychology. As in other areas of psychology, it is important that the clinical neuropsychologist be trained as a scientist-practitioner in order to meet the challenges confronting the field. The field of clinical neuropsychology has witnessed a rapid growth during the decade of the 1980s. Education for competency assurance in clinical neuropsychology has been, and continues to be, an important issue (Meier, 1981; International Neuropsychological Society Task Force, 1981). In the mid-1980s, several reports appeared evaluating the educational background and specialty training of instructors of clinical neuropsychology in graduate training programs (McCaffrey & Isaac, 1984), the educational backgrounds of the clinical neuropsychologists in APA-approved internship sites (McCaffrey, 1985), internship opportunities in clinical neuropsychology emphasizing recent INS training guidelines (McCaffrey, Malloy, & Brief, 1985), and the availability of neuropsychological training in APA-approved counseling psychology programs (Solomon, Hale-Fiske, McCaffrey, & Orabona-Roman, 1985). Results of these surveys indicated that there was a growing demand for training in neuropsychology at both the graduate training level and the internship level. Unfortunately, the educational background and specialty training of instructors in both graduate programs and APA-approved internship sites lagged far behind the minimal criteria as outlined by Meier (1981). The results of a recent national survey of psychologists who offer neuropsychological services found that the modal psychologist is only tangentially involved in neuropsychology (Guilmette, Faust, Hart, & Arkes, 1990). Distressingly, the modal practitioner performs less than one neuropsychological assessment a month and his/her formal educational background in specialty training falls far short of the INS/Division 40 Task Force recommendations for neuropsychologists.

Despite the fact that the types of surveys summarized above may be criticized based on methodological grounds, it nonetheless appears that we have failed to see an implementation of the INS/Division 40 guidelines for training in clinical neuropsychology during the decade of the 1980s. The training of clinical neuropsychologists in a scientist-practitioner model remains a problem in need of solution for the decade ahead.

The issue of diversity in understanding patients in the context of their lives will require an effort on the part of the clinical neuropsychologist to develop norms for diverse populations. Along these same lines, it will be necessary to develop flexible clinical neuropsychological assessment batteries and individual assessment instruments that are adaptable to individual patients and not necessarily specific to particular disorders. In addition, there is likely to be increasing pressure from third-party insurance carriers requesting that rehabilitation programs be based on an individual case-by-case approach guided by firm scientific data as to the efficacy of various rehabilitation or remediation therapies (see McCaffrey & Gansler, in press).

Another important issue is the further development of neuropsychological assessment instruments designed specifically to evaluate patients in the context of their developmental period, current life and related factors, in order to increase the generalization of neuropsychological assessment findings. Moreover, it will be necessary to continue to develop, validate, and evaluate new assessment procedures and approaches for use by clinical neuropsychologists with diverse populations. For example, there are few neuropsychological assessment procedures for evaluating executive functioning.

CONCLUSION

The goal of this volume has been to sensitize clinical neuropsychologists to a host of contextual variables in neuropsychological assessment. We anticipate that the major variables have been covered in some fashion in these chapters. Nevertheless, it is anticipated that other variables will eventually warrant further evolution and consideration. What will not change, however, is the importance of assessing the client in a comprehensive biopsychological framework.

REFERENCES

Boring, E. G. (1950). *A history of experimental psychology* (2nd ed.). New York: Appleton–Century–Crofts.

Costa, L. (1988). Clinical neuropsychology: Prospects and problem. *Clinical Neuropsychologist, 2*, 3–11.

Faust, D., & Ziskin, J. (1988). The expert witness in psychology and psychiatry. *Science, 241*, 31–35.

Franzen, M. D. (1989). *Reliability and validity in neuropsychological assessment*. New York: Plenum Press.

Guilmette, T. J., Faust, D., Hart, K., & Arkes, H. R. (1990). A national survey of psychologists who offer neuropsychological services. *Archives of General Neuropsychology, 5*, 373–392.

International Neuropsychological Society Task Force. (1981, February). Report of the Task Force on Education, Accreditation and Credentialing of the International Neuropsychological Society. Atlanta, Ga. *Neuropsychological assessment* (2nd ed.). New York: Oxford University Press.

Jones, J. (in press). Race. In B. Hammonds (Ed.), *APA master lectures*. Washington, D.C.: American Psychological Association.

Lezak, M. (1988). *Neuropsychological assessment* (2nd ed.). New York: Oxford University Press.

Matarazzo, J. D. (1990). Psychological assessment versus psychological testing: Validation from Binet to the school, clinic, and courtroom. *American Psychologist, 45*, 999–1017.

McCaffrey, R. J. (1985). Educational backgrounds of clinical neuropsychologists in APA-approved internship sites. *Professional Psychology: Research and Practice, 16*, 773–780.

McCaffrey, R. J., & Isaac, W. (1984). Survey of the educational backgrounds and specialty training of instructors of clinical neuropsychology in APA-approved graduate training programs. *Professional Psychology: Research and Practice, 15*, 26–33.

McCaffrey, R. J., & Gansler, D. A. (in press). The efficacy of attention-remediation programs for traumatically brain injured survivors. In C. J. Long & L. K. Ross (Eds.), *Head trauma: Acute care to recovery*. New York: Plenum Press.

McCaffrey, R. J., Malloy, P. F., & Brief, D. J. (1985). Internship opportunities in clinical neuropsychology emphasizing recent INS training guidelines. *Professional Psychology: Research and Practice, 16*, 236–252.

Meier, M. J. (1981). Education for competency assurance in human neuropsychology: Antecedents, models, and directions. In S. B. Fiskov & T. J. Boll (Eds.), *Handbook of clinical neuropsychology* (pp. 754–781). New York: Wiley.

Moccaci, L. (1984). Looking for the social and cultural dimensions of the human brain. *International Journal of Psychophysiology, 1*, 293–299.

Mountz, J. M., Modell, J. G., Wilson, M. W., Curtis, G. C., Lee, Y. L., Schmaltz, S., & Kohl, D. E. (1989). Positron emission tomographic evaluation of cerebral blood flow during state anxiety in simple phobia. *Archives of General Psychiatry, 46*, 501–504.

Puente, A. E. (1989). Historical perspectives in the development of neuropsychology as a professional discipline. In C. R. Reynolds & E. Fletcher-Janzen (Eds.). *Handbook of clinical child neuropsychology*. New York: Plenum Press.

Reynolds, C. R., & Fletcher-Janzen, E. (Eds.). (1989). *Handbook of clinical child neuropsychology*. New York: Plenum Press.

Solomon, G. S., Hale-Fiske, F. R., McCaffrey, R. J., & Orabona-Roman, L. (1985). Neuropsychological assessment training in APA-approved counseling psychology programs. *Professional Psychology: Research and Practice, 16*, 22–25.

Squires, L. R. (1987). *Memory and brain*. New York: Oxford University Press.

Tarter, R. E., Van Thiel, D. H., & Edwards, K. L. (Eds.). (1988). *Medical neuropsychology*. New York: Plenum Press.

Index